JOLLY'S DISEASES
OF CHILDREN

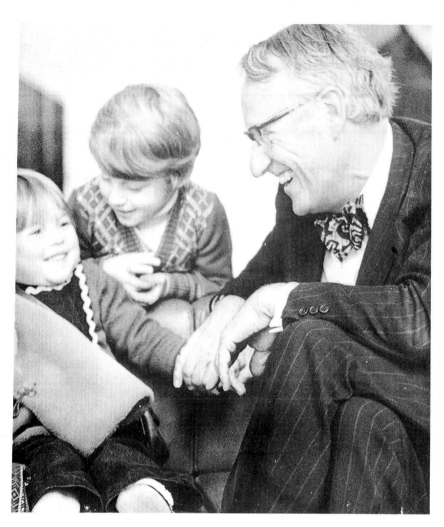

Hugh Jolly
5.5.18–4.3.86

JOLLY'S DISEASES
OF CHILDREN

EDITED BY

MALCOLM I. LEVENE
MD FRCP
Professor of Paediatrics and Child Health
The University of Leeds
Clarendon Wing
The General Infirmary
at Leeds

SIXTH EDITION

OXFORD

BLACKWELL SCIENTIFIC PUBLICATIONS

LONDON EDINBURGH BOSTON

MELBOURNE PARIS BERLIN VIENNA

First published 1964
Reprinted 1966
Second edition 1968
Reprinted 1971, 1973, 1974
ELBS editions 1971, 1973, 1975
Third edition 1976
Reprinted 1979
ELBS editions 1976, 1978
Spanish edition 1977
Fourth edition 1981
Reprinted 1983, 1984
ELBS editions 1981, 1983
Fifth edition 1985
Reprinted 1988
Sixth edition 1991
ELBS edition 1991

Set by Best-set Typesetter, Hong Kong
Printed and bound in Great Britain by
William Clowes Limited
Beccles and London

DISTRIBUTORS

Marston Book Services Ltd
PO Box 87
Oxford OX2 0DT
(*Orders*: Tel: 0865 791155
          Fax: 0865 791927
          Telex: 837515)

USA
Mosby–Year Book, Inc.
11830 Westline Industrial Drive
St Louis, Missouri 63146
(*Orders*: Tel: 800 633–6699)

Canada
Mosby–Year Book, Inc.
5240 Finch Avenue East
Scarborough, Ontario
(*Orders*: Tel: (416) 298–1588)

Australia
Blackwell Scientific Publications
(Australia) Pty Ltd
54 University Street
Carlton, Victoria 3053
(*Orders*: Tel: (03) 347–0300)

British Library
Cataloguing in Publication Data

Jolly, Hugh *1918–1986*
   Jolly's diseases of children.—6th. ed.
   1. Children. Diseases
   I. Title   II. Levene, Malcolm I. (Malcolm Irvin)
   III. Jolly, Hugh *1918–1986. Diseases of children*
   618.92

   ISBN 0-632-02723-1

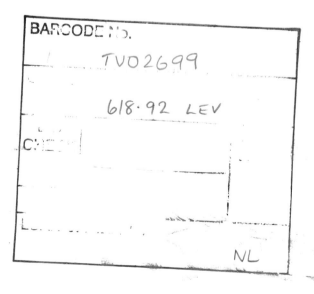

CONTENTS

List of Colour Plates, vii

List of Contributors, viii

Preface to the Sixth Edition, ix

Acknowledgements, x

Preface to the First Edition, xi

1   History Taking and Examination, 1
    MALCOLM LEVENE

2   Child Care in and out of Hospital, 15
    MALCOLM LEVENE

3   Minor Disorders of Children, 23
    MALCOLM LEVENE

4   Growth and Development, 37
    MALCOLM LEVENE

5   Normal Newborn Infant, 52
    MALCOLM LEVENE

6   Infant Feeding, 63
    MALCOLM LEVENE

7   Special Care of the Sick Newborn Infant, 77
    MALCOLM LEVENE

8   Inherited Disorders and Genetic Counselling,
    116
    IAN YOUNG

9   Congenital Abnormalities Apparent at Birth,
    136
    MALCOLM LEVENE

10 Disorders of the Ear, Nose and Throat, 152
    MALCOLM LEVENE

11 Respiratory Disorders, 165
    NICK ARCHER

12 Disorders of the Gastrointestinal System, 191
    NIGEL MEADOWS

13 Disorders of the Cardiovascular System, 214
    NICK ARCHER

14 The Critically Ill Child, 240
    NICK ARCHER

15 Disorders of the Urinary Tract, 246
    ALAN WATSON

16 Fluid and Electrolyte Problems, 273
    ALAN WATSON

17 Disorders of the Nervous System, 279
    MALCOLM LEVENE

18 Disorders of the Special Senses, 307
    MALCOLM LEVENE

19 The Child with a Handicap, 319
    MALCOLM LEVENE

20 Emotional and Behavioural Disorders, 334
    RORY NICOL

21 Immunization and Infectious Diseases, 351
    PETER RUDD

22 Metabolic Disorders, 370
    MALCOLM LEVENE

Contents

23 Endocrine Disorders, 382
    PETER SWIFT

24 Haematological Disorders, 423
    ELAINE SIMPSON

25 Cancer in Children, 442
    ROSS PINKERTON

26 Disorders of the Bones and Joints, 474
    JOHN OSBORNE

27 Skin Disorders, 486
    TONY BURNS

28 Sudden Infant Death, Accidental Injury and
    Child Abuse, 510
    MALCOLM LEVENE

29 Paediatrics in Developing Countries, 529
    JOHN AXTON

    Index, 576

LIST OF COLOUR PLATES

1 Harrison's sulci and prominent sternum secondary to chronic severe upper airway obstruction.
2 Jejunal biopsy under the dissecting microscope.
3 Small bowel histology in a normal child and a child with coeliac disease.
4 Small bowel biopsy in a child with cow's milk protein intolerance.
5 Sunsetting.
6 Typical rash of measles.
7 The erythematous 'slapped cheeks' of Fifth disease.
8 Eczema herpeticum.
9 The typical facial rash of scarlet fever.
10 Skin lesions of dermatomyositis.
11 Dermatomyositis.
12 Systemic lupus erythematosus.
13 Child's hands with Kawasaki's disease.

Plates 1–13 appear between pages 212 and 213

14 Typical plaques of psoriasis.
15 Guttate psoriasis.
16 Pink macule seen in pityriasis rosea.
17 Ichthyosis.
18 Collodian baby.
19 Flexural involvement in atopic eczema.
20 Eczema herpeticum.
21 Napkin psoriasis.
22 Irritant napkin dermatitis.

23 Juvenile plantar dermatosis.
24 Mosaic plantar warts.
25 Plane warts.
26 Molluscum contagiosum.
27 Impetigo
28 Scalp ringworm.
29 *M. canis* ringworm under Wood's light.
30 Kerion.
31 Tinea corporis produced by *M. canis*.
32 Scabies burrow.
33 Scabies in an infant.
34 Scabies mite and eggs.
35 Papular urticaria produced by arthropod bites.
36 Acquired syndactyly in recessive dystrophic epidermolysis bullosa.
37 Bullae on the vulva in chronic bullous dermatosis of childhood.
38 Infantile acne.
39 Alopecia aereata.
40 Urticaria.
41 Urticaria pigmentosa.
42 Target lesions in erythema multiforme.
43 Granuloma annulare.
44 Warty epidermal naevus.
45 Sebaceous naevus.
46 Strawberry naevus.
47 Mongolian spots.
48 Neonatal syphilis.
49 Pellagra involving the forearm and the face.
50 Cervical adenitis due to primary tuberculosis.

Plates 14–50 appear between pages 500 and 501

LIST OF CONTRIBUTORS

NICK ARCHER MA, MRCP, *Consultant Paediatric Cardiologist, John Radcliffe Hospital, Oxford OX3 9DN*

JOHN AXTON MD, FRCP, DCH, *Consultant Paediatrician, Derbyshire Children's Hospital, Derby DE1 3BA*

TONY BURNS FRCP, FRCP (Edin), *Consultant Dermatologist, Leicester Royal Infirmary, Leicester LE1 5WW*

MALCOLM LEVENE MD, FRCP, *Professor of Paediatrics and Child Health, Leeds General Infirmary, Leeds LS2 9NR*

NIGEL MEADOWS MD, MRCP, *Consultant Paediatrician, Whipps Cross Hospital, London E11 1NR*

RORY NICOL FRCP, FRCPsych, *Professor of Child Psychiatry, University of Leicester, Westcotes House, Leicester LE3 0QU*

JOHN OSBORNE MD, FRCP, *Consultant Paediatrician, Royal United Hospital, Bath BA1 3NG*

ROSS PINKERTON MD, DCH, FRCPI, *Consultant Paediatric Oncologist, The Royal Marsden Hospital, Sutton SM2 5PT*

PETER RUDD MA, MB, BChir, MRCP, MD, *Consultant Paediatrician, Royal United Hospital, Bath BA1 3NG*

ELAINE SIMPSON MRCP, MRCPath, *Consultant Haematologist, Royal Hospital for Sick Children, Glasgow G3 8SJ*

PETER SWIFT MA, FRCP, DCH, *Consultant Paediatrician, Leicester General Hospital, Leicester LE5 4PW*

ALAN WATSON FRCP, *Consultant Paediatric Nephrologist, Nottingham City Hospital, Nottingham NG5 1PB*

IAN YOUNG MD, FRCP, *Clinical Geneticist, Senior Lecturer in Child Health, University of Leicester, Leicester LE1 5WW*

PREFACE TO THE SIXTH EDITION

It is now 5 years since the publication of the fifth edition of *Diseases of Children* and 3 years since the death of Hugh Jolly. The first edition of *Diseases of Children* was published in 1964 and instantly became a successful undergraduate text which I myself used as a basic source for learning paediatrics. Many have commented on the readability of earlier editions and the individual approach to the child seen firmly in the context of his or her family.

Paediatrics has changed enormously since 1964 and today most children are managed out of hospital. The spectrum of infectious disease in developed countries has receded and major advances in high technology medicine can now cure children who, 10 years ago, died of congenital abnormalities, malignancy and extreme prematurity. Other changes have occurred, including increasing recognition of child abuse and in particular sexual abuse of both girls and boys. Because of these major changes, the sixth edition of Hugh Jolly's book has been completely rewritten by a team of authors — all young British paediatricians or specialists experienced in the problems of children. Every effort has been made to retain the 'readability' of the book, but those who have read previous editions will notice a change in emphasis away from disease orientation to problem or symptom orientation. The child usually presents to the doctor with a problem and the diagnosis or diagnoses must be arrived at after taking a careful history, performing a complete physical examination and undertaking appropriate investigations. Most chapters consider the major presenting symptom and then discuss the disease entities.

No one textbook can serve as the standard work for undergraduates, postgraduates, general practitioners and specialists developing a major interest in disorders of children. In most medical schools the undergraduate course in paediatrics has contracted in recent years in competition with other specialties. This book provides additional background information for the medical student and will give a very good basic ground work for the postgraduate student who is working for specialist disciplines. The book is also intended as a source book for general practitioners who may see rare conditions very infrequently in their professional life and who need succinct and accurate information on these disorders.

Previous editions of *Diseases of Children* have been widely read in developing countries and in the sixth edition we have devoted an extensive chapter to the problems of child health and disease in these countries. In some developing countries the gap between high technology Western medicine and local facilities is becoming wider and a separate section is felt to be necessary. The standard of child health in most developing countries is improving, but it is of some concern that increasing urban deprivation in so-called developed Western countries is causing the reappearance of disease and deficiency states once thought to have been conquered, particularly in the rundown inner city areas.

Throughout this book the child is referred to as

male. The term he or him or his is not in any way to be interpreted as a neglect of the female sex, but brevity and convenience dictates the use of these pronouns. In mitigation of this usage, female infants and children have lower mortality than males, and the incidence of many disease states is lower than in males; the superiority of the female in this respect encourages one to refer to the patients as males.

Acknowledgements

I am indebted to Per and Peter Saugman for their confidence and support which enabled me to undertake the task of editing the sixth edition. I am also grateful to Geraldine Jolly for her encouragement to take the book into its third decade. I am grateful to Drs Tudehope and Theale for permission to reproduce some illustrations first published in our book *Essentials of Neonatal Medicine* and to the Department of Medical Illustration at the Leeds General Infirmary and University of Leeds. Christine Hildyard has been unstinting of her time in the preparation of the manuscript and I am extremely grateful to her for her unflagging energy and enthusiasm.

Malcolm I. Levene

PREFACE TO THE FIRST EDITION

This book is intended for medical students and general practitioners. Emphasis has been laid on the common disorders of childhood, but rare conditions are included so that it can be used for reference. The care of sick children is essentially a matter of teamwork, therefore the advice the doctor should give the nurse who is assisting him has been included. It is hoped that nursing tutors will also find this of value.

The steady improvement in the mortality rates for infants and children should not lead the student to spend less time learning about normal and sick children. Most paediatric centres now report increasing pressure on their beds and out-patient clinics. Amongst other reasons, this is related to a greater emphasis on special-care units and the needs of premature infants, a more active approach to the management of congenital malformations, and a wider recognition of the needs of the emotionally disturbed child. Further factors increasing the demand for hospital beds are the loosening of family ties, whereby a grandmother is no longer available to nurse the sick child at home, and the frequency with which mothers go out to work.

A wide knowledge of the child in health and disease is essential for the family doctor, a large proportion of whose patients will be children. An ability to look after children is one of the keys to successful general practice, reputations being made more rapidly by success with children than in any other way. The problems of sick children in general practice and the needs of the general practitioner have been largely derived from 9 years experience as a consultant paediatrician in a large provincial area where it is possible to achieve a closer relationship between consultant and general practitioner than in a teaching hospital.

Paediatrics is changing fast, so that there is now much greater emphasis on the neonatal period, this being reflected in the number of pages devoted to this age group. The pattern of disease is also changing in older children; for example, in children over 1 year of age accidents are the most frequent cause of death, while cancer, although rare, is now the most common natural cause of death.

The sick child must be studied within the context of medicine as a whole; this book anticipates a knowledge of general medicine in its readers. Stress is laid on the frequent occasions when the child's reaction to disease differs from that of the adult. The fact that the temperature of a newborn baby with infection is as likely to fall as to rise is an example of such a difference.

There is no separate chapter on tropical diseases. Many of the diseases of the tropics are the same as those in temperate climates, but their pattern is different because of alterations in the environment or in the response of the individual to disease. Other diseases, which used to be confined to tropical areas, and were often, therefore, left out of textbooks designed for use in temperate climates, have been incorporated within the systems affected. Nowadays, immigration and the speed of travel requires that every practitioner should be competent to recognize and treat these disorders. For the same reason a geographical history is described as part of normal history taking.

The more frequent references to West Africa, particularly Nigeria, than to other tropical areas result from a year spent working there. For the same reason a number of illustrations are of African children. It is hoped that an approach to paediatrics through a study of sick children both in temperate and tropical countries will assist students and doctors in both areas.

Hugh Jolly

1
HISTORY TAKING
AND EXAMINATION

In clinical medicine, history taking and physical examination are the keystones of diagnosis. When the patient is a child, the doctor's approach is of special importance and techniques must be altered in light of the patient's age. In general terms the history is taken from the parent, but even in young children direct questions may be put to them in order to elicit further information. When taking the clinical history, the doctor must decide whether it would be better for the child to go out of the room to play rather than to hear himself discussed. However, he should always come into the consulting room in the first place to prevent fear of the unknown while waiting to be called. A sensitive doctor will often anticipate the parents' wish to talk on their own. Some parents feel too embarrassed to make the request with the result that they may withhold important information.

The child needs to be put at his ease and made to feel welcome. He is usually greeted first, provided this is unlikely to embarrass him. The greeting sometimes takes the form of a complimentary remark about his clothes or showing him a special toy. It may be appropriate to tell the child your name and then to ask his. Alternatively, a question such as 'do you go to school?' may be easier for him to answer. The aim is to become friends and help the child to make contact with the doctor.

History taking

In children, and perhaps adults, the medical history often provides more information on which to make a diagnosis than the clinical examination. The aim of the history is to build up a picture of the child, his problem(s), his family and his environment and a structured approach to the history taking is important. Asking questions in a fixed sequence is necessary in order to avoid forgetting things, but this must not become too rigid as sometimes it is necessary to pursue a different line in questioning to arrive at important information. Table 1.1 suggests a protocol of sub-headings to be used in history taking and this should be memorized. At the end of the first meeting with the patient and his family, a problem list should be drawn up. This is different to the presenting complaint and should include family, social, school and emotional problems. An example of a problem list might look like this:

1 Intermittent wheezing.
2 Poor school attendance.
3 Parental anxiety.
4 Headaches.
5 Systolic cardiac murmur.

It is important to list the problem as the child or parent sees it. If intermittent wheezing is the problem, the diagnosis may be asthma. Problems 1–4 are probably closely connected and may all improve with treatment directed at one of them. Problem 5 may be quite unrelated, and may require separate investigation. If the murmur eventually turns out to be innocent, the problem becomes inactive.

Vague data should not be accepted, particularly words which could have many meanings. This is especially the case when a technical word is used

Table 1.1 A framework for taking and recording the history.

Presenting complaint

Family history
   Father: age and occupation
   Mother: age and occupation
   Children in chronological order with names and ages
   Deaths of close family members including
      miscarriages, stillbirths and terminations
   Family illness and allergies
   Housing

Previous history
   Place of birth
   Pregnancy, labour, birthweight
   Perinatal problems
   Feeding methods
   Developmental history and school progress
   Immunization
   Allergies
   Previous illnesses
   Geographical history

such as bronchitis or dermatitis which must be defined by the patient or parent. This is also important for everyday words such as diarrhoea or constipation which may have very different connotations according to the user's experience. Ask the patient or parent 'what do you mean by such a term?'.

Leading questions and jargon must be avoided and, although it is important not to rush the patient or parent, it is essential to control the interview so that the parent (or patient) does not ramble on irrelevantly. Often a question such as 'what worries you most about the child?' or 'what single complaint do you want to tell me about?' may cut throught a lot of extraneous information.

Interviewing parents whose first language is not English may be difficult and confusion easily arises. Ask the parents to bring a relative or friend who does speak English (or the same language as the doctor). Often a nurse or hospital worker may be able to translate but always be suspicious when the interpreter translates monosyllabically after a lengthy conversation in the foreign language. Ask the interpreter exactly what was said and ask him or her to translate in full what you say to the parent or patient.

If a question to the parent causes apparent distress, then it is essential to enquire further as it may have touched the core of the problem. This must be done in as sensitive a manner as possible and a direct question such as 'why have I made you cry?' should be avoided. It is better to say 'something I have said has caused you some distress, could you tell me what it was?' No verbal or non-verbal clue should be ignored. Parents often bring up subjects because they want to talk about them but are unable to say so directly. If a patient said that he felt low it would be appropriate to ask how this affected him or exactly what he meant. It is also important to establish how this affects the rest of the family.

Sometimes formal history taking and examination are irrelevant such as when a sick child is seen in the Accident and Emergency department. Examination of the sick child must precede detailed history taking and this is discussed on p. 240. Routine examination of the normal newborn is discussed in Chapter 5.

The description that follows is intended for those who see children referred by family doctors or general practitioners (GPs). Under such conditions the consultant, registrar (resident) houseman (intern) or medical student is without the GPs advantage of knowing the family background and the child's social and home circumstances. The vital link for bridging this gap is the GPs letter or telephone call which should give the reason for referral, the results of any investigations performed and the treatment including dosage of medicines prescribed. It is helpful to be told whether it is the parents who have made the initial request for a second opinion. The letter need not give lengthy details about symptoms since the hospital doctor will check these himself.

Before the child is seen by a doctor he should first have been weighed, measured and had his urine checked. This is particularly important on the first visit. The child should be undressed for these measurements but allowed to redress afterwards whilst waiting to see the doctor. Sometimes undressing the child may cause him considerable upset and it may be best to leave it until after he has been seen by the doctor. The doctor should plot the height and weight on a centile chart prior to calling the patient into the room (p. 39). It is particularly important to screen the urine for the presence of blood, protein and glucose.

Presenting complaint

This may be an obvious condition such as skin rash, swollen joint or wheezing, but a child's complaint may be the presenting symptom of major family pathology. It is therefore important to try to elicit what it is that the parent is worried about and record that. It may be necesssary to list more than one presenting problem, but in general the more there are, the more likely it is that the child is representing the focus of anxiety in a complicated family situation (see Chapter 20).

Record the chronology of the presenting complaint in a systematic manner with a heading for each date line:

4 weeks ago: onset of cough
3 days ago: sore throat
yesterday: rash
today: convulsion.

Never write the days of the week in the history since they give no indication of the duration of the disease. It is important for the person taking the history to have a clear idea in his or her own mind of the chronology of the presenting complaint. If you are confused, ask direct questions to clarify the points.

Previous medical history

This includes a series of categories which should be specifically inquired after.

BIRTH HISTORY

The amount of time given to antenatal and birth history will depend on the child's age and complaint and is particularly relevant if the child presents with mental retardation, cerebral palsy, weakness, convulsions or congenital malformations. Enquire about drugs taken by the mother during pregnancy. Record the number of pregnancies, miscarriages, terminations of pregnancy and stillborn children. Draw a family tree to indicate birth order.

Ask about labour, requirements for forceps or operative delivery and birth weight. Condition of the infant at birth is important and direct questions are often necessary. Enquire whether the baby was taken away for special treatment, and when did the mother first see him. If the baby was taken away to a neonatal unit was he nursed in an incubator and if so for how long. When did he first take bottle feeds or how long did he require oxygen. This information will allow the clinician to get an impression as to how sick the newborn infant was. Record whether the mother breast fed and for how long. With babies a feeding history is important. What type of milk, how much and how often? Ask when mixed feeding was introduced.

DEVELOPMENTAL HISTORY

The details of developmental history depend on the presenting complaint. If the child has a neurological problem, failure to thrive or the possibility of a degenerative condition, a detailed developmental history is required. Developmental milestones are discussed in Chapter 4 and summarized in Table 4.2.

SCHOOL PROGRESS

Record the name of the school that the child attends and whether he requires remedial help. If there appears to be a school-related problem, a letter to the headmaster enquiring as to his progress may be helpful, but this should only be done with the consent of the child or his parent.

IMMUNIZATIONS

These should be recorded in as much detail as possible. Do not accept from the parent that the child as 'fully immunized'. Ask specifically whether this includes pertussis and measles and whether the boosters are up to date. See Chapter 21 for immunization details.

PREVIOUS ILLNESS

An enquiry should be made into previous illnesses and, if necessary, specifically about the infectious fevers such as measles, rubella and others. These are often forgotten by the mother or merely recorded by the doctor as 'usual childhood complaints'. An absence of this detailed information is particularly irritating in the case of children in hospital when another patient in the ward develops an infectious fever. If this happens it is necessary to know at once which of the other patients are at risk and need to be isolated. A direct question should be asked as to whether the child has had any operations including tonsillectomy and/or adenoidectomy.

ALLERGIES

It is important to ask about allergies, particularly drugs such as penicillin, and whether the child is on any regular medication. Since some parents associate 'drugs' with narcotics it is better to ask about medicines, tablets or pills.

GEOGRAPHICAL HISTORY

World-wide travel is common today even for small children. Record where the child has been and whether he had been ill overseas. This is particularly important if he has been to underdeveloped parts of the world. It is possible that a child who has not travelled abroad may have picked up a 'tropical' or unusual disease from a relative or contact who has returned from such a country.

System review

It is customary to enquire from the child or parent whether there have been any symptoms related to specific systems. Hopefully any important ones would already have come to light but asking specifically about problems related to vomiting, bowel habit, micturition, abdominal pain, headaches,

limb pains, rashes may elicit some further important information.

Clinical examination

The approach to the clinical examination depends on the age and co-operation of the child. Older children are examined in a manner very similar to the adult: by organ system in a systematic manner. The young child, particularly if fretful or anxious must be approached quite differently. Any uncomfortable procedure such as examination of ears and throat should be left to last in order to avoid upsetting the child as much as possible. Time spent initially gaining the child's confidence is never wasted. Examination of the nervous system of a baby is best preceded by a period of observation and watching him play. Before using a stethoscope on the child it is often helpful to put it first on the chest of the mother or a teddy bear to show the child that it is not frightening. Pre-warm the stethoscope as cold steel on the child's back or chest may cause discomfort. Inside the consulting room the mother should be left to undress the young child since he is liable to be nervous of a stranger doing this. The doctor must be prepared to vary his routine to suit the child, and it may be necessary to examine the back of the chest before the front, or the abdomen before the chest. This variable routine has the disadvantage that parts of the examination may be left out, but this can be prevented by a strictly systematic method of recording so that it is immediately obvious if any part of the examination has been overlooked.

Small children should, as far as possible, be examined on their mother's lap. The child can always be moved to the couch for further examination but this may make him cry. If the child is asleep in his mother's arms much of the examination should be completed before he is woken up. The sleeping child may give the doctor the best chance to examine the heart, respiratory system, abdomen and possibly fundi.

A young child may be put at his ease if the doctor keeps up a 'running commentary' during his examination. The doctor asks questions as he goes along but if the child fails to answer he

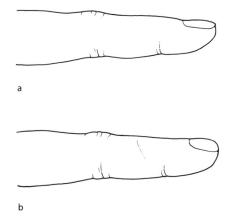

a

b

Fig. 1.1 Profile of nailbed angle: (a) normal, and (b) clubbing.

should immediately pass on to another. A child can become acutely embarrassed by the silence after a doctor's question, whereas he may be reassured by the doctor's ceaseless chatter.

Examination of the normal newborn is discussed in Chapter 5. A system-orientated approach to the clinical examination is described here and is directed towards younger children in whom the detection of physical signs may be more difficult.

Observation

Watch the way the child plays. Is he inquisitive to explore the consulting office? Does he play purposefully or does he wander from one toy to the next with little real interest in any. How does he react with his parent(s) and how does the mother react to her child.

A good introduction to the physical examination is to examine the child's hands. Observe the hands for colour (cyanosis, anaemia), palmar creases and for the presence of clubbing. The most sensitive way to detect early clubbing is to look at the profile of the nailbed as the normal angle is lost very early in the clubbing process (Fig. 1.1).

Next observe the child's facies. Is there any evidence of dysmorphic features or weakness? Look at the lips and tongue for central cyanosis.

Nervous system

In infants, palpation of the fontanelle may yield useful information. When the child is quiet, the fontanelle is normally seen to pulsate. The fontanelle tension cannot be assessed in crying children. In all children the maximum occipito-frontal head circumference should be measured by the examining doctor and plotted on an appropriate growth chart.

It is not possible to systematically examine the cranial nerves in infants or young children. Ocular movements can easily be assessed by getting the child's visual attention and observing his range of eye movements as he tracks the object through 360 degrees. Check the pupils for size, shape and reaction to light. Facial palsy should be obvious when the child cries. Look for inability to close the eye on the affected side as well as distortion of the mouth. Hearing can be tested even in the youngest of children (see Chapter 18) and the method of testing hearing by distraction is discussed on p. 308. The higher cranial nerves are more difficult to assess, but testing for a gag reflex and watching the child feed is useful in assessing the vagus nerve. Fundi should be examined, but this may be difficult in toddlers and is best left to near the end of the examination. Testing for a squint is described on p. 313.

Tone should be assessed both passively and actively. Passive tone is examined by observing the child's response to gravity. Young babies are held in the ventro-suspended position (Fig. 1.2) to observe back, neck and limb tone. Pulling the infant to sitting gives information on trunk and back tone. Active tone is assessed by moving the limbs through extension/flexion, and pronation/supination as appropriate. Tone is assessed by experience of the normal and it is particularly important to examine the arm flexors and extensors (biceps and triceps), supinators and pronators (brachioradialis) and hip adductors, leg extensors (quadriceps) and flexors (hamstrings) as well as ankle extension (gastrocnemius). The movements to be made on the child are shown in Figures 1.3–1.6.

Motor function is best tested by observation and

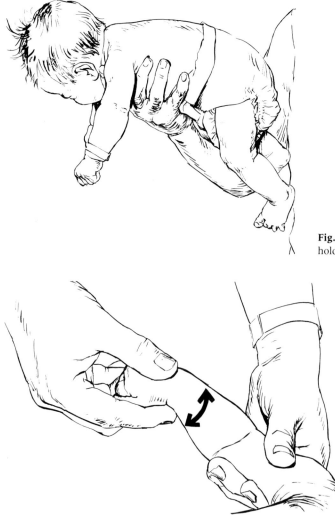

Fig. 1.2 Examination of trunk and neck tone by holding the infant in ventro-suspension.

Fig. 1.3 Eliciting tone in the pronator and supinator muscles of the forearm. The upper arm is held in a fixed position and the forearm is rapidly supinated and pronated.

particular attention is paid to symmetry. Sensation should also be carefully assessed but only responses to painful stimuli can be confidently elicited in small children. Tendon jerk reflexes should always be elicited and Table 1.2 refers to the root values associated with each reflex. The presence of persistent primitive reflexes should be examined. If detected after 6 months of age they are always abnormal. Table 1.3 lists the more common primitive reflexes and their average age of extinction. The parachute reflex is an important protective reflex that should always be assessed in young children. It develops at approximately 9 months and is elicited by tipping the child head downward towards the tabletop (Fig. 1.7). Absence or asymmetry may indicate an upper motor neurone lesion (see Chapter 19).

Table 1.2 Root values corresponding to tendon reflexes.

Biceps	C5,6
Supinator	C5,6
Triceps	C6,7
Knee	L2,3,4
Ankle	S1,2
Plantars	L5, S1

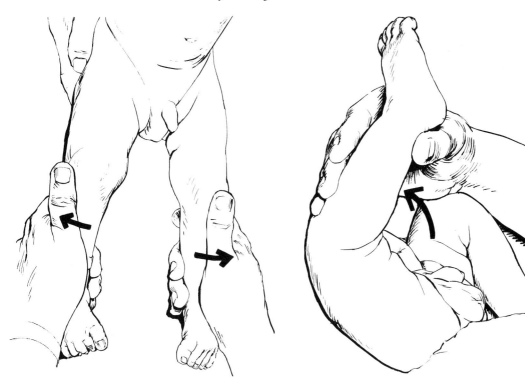

Fig. 1.4 Tone in the hip adductors. The arrows indicate the direction of movement to elicit tone.

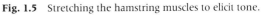

Fig. 1.5 Stretching the hamstring muscles to elicit tone.

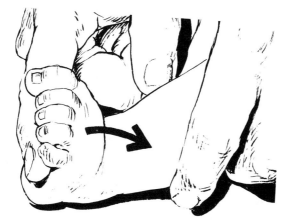

Fig. 1.6 Dorsiflexion of the foot to elicit tone in the gastrocnemius muscle.

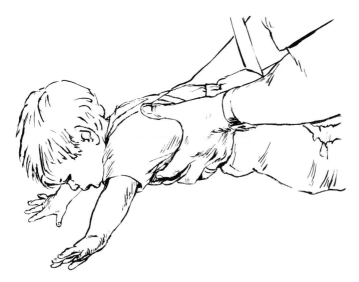

Fig. 1.7 Demonstrating a normal parachute reflex.

Table 1.3 Final age by which primitive reflexes should have disappeared.

Moro reflex (p. 43)	6 months
Palmar grasp	2 months
Plantar grasp	10 months
Stepping	2 months
Placing	1 year
Asymmetrical tonic neck reflex (p. 43)	6 months

Cardiovascular system

The presence of breathlessness, cyanosis and clubbing should all be noted on inspection. A peripheral pulse (radial or brachial) is palpated for rate, rhythm and character of the impulse. Irregularity of the pulse is not uncommon in children and is usually due to innocent extrasystoles. A collapsing or waterhammer pulse is characteristic of patent ductus arteriosus or aortic incompetence. There is a very rapid upstroke to the pulse and a wide pulse pressure when blood pressure is measured. A weak pulse may be felt with hypotentsion, aortic stenosis or hypoplastic left heart syndrome. The femoral pulses should always be palpated and any delay between the femoral and radial impulse noted (see Coarctation of the aorta p. 232).

Examination of the jugular pulse at the neck is not possible in small children but may be of value in older ones. Cardiomegaly may be assessed by percussion and palpation. The apex beat is detected by one finger laid over the praecordium and is normally felt in infants in the anterior axillary line, fourth intercostal space. By 7 years the normal position is in the fifth intercostal space. If it is palpated lateral to this it implies left ventricular hypertrophy. Right ventricular hypertrophy is detected by feeling for a parasternal heave. The hand is placed over the chest as shown in Figure 1.8 and if present a heaving impulse is felt over the heel of the hand. In infants percussion of the heart is of little value. The chest is also palpated for thrills. These are palpable murmurs and the four areas shown in Figure 1.9 should be palpated separately.

The chest should be auscultated carefully with both the bell and diaphragm of the stethoscope. The bell is particularly important to pick up low pitched murmurs. The examiner must discipline himself to listen first for the heart sounds and then for murmurs. The chest should be auscultated in five areas. The four praecordial areas are shown in Figure 1.9 as well as the back. The first heart sound comprises closure of the mitral and tricuspid valves. The second sound occurs with closure of the aortic and pulmonary valves. These two valves do not close simultaneously. On inspiration, blood is sucked into the right side of the heart and

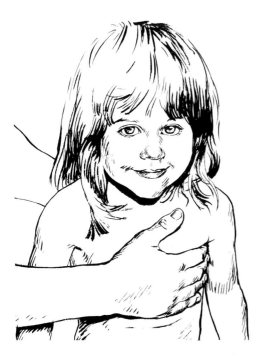

Fig. 1.8   Detecting a parasternal heave. The impulse is detected over the heel of the hand.

right ventricular ejection is prolonged causing the pulmonary valve to close slightly after the aortic valve. During expiration the two valves close together. Normally splitting of the second heart sound is heard in inspiration in the pulmonary area. Fixed splitting of the second heart sound (does not vary with respiration) is due to overfilling of the right ventricle usually due to an atrial septal defect (p. 228) or pulmonary stenosis (p. 233). A loud and single second heart sound is heard when pulmonary vascular resistance is raised, usually due to a large left to right shunt such as occurs with a big ventricular septal defect (p. 229). A single second heart sound may also be heard in aortic stenosis. A third heart sound is heard in up to a quarter of normal children and is due to rapid filling of the ventricles. An ejection click occurs due to aortic or pulmonary valve stenosis.

Murmurs are due to turbulence of blood flow and may be innocent or associated with cardiac pathology. In infants there may be no murmur despite major cardiac anomalies. The loudness of the murmur does not correlate with the severity of the lesion. The murmur may occur during systole or diastole. Diastolic murmurs usually denote definite cardiac pathology. Systolic murmurs may be either ejection (diamond-shaped) or pansystolic (Fig. 1.10). In the latter case this term may be misleading as the murmur does not always occur

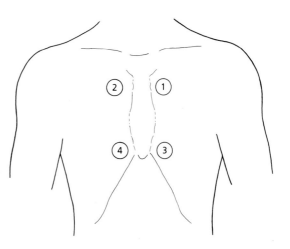

Fig. 1.9   The four anterior chest positions for detecting murmurs and thrills. **1** Pulmonary, **2** aortic, **3** mitral, and **4** tricuspid.

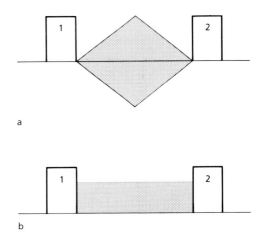

Fig. 1.10   Timing of murmurs. (a) Ejection systolic murmur, and (b) pan-systolic murmur. **1, 2** A first and second heart sound.

throughout systole. Diastolic murmurs may be due to:

1 Increased blood flow through normal atrioventricular valves.

2 Narrowing (stenosis) of atrioventricular valves.

3 Incompetence of the pulmonary or aortic valves.

These conditions are discussed in Chapter 13. The distinction between in innocent murmur and one due to cardiac pathology is described on p. 224. A vibratory murmur heard in mid-systole is very common and is innocent. If the child leans backwards with the neck extended the murmur usually disappears and thus can be distinguished from a sinister murmur which does not vary with movement. A venous hum is due to blood flow in the neck veins and is often continuous and heard in the supraclavicular fossa. It can be abolished by jugular venous compression.

Blood pressure should be measured in all new patients. An appropriately sized cuff must be used. It should be wide enough to cover two-thirds of the upper arm and the bladder should competely encircle the arm. It is important to have a range of cuff sizes available in every paediatric clinic. It may be necessary to use a Doppler probe to detect systole in very young children. Another method is the flush technique. The cuff is applied and the child's hand and lower arm wrapped in a bandage or squeezed by hand. The cuff is then inflated to above the expected systolic pressure. The bandage is removed and the child's hand will look white as the blood has been squeezed out. As the cuff is gradually deflated the colour will suddenly flush back when systolic pressure has been reached. See p. 271 for the normal range of blood pressures in paediatric age groups.

Respiratory system

Signs of respiratory distress should be noted during the period of observation. Respiratory rate, use of accessory muscles, nasal flaring or recession are easily seen. Recession may be subcostal, intercostal, supraclavicular or suprasternal.

The shape of the chest must be carefully observed. A barrel chest implies air trapping with overexpansion. The antero-posterior (A–P) diameter is increased and this is best observed by looking at the chest from the side. Various types of chest deformities are described on p. 171. Pectus excavatum (funnel chest) is also a common deformity and may be without significance.

The movement of the chest wall should be assessed. On inspiration the ribs move in two directions and these movements can be described as pump handle and bucket handle. The pump handle represents the increased A–P diameter on inspiration. The bucket handle movement describes both the A–P and lateral expansion. This can be best assessed by placing the examiner's hands on the chest with the thumbs just touching each other at the sternum and the fingers lightly resting on the skin over the ribs (Fig. 1.11). The child is asked to take a deep breath and the distance the thumbs moves apart determines the degree of bucket handle movement.

The chest is percussed to assess its degree of resonance. The middle finger of the left hand (if the examiner is right handed) is placed along the line of a rib and is then struck with the first finger of the right hand as if hammering in a small nail. The quality of the resonant note is compared with other parts of the chest. The entire chest, back and front, should be percussed in a systematic way. The resonance is increased with overexpansion and diminished when the underlying lung is more solid (less air) than usual. The degree of resonance reduces over the anterior part of the right chest at a higher position than the left due to the presence of the liver. It is important to percuss out the position of the liver and this is described below. In small children the heart may not affect the degree of resonance.

The lungs should then be auscultated. Start at the top of the chest anteriorly, comparing one side with the other, then turn the child around and auscultate the back in a similar manner. There are two main types of breath sound: *vesicular* and *bronchial*. Vesicular sounds are heard when air enters and leaves normal lung tissue. The sound is continuous. Bronchial breathing is normally heard over the trachea and there is a distinct interval between the inspiratory and expiratory sound. The

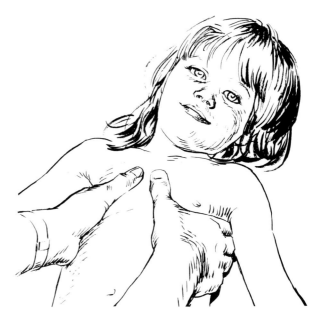

Fig. 1.11 Assessment of 'bucket handle' chest expansion.

sound is harsher than that heard in vesicular breathing. Adventitious sounds are then described. These are described as wheezes or rhonchi (musical sounds) or crepitations (crackling sounds). Wheezes may be inspiratory or expiratory and indicate bronchial narrowing. Crepitations are discontinuous noises that sound like rustles or crackles and may be normal, often cleared by coughing if the child is old enough to co-operate. The detection of vocal resonance is only of value in the older co-operative child.

In young children, sounds transmitted from the upper airway may be confused with lower respiratory sounds, particularly rhonchi. It is important to listen first without the stethoscope to the noise the child is making. Sometimes, when the upper airway sounds are soft, applying the stethoscope close to the child's mouth, nose or larynx may help to clarify the nature of the upper airway noise to avoid confusing it with the noises coming from the chest itself.

Abdomen

The abdomen can only be examined with the child lying on his back, although in small children this may be on the mother's lap. Observe the abdomen and describe its shape. Distention (either generalized or localized) and visible peristalsis should be noted particularly. Enquire of the child whether the abdomen is tender. Initially palpate the abdomen lightly with two to four fingers depending on the size of the child. All four quadrants should be palpated for tenderness or masses. If the abdomen is not tender then re-examine with deep palpation.

The major intra-abdominal organs should be palpated separately. The liver enlarges downwards to the right iliac fossa, thus to examine it the palm of the extended hand is placed on the right lower quadrant. The patient should be examined from the right with the right hand if right handed. The liver is palpated with the lateral aspect of the whole right index finger (Fig. 1.12) and the examining hand is gradually moved up to the right costal margin until the liver edge is felt. In infants the liver edge is normally easily palpable 1 cm below the costal margin and is smooth and soft. When a child is fretful and does not permit thorough palpation of the abdomen, he can often be persuaded to co-operate if the doctor places the child's hand on the abdomen and then, covering it with his own hand, palpates through it.

The spleen enlarges towards the right iliac fossa

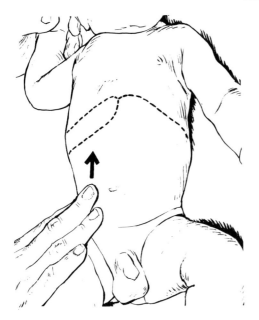

Fig. 1.12 Examination to detect the liver edge. The hand should be moved upwards in the direction indicated.

and is examined with the hand initially in the right iliac fossa. It is progressively moved up towards the left costal margin (Fig. 1.13). It is felt on inspiration as the diaphragm contracts and pushes it down towards the examiners hand. Sometimes a modestly enlarged spleen may be difficult to palpate. Detection is aided by placing the left hand on the left loin and pushing the spleen up towards the palpating right hand. Another method is to turn the child onto his left side whilst palpating with the right hand so that the spleen drops towards it. The spleen, if enlarged, may be very soft and the examiner must be aware that the sensation may be a subtle one. The kidneys are examined by bimanual palpation. One hand in the loin pushing up and the other on the anterior aspect of the flank pushing down. The kidney will be felt between the two hands.

The abdomen should then be percussed for resonant note. The liver edge may be palpable and apparently enlarged because the lungs are overexpanded so it is important to delineate the upper position of the liver by its dullness over the chest. A distended bladder will also be dull to percussion. The hernial orifices should be inspected and examined. Rectal examination is not mandatory but if required should be left to last and in carrying this out, the tip of the index finger should be pressed flat against the edge of the anus before insertion. This method causes much less discomfort than insertion direct into the centre of the orifice.

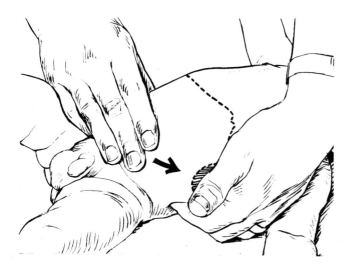

Fig. 1.13 Bimanual examination to detect the spleen. The right hand palpates towards the left costal margin whilst the left hand lifts the spleen towards the examining right hand.

Hips

Routine examination of the hips is essential as part of the newborn examination (p. 59). In all children examined at 1 year or less, it is important to check that both hips abduct normally and symmetrically to ensure there is no late dislocation.

Genitalia

The genitalia should always be examined in children. In boys inspect the scrotum and palpate the testes. The urethral orifice must be identified and the development of the scrotum noted. The testes may be retracted in some children. Patience is needed to gradually milk the retracted testes down into the scrotum. If in doubt re-examine later. In the female, the vulval lips should be gently parted to exclude an abnormality of the lower vagina.

Reticuloendothelial system

Enlarged lymph nodes should be detected by systematic examination of the neck (anterior and posterior triangles), supraclavicular fossae, axillae and groin. In children it is very common to detect small pea-like nodes in the neck or groin. They are mobile and hard and of no significance. If a node is detected, record its size, position and whether it is freely mobile. Immobile or matted nodes are very suspicious.

Ears and throat

This should be left to last as their examination is likely to distress the child. To examine the ears, the young child should be held firmly by the mother in the manner shown in Fig. 10.1. with one hand securing the child's chest against the

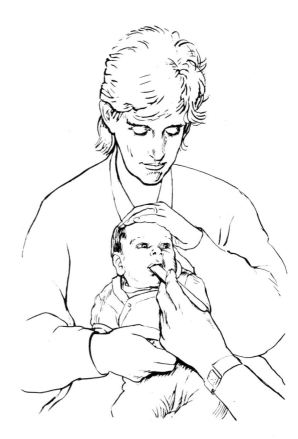

Fig. 1.14 Position to hold a young child for examination of the throat.

mother's chest. This position must be reversed to examine the other ear. The external auditory meatus is straightened by pulling up on the pinna and the largest aural speculum suitable for the size of the child used. The appearances of the normal tympanic membrane should be well known to the observer (p. 153) and abnormalities are discussed in Chapter 18. To examine the throat the child is held facing the examiner by the adult as shown in Fig. 1.14. If the child is co-operative he will voluntarily open his mouth. If this is not the case the wooden spatula is gently used to open the mouth and the tongue depressed. If the child cries, this facilitates the examination.

2

CHILD CARE

IN AND OUT OF HOSPITAL

The health of children in Britain can be measured on a number of different yardsticks. Towards the end of the twentieth century, fewer children die than at any time in the last 100 years (Fig. 2.1). It is clear that early childhood mortality has been declining since 1870 and this preceded an improvement in infant mortality by 30 years. The causes of the very high mortality rates were mainly infectious diseases, which are now very rare causes of death. Today, in Britain the commonest cause of death in infancy (1 month to 1 year) is the suddden infant death syndrome and this is discussed on p. 510. Table 2.1 lists the commonest causes of death in children aged 1–4 years. Accidental death is the most important cause of death in this age group, followed by respiratory disorders and malignancy. These conditions are discussed in much more detail in the relevant chapters.

Mortality rates are widely used as indices of the quality of care in a community, hospital or country. The World Health Organization recommends the perinatal morality rate as an index of the quality of perinatal health services.

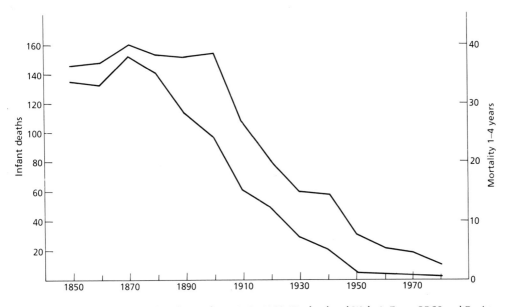

Fig. 2.1 Infant (upper line) and childhood mortality, 1850–1980 (England and Wales). From OPCS and Registrar General's annual reports. Infant death rates are per 1000 live births and mortality rates are per 1000 population.

Table 2.1 Causes of death in children aged 1–14 years in the UK. (Source OPCS.)

Disease classification	Proposition of deaths (%)
Accidents, poisoning and violence	27.0
Respiratory disorders	16.6
Malignancies	16.2
Congenital abnormalities	11.7
Miscellaneous	9.4
Infection (specific)	8.1
Nervous system disease	7.3
Allergic and endocrine	2.2
Circulatory	1.5
Total	100.0

Table 2.2 Mortality rates (1982) in England and Wales. (Source OPCS.)

Stillbirth rate	6.25
Perinatal mortality rate	11.25
Neonatal mortality rate	6.27
Infant mortality rate	10.82

Definitions

1 Perinatal mortality rate. The number of still-births and neonatal deaths in the first week of life per 1000 live births and stillbirths. The causes of perinatal mortality are discussed in Chapter 7.
2 Infant mortality rate. The number of deaths of all live-born infants in the first year of life per 1000 live births. This can be subdivided into:
(a) Neonatal mortality rate. The number of deaths of live-born infants in the first 28 days of life per 1000 live births.
(b) Post-neonatal mortality rate. The number of deaths of live-born infants dying after 28 days but before 1 year of age per 1000 live births.
These rates are shown for 1982 in Table 2.2.

Although the mortality rates in Britain are relatively low they belie the heterogeneous nature of the population. Britain is a multiracial society, and 7% of the population of children aged 0–16 years are born to mothers of non-Caucasian ethnic origin. Table 2.3 shows the perinatal and infant mor-

Table 2.3 Perinatal mortality and infant deaths by mother's country of birth. This data refers to women living in the UK. (Source OPCS.)

	Perintal mortality rate (per 1000 total births)	Infant mortality rate (per 1000 live births)
UK	12.9	11.6
Australia, Canada, New Zealand	8.0	9.6
Bangladesh, India	15.7	12.8
West Indies	17.9	15.4
Pakistan	26.3	22.0

tality rates for the mother's country of birth. It is clear that infants born to Pakistani mothers have a twofold increased chance of death compared to those born to mothers who themselves were born in Britain. The risk of death is also higher for mothers born in the West Indies and India. Social class, maternal age and parity are also important variables for risk of death. Table 2.4 shows the perinatal and infant mortality rates for the five social classes. Those infants born into the lowest social class have a 1.5 increased risk of dying compared to an infant born into a social class 1 family.

Children are a particularly vulnerable group in society, and in Britain the Welfare State provides a variety of agencies to protect them. Inevitably there is some overlap, but this is less of a problem than when the services do not reach those who need them most; often the poor, members of ethnic minority groups and those living in derelict inner cities. In 1976, Professor Court chaired the Committee on Child Health Services which published a report called *Fit For the Future*, commonly known as the 'Court Report'. His aim was to review the provision made for health services for children up to and through school life. The report recommended an integrated service to facilitate the abilities of parents to care for their children. Particular emphasis was put on prevention and urging better liaison between primary and secondary care. It was recommended that some health visitors should specialize only in the needs of children and some GPs should be especially trained

Table 2.4 Perinatal and infant mortality rates for England and Wales by social class. (Source OPCS, 1980–81.)

Social class	Perinatal mortality	Infant mortality
1	71	73
2	83	76
3	95	89
4	112	115
5	129	139

for a primary health role directed at children. In addition, consultant community paediatricians would be appointed who were specialists in prevention and in the care of children outside hospital. Unfortunately, few of these recommendations have been taken up through the country, but the Court Report still points the way forward for the integration of child health facilities in Britain.

Currently, the services for children are under the control of different national and local government agencies and these are summarized in Figure 2.2. Health care is organized in a tripartite manner: primary (based on the GP), community and hospital. These agencies are also responsible for providing medical, dental and nursing input into schools. The Social Services, organized by local government agencies, are community based but provide hospital liaison via hospital social workers. The local Education Department provides the school psychological services with a role in assessing the educational needs of children with learning difficulties or more severe handicap. In addition the child may come in contact with other agencies such as the police or probation services, and this may impinge on others providing child health care.

A particularly important role of the plethora of agencies involved in child health is in making

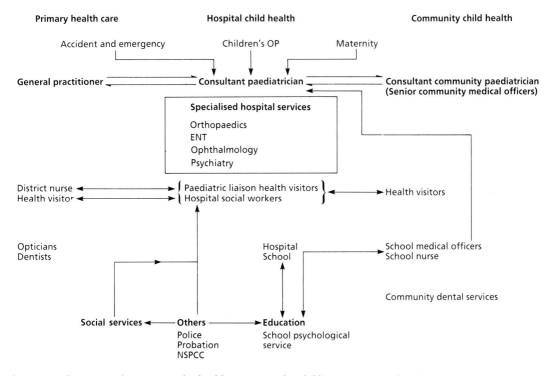

Fig. 2.2 A diagram to demonstrate the health provisions for children in Britain. This does not refer to handicapped children, who are considered in Chapter 19.

provision for the assessment and management of handicapped children. The Court Report identified this as an area where the various services needed to work more closely together. This is discussed in detail in Chapter 19.

Primary health care

The British National Health Service (NHS) provides local health care through two main bodies: the Family Practitioner Committee (FPC) and the District Health Authority (DHA). The FPC is responsible for administering primary health care in the form of general practitioners (family doctors), dentists, opticians and dispensing chemists. The GP is self-employed and contracted to provide general medical services to patients living in their practice area who register with them. They are supported by health visitors, district nurses and community midwives.

Health visitors. The health visitor is a state-registered nurse with training in obstetrics and further special training in child development and community health in general. She is employed by the DHA and may be attached to a group General Practice or hold responsibility for a geographical area. Although not responsible for children alone, she has an important role in visiting at home every newborn baby at least once and more often at her discretion. The health visitor continues her responsibility to the child until he reaches the age of 5 years or enters full-time education. She provides an important function in giving advice to mothers about their children (feeding, sleeping problems, play, etc.) and can arrange for a doctor (GP or community paediatrician) to see the child for further advice or investigation. Developmental surveillance of all children is another important role for the health visitor and this includes screening for hearing impairment at 7–9 months. Specialist health visitors exist for the needs for handicapped children.

District nurses. The district nurse is also attached to the primary health team of the GP and health visitor. Her role is to visit children (and adults) who require nursing care at home. There are provisions for district nurses to visit at night if necessary. Many children with chronic medical problems can be nursed at home, even those requiring tube feeds, intramuscular medication and other specialized forms of treatment. The district nurse therefore plays a particularly important role in keeping sick children out of hospital.

Community child health care

Community services for children are organized by the local District Health Authorities and have been subject to changes in recent years with the patchy introduction of recommendations from the Court Report. Previously, services were organized by the senior community medical officer (child health) but there are now an increasing number of consultant community paediatricians with a similar role.

The child health clinics are organized by either the community health services or GPs and provide facilities for screening all children at particular ages. Careful liaison is important to avoid reduplication of efforts. In many districts children are seen at 6 weeks, 7.5 months and 3.5 years for developmental screening and this may be done either by the doctor or health visitor. The community child health clinics are run by health visitors, with medical officers in attendance. In many districts the community paediatric services organize a comprehensive vaccination programme. This is computerized for the district so that the parents of all children are notified by post prior to the immunization date. The injection may be given in child health clinics or GP surgeries by either health visitors or GPs.

Unfortunately, in some areas, particularly in the deprived inner cities, there is poor uptake of these services. Health education has an important role in advertising these services to those families who need them most.

School medical services

The community paediatric services also provide staff for the school medical services. School doctors are community medical officers and work together with school nurses. Every school has a named doctor and nurse and each child within the school is offered a physical examination during their first term of full-time education (from the age of 5 years) and this is repeated at 10 and 13 years. The parents are invited to attend for the examination but also have the right to decline examination for their child. A dentist (from the community dental service) examines the mouth and teeth of all schoolchildren on an annual basis and if treatment is necessary refers the child to the community dental service clinic or their own dentist.

Hospital health care

Children are referred to hospital by GPs or community paediatricians. They may be referred to either the children's out-patients for a consultant opinion, or to non-paediatric consultants for an ophthalmic, surgical, ear, nose and throat, orthopaedic or psychiatric opinion. It is essential that the GP writes a good referral letter to the hospital including social details, current and previous medication and what has been said to the parents about the nature of the problem and the reason for referral.

In general it is best for the consultant paediatrician to be the first line of referral and for him or her to decide on any other consultant opinions to be sought. This is to avoid the child being treated as a series of organ-related symptoms. The problems of children should be viewed as a whole and within the context of the family and very important aspects of this may be missed by 'organ specialists' who do not have a major interest in children.

This is particularly important if a child is admitted to hospital. There has been much improvement in recent years in the services for children in hospital. Children should never be nursed on adult wards and facilities for children should be based around a floor or separate ward area. 'Adult' consultants should come to visit their patients on the children's wards and not expect the children to be nursed on their own wards for their convenience.

When a young child has to be admitted to hospital, his mother should be encouraged to stay. Many hospitals now have facilities for the mother to sleep in the same cubicle as the infant or elsewhere on the ward nearby her child. All children's wards should have unrestricted visiting for parents. Grandparents and siblings should also be encouraged to visit but this may put a strain on the ward facilities and many hospitals limit the number of visitors with the child at any one time to two. It must be realized that unrestricted visiting places a considerable strain on the mother, who may feel that she must spend all day with her young child. The strain is reduced if a rest room for parents is provided, where they can make themselves a cup of tea or coffee and sit in comfortable chairs. Mothers may also feel torn by the needs of their child in hospital and the opposing needs of their other children at home. This problem may be eased if a visitors' playroom is run by the hospital for the accommodation of child visitors for a part or the whole of a day. The room should be staffed by play therapists, nursery nurses or volunteers.

For nurses, unrestricted visiting brings a problem in that nursing procedures will be carried out in front of the parents. Ward staff should not make the mistake of sending the mother out when they come to do some special procedure on her child. There are very few procedures that the mother cannot witness; if the mother is handled wisely, her confidence in the staff will increase from knowing what is going on. At the same time the child is given greater security by having his mother with him on such occasions. If properly instructed a mother will be able to undertake much of the nursing required for her child.

Children are subjected to many painful and frightening experiences in hospital and the ward staff must work to reduce the child's feelings of anxiety. This is done by explaining in advance what is to happen. It is absurd to say to a child that a venepuncture will not hurt, but if it is explained that it will be a 'little scratch' then the child may trust the doctor on the next occasion.

Some hospitals have the skills of a play therapist available to facilitate this role. The work requires a deep understanding of children and a detailed knowledge of their development and psychology. She must also know a reasonable amount about children's illnesses and the practical aspect of the investigations ordered.

Staff must be particularly careful not to talk about a child's illness in his hearing. At the same time they must explain in simple language what is happening to him. There are some occasions when it is right to tell a child that he has a fatal illness. This depends on the questions he is asking and staff must be alert to their meaning and must provide the sympathetic atmosphere for parents to be able to talk out their feelings. Children are more frightened about how they will actually die than of no longer existing. Studies have shown that they believe death itself will be painful. Since a child has had honest answers from his parents to all previous questions, he has the right to expect an honest answer to the most crucial question of all, 'am I dying?'. Parents may find it easier to leave the telling to the consultant or favourite nurse.

Day cases

Many children requiring cold surgery such as hernia repair or circumcision can be admitted for the day of operation only. Apart from the obvious advantage to the child and his parents there is the advantage to the hospital in the saving in beds. Much of the success of the method depends on careful selection of the mothers concerned who must be told beforehand that they will be expected to spend all day in the hospital with their child.

Admission as day cases can also be used for the investigation and management of certain medical problems, for example, the infant who is failing to thrive or the baby with a feeding problem. The investigation of many handicapped children can also be undertaken as day cases. The work of a children's unit should no longer be measured by its number of beds. By integrating its out-patients, in-patient beds and the community services, a higher output of work can be achieved from a smaller number of beds.

Hospital–community liaison

Close communication with the primary health services are vital when a child is in hospital. Often a liaison health visitor is attached to the children's department who can communicate with the child's health visitor. Once the child is home, this link is very helpful in sorting out minor problems or to relieve misunderstandings. In addition, the hospital will have designated social workers, and hopefully a hospital paediatric social worker. He or she will liaise with the community social services and ensure that any social needs are being met. At discharge from hospital a discharge letter or note must rapidly be sent to the GP and community paediatricians giving details of the illness, medication used on discharge and dates of follow-up appointments.

HOSPITAL SCHOOLING

Every hospital with a children's ward has a statutory responsibility to provide education for school-age children. The hospital school teacher is a fully trained teacher, working in the hospital, and paid by the education department. For children who are likely to be admitted for a long time (lower limb fractures for instance), the hospital teacher should contact the child's teacher at school in order to learn more about the child in general and to discuss what teaching should be continued in hospital.

Accident and Emergency department

The Accident and Emergency department of any hospital is often an area of great activity with frequent scenes of human suffering. It is not a place conducive to the needs of children. If a paediatric Accident and Emergency department is not feasible, then a special area within the main department is necessary for children. This should be physically separate from the main department so that the child is not exposed to the sounds and sights of the adult department.

The department should be bright with a variety of toys and separate cubicles for private interviews. It is very helpful if one of the consultant doctors in Accident and Emergency has a strong interest in children. The junior doctors in the department must be aware of the variety of presentations of childhood illness, particularly non-accidental injury.

Neonatal wards

The newborn nursery should have open visiting for parents and siblings; grandparents and friends should also be encouraged to visit at prearranged times. The parents must be made to feel at home on the newborn unit and to feel that it is their baby and not the property of the medical and nursing staff. Mothers should be encouraged to express milk for their infants as this is a tangible contribution the mother is making in the treatment of her child. Whenever possible the baby should be taken out of the incubator and given to the parents to hold. It is possible to do this for short periods even with ventilated babies. Rooms should be available for the mother to live in with her baby prior to going home. This gives her confidence, particularly if the baby has been very ill for a long time. The parents must know that they can telephone the unit at any time, day or night, to find out how their baby is getting on.

Communication with other agencies is important and this can be achieved by the liaison health visitor and hospital social worker attending rounds at least once a week. In the event of the baby's death the consultant obstetrician and mother's GP should be telephoned so that they are aware of this information before saying anything to the parents.

Social Services

The Social Services provide social workers who have responsibilities for the protection of children. In particular they are responsible for taking children into care. This may be undertaken at the parent's wishes (voluntary care) or in an emergency a 'Place of Safety Order' is obtained from a magistrate which allows the child to be removed from the parents or guardian for up to 28 days and detained in a place of safety. It is necessary to have reasonable cause to suspect that the child's physical or emotional health is being neglected or he has been, or is, at risk of being ill-treated. In addition, truancy or lack of parental control may be grounds for taking a place of safety order. The law also protects the child by other means. The Social Services can apply for a Supervision Order, a Care Order, or the child may be made a ward of Court. In effect the Social Services must then ensure that the child is looked after in a safe environment. This may allow the child to be returned to his home, or to a foster home. The Social Services are usually responsible for running adoption agencies, family centres, children's homes, day nurseries and supervizing child minders. Liaison between the hospital and Social Services is effected by hospital social workers and they are closely involved with the social problems of children admitted to neonatal nurseries or children's wards.

Education

The Education department is of course responsible for providing appropriate education for all children of 5 years and over. This includes the provision of schooling for handicapped children and long-stay children in hospital. The role of school nurses and medical officers has been described above.

The school's psychological services provides assessment for children with learning problems and gives advice as to their appropriate educational placement. The child guidance service provides psychiatric input to children with severe emotional or behavioural problems.

Other services

Children may become involved with other services quite commonly. The police are often involved in cases of non-accidental injury and may interview the child and his parents. This is best done by a small team of experienced police officers who are sensitive to the needs of children. Police may become involved with delinquent children from unhappy families and there may be associated medical or psychiatric problems. Probation officers are another professional group with overlap into the health services for children.

Amongst the non-government services for children, the best known is the NSPCC (National Society for the Prevention of Cruelty to Children). The NAWCH (National Association for the Welfare of Children in Hospital) is another important voluntary group working to improve the well-being of children in hospital.

The aims of the NSPCC are to prevent the public and private wrongs of children, and the corruption of their morals; to take action for the enforcement of laws for their protection. The organization provides trained personnel to prevent and treat child abuse in the form of child protection teams as well as playgroups and day-care centres for family orientated support of abused or deprived children.

3

MINOR DISORDERS OF CHILDREN

All children suffer from minor ailments or disorders at sometime during childhood, but these complaints may cause major distress to inexperienced parents. This chapter deals with those conditions not usually referred to hospital but which commonly come to the attention of the GP or health visitor. Sometimes the complaint is a symptom, such as excessive crying, and the doctor must be able to approach the problem in a logical manner. In the majority of cases the cause of the crying is innocent and self-limiting but occasionally the underlying condition is much more serious and requires admission to hospital for further investigation or treatment. The more serious disorders are discussed in detail elsewhere in this book.

Behavioural disorders

The child who refuses food

One of the commonest causes of maternal anxiety is the child who will not eat. The primary error is often the mother's belief that her child must eat a fixed amount of food. The fear that her child may starve to death is very real, even if not expressed. Such fears and the resultant error of forcing the child to eat may be particularly strong if there are extra reasons for parental anxiety. There is no fixed amount that a child should eat; mothers should allow their own common sense to tell them whether their child is well, not permitting the figure on a weight chart to dictate to them. There is no such thing as a 'normal' weight for a

child; charts may show average weight for a given age-group but parents are liable to mistake the average weight for the 'normal' weight. This error in concept can only be corrected by parent instruction.

Parents must understand that a normal child gains weight erratically, in a step-ladder fashion, rather than as a simple steady gain. The child of small build is likely to put on weight at a slower rate than one who is of heavy build. Yet, it is the mother whose child is of light build who is likely to be the one to become concerned by a slow weight gain and mistakenly to compare adversely his rate of weight gain with others of a larger build.

Weight is a very poor indication of health, whereas energy is an excellent guide. The child who is starved is relatively inert, conserving energy. By contrast, the child who is energetic has a sufficient intake of calories even though his mother insists that he does not eat anything. Mothers must be helped to accept the fact that a child who is thriving is getting enough to eat, no matter how small his appetite.

In some families, the meal-time becomes a battleground with the child refusing to eat and the parents pleading, forcing or entertaining the child to distract him from clenching his teeth in a desperate attempt to avoid food. This pattern of behaviour is very common and reflects the normal negativistic phase children go through. Unfortunately the inexperienced parent may interpret this as the child being 'difficult' or spoilt and persist in battling with him in an effort to make him change

23

his behaviour pattern. This reinforces the child's negative behaviour and exacerbates the family tension.

An explanation for the child's behaviour must be given to the parents so that they can understand the reasons that the child behaves in the way he does. These children should be offered helpings of the food the rest of the family eats. If he refuses it is withdrawn until the next mealtime and a portion of the family meal is again offered. The child should not be admonished for not eating, but snacks between meals must not be offered. The success of this regime depends on the level of anxiety within the family. If the parents do not understand, or will not accept, the explanation for the difficulties then this form of treatment is unlikely to be successful.

Possetting

This refers to the regular habit of dribbling semi-digested milk after a feed. It is very common, but some babies possett to such an extent that the parents carry a towel over their shoulder everywhere they go. The baby smells of vomit and the mother may become very concerned or irritated by the habit. It is due to gastro-oesophageal reflux and is usually self-limiting. By the time the child is 6 months old and on a more solid diet it has largely resolved.

Some infants possett so much that they fail to gain weight normally and some therapeutic measures may be necessary. The mother should keep her baby upright as much as possible during feeds, and elevate the head of the cot so that the effect of gravity is to retain the milk in the stomach. Thickening the feeds with a substance such as Nestargel or Carobel may also cause symptomatic improvement.

Food fads

Some children exist on a diet of crisps and cola drinks. Others will only eat one particular type of food meal after meal. This pattern of behaviour, common in toddlers, often occurs in those children who had previously show negativism and

food refusal. The parents have given in to the child and provided him with foods they know he will consume and he then refuses everything else. Treatment again depends on the parents understanding the reasons for this form of behaviour. Behaviour modification is possible if the parents are prepared for the child initially to refuse food not to his liking.

Thumb-sucking

This is a normal activity. Most newborn babies thumb-suck, but this is not a purposeful activity. It results from random movement of the hand close to the face in the presence of a very active rooting reflex. By 4–6 months, babies start to suck their thumb or finger as a purposeful activity. This is the start of the oral phase of their development when the mouth is the centre of sensory input and this lasts for several months. Approximately one-half of babies suck a finger or thumb at 1 year of age and this persists for much of the second year of life. Thumb-sucking at this age is often used as a self-comforting activity and is commonly seen with tiredness, anxiety, boredom, hunger and teething. Many children fondle a favourite piece of material, blanket or other treasured object whilst thumb-sucking. Few children continue to thumb-suck after 5 years of age.

Malocclusion of the front teeth is commonly thought to result from thumb-sucking, but this is probably quite unusual and if it occurs is only likely to affect the primary dentition. A cure for thumb-sucking should not be sought, as it is not an illness. Parents should be discouraged from repeatedly drawing the child's attention to it and not to paint or otherwise treat the offending thumb.

Masturbation

After discovering the mouth, the developing child reaches the age at which he discovers that handling his genitalia gives him greater pleasure than any other part of the body. This phase is common to all children but if parents are unaware that this is normal, they may have intense reactions to the situation. Such a reaction increases the child's interest in this area, causing him to carry on the practise more often when his parents are not present. Parents must therefore be educated to understand that handling genitalia is a normal phase of development, similar to thumb-sucking. It is only perpetuated if they draw attention to the situation, thereby increasing their child's interest. Some children appear to masturbate because of genital irritation. Vulvovaginitis should be excluded in girls who appear to start the habit suddenly.

Masturbation in young children is usually achieved by rubbing the thighs together and sometimes by rocking the body. During the act the child may appear to be in a trance, going red in the face with audible breathing. In extreme cases this may be mistaken for a convulsion. Masturbation as a form of sexual exploration in older children is more common in boys than girls, particularly between the ages of 10 and 15 years, and this again is entirely normal behaviour.

Nail-biting

Approximately one-half of children bite their nails at some time, and it is commoner in girls than boys. In some children it results from increased nervous tension and it is this that should be relieved rather than any direct attack on the nails.

Head-rolling and head-banging

Head-rolling is very common in infants and young children. Young children often have a bald patch over the occiput as a result of this habit. It is of little consequence and the children often head-roll as a way of rocking themselves to sleep. The habit usually disappears by 3 years of age.

Head-banging occurs at an older age (6−10 years) and has been reported to occur in 7% of children of this age group. The child usually bangs his head up and down onto the mattress or floor whilst lying prone. Some bang their head sideways against a wall whilst asleep, awakening the whole house with the noise. Moving the bed away from the wall solves the problem. Head–banging is considerably more common in mentally retarded

children and there are reports of an increased risk of cataracts in autistic children who head-bang. There is no reason to believe that this is a risk in normal children.

Parents may become extremely alarmed by head-banging activity for fear of self-inflicting brain injury. They can be reassured that this does not appear to happen. There is no cure for the habit and it should not be regarded as a disorder.

Sleeplessness

This is one of the commonest complaints made by parents about their children. The problem commonly starts around 9 months of age when the child becomes conscious of being left alone. Anxiety is increased by the misconception, held by many parents, that children require a specific number of hours of sleep according to their age.

The sleep needs of children vary enormously; the bright active infant often sleeping less than the more placid one and requiring less sleep than his parents. It is most unreasonable to expect anyone to go to sleep when they are not tired; all the more so a young child. Sleep patterns are dependent on the physical size of the child (how long he can go between feeds) and brain maturation. Children with brain damage have more disturbed patterns of sleeping. Over the early months of life, the child acquires a night-sleeping pattern and three-quarters of infants at 3 months of age take the majority of their sleep at night. Sleep problems can be divided into a number of groups:

THE CHILD WHO WILL NOT GO TO BED

This is an example of negativistic behaviour. It is reinforced by parents who resist putting the child to bed and leaving him. The parents should agree on a definite bed-time which is adhered to every night with no exceptions. This may be earlier or later depending on the sleep requirement of the child. The child will often cry when the parents leave the room. He should be left to cry providing there is no risk of him hurting himself. The crying may last for up to half an hour, but will become progressively less night after night and within a week the habit is broken in most children. It is not necessary for the child to go to sleep when he is placed in his cot, and he should be encouraged to play until he falls asleep. Plenty of toys should be left with him and he can play with these when he wakes in the morning.

THE CHILD WHO WAKES IN THE NIGHT

Sleep patterns vary through the night from light to deep. Children are more likely to wake from light sleep, particularly if disturbed by noises or discomfort such as being wet. There is some evidence that infants who wake at night spend more of their night-time in light sleep. In other children, conditions such as upper respiratory tract infections, eczema or cough may cause them to wake. Waking at night occurs very commonly (15% of 3-year-olds and 3% of 8-year-olds). Often the child will sing or play by himself, but some parents mistakenly feel it is necessary to play with the child in the night. If the child wakes crying, he should be checked to ensure that he is not unwell, uncomfortable or otherwise distressed. He may be given a brief cuddle and should then be then put down. If he knows that the parent will take him into their bed this will reinforce the waking behaviour. Similarly, hot drinks, stories and other bribes should be resisted as a nightly ritual otherwise they will rapidly become a habit.

Crying at night may be a very difficult habit to break if it is well established. Parents find themselves exhausted and there may be additional considerations such as the worry of waking other children or intolerant neighbours. In co-operative children, a reward system such as positive reinforcement (see Enuresis) may be successful. Sometimes it is necessary to give the child a hypnotic at night to break the habit. Vallergan (trimeprazine) or chloral are very effective and the dose increased until it has the desired effect. Drugs should only be used for a week to 10 days in an attempt to break the habit and must not be used long-term.

THE CHILD WHO WAKES EARLY

This is a common problem and there is no way of making them go to sleep again. The parents of such children can only hope to obtain peace for themselves by surrounding the child with lots of toys to occupy him in the early mornings.

Night terrors

These occur during periods of deep sleep, 15–90 minutes after falling asleep. They are usually seen in children over the age of 5 years and may be familial. The child awakes from sleep screaming and cannot be comforted. He is often in a confused state, unaware of his parent's presence and there is usually no recollection of the event in the morning.

Nightmares, which are different to night terrors, occur in younger children and no explanation for the terror may be given. The child should be reassured and comforted until he falls back to sleep.

Sleep-walking

This occurs in up to 10% of children and may be accompanied by sleep-talking but usually they have no recollection of walking in the morning. Injury during sleep-walking is unusual but if the child sleep-walks regularly, a stair-guard will prevent him falling down the stairs.

Enuresis

Enuresis refers to incontinence of urine or more particularly bed-wetting and is a common problem in children. The child develops control over his bladder gradually. By about 18 months he is able to indicate that he has passed urine and by 2 years may be able to give his mother enough warning that she can get a potty. By 2.5 years the child should be able to toilet himself and is often dry during the day. A child is not capable of being dry at night until he has sufficient bladder capacity to hold the urine for an 8-hour period. Most children are dry during the day and most nights by 3 years of age, although a number have achieved this well before then. Approximately 15% of otherwise normal 5-year-olds and 7% of 10-year-olds wet the bed. Enuresis commonly runs in families and its cause is probably due to delayed development

Table 3.1 Causes of enuresis. These conditions will usually cause wetting both day and night.

Urinary tract infection

Polyuria
    Diabetes mellitus
    Diabetes insipidus

Constipation

Anatomical abnormality
    Ectopic ureter or urethra
    Ectopia vesica
    Epispadias
    Prune belly syndrome

Neurological abnormality
    Spina bifida cystica
    Sacral agenesis
    Diastematomyelia
    Spinal cord tethering

of bladder control. The majority of children with this problem are psychologically normal.

Enuresis is either primary (the child has not acquired bladder control by 3 years) or secondary (enuresis occurs after acquisition of normal bladder control). If a child presents with enuresis (primary or secondary) he should be carefully examined and organic causes considered. If the child does not have a good stream of urine or dribbles urine this is particularly suggestive of urinary obstruction (p. 252). Table 3.1 lists important causes of enuresis. It is essential to examine the urine for micro-organisms, white cells and glucose.

Treatment

Assuming no cause for the enuresis can be found, the management is aimed at encouraging the development of normal control and removing any contributory emotional factors. It is often helpful to lift the child before the parents go to bed and place him on the potty. The sensation of the rim of the potty on his thighs usually causes reflex micturition. It is sensible not to give the child a drink immediately prior to putting him down for the night.

The principles of positive reinforcement must be

explained to the parents. They should not scold or chastise the child when he is wet. Praise for dry nights and no comment for wet ones is required. A 'star chart' system may be very useful in this context. The child keeps a dry bed diary in a prominent place. He is given a red star for each dry night and a gold star for 3 or 5 consecutive dry nights. He is rewarded by a small present once he has collected four or five gold stars. This system is only successful if the child understands the reward system and is constantly encouraged. This is aided by involving everyone in the house so that it becomes a family effort.

A buzzer alarm may also be successful in some families, but is not recommended in children below 5 years of age. The child lies on a sheet with a moisture-sensitive pad underneath. When the child wets the bed the pad registers the moisture and sets off an audible alarm. This works by strengthening the inhibitory reflex and eventually the child is inhibited from micturating in the bed. This device should only be used under medical supervision and if not successful after 3 months it should be withdrawn.

Imipramine (a tricyclic antidepressant) has also been widely used to treat enuresis. A dose (25–50 mg) is given prior to bed and is often successful in preventing enuresis, but there is a very high relapse rate after cessation of the drug. It probably works by causing the child to sleep less deeply and being more aware of bladder filling.

Some children continue to bed-wet despite all treatment. In these families I usually try to defuse the cycle of anxiety that has developed and recommend no further treatment for at least 6 months. If enuresis remains a major problem, referral to a psychologist or psychiatrist may be helpful (p. 349).

Encopresis

Encopresis refers to incontinence of stool or faecal soiling and is a very common problem in childhood. Acquisition of stool continence follows a similar pattern to that of bladder control, but bowel control is usually acquired before bladder control.

Encopresis may be considered to develop in one of the following two ways.

STOOL-HOLDING

This is a very common activity amongst children of the age of 3–5 years. They adopt a characteristic posture standing with their legs crossed and often going red in the face. The reason for this may be that they are too busy playing a game to go to the toilet or that they get some pleasurable sensation from doing it. The unwary parent may think that the child is straining to pass the stool and draw attention to the child's bowel habit. During the negativistic phase of development this makes the child aware of the power he has over his parents by refusing to go to the toilet when requested. Many parents have been brought up to believe that a regular bowel habit is essential to health and take an inordinate interest in the bowel habit of their children.

Stool-holding may therefore be a normal phase that many children go through and it may lead to encopresis by one of two means. Stool-holding may cause constipation with the child eventually passing a large stool which is painful and may cause some fissuring of the anal mucosa. The memory of pain and discomfort reinforces his stool-holding behaviour and constipation with soiling commonly develops. Secondly, the child may react against the wishes of his parents to 'perform' regularly and deposit stool everywhere other than where his parents wish it to be. Many children are sat on the toilet or potty for long periods by their parents, only to soil their pants as soon as they get off. This is one of the most effective weapons children have in the guerilla warfare that goes on in many homes. This problem is dealt with in detail in the chapter on emotional disorders (p. 348).

CONSTIPATION

Constipation may be psychogenic and develops in the ways detailed above, or may be due to a variety of organic causes. The problem of constipation is discussed fully in Chapter 12. Neonatal constipation is discussed on p. 140.

Habit spasm (tic)

These are common in nervous children, often starting by the perpetuation of a simple habit. For example, a lock of hair which falls in front of the eye may be tossed back by a movement of the head and this can become a habit. The head and shoulders are principally involved, the abnormal movements including blinking, wrinkling of the forehead, grimacing, head shaking and shrugging of the shoulders.

The movements must not be mistaken for chorea (p. 293). They are repetitive and can be repeated on request, whereas in chorea they are always changing. A habit spasm can be controlled for a time when asked, whereas choreic movements become exaggerated by such a request.

Treatment

The reason for the increased tension must be discovered but no attention should be drawn directly to the symptom. The child must never be told to stop making the movement, but he should be told it is not his fault and that it will eventually disappear.

The crying infant

Crying is an entirely normal feature of infants and toddlers. Most newly born babies greet the world with vigorous crying and a mother can recognize the cries of their own infant within a day or two of birth. The cry is the young child's method of communicating with the world and experienced or sensitive parents can 'understand' what their baby is asking for when he cries. Nevertheless many parents become very frightened by the incessant crying of their infant and this may be a major problem if it occurs for long periods at night. The worry of many parents is that the child is crying because he is in pain and the doctor may be called for this reason.

Normal children cry for a number of reasons; discomfort (wet or soiled nappy), boredom, frustration, separation from the mother, hunger, thirst or loneliness. By 6 months the child is developing

Table 3.2   Organic causes of crying in infancy.

Infection
    Non-specific fever
    Otitis media
    Meningitis
    Urinary tract infection

Neurological abnormality
    Post-asphyxial irritability
    Raised intracranial pressure
    Cri du chat syndrome
    Inborn errors of metabolism
    Autism

Gastrointestinal abnormality
    Colic
    Bowel obstruction
    Intussusception
    Strangulated hernia
    Failure to thrive

Others
    Torsion of the testicle
    Withdrawal from maternal opiate addiction

a sense of his own individuality and realizes that crying is an effective method of getting attention. This is entirely normal, but many parents are frightened of spoiling the child by giving them too much attention. Once a child is sitting he may resent being laid down particularly when he wants to play. The parent should be encouraged to listen to what their child is trying to tell them. Consolability is a very important feature of the normal crying child. If the cause of the discomfort can be relieved, cuddling or feeding will settle the child rapidly. This is not possible in infants with an organic problem. If a normally placid baby starts to cry for no apparent reason, pain or occult infection should be suspected.

Crying may certainly be due to disease; either a feature of pain or neurological abnormality. Table 3.2 lists the causes of crying as a result of a disease state. It must however be emphasized that the commonest reason for a child crying is non-organic. In contrast to a normal child who can be consoled when crying, an infant who cries because he is irritable due to a neurological reason or because he is in pain cannot be consoled in the same way. This is the most important factor in assessing the crying infant.

All parents know that sometimes a baby cries incessantly for no apparent reason, but this is nevertheless a most uncomfortable and potentially worrying situation. Babies pick up anxiety from their parents and may cry more incessantly, thereby causing more anxiety. It is easy to understand how a young (often unsupported) mother cannot cope with her crying baby. She may be socially isolated, perhaps living near the top of a high rise, high density, block of flats with unsympathetic neighbours. Simply telling her that there is no medical cause for her infant crying is not relieving the situation. The infant may be at risk of emotional or physical abuse and the mother must be given adequate support. This may be best done by the health visitor, or a social worker may be able to provide support. Nevertheless it is sometimes necessary to admit a crying baby to hospital in order to relieve the mother of the situation. It is of interest that these children are often not thought to cry excessively in the hospital ward and the mother may be encouraged to see her baby transformed by a short admission that breaks the cycle of anxiety.

Minor disorders of the gastrointestinal tract

Teething

Teething is a normal process and does not cause any illness. The greatest danger is that symptoms are incorrectly ascribed to teething so that serious underlying disease is overlooked. Convulsions should never be regarded as the result of teething and nothing is more dangerous than to consider teething to be the cause of failure to thrive.

Rarely babies are born with teeth (natal teeth). If they are loose they should be removed. The timing of normal dentition is described in Chapter 4. There is a very wide range for normal dental eruption and the first tooth may not appear until after the first birthday.

It is clear that teeth erupt in a sequential fashion for most of the first and second year of life. The only symptoms usually associated with this are ex-cess salivation, rubbing of the gums and a desire to gnaw. Some children are a little more fretful dur-ing eruption but it is not a cause of incessant crying.

Mouth breathing

Small babies are obligate nose breathers; they can-not breath through the mouth. As they mature, mouth breathing becomes possible but is only prominent if the child develops nasal or postnasal obstruction. Enlarged adenoids are the commonest cause of mouth breathing. Breathing through the mouth may develop as a habit and this is particu-larly common in mentally retarded children.

Pica

Pica refers to dirt eating but may refer to other abnormal substances taken by mouth. Children, usually toddlers, who develop this habit acquire a perverted taste, choosing to eat dirt, coal, paper, hair and bits of toys. It is more common in men-tally retarded children and there is often a family history on the mother's side. There is a risk that their abnormal eating habits may lead them to chew objects containing lead, so causing lead poisoning. Iron deficiency anaemia is another cause of pica.

Trichobezoar refers to a hair ball obstructing the stomach due to plucking hair (trichotillomania) and swallowing it. It usually occurs in mentally retarded or emotionally disturbed children. The hair ball may be enormous and require lapar-otomy to remove.

Toddler's diarrhoea

Toddler's diarrhoea is seen in well children be-tween the age of 6 months and 5 years. They present because the parent is concerned that the child has never had a formed motion and un-digested food (peas and carrots) are seen in the motion. Its cause is not clear but the child thrives, although weight gain may be suboptimal in some.

Diagnosis is by exclusion and improvement may be obtained by introducing a higher unsaturated fat diet than they had previously received. Loper-amide may give symptomatic relief.

Anal fissure

This results from a mucosal tear due to the passage of hard stool and is commonly associated with a sentinel pile. It is the commonest cause of rectal bleeding (p. 203). Healing is usually rapid once the constipation has been successfully treated. Digital dilatation of the sphincter reduces spasm and this can be combined with the local application of lig-nocaine ointment for the relief of pain.

Minor disorders of the genito-urinary system

Phimosis and paraphimosis

The penis, including the prepuce (foreskin), de-velops *in utero* as a solid bud; the urethra being formed as an infolding of its under surface. Not until late in fetal life does cleavage begin, delineat-ing the future prepuce from the future glans. At birth this plane is a visible division but not a free space. Separation of the glans from the foreskin is not complete until some time between 9 months and 3 years. Until this has occurred, the foreskin can be retracted only with force which tears through the cellular link between them, leading to fibrosis with an adherent foreskin. Mothers should be warned against trying to retract the foreskin in their young sons. Provided the child can pass a normal stream of urine, congenital phimosis does not exist.

Paraphimosis refers to retraction of the foreskin over the glans beyond the penile corona. This causes obstruction to the venous return of the glans with swelling and pain. Manual reduction should be attempted initially and the injection of 1−2 ml of hyaluronidase into the swollen tissue will reduce the swelling. Definitive treatment is a dorsal slit under general anaesthetic with later circumcision.

Balanoposthitis

This refers to inflammation of the glans penis (balanitis) and foreskin (posthitis) due to retention of smegma within the preputial sac. It occurs after 3 years of age and is associated with phimosis. Retraction of the foreskin is usually impossible due to oedema and there is a purulent offensive discharge from the sac.

Treatment

This is with systemic antibiotics and local toilet. Once the swelling has settled, circumcision should be undertaken to prevent recurrence.

Meatal ulcer

This condition is seen only in circumcised boys, usually in association with ammonia dermatitis (p. 492). The ulcer is situated on the glans at the edge of the urethral meatus and extension of the ulcer may involve the urethral mucosa. Considerable pain is experienced every time urine is passed and healing is retarded by its repeated passage. Fibrosis may occur causing meatal stenosis.

Treatment

An antiseptic tulle gras dressing should be placed over the glans and local anaesthetic cream used for pain relief. Benzalkonium chloride ointment may be used on a solid ophthalmic glass rod to reach the meatal extension of the ulcer. This also has the function of dilating the urethral meatus.

Vaginal discharge

A thick white secretion from the vagina is commonly seen in newborn infants. This may persist for up to 14 days and may be lightly blood-stained. It is entirely normal and is due to withdrawal of maternal oestrogens and invasion of the external genitalia with colonizing organisms.

VULVOVAGINITIS

This occurs in older girls and the discharge is always offensive. The skin of the vulva is usually red and sore. It may be due to poor hygiene, masturbation, a foreign body in the vagina or possibly threadworms. Culture of the discharge usually shows a mixed growth of staphylococci, streptococci, diphtheroids and coliform organisms. Gonococcus is a rare isolate, but if found it is very suggestive of sexual abuse (p. 524).

Treatment is with appropriate antibiotics and local toilet or sitz baths. The presence of a foreign body must be excluded.

Pain in the scrotum

This is usually a serious symptom and torsion of the testicle (p. 394) must be excluded as a matter of some urgency. Table 3.3 summarizes the causes of a painful scrotum.

Pain on micturition

The commest cause is urinary tract infection (p. 257), particularly in girls. Girls may, however, have dysuria without any evidence of infection and alkalinizing the urine may be a successful treatment. Local inflammation (vulvovaginitis or meatal ulcer) may also cause pain on micturition.

Neurological disorders

Breath-holding attacks

These commonly occur between the ages of 1 and 5 years. A typical episode is initiated by a precipitating factor which causes the child to cry. This may be temper at being told off, an altercation with another child or a painful insult. The child starts to cry and after two or three breaths, holds his breath at the end of expiration. The child goes

Table 3.3 Causes of a painful scrotum.

Trauma
Torsion of the testicle
Inguino-scrotal hernia
Epididymitis
Orchitis (mumps)
Oedema

red in the face and then blue. The attack may be self-limiting at this stage or may continue. After 15–20 seconds the child goes limp and faints. In some, this is followed immediately by a brief convulsion presumably due to cerebral hypoxia. The child then rapidly recovers but may be confused for a short time. A rarer variety is associated with pallor rather than cyanosis and he becomes limp and falls (p. 289).

Breath-holding attacks are very distressing to parents, particularly if associated with a fit. The distinction between this form of attack and epilepsy is only possible on taking a careful clinical history of the attacks. The child may realize the fear these episodes induce in the parents and use them as a form of manipulative behaviour. For this reason the child should not be allowed to have his own way as a result of the threat of an attack. The parent should try and avoid situations likely to precipitate breath-holding attacks but this is not always possible. A variety of distraction techniques can be used during an attack. These include blowing hard on the child's face, hooking a finger around the back of the tongue and drawing it forward, or splashing cold water onto him. The prognosis is excellent and the child usually grows out of the habit by 5 years, and often somewhat sooner. Anticonvulsant drugs have no place in the treatment of this condition.

Faints

These are most common during the second half of childhood. The attacks usually occur only when standing up, particularly in crowded or stuffy places such as school assembly. The child initially feels faint, thinks he is going to be sick, goes deathly pale and sinks to the floor. Convulsive movements rarely occur and there is no incontinence. Children who apparently faint whilst sitting or playing are more likely to have epilepsy as the cause of the episode. Other conditions that can cause episodes similar to fainting are epilepsy (p. 341), hysteria (p. 284) and cardiac arrhythmias (p. 226).

Treatment of a simple faint is to lie the child flat, loosen his collar and elevate the legs above the level of the head. The child should recover very rapidly.

Minor infections

Recurrent mild infections

Recurrent upper respiratory tract infections (URTI) are very common in children, particularly toddlers when they first start playgroup and 5-year-olds when they enter school. They are then exposed to a large number of viral organisms for which they have no immunity. The mother describes her child as having one cold after another. URTI are commonly associated with cough and the child may be given frequent courses of antibiotics. Mothers (and doctors) must understand that frequent mild infections in these young children are common and benign. They do not need antibiotic cover for each episode.

Newborn babies are not particularly susceptible to colds as they have passive immunity from maternal transplacental IgG antibodies. Breast feeding also reduces the risk of minor infections. Once the child is 3–6 months, frequent URTI may start and this is much more likely if there are older siblings at home who expose the baby to new viral agents.

ACUTE CORYZA (COMMON COLD)

The commest cause of coryza is a rhinovirus but a number of other viruses can produce a similar spectrum of illness. In young babies nasal obstruction is usually the most troublesome problem associated with the common cold. The use of 0.5% ephedrine nasal drops (two drops each nostril) immediately before feeds is good symptomatic treatment. Ephedrine should not be used for more than a week at a time.

Lymphadenopathy

Enlargement of lymph nodes in children is particularly common and is usually benign. If there is generalized lymphadenopathy or if a mass of nodes are matted or immobile then this is a very serious sign and is discussed in Chapter 24.

Enlarged glands in the neck are found at some time in most children. The primary source of the infection is most often in the tonsil but may be the adenoids, middle ear or teeth. The tonsils may look diseased but are just as likely to look entirely normal. Many children have pea-sized highly mobile nodes in the neck or groin and these represent chronically activated lymph glands in healthy children and are of little significance.

Children with lymphadenopathy should be carefully examined. Neck, suboccipital, submental, axillary and groin sites should be palpated and the presence of a spleen investigated by careful palpation. Fixed, matted or large lymph glands should be referred to a paediatrician.

Infestation with threadworms

There are a large number of parasites that cause infestations in children. The majority are discussed in Chapter 29.

Threadworms are the commonest worms in temperate climates, being most widespread where there is poor hygiene and overcrowding. The worms infest the large bowel, especially the caecum and appendix. The fertilized female emerges from the anus to lay her eggs on the perianal skin. This causes irritation and the consequent contamination of the hands from scratching results in reinfection of the host and transfer to others by direct contact or through food.

The symptoms are largely the result of perianal irritation and, since this is most marked at night, it can cause sleeplessness and sometimes enuresis. The worms may enter the vagina to cause vulvovaginitis. Acute appendicitis is not caused by threadworms although they are commonly found in the appendix.

Adult worms look like threads of cotton and are easily identified. Ova can be demonstrated by placing a short strip of sellotape on the perianal skin in the morning before bathing or defaecation. The ova adhere to the tape which is then mounted on a slide with deci-normal sodium hydroxide solution and examined under the microscope.

Treatment

Piperazine is an effective drug and acts by paralysing the worms. It can be given as a single-dose preparation (Pripsen one-half to one sachet) with a second dose 2 weeks later to deal with worms maturing from ova ingested after the time of the first dose. Mebendazole, a single-dose antihelmintic, is possibly the most effective drug, but should not be used in children below 2 years of age. All members of the family should be treated since it is likely that more than one is infected, even if worms are not seen.

Orthopaedic abnormalities

There are a number of minor abnormalities affecting the limbs which cause anxiety but require little or no specific therapy. The more severe disorders are discussed in Chapters 9 and 26.

Bow legs

A certain amount of bowing of the legs is normal, particularly in the toddler age group. This is a physiological state which improves spontaneously from the age of 2 years, although it may persist until the fifth year. If the degree of bowing is marked, rickets must be considered as a cause (p. 549).

Knock knees (genu valgum)

There should normally be about 2 cm of separation between the medial malleoli of the ankle when the patient is standing upright with the knees together. When lying down, a distance of up to 9 cm between the malleoli is acceptable. An increase in this space represents genu valgum and is mainly seen in association with obesity. Weight reduction is essential to correct the abnormality.

In-toeing (pigeon toes)

It is common for young children to walk with their feet turned inwards. This is usually due to femoral anteversion which can be regarded as

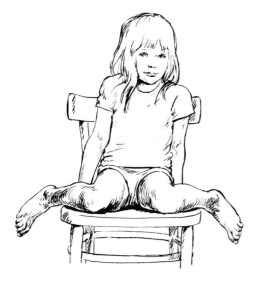

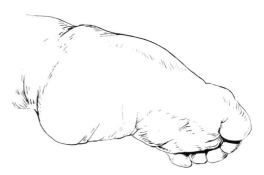

Fig. 3.2 Metatarsus varus.

Fig. 3.1 Femoral anteversion demonstrated by a child sitting in the 'W' position.

physiological during the first 5 years. These children sit in the 'W' position (Fig. 3.1) with hips internally rotated and the legs out sideways. Eighty per cent apparently correct by the age of 8 years, often with compensatory external tibial torsion. In-toeing from this cause must be differentiated from abnormality of the feet, particularly metatarsus varus (see below). Medial tibial torsion which may be associated with bow legs also causes in-toeing.

Femoral retroversion

Children with this condition splay their feet out and walk like Charlie Chaplin. It is particularly common in children who have been born prematurely. The infant lies prone in his incubator causing the femora to be rotated laterally. In these infants it is self-limiting and requires no treatment. Congenitally dislocated hips cause femoral retroversion and this should be excluded in every case.

Metatarsus varus

This refers to medial curvature of the midpart of the foot with no equinus of the heel (Fig. 3.2). It is

a common isolated abnormality but may also be seen with talipes. In 90% of cases, spontaneous resolution occurs by 3–4 years and it requires no specific treatment. If still present by school age, the child should be referred for an orthopaedic opinion.

Pes planus (flat foot)

During the first year of life, the foot looks flat owing to the normal pad of fat in the sole obscuring the outline of the arch. During the first 5 years the foot, as indicated by the footprint, is always flat. The majority of feet believed to be flat in the early years are normal, or will become so during the first 7 years. The arch is restored in such children when standing on tiptoe and only if this is not so or there is pain in the foot, especially at the end of the day, is there any problem. In such patients the foot, though of normal appearance when not weight bearing, rolls into valgus on standing so that, viewed from behind, the navicular is unduly prominent on the inner side. There is excessive wear of the heel of the shoe on that side. For these patients an inside heel wedge of 5 mm should be applied to well-built shoes, or they may be given a shoe with a built-in inner raise.

Bowing of the tibia

Lateral bowing of the tibia is normal up to the age of 2 years and may be associated with medial tibial torsion. It usually corrects spontaneously but some children may be left with genu valgum.

Abnormality of the toes

POLYDACTYLY

One or more extra toes or fingers are common and is often familial. If the digit is vestigal with a narrow base it may be tied off with cotton thread, otherwise surgical removal is recommended.

SYNDACTYLY

Fusion of two toes (or fingers) is common. It is usually bilateral and often familial. No treatment is necessary.

CURLY TOES

The affected toe lies curled under its medial neighbour and the extent to which it occurs determines the need for surgery. The child should be examined weight bearing and if the abnormality is mild, no treatment is necessary other than wearing well-fitting shoes. Strapping is of little value, and surgical treatment involves transplantation of the long flexor tendon into the extensor tendon.

OVER-RIDING OF THE TOES

The fifth toe is most commonly involved, but any toe with a medial neighbour may be affected. They lie on the upper and outer aspect of the neighbouring toe, and are rotated laterally. If this causes abrasion from a well-fitting shoe, surgery is recommended.

Skin

Nappy rash

A rash in the napkin area, involving the genitalia, buttocks and inner aspects of the thighs is extremely common owing to prolonged contact between skin and urine or stool. Additional factors are infrequent napkin changes, wearing of plastic pants and use of biological washing powders. The perianal region and buttocks are often erythematous, sometimes with a vesicular or papular eruption. The groin creases are usually spared but the foreskin may be severely involved. Some children with long-standing nappy rash develop thickened and cracked skin.

Successful treatment of the condition depends on the underlying cause and this should be considered in every case. Napkin dermatits is discussed in detail in Chapter 27.

AMMONIA DERMATITIS

Ammonia is liberated from urine by the action of bacteria in the stools. The ammonia irritates the skin causing erythema. The role of ammonia in producing the rash has been disputed and it is likely that the action of urine-soaked nappies, particularly when plastic pants are used, is enough on its own to cause the excoriation. Chronic nappy rash causes the thickened paper-like skin referred to above.

Treatment involves meticulous attention to detail. Wet nappies must not be allowed to remain in contact with the skin and frequent changing is required. Whenever possible the nappy area should be left exposed to the air, with the child lying on the nappy. Plastic pants should be avoided. Thoroughly wash the affected area with a pure soap whenever soiled. Creams which form a barrier to the skin can be used to protect the skin if exposure is impracticable. Substances such as zinc and castor oil ointment or metanium are effective but must be re-applied with each nappy change.

SEBORRHOEIC DERMATITIS

A seborrhoeic nappy rash is extensive and of a brownish-red colour. This condition is discussed in detail on p. 492. The diagnosis is made by the presence of other seborrhoeic lesions of the scalp (see p. 36).

CANDIDA (THRUSH)

This is a common cause of nappy rash. Initially the lesions are vesicular on an erythematous base and originate around the anus. They are weepy as if the tops have been sliced off. The rash may not be confined to the nappy area, and may extend up the anterior abdominal wall. More severe cases present with a generally red and sore looking nappy area. It is often accompanied by oral thrush (white plaques in the mouth that are difficult to scrape away). Thrush should be suspected in any case of nappy rash not responding to the measures outlined above.

The diagnosis can be confirmed by examining scrapings from the affected skin for budding hyphae. Treatment is by an anti-fungal cream (nystatin or Daktarin) applied with every nappy change. Oral thrush should be treated simultaneously with nystatin or Daktarin drops or gel.

Seborrhoeic dermatitis ('cradle cap')

In young babies seborrhoeic dermatitis is most commonly seen as a thick brown layer of crusts over the scalp, sometimes called cradle cap. It may also be present behind the ears. It is often associated with inadequate washing of the head. The crusts can sometimes be removed with olive oil or by washing the hair with a medicated shampoo. Eczema (p. 490) may cause an appearance similar to cradle cap and may require specific treatment.

Pigmented naevus (mole)

This consists of a localized deposit of melanin which may be flat or papillomatous and may or may not be hairy. They are very common, the vast majority causing no trouble except that they may be disfiguring so that removal by plastic surgery is required. Malignant change in the paediatric age group is extremely uncommon but moles on the scrotum, soles of the feet or palms must be referred to a dermatologist as these are most likely to become malignant.

Intertrigo

This is a condition particularly seen in the tropics, but in Britain is principally associated with obesity. It occurs in flexures and is particularly seen between rolls of fat in the groin or neck. The skin becomes macerated and is red and weeping. Treatment is with an anti-fungal dusting powder (Cicatrin) and once cured, meticulous attention must be paid to hygiene in order to prevent recurrence.

Folliculitis and furunculosis (boils)

Folliculitis is a superficial infection of the hair follicle which, if neglected, gives rise to a number of similar lesions or goes on to form a furuncle or boil in which the infection is at the base of the hair follicle. Alternatively the infection may start in the depths of the follicle as a boil. Staphylococci are the usual infecting organisms. Boils are extremely painful during the course of formation but once they have discharged their pus and the pressure is reduced, pain is relieved. In cases of recurrent boils diabetes mellitus should be excluded.

Treatment

A warm compress is useful for encouraging a ripe boil to decompress. If the boil becomes large, an abscess may develop and surgical drainage is necessary when it begins to 'point'. Extensive boils may be treated with systemic flucloxacillin.

Chillblain (erythema pernio)

These are due to arteriolar spasm in response to cold. The lesions occur on the extremities, often the extensor surfaces of the fingers, and consist of painful and irritating red swellings. The surface may break down to form indolent fissures. The treatment involves keeping the limb warm and antipruritic ointment rubbed well in.

Milia

These are yellowish-white opalescent spots seen particularly on the nose in many normal babies. They are due to blockage of the openings of the sebaceous glands and disappear spontaneously.

MILIARIA RUBRA

This refers to heat rash (prickly heat) which is seen in tropical countries. In this condition the child develops erythematous, itchy papules and vesicles situated at the openings of the sweat glands.

4
GROWTH AND DEVELOPMENT

Growth and development are intimately related but are not necessarily dependent with one another. Growth is a combination of increase both in the number of cells (hyperplasia) and the size of the cells (hypertrophy). Development is increase in complexity of the organism due to maturation of the nervous system. A child may develop normally, but be retarded in growth and although many severely retarded children are small, brain injury does not necessarily caused impaired growth. Growth can be measured accurately but the measurement of development is much more difficult to quantify.

Growth

Growth is influenced by a number of semi-independent factors. Children are born with genetic growth potential related to parental size. Normal growth before and after birth is dependent on adequate nutrition and is regulated by trophic hormones (mainly thyroxine for early growth, and growth hormone later). The sex hormones play an important part in the pre-pubertal growth spurt. External factors such as illness or socio-economic class also have an important influence on growth.

During a period of illness or starvation the rate of growth is slowed, but after the incident the child grows more rapidly than usual so that he catches up towards, or actually to, his original growth curve ('catch up growth'). The degree to which this catch up is successful depends on the length of time growth has been slowed. This is particularly important in infants who have suffered intra-uterine growth retardation (p. 77). If growth has been slowed for too long or into puberty, complete catch up is not achieved and there are important therapeutic implications in the early detection of children with abnormal growth velocity patterns. They may require replacement hormone therapy to achieve acceptable adult height (p. 391).

Not all body systems grow at the same rate and in some respects the growth rates of some organs are independent of others.

Brain growth

The human growth spurt begins early in pregnancy and is largely completed by 3 years. Neuronal development is complete by 20 weeks following conception and glial cell growth occurs between 24 and 34 weeks after conception. Myelination is not complete until early in the second decade. This has important implications for the management of under nutrition. As brain growth is very rapid early in development, adequate nutrition, both before the birth and in the few years after the birth, is essential for normal development. Children who are chronically malnourished in the early years may have permanent impairment of intelligence and neurological function in later life.

Lymphoid tissue growth

Lymphoid tissue shows an entirely different growth pattern to other organs. It grows progressively throughout childhood, but ceases at the age of 10–12 years; before the pubertal growth spurt. Moreover, the maximal growth is followed by regression so that the amount of lymphoid tissue in the body actually decreases. These changes can be watched in the tonsils which are barely visible at birth, become very obvious by the age of 4–5 years and get smaller in the early teens.

Adipose tissue growth

Fat increases rapidly during the first year, followed by a small steady loss until the age of 7 years. Thereafter the amount of fat remains constant until the pre-pubertal growth spurt, when there is a rapid increase. Fat children are generally taller than their non-obese peers. Obese children have greater numbers of adipose cells as well as the fat cells being larger than the non-obese children.

It is sometimes said that fat infants become fat adults but it is not clear that 'overfeeding' in the first few months of life causes obesity in later life. Infants have vastly different nutritional needs and will take as much as they require, provided they are not forced to finish all their feeds. Genetic factors may also be very important for the later development of obesity. Obesity is fully discussed in Chapter 23.

Skeletal growth

The newborn infant is born with relatively less muscle than an adult. At birth, skeletal muscle accounts for only 25% of the infant's weight, compared to 40% of the adult weight.

Bone development proceeds in a regular sequence. In the fetus the shaft of the long bones (diaphysis) ossifies first leaving the cartilaginous ends of the bones (epiphyses) to elongate. The epiphyses begin to ossify shortly before birth and this proceeds rapidly in the next few years. Ossification centres seen on X-ray examination of the wrist, hand, foot, knee or elbow can be compared with appearances in standardized atlases (Fig. 4.1) to assess the skeletal maturity of a child. This is of importance in assessing the child of short stature (p. 387).

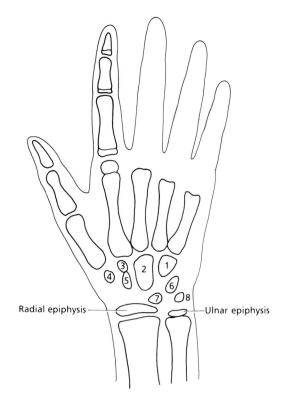

Fig. 4.1 Ossification centres in the wrist. The epiphyseal centres of the phalanges appear between 6 and 24 months and the metacarpals between 10 and 24 months. The radial epiphysis appears at 3–18 months and the ulnar epiphysis at 4–9 years. The mean age at which the carpal bones appear are: hamate **1** 2 months, capitate **2** 2 months, trapezoid **3** 5 years, trapezium **4** 4 years, navicular **5** 5 years, triquetrum **6** 2 years, lunate **7** 3 years, pisiform **8** 12 years.

Somatic growth

The rate of growth in the first year of life is more rapid than at any other age. Between birth and 1 year of age, children on average increase their length by 50%, and triple their birth weight. The head circumference increases by a third. Growth rates decrease until the pre-pubertal spurt which starts at about 11 years in girls and 12 years in boys.

The increase in skull size is usually dependent on brain growth. If the brain fails to grow, the child becomes microcephalic. Excess fluid in the brain (hydrocephalus) causes the head size to be large.

Changes in weight may be due to acute loss of water (dehydration) or accumulation of water (oedema) and may be an unreliable estimate of growth. Increase in linear size is the most sensitive estimate of growth in children.

ASSESSMENT OF SOMATIC GROWTH

Measurement of somatic growth is a precise science and care should be taken to ensure accurate measurements in every child. Inaccurate measurements of growth are worthless. Premature infants should have their measurements corrected for their gestational age. At 3 months from birth, a baby born at 28 weeks gestation will have his height and weight plotted at 40 weeks post-conceptual age. Prematurity should be taken into consideration for the first 2 years when plotting growth data.

HEIGHT

The measurement of height should be precise and is only accurate if made with care. Descriptions of how to make these measurements accurately are described in Chapter 23.

A child's length or height is plotted on a height chart (Fig. 4.2) and his growth followed along a centile line. The rate of growth is an important measurement in children whose growth is sub-optimal. Height velocity charts are available for plotting the rate of growth of a child per unit time (see Fig. 23.5).

After the first 6 months of life, a child should continue to grow along the same centile although infants in the first few months of life may follow a centile quite different to their subsequent growth centiles. It is important to record the relative height compared to weight and head circumference centiles. This gives an idea of the build of the child. In compromised children, weight falls before height is impaired and head growth is the last to be affected.

When comparing the growth of an individual child with that of a standard, the standard used should have been made from a sample similar to that of the child in question as regards sex and race. Unfortunately, in Britain we do not yet have growth charts for ethnic minority groups, but it is likely that successive generations of ethnic minority groups living in Britain will grow towards the ethnic majority standard. The experience of successive generations of Japanese living in the USA supports this pattern. Heredity is a very important factor in the variation of growth seen in children. Recordings of accurate height for both parents are important when assessing a child of short stature. Special charts which allow for 'mid-parental' height (average of father's and mother's height) are available (p. 387).

WEIGHT

During the first weeks of life the average baby gains 150–190 g a week, doubling his birthweight by about 4 months of age. However, many perfectly normal babies gain less than this and mothers should be reassured that, provided the baby is contented, a slower weight gain is normal. At 1 year he will weigh on average about 10 kg, at 2 years 12 kg and at 3 years 15 kg. From the age of 3 to 7 years he gains an average of 2 kg a year and from 8 to 12 years about 3 kg a year.

As mentioned above, weight may be influenced by acute changes in total body water. Weight may also reflect the amount of adipose tissue in the body. Fat is better and more directly measured by skinfold thickness. The folds over the triceps muscle and in the subscapular area are picked up between the finger and thumb and measured with skinfold thickness calipers. This instrument exerts a constant pressure on the skinfold and measures the thickness in millimeters.

HEAD CIRCUMFERENCE

This is usually a measure of brain size and the causes of both microcephaly and macrocephaly are described elsewhere. There is only one maximum measurement of occipito-frontal head circumference and this should be made with a

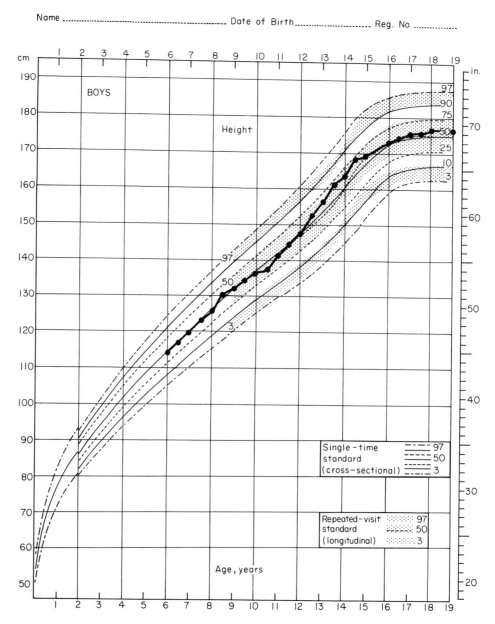

Fig. 4.2 Height chart for boys. The growth of one child is plotted between the ages of 6 and 19 years, showing his pubertal growth spurt between the ages of 12 and 15 years.

non-stretchable tape and the average of three recordings plotted on an appropriate centile chart.

The greatest increase in head circumference takes place in the first year of life, when it ad-vances from an average of 33 cm at birth to 46 cm at 12 months. At the age of 14 years it is 53 cm which represents an advance of only 7 cm in 11 years as compared with 13 cm in the first year.

Table 4.1 Age at which first (deciduous) and permanent dentition occur.	Deciduous dentition		Permanent dentition	
	Incisors	6–9 months	First molars	6 years
	First molars	12–14 months	Incisors	7–8 years
	Canines	18 months	Premolars	10–11 years
	Second molars	2–2.5 years	Canines	9–12 years
			Second molars	10–13 years
			Third molars	12–25 years

Dental maturation

Maturation of teeth can be affected by the same influences as those affecting skeletal maturity, though some variations in skeletal maturity are seldom accompanied by such marked changes in dental maturity. Moreover, illness does not retard dental maturity as it does skeletal maturity. There is a very wide normal range for tooth eruption and the first tooth to appear is a central incisor, usually the lower, and the first dentition is completed with the eruption of the second molars by the end of the second year. The first tooth of the permanent dentition is the first molar which appears at the end of 6 years. The average times of tooth eruption are shown in Table 4.1.

Puberty

Puberty describes the process of becoming functionally capable of procreation and usually occurs over a period of 4 years. It is dependent on the gonads changing from infantile to an adult state and this process affects most of the organ systems within the body. The onset of puberty is accompanied by a growth spurt and this occurs 2 years earlier in girls than in boys. During the twentieth century, the age of puberty in girls (denoted by menarche) has fallen from 16 years in 1900 to 13 years in 1980.

Details of the development of secondary sexual characteristics during puberty is discussed in Chapter 23.

Neurological development

The neuronal complement of the brain is fully developed well before birth, but the infant is born in a very dependent state, completely unable to attend to his most basic needs. In the human, independence is not achieved for many years. During the period of neurological development, two major structural changes are occurring in the brain; synaptic branching and axonal myelination. These developments permit the brain slowly to gain control over its environment as well as acquiring and synthesizing knowledge, a process known as learning.

An assessment of development must be accompanied by careful clinical assessment of the nervous system. A child with cerebral palsy may not be able to perform a variety of motor tasks such as reaching or walking and if very severe, speech may be impaired due to bulbar palsy. The child's developmental assessment will clearly be impaired by any motor disability, yet his intellectual function may be normal. This is discussed in more detail in Chapter 19.

Assessment of an infant's neurological maturity is made from a study of his behaviour and his reaction to standard stimuli, so that comparisons can be drawn. This comparative assessment can be made from the age of 1 month and gives the developmental quotient (DQ). This is calculated as:

$$DQ = \frac{\text{developmental age in months} \times 100}{\text{chronological age in months}}$$

Specific tests of intelligence can be carried out from the age of 3 years and give the intelligence quotient (IQ). The DQ is not a measure of intelligence although those children with a low DQ often subsequently show a low IQ. The exception may be children with severe disability of their motor system. Advanced DQ in the first 2 years of life shows very poor correlation wih high IQ.

Table 4.2   Milestones in development. It must be emphasized that these ages are very approximate and there are wide variations between normal babies.

Age	Social	Speech and language	Gross motor	Fine motor
1 month	Quietens when talked to	—	Holds head up momentarily	Fists clenched at rest
2 months	Smiling with good visual interest	Listens to a bell	Chin off couch when prone	Hands largely open
3 months	Follows objects through 180°	Vocalizes when talked to	Weight on forearms when lying prone	Holds objects placed in hands
4 months	Laughs aloud	—	Pulling to sit—no head lag	Hands come together
6 months	Imitates	Localizes sound	Lying prone, pushes up on hands	Reaches for objects
7 months	Feeds himself with biscuit	Makes four different sounds	Sits unsupported	Transfers from hand to hand
9 months	Waves bye-bye	Says 'mama'	Stands holding on	Pincer grasp
12 months	Plays 'pat-a-cake'	2–3 words	Walking unsupported	Gives objects
15 months	Drinks from a cup	4–5 words	Climbs up stairs	Tower of 2 cubes
18 months	Points to three parts of body	8–10 words	Gets up and down stairs	Tower of 3–4 cubes
21 months	Dry (mostly) during day	2-word sentences	Runs	Scribbles circles
24 months	Puts on shoes	2–3-word sentences	Walks up and down stairs	Tower of 6–7 cubes
2.5 years	Recognizes colours	Knows full name		Copies with pencil −1
3 years	Dresses and undresses fully	Tells stories		Copies with pencil +0

Development is a continuous process from conception to maturity but its rate varies greatly in different, though still normal, children. There are also racial differences; the Afro-Caribbean baby at birth is developmentally more mature than the European and remains ahead for the first year.

Development is not a smooth continuous process but made up of lulls and spurts. Moreover, having achieved a skill, this may go into abeyance while another is being learned. Some skills develop separately, becoming co-ordinated later. The achievement of a new stage is dependent on the growing maturity of the nervous system so that development cannot be accelerated from outside sources, but external factors, particularly environmental and to a lesser extent illness, can retard it.

It is convenient to divide development into four major areas: (a) social, (b) speech and language, (c) gross motor, and (d) fine motor and important

milestones (summarized in Table 4.2). Delay in all four areas of development usually denotes mental retardation, unless it is due to severe emotional deprivation, but an isolated delay in any one area may not be abnormal. Delay in walking alone is common and may have been present in previous generations. Some children (especially boys) become adept at getting about by bottom shuffling; the need to walk being relatively unimportant as he has an effective method for locomotion. A history of bottom shuffling can often be obtained from at least one family member. Acquisition of speech is another common isolated delay. It is particularly seen where the child is exposed to more than one language at home, when the child's gestures are interpreted by overzealous parents thereby reducing his need to communicate verbally and in twins who share private non-verbal methods of communication. In all children with speech delay, deafness must be excluded.

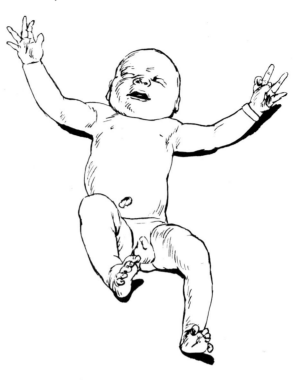

Fig. 4.3 The abduction phase of the Moro reflex.

Reflex development

Infants are born a 'bundle of reflexes' and it is necessary for these to disappear before normal motor development can occur. The grasp reflex of a normal newborn infant is very inhibiting if still present at 6 months when an infant is trying to manipulate objects. Persistence of primitive reflexes indicates severe neurological abnormality and three of the more important and complicated reflexes are briefly described here.

Moro reflex. This is elicitied by gently letting the infant's head drop back about 30 degrees, but may occur spontaneously or in response to tactile or painful stimuli. Initially the arms abduct with extension and opening of the hands (Fig. 4.3), followed by adduction with flexion as if to clasp the arms over the chest. In premature infants the complete movement is not always seen and consists mainly of abduction with extension. Persistence of the Moro reflex beyond 6 months is always abnormal.

Asymmetrical tonic neck reflex. This is elicited by laying the infant supine with the face in the midline. When the head is turned to one side, the arm on the side to which the head has been turned extends, with variable extension of the leg on the same side. There may be flexion of the opposite arm (Fig. 4.4). Although not often present at birth, it is seen in the majority of normal infants at 1 month of age. The presence of this reflex after 24 weeks of age is definitely abnormal.

Palmar grasp reflex. A powerful grasp reflex is present at birth. It usually disappears by 8 weeks and voluntary grasp develops at 4–5 months.

Developmental assessment

It is necessary to memorize a number of normal developmental milestones for different age groups and Table 4.2 summarizes some of the most important. Although development is assessed in four categories, it is always important to note how the

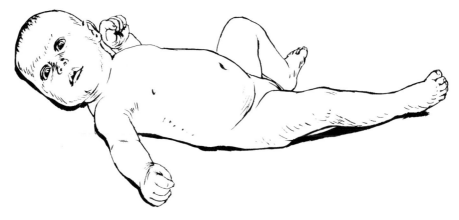

Fig. 4.4   Asymmetrical tonic neck reflex.

child is functioning overall. It is important that his brain integrates all the activities in a functional manner appropriate to the child's age.

Social

This is an assessment of how the child interacts with the people around him. Sights and sounds are the most important stimuli that elicit reactions in the child. By 4 weeks he will become quiet, or open his eyes widely in response to a spoken word. At 6 weeks the baby smiles responsively. For this to be considered a social reaction the child must smile in response to the examiner's (or parent's) smile. Failure to smile by 8 weeks is definitely abnormal. By 12 weeks the baby squeals with pleasure, and by 16 weeks laughs out loud. By 20 weeks the child will smile at himself in a mirror.

A very important stage in social development is the concept of 'permanence of objects'. At this stage an infant will search for an object that drops from his view and this usually develops at about 20–24 weeks. This is also the age when the child starts to be wary of strangers and may become upset by being picked up by the examiner. By 8 months he should understand the meaning of the word 'no'. By 9 months he waves bye-bye and by 11 months plays 'peek-a-boo' and at 12 months plays 'pat-a-cake'. At 11 months he will start to take an interest in picture books and gestures

appropriately to various actions in the story. At 12 months the child is capable of demonstrating memory and may respond appropriately to already learned commands such as 'where is the dolly?'

At 15 months he drinks from a cup and points to objects he wants. It is at this stage that he starts to show negativistic behaviour (p. 51).

At 18 months he can point to at least three parts of his body, and will point on request to named objects in books (e.g. cat or house). He will also follow simple commands such as 'give me the cup'.

At 21 months the child indicates his toilet needs and knows four parts of his body.

By 2 years he tries to put on his shoes and will fetch familiar objects. He is wary of playing with other children but will play near them and watch them.

Speech and language

Speech delay is relatively common and as an isolated finding is not significant but understanding should be present.

At 3 months the child should start to vocalize and enjoy playing with his voice. By 7 months he should be making four different sounds such as 'da', 'ba', 'ma' and 'ka', and by 8 months combining these sounds together in repetitive utterances.

At 11 months the child starts to use his first word and by 12 months he has two or three

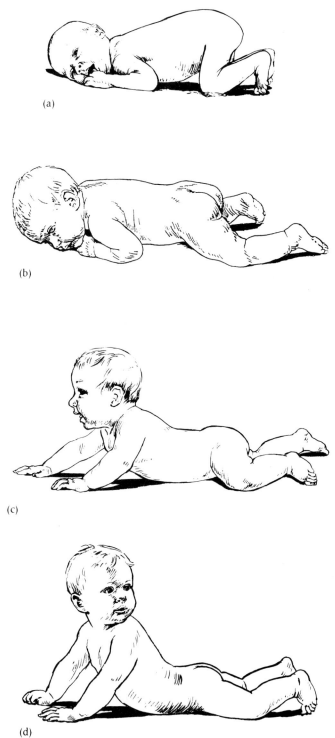

Fig. 4.5 Gross motor development in prone
position. (a) Birth; (b) 6 weeks; (c) 4 months;
and (d) 6 months.

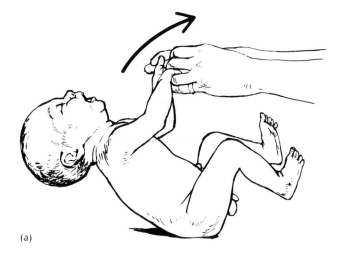

(a)

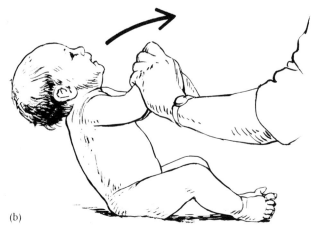

(b)

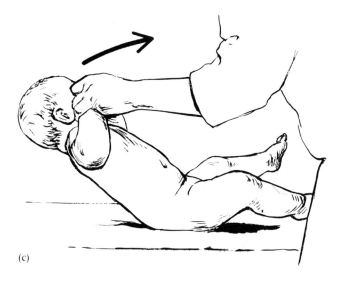

(c)

Fig. 4.6 Pulling to a sitting position at various developmental ages. Note the relationship of the head to the back. (a) Birth; (b) 6 weeks; and (c) 6 months.

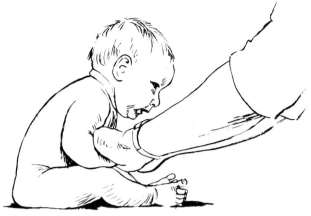

(a)

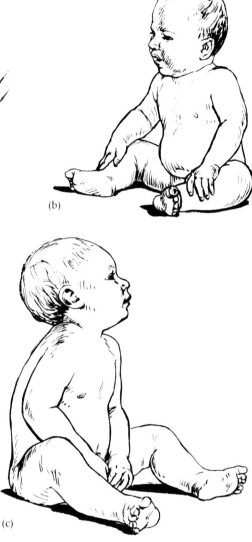

(b)

(c)

Fig. 4.7 Acquisition of sitting. (a) Curved back needs support from an adult at 6 weeks; (b) sits with some self-propping at 7 months; and (c) sits and pivots at 11 months.

which he uses with some meaning. The words may be indistinct but the mother can understand what her child says.

At 15 months he may have four to five words with meaning and talks incessantly in jargon or nonsense language. At 18 months he uses eight to 10 words and by 21 months starts to use two words together in little sentences, e.g. 'Dadda gone', 'nice dolly'.

By 2 years he is using personal pronouns such

as me and mine and talks in two to three word sentences.

Gross motor

At birth the infant assumes a naturally flexed posture and when prone flexes his hips and tucks his bottom up. By 6 weeks his pelvis is flatter on the table, but by 4 months he lifts his head and shoulders off the couch. By 6 months his arms are held

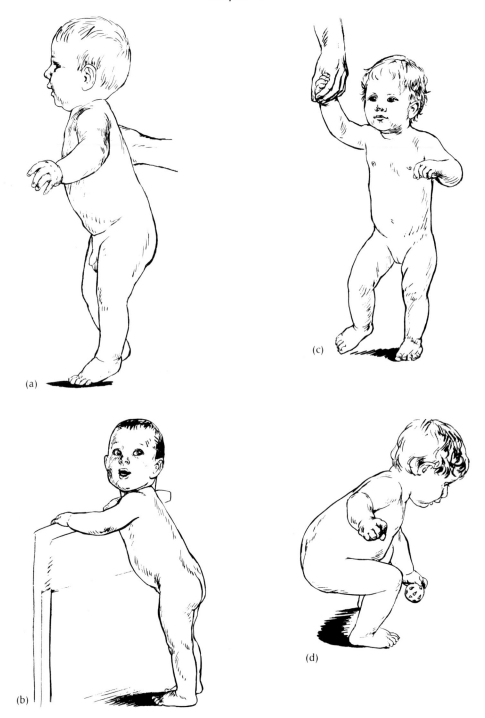

Fig. 4.8 Gross motor development showing the acquistion of walking skills. (a) 6 months, stands with support; (b) 9 months, pulls to standing and stands holding on; (c) 12 months, stands and walks with one hand held; and (d) 14 months, walks independently and stoops.

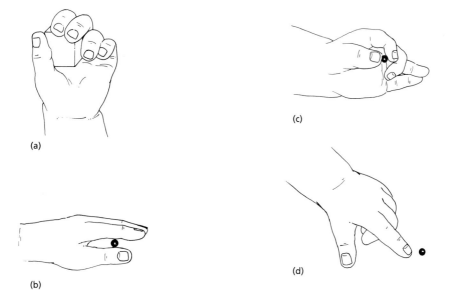

Fig. 4.9 Development of fine motor hand control. (a) Whole hand grasp at 5 months; (b) scissor grasp at 8 months; (c) neat pincer grasp at 10–11 months; and (d) pointing at bead at 10–11 months.

extended supporting the chest off the couch (see Fig. 4.5).

The sitting position is achieved gradually with progressive improvement in neck and trunk tone. On pulling the child to a sitting position the degree of head lag is less with advancing age (Fig. 4.6). The average age for sitting independently is 7 months and at this age the child needs his hands for support (Fig. 4.7b). By 9 months he sits without support and by 11 months can pivot (Fig. 4.7c). The child moves from a sitting to a crawling position at 9–10 months, pulling to standing by 10 months and walking around the furniture by 11 months. Figure 4.8 summarizes acquisition of walking skills. At 12 months he can walk with one hand held and can stand unsupported. As mentioned above, the age at which walking starts is very variable but it is often at 12–13 months. At 15 months he can get to a standing position without climbing up an object and can clamber up stairs. By 18 months he walks up stairs holding the banister and is very steady on his feet. He can throw a ball without falling over. By 21 months he runs without falling. By 2 years he walks up and down stairs confidently, two feet at a time.

Fine motor

At 1 month the infant's hands are closed most of the time but by 2 months the hands are largely open. By 3 months the grasp reflex has disappeared and he holds objects in the mid-line and he will shake a rattle purposely. At 5 months he starts to reach for objects initially with both hands embracing them towards his body and by 6 months starts to use his hands independently. At 7 months he has achieved finger-thumb apposition hand to the other. At this age he will feed himself with a biscuit.

By 9 months the hand and finger movements become more refined. At 7–8 months he has a raking grasp, by 8–9 months he has a scissor grasp using the thumb and first finger and by 9–10 months he has achieved finger-thumb apposition (summarized in Fig. 4.9).

By 1 year, the baby will give a block to the examiner and release it into his hand. He builds a tower of two wooden cubes at 15 months and three to four cubes at 18 months. At this age he scribbles with a pencil and turns the pages of a book. He brings a spoon to his mouth but usually

Table 4.3 Summary of the development of social interaction.

0–2 months	Environmental effects on the establishment of behavioural states
2–5 months	Visual engagement
5–8 months	Manipulative interaction
8–18 months	Exploration
18+ months	Dialogue

drops much of what is on it. By 21 months he can place five or six cubes on top of each other. By 2 years of age he builds a tower of six to seven cubes and can unscrew a lid on a container.

Social interaction and development

Humans are social creatures who interact in complicated ways in most everyday activities. The newborn infant is born into a social world and learns to interact initially with his mother, then other close relatives and eventually with other adults and children. Social development is dependent on achieving important neurodevelopmental landmarks which gives him contact with the outside world.

Early social development is divided into discrete periods of time corresponding to developmental landmarks and each period can be considered to have an important milestone in the development of the child into a social being (Table 4.3).

0–2 months

The infant is born with a variety of needs which must be met by the parents, usually the mother. In the first 2 months the baby starts to adapt his behaviour into states of arousal. Sleep and waking cycles begin to emerge and this is influenced by the routine in the house. The longest period of sleep usually occurs in the night. It has been shown that infants who sleep in the same room as their mothers in the first nights after birth establish this diurnal rhythm earlier than those looked after in the hospital nursery.

During the appropriate state the infant shows a great degree of alertness and is paticularly attracted by the human face and the spoken word. He achieves contact with his mother particularly during feeding when patterns of interaction occur. The mother and baby co-ordinate their behaviour and take turns to initiate contact by means of alternating sucking with pauses for eye contact. It appears that the infant is programmed to respond to his carer in particular ways and in turn the carer is profoundly influenced by her own programming to stimulate her infant in certain ways and to respond to his contact. During the first 2 months the baby emerges from his state of inaccessability to react and respond to his parents as a social being.

2–5 months

The major developmental change that occurs at about 2 months is the infant's visual development. At 2 months he can sustain eye contact and this is the first evidence that the baby shows to his mother of individuality. This is clearly a vital stimulus for the parents to interact with *their* child. With increasing development the infant shows progressively more gaze interaction. He develops patterns of gaze and looking away and the mother responds to her infant's gaze with stereotyped facial movements, speech and intonation patterns.

Another important aspect of this stage of development is the beginning of vocalization. When the child starts to babble the parents respond in an interactive verbal manner almost as if engaging in a conversation with the child. The baby may initiate vocalization and the mother responds by questioning or talking to the infant with pauses for the baby's responsive babble. Although the infant clearly does not understand the meaning of his parents' speech, its pattern and interaction with him is essential for his own speech and social development. The parents are sensitive to the needs of the baby and it has been shown that if the mother does not respond appropriately to her infant at this age by smiling and talking when in an *en face* position, the baby becomes distressed and may withdraw from further interaction. The mother's sensitive responses to her baby at this age are essential for his normal social development.

5–8 months

At this age the child transfers his attention from mother to objects. The child must be able to reach for toys in order to explore the inanimate world. The mother interacts with her child through the object rather than directly. At this stage simple play patterns start to emerge. At 6 weeks of age the baby spends approximately 70% of his contact time regarding his mother but by 6 months two-thirds of his time is taken up with looking at the rest of his world.

The baby begins to initiate contact with an object by gaze and later pointing which his mother then follows. Later the child will be directed to an object by observing the direction of the parents gaze. At this stage the infant is transforming from a completely egocentric creature to one who realizes he lives in a world which he shares with many objects and people.

8–18 months

This is the age that mobility is rapidly developing and the child starts to leave the safety of his mother to interact further with his environment. The child begins to initiate contact rather than simply reacting to it. It is at this age that the concept of reciprocating begins to emerge. The child can initiate an enjoyable game such as 'peek-a-boo' and can control the game by reciprocating his response to that of the adults. He is 'learning the rules' both of the game and of social interaction in general. The child begins to be able to use the adult to obtain desired objects and can also manipulate objects to attract the attention of the adult.

The child associates his cry with response and knows that if he is uncomfortable with a wet nappy his mother will provide relief. Babies who are institutionalized become apathetic if their cries are unanswered; its communicative role is extinguished.

In the first half of the second year the baby will begin to take more interest in other children. Initially they play side-by-side occasionally sharing a toy and by 18 months they may play together, but there is much less vocal contact than the child has with an adult at that age. The adult, particularly the parent, is the main influence in social training at this age.

After 18 months

By 18 months the child is a highly integrated individual capable of verbal communication and exploration. He understands the communicative role of speech and engages in endless naming of objects. He understands the role of symbolic play. A doll may represent a baby to be fed or a box a garage for his cars. By these means the child becomes a social individual by his interaction with the adult world. The way in which he learns this is not clear but it is most likely that his parents direct by controlling his behaviour towards socially acceptable and away from less acceptable activities. This is much more successful if direct conflict is avoided but a clash of wills is common at this stage because of the development of negativistic behaviour. The parents who are successful at rearing a normally social child are the ones who have themselves been successfully socialized from birth.

Reading list

Illingworth RS. *Basic Developmental Screening: 0–4 years*, 3rd Edn. Blackwell Scientific Publications, Oxford 1982.
Lingham S, Harvey DR. *Manual of Child Development*. Churchill Livingstone, Edinburgh 1988.
Schaffer HR. *The Child's Entry into a Social World*. Academic Press, London 1984.

5

NORMAL NEWBORN INFANT

As a consequence of improved results in the management of disease in older children, the emphasis in paediatrics has now swung towards the prevention and management of disease in infancy, particularly the newborn baby whose problems are now subjected to careful statistical analysis. For a proper understanding the following definitions must be stated:

1 Duration of pregnancy. This is calculated from the first day of the last normal menstrual period. This assumes both a regular 28-day cycle and that ovulation occurred 14 days after bleeding commenced. By this reckoning the duration of pregnancy (really the period of amenorrhoea) is between 37 and 42 weeks (259–294 days).

2 Full-term delivery. This occurs between 37 and 42 weeks from the date of the last menstrual period.

3 Pre-term delivery. This occurs if the infant is born less than 37 weeks (259 days) from the first day of the last normal menstrual period.

4 Post-term delivery. This occurs if the infant is born after 42 completed weeks (294 days) from the first day of the last normal menstrual period.

5 Low birth weight (LBW). This refers to any infant who weighs 2500 g or less at birth. In Britain approximately 7% of infants are LBW. These babies are born either too early (pre-term), or have grown inadequately *in utero* and are described as 'small for gestational age'. Some LBW infants may be both pre-term and small for gestational age.

6 Very low birth weight (VLBW). These are infants who weigh 1500 g or less at birth. Approximately 1% of births in the UK are VLBW.

7 Extremely low birth weight (ELBW). These are infants who weigh 1000 g or less at birth. Approximately 0.5% of births in the UK are ELBW.

8 Small for gestational age (SGA). This describes those infants whose birth weight falls below the 10th centile for gestational age. Infants whose birth weight falls below the 3rd centile are sometimes referred to as severely SGA.

9 Live birth. This is one in which there are signs of life (gasping, heart beat or spontaneous movement) after complete expulsion from the mother, irrespective of gestational age.

10 Stillbirth. A stillborn infant is one expelled from the birth canal after 28 weeks of pregnancy who shows no signs of life and has no heart beat. This definition varies in different countries and comparison of figures may be misleading. The stillbirth rate is expressed as the number of infants born dead after 28 weeks gestation per 1000 live births and stillbirths. In the UK the stillbirth rate is approximately 5 per 1000.

11 Perinatal mortality rate (PMR). This refers to the number of stillbirths and neonatal deaths in the first week of life per 1000 live births and stillbirths. In the UK the PMR is approximately 10 per 1000. The World Health Organization recommends this rate as an index of the quality of perinatal health services.

The definitions of neonatal mortality, postneonatal mortality and infant mortality rates are given in Chapter 2.

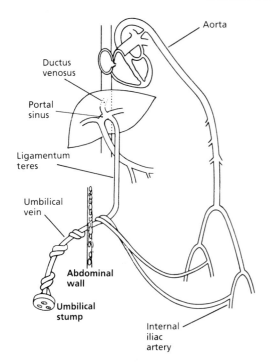

Fig. 5.1 Diagram of the fetal circulation.

Adaptation of the fetus to birth

The fetus occupies an aquatic environment and receives oxygen and nutrition from the placenta. The lungs contain fluid but have no respiratory function whilst the fetus remains *in utero*. Oxygenated blood flows from the placenta via the umbilical vein through the ligamentum teres into the inferior vena cava and to the heart (Fig. 5.1). Because the lungs are unexpanded there is a high pulmonary vascular resistance and oxygenated blood is diverted away from the right ventricle through the foramen ovale. In addition the ductus arteriosus provides a further right to left shunt of blood away from the lungs. Less than 10% of the blood ejected from the heart enters the lungs (Fig. 5.2). The pressure in the right heart *in utero* is higher than that in the left chambers. Systemic blood flow is preferentially diverted to the head and desaturated blood returns to the placenta via the umbilical arteries which arise from the internal iliac vessels. Fetal blood is considerably less saturated than that of the newborn (70% saturation in

the umbilical vein compared with 50% in the descending aorta). The fetus is well adapted to this low oxygen saturation by virtue of fetal haemoglobin which has a higher oxygen affinity than adult haemoglobin. The oxygen dissociation curve of fetal blood varies from that of the adult by being shifted to the left so that for any given pO_2, fetal blood contains a larger quantity of oxygen per gram of haemoglobin than does maternal blood.

At birth the infant gasps and expands his lungs. The pulmonary vascular resistance falls rapidly to below systemic levels and the pressure in the right side of the heart falls. When the cord is ligated the low resistance placenta is removed from the circulation and the systemic resistance increases. These changes in resistance between lung and systemic circulation cause a dramatic change in the blood flow through the lungs and the ductus arteriosus. Left atrial pressure will increase and functional closure of the foramen ovale occurs. With the start of breathing, arterial blood becomes fully saturated and this is the stimulus for the ductus arteriosus to close within the first few hours of life. Prostaglandins are necessary to maintain the ductus physiologically closed and anatomical obliteration occurs by 2 weeks from birth.

Immediate care of the newborn

The majority of newborn infants do not require formal resuscitation, but measures should be taken to ease the transition from intra- to extra-uterine life. As the head is delivered, gentle suction of the baby's mouth should be performed. The normal baby requires minimal interference and should be placed in the mother's arms immediately after delivery and the cord cut when it stops pulsating. Whilst the cord is attached, the baby should not be raised or lowered from the level of the placenta, otherwise blood transfusion occurs from the baby to the placenta or vice versa with the risk of anaemia or polycythaemia respectively. It is not necessary under normal circumstances to separate the baby from his parents for at least an hour after delivery. At this time, newborn infants are usually very visually attentive and the parents will enjoy getting to know their new baby.

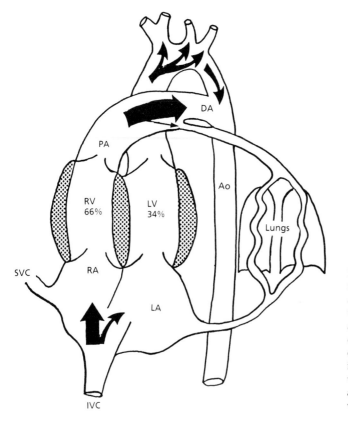

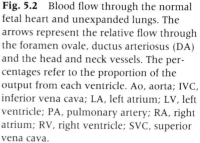

Fig. 5.2 Blood flow through the normal fetal heart and unexpanded lungs. The arrows represent the relative flow through the foramen ovale, ductus arteriosus (DA) and the head and neck vessels. The percentages refer to the proportion of the output from each ventricle. Ao, aorta; IVC, inferior vena cava; LA, left atrium; LV, left ventricle; PA, pulmonary artery; RA, right atrium; RV, right ventricle; SVC, superior vena cava.

Approximately 1% of newborn infants suffer intrapartum asphyxia. The asphyxiated fetus follows a predictable sequence of physiological responses involving both the respiratory and cardiovascular systems.

The initial response to placental hypoperfusion is for the fetus to increase respiratory activity which is then followed by a period of apnoea (primary apnoea). If no intervention occurs, the fetus starts to gasp after a short period of primary apnoea. The gasping reduces in frequency until secondary (or terminal) apnoea occurs. The infant may be born in either the primary or secondary apnoeic state. During primary apnoea the circulation is still vigorous and the infant maintains a good cardiac output with an accelerating heart rate. The infant looks cyanosed in the stage of primary apnoea. During the gasping stage, the blood pressure starts to fall until the stage of

secondary apnoea occurs. At this time the infant is pale and limp due to circulatory compromise. Primary and secondary apnoea can therefore be distinguished clinically on the basis of the infant's colour. The baby with secondary apnoea will not recover without vigorous resuscitative measures. It may be difficult to distinguish these two stages of apnoea in the delivery room and in practice, active resuscitative efforts should be started on all apnoeic, newborn infants, particularly if born prematurely.

Assessment of the infant at birth

In 1953, Virginia Apgar, introduced a scoring system (the Apgar score) to describe the condition of the infant at 1 minute of age. The infant may be scored again at 5, 10 or more minutes from birth if he has not reached optimal condition by that time.

Table 5.1 The Apgar score; maximum is 10 and minimum 0.

Sign	0	1	2
Heart rate	Absent	≤ 100 b.p.m.	> 100 b.p.m.
Respiratory effort	Absent	Gasping or irregular	Good
Muscle tone	Limp	Floppy	Normal
Reflex irritability (response to stimulation of foot)	No response	Some movement	Vigorous withdrawal
Colour	White	Blue	Pink

b.p.m, beats per minute.

The Apgar score must be done accurately and objectively for each of the five items shown in Table 5.1. A useful way of deriving an Apgar score is to delete points from 10 for a baby born in relatively good condition, and allocate points from 0 for a baby born in depressed state.

Resuscitation

Depression of the newborn infant may be due to a number of conditions including prematurity, intrapartum asphyxia, birth trauma and analgesic or anaesthetic agents given to the mother. The paediatrician should get as much information as possible about the pregnancy and labour prior to the delivery and specifically enquire as to whether opiate analgesia has been given within the previous 4 hours. The doctor must check the equipment prior to delivery. It is particularly important to have adequate suction, air and oxygen supply, bag and mask and a laryngoscope with functioning light.

At birth the infant is suctioned through the mouth and nostrils as described above. The stimulus of the catheter may be sufficient to establish spontaneous respiration. If the baby fails to make adequate respiratory efforts he should be placed on his back in a head-down position on the resuscitaire.

If the infant has not established adequate respiratory efforts by 1 minute, then ventilation with oxygen will be necessary in addition to the more basic methods described above. All staff re-sponsible for supervising delivery should be able to actively resuscitate a baby with a bag-and-mask.

BAG-ANG-MASK RESUSCITATION

A well fitting soft face-mask should be placed over the mouth and nose of the infant, but it is important to avoid obstructing the nares. The infant's jaw is held forwards as the operator squeezes the bag at a rate of 30–40 per minute (Fig. 5.3). Ensure that there is adequate expansion of the chest with each inspiratory breath and the infant's colour and heart rate should rapidly improve. It should be possible to maintain good ventilation with a bag and mask until the infant recovers or someone arrives who can intubate the infant.

INTUBATION

This should be performed only by experienced staff. The indications for intubation are:
1 Failure of bag-and-mask resuscitation.
2 Severe depression at birth with poor circulation.
3 The need for intermittent positive pressure ventilation during transfer to a neonatal unit.

Intubation may be through the nose (naso-tracheal) or the mouth (orotracheal) and requires the use of a laryngoscope to visualize the glottis.

DRUG TREATMENT

An infant who may be under the influence of opiates given to the mother for pain relief should

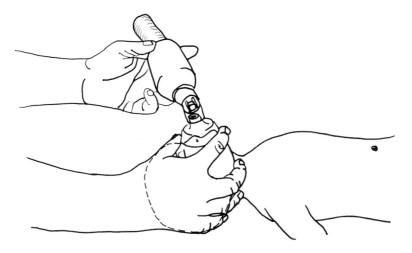

Fig. 5.3 Method of bag-and-mask resuscitation. Note that the neck is slightly extended and the jaw pulled forward with a good seal of the mask around the infant's face.

be given intramuscular naloxone (Narcan) which is a specific opiate antagonist and this reverses the respiratory depressant effects.

If the infant has a poor cardiac output, a drug such as adrenaline given intravenously is a useful cardiac stimulant. Calcium gluconate and isoprenaline may also be useful for resuscitation of infants with severe cardiopulmonary collapse.

Examination of the newborn

All newborn infants should be carefully examined within 24 hours of birth. The mother should be present during the examination and she should be given an explanation of what is being done. The examination should be performed in a systematic manner to avoid forgetting things. It is easy, when examining many infants, to mentally switch off and this negates the point of the examination. The examiner should especially concentrate on the less obvious but potentially more important abnormalities which should be particularly searched for in newborn infants. These include cataracts, cardiac murmurs and dislocation of the hip. Either before or after the examination, the infants length, weight and occipito-frontal head circumference should be carefully measured (p. 39) and plotted on a centile chart.

Observation

The colour should be noted. Normal infants may show peripheral cyanosis of hands and feet (acrocyanosis) and this is not abnormal providing the lips and tongue are pink. A transient colour change is often seen in babies, one half of the body becoming pale and the other half remaining pink. Often a clear cut demarcation line runs down the midline and this is referred to as *harlequin colour change* and is not abnormal.

Note any signs of respiratory distress (p. 85) including tachypnoea, grunting or recession. Examine the infant's facies which may be typical of a number of syndromes (see Chapter 8). The infant's posture and spontaneous movements should be observed and may give clues suggesting neurological abnormality. Supernumerary nipples are relatively common and may extend to the groin.

Head

Note the shape of the head and the size of the fontanelles. Two fontanelles can usually be palpated, the anterior and the posterior, and there is normally considerable variation in their size. The anterior fontanelle can usually be seen to pulsate and this is entirely normal.

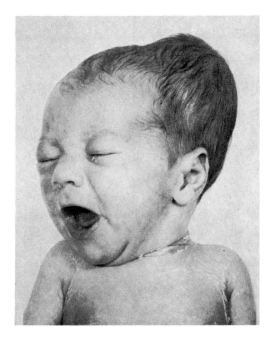

Fig. 5.4 Left parietal cephalhaematoma.

CEPHALHAEMATOMA

This is a localized fluctuant swelling usually seen over a parietal bone (Fig. 5.4). It is due to subperiosteal bleeding and is a benign condition. Parietal cephalhaematomata never cross the midline, but the rare cephalhaematoma of the occipital bone is seen posteriorly in the midline. The lesion may take 6–12 weeks to finally resolve but requires no specific treatment.

CRANIOTABES

This refers to softening felt over the parietal bone when pressed. The bone momentarily indents before popping out again much like a ping-pong ball does. It is not usually abnormal but in some babies may suggest rickets.

Eyes

In most infants vision can be detected by getting the baby's visual attention and observing his eye movements in response to the examiner moving his own head (p. 312). Abnormalities of the eyes to note particularly are:

1 Subconjunctival haemorrhage. These are common but have little significance. The mother should be reassured.

2 Coloboma. This refers to a notch or wedge defect of the iris (Fig. 5.5) and more rarely involving the eyelid. If present, a careful examination of the fundi should be made to exclude a full thickness coloboma of the choroid which may be associated with severe visual impairment (p. 317).

3 Cataracts. This should be carefully excluded in every infant. A red reflex is normally seen on shining a light into the infant's eye. This refers to the red reflection off the retina. If a white reflection is seen, then a cataract should be suspected (p. 315).

Mouth

The palate should be carefully examined for a cleft. Cleft palate (p. 138) may be diagnosed by observation when the infant cries or by palpation with the soft tip of a clean finger. Cleft palate is often associated with cleft lip but this is of course immediately obvious.

EPSTEIN'S PEARLS

These are small inclusion cysts in the midline of the hard palate and are normal. They disappear spontaneously with no treatment.

MICROGNATHIA

This refers to a small jaw and may be a feature of Pierre Robin syndrome (p. 138).

RANULA

These are round cystic swellings seen in the floor of the mouth and require no treatment.

Chest

After observation, the chest should be auscultated. Breath sounds should be symmetrical and crepitations may be heard normally in the first few hours

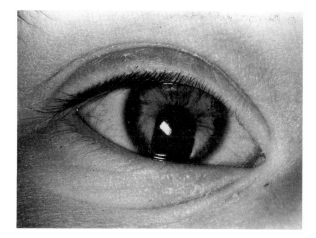

Fig. 5.5 Coloboma of the iris. A coloboma of the choroid was also present.

of life. Asymmetrical breath sounds should suggest diaphragmatic hernia or pneumothorax, but both are associated with respiratory distress.

BREAST ENGORGEMENT

This is common in full-term babies from the fourth to tenth day, and occurs equally in either sex (Fig. 5.6). It is hormonal in origin and 'milk' may be secreted from the nipple.

Cardiovascular system

The normal heart rate can vary between 100 and 170 beats per minute, but may fall below this during sleep. The brachial and femoral pulses should be routinely palpated. Delay or absence of the femoral pulsation suggests coarctation of the aorta (p. 232). Collapsing pulses suggest patent ductus arteriosus (p. 230).

On auscultation the heart sounds should be carefully assessed and any murmurs noted. The distribution of a murmur over the praecordium should also be noted.

Abdomen

The shape of the abdomen should be noted. Distension suggests bowel obstruction or intra-abdominal mass. A scaphoid abdomen suggests diaphragmatic hernia. The liver is normally palpated 1–2 cm below the right costal margin and the

spleen tip may be palpated in about 25% of normal infants. Splenomegaly suggests infection or haemolysis.

The kidneys should be carefully examined and the lower pole particularly on the right side is

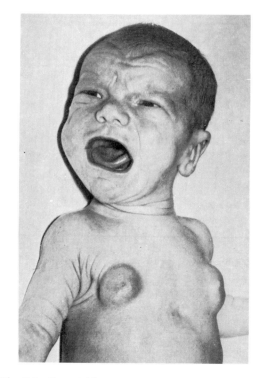

Fig. 5.6 Neonatal breast engorgement.

commonly felt in normal infants. The bladder should not normally be palpable in infants and if present suggests bladder neck obstruction (p. 255).

The anus should be patent and tested with a rectal thermometer.

Umbilicus

The three vessels of the umbilical stump should be counted. Approximately 1% of infants have a single umbilical artery and other congenital abnormalities may be seen in a very small proportion of these. It is unnecessary to investigate the renal tract of all infants with a single umbilical artery to detect the very few with anomalies.

The cord usually separates by 10 days leaving a yellow odourless eschar. Reddening of the skin around the umbilicus suggests infection and if present a swab should be taken. The need for systemic antibiotics must be carefully considered in cases of suspected umbilical sepsis.

Genitalia

PENIS

The urethral orifice should be identified. If it is not situated at the tip of the glans the infant has *hypospadias*. Hypospadias refers to the urethral orifice opening on the ventral surface of the penis. Glandular hypospadias (see Fig. 9.8) is only of importance for cosmetic reasons. The mother should be strongly reassured that mild degrees of hypospadias will not affect the child's ability to urinate standing up or his ability to procreate. These infants should be referred to a surgeon. Epispadias occurs when the urethra opens on the dorsal surface of the penis. Severe hypospadias may cause confusion as to the infant's true sex and this is discussed in Chapter 23.

SCROTUM

The testicles are descended into the scrotum at term in 98% of infants. Undescended testicles are discussed in Chapter 23. Scrotal swelling may be due to a hydrocele or an inguinal hernia, although the latter is rarely seen at birth.

VULVA AND VAGINA

Hymenal skin tags are common and are associated with redundant vaginal mucosa. The condition usually regresses over the first few weeks of life and requires no treatment.

The size of the labial folds depends on the gestational age of the infant, but at full-term the labia majora should completely cover the labia minora.

Limbs

The joints should be put through the normal range of movements to exclude congenital contractures. The fingers and toes are examined for polydactyly or syndactyly (p. 35).

TALIPES

Mild positional deformities may be present, but are not of any concern if the infant's foot can be put through a normal range of movements. Abnormalities include talipes equino varus (p. 149), talipes calcaneo valgus (p. 149) and metatarsus varus (p. 34).

Hips

Examination of the hips is a very important part of the newborn examination and should be left to last as it often makes the baby cry. Examination should start with observation for signs of established dislocation such as unequal leg length and asymmetry of the thighs. The physical examination should be undertaken in two parts.

ORTOLANI'S (REDUCTION) TEST (Fig. 5.7)

This test establishes whether the hip is dislocated. With the baby relaxed on a firm surface the hips and knees are flexed to 90 degrees. The examiner grasps the baby's thigh with the middle finger over the greater trochanter and lifts the thigh to bring the femoral head from its dislocated posterior

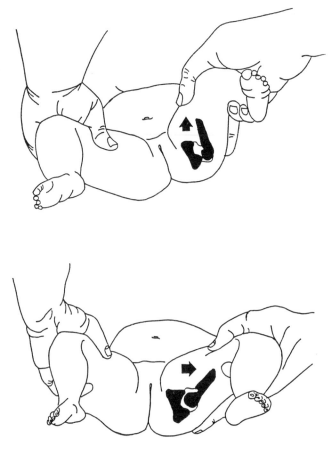

Fig. 5.7 Ortolani's test. The hip cannot be abducted due to posterior dislocation of the femoral head. The hip is pulled upwards (upper) and the head clunks into the acetabulum permitting abduction (lower).

position to opposite the acetabulum. Simultaneously, the thigh is gently abducted, reducing the femoral head over the posterior lip of the acetabulum. In a positive case the examiner senses the reduction by feeling a 'clunk' and there is a forward movement of the head of the femur.

BARLOW'S (DISLOCATION) TEST (Fig. 5.8)

This is really the reversal of Ortolani's test and assesses whether the hip can be dislocated. One hand fixes the pelvis with the thumb anteriorly over the symphysis pubis and the other fingers posteriorly over the coccygeal region. The other hand grasps the baby's thigh and adducts it gently downwards. Dislocation is palpable as the femoral head slips over the posterior lip of the acetabulum.

Using these two manoeuvres and by carefully examining each hip separately, infants with congenital hip dislocation or subluxation will be detected. The management of this condition is described in Chapter 9.

Neurological system

There are only a few items on the standard neurological assessment of newborn infants which gives useful information on higher cerebral function. Infants born with little or no cerebral cortex may show normal neonatal reflexes and appropriate tone. A normal infant should vary in his state of arousal from quiet sleep to crying and includes active sleep, semi-wakefulness, alert state and restlessness. A normal infant is able to be consoled

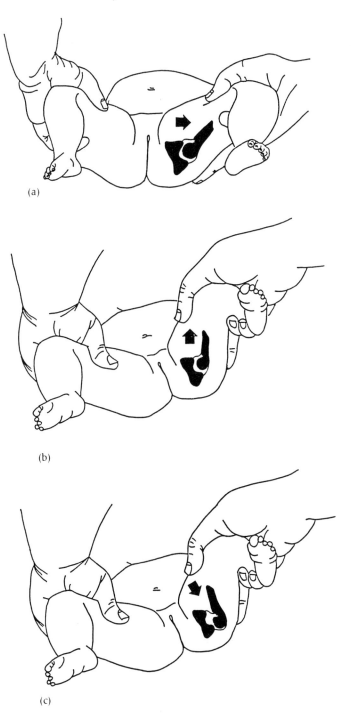

(a)

(b)

Fig. 5.8 Barlow's test. The hip is abducted to establish that it is not dislocated (a). The adducted hip is then pulled upwards (b) and then the femoral head pushed downwards and laterally to see whether it is dislocatable (c).

(c)

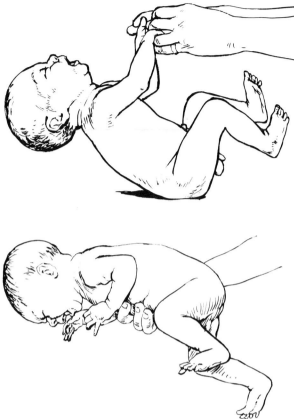

Fig. 5.9 Normal trunk and neck tone in response to gravity. (a) Pulling to sitting. Note arm tone as well as neck; and (b) ventrosuspension.

when he cries, but neurologically abnormal infants are very difficult to console.

Note the infants spontaneous movements. They should be relatively smooth, but spontaneous startles are not uncommon. Tone should be assessed actively by moving the limbs through a range of movements and his posture in response to gravity should also be observed (Fig. 5.9). A hypotonic baby lies in a frog-like posture with arms and legs flexes and abducted. A hypertonic baby is stiff and in a state of excessive limb flexion, often with extension of the back and neck.

Neonatal reflexes should be elicited, including tendon jerks, palmar grasp, rooting, sucking, walking and the Moro. The Moro reflex is described on p. 43.

Higher cerebral function may also be assessed by observation of vision and hearing. In an appropriately alert state, the infant will fix on an interesting object such as the examiner's face or a red woollen ball and will track the object both horizontally and vertically. Hearing can be assessed by sounding a loud rattle outside of his range of vision and noting the infant's response to it. This should include stilling to the noise, and sometimes an effort to turn the head towards the sound.

Further reading

Levene MI, Tudehope DI, Thearle MJ. *Essentials of Neonatal Medicine*. Blackwell Scientific Publications, Oxford 1987.

Roberton NRC. *A Manual of Normal Neonatal Care*. Edward Arnold, London 1988.

6
INFANT FEEDING

Milk is the food of the newborn baby and it is capable of sustaining all the infant's nutritional needs for the first 4–6 months of life. Breast milk is the natural food for babies but very adequate alternative formula feeds are now available. Although the aphorism 'breast is best' holds largely true there are some exceptions and these are discussed in this chapter. Table 6.1 compares the constituents of breast milk with a modern formula feed.

Nutritional requirements

Water

Over 70% of the weight of a newborn infant is represented by water compared with 60% of the adult weight. Infants are less able to conserve water and consequently their fluid requirements are considerably higher than that of older children. In addition, the fluid loss through the immature skin and kidneys of very premature infants is considerably higher than that of the full-term infant and their requirements will be yet higher. Table 6.2 summarizes the fluid requirements of both premature and full-term infants.

Energy

The energy requirements of premature and growth-retarded infants are higher than those born at full-term. In addition the sick infant will also require more energy to overcome increased

Table 6.1 Comparison of various constituents of pooled expressed breast milk, unmodified cow's milk and a modern formula feed. All values are per 100 ml of milk.

	Breast milk	Cow's milk	Formula milk
Energy (kcal)	70.0	66.0	65.0
Protein (g)	1.07	3.5	1.8
Fat (g)	4.2	3.7	3.5
Carbohydrate (g)	7.4	4.9	6.9
Sodium (mEq)	0.64	2.2	1.0
Potassium (mEq)	1.5	3.5	1.6
Chloride (mEq)	1.2	2.9	1.55
Calcium (mg)	35.0	117.0	47.0
Phosphorus (mg)	15.0	92.0	37.0

catabolism. The newborn infant requires approximately 110 kcal/kg/day for normal growth and these energy requirements are provided by fat, carbohydrate and protein.

FAT

Fat is the most important source of energy in milk and provides approximately one-half of the infant's requirements. Human milk fat is more easily absorbed than fat in cow's milk preparation which is usually of vegetable origin. Unsaturated fatty acids are better absorbed than saturated ones and medium chain triglycerides (present in some commercially available milks) is better absorbed than long chain fats. Infants require 4–6 g fat per day.

	Day 1	Day 2–3	Day 4–5	Day 6–7	Day 14
Volume (ml/kg)	40–60	80–100	120–140	150–160	150–200

Table 6.2 Guidelines for the volume of milk a healthy infant should take in a 24-hour period.

CARBOHYDRATE

Almost all the carbohydrate in both human and formula milk is lactose and about 40% of the total energy requirements comes from carbohydrate sources.

PROTEIN

Milk protein can be divided into curd and whey. Curd is predominately casein and precipitates in the stomach. It may be important as a regulator of gastric emptying. The whey component contains mainly lactalbumin and lactoferrin. Human milk protein is composed of 40% casein and 60% whey (lactalbumin) compared to cow's milk which contains 80% casein. In early human milk (colostrum) there is a very high concentration of immunoglobulins which contribute to the total protein load.

AMINO ACIDS

An appropriate balance of essential amino acids are necessary for normal development. Too little may produce deficiency symptoms and too much may cause neurological toxicity. The amino acid requirements of infants is considerably higher than that of older children.

MINERALS

There is a large variation between the relative proportion of minerals in different types of milk. The mineral constituent of breast milk also varies depending on the gestational age and post-natal age of the infant. The calcium to phosphorus ratio is important for absorption of these two minerals. High phosphorus intake (as occurs if unmodified cow's milk formulas are used) will cause renal excretion of calcium with hypocalcaemia possibly leading to tetany or convulsions.

VITAMINS

All modern milk formulae are fortified with vitamins to the recommended values. Surprisingly, breast milk is deficient in two vitamins; vitamin K and D. All newborn infants should be given vitamin K at birth to prevent haemorrhagic disease of the newborn (p. 110). All breast-fed babies should be given vitamin D supplements until they are on a mixed weaning diet as, although breast milk contains water soluble vitamin D, it does not appear to have antirachitic properties. Breast-fed babies should be given daily vitamin A (200 μg), vitamin C (20 mg) and vitamin D (7 μg).

IRON AND TRACE ELEMENTS

There are a large number of essential trace elements present in milk which are essential for normal growth and development.

Breast milk contains sufficient iron for the requirements of infants born at full-term until mixed feeding is introduced. Premature infants require supplemental iron from 1 month of age (4 mg elemental iron or 45 mg of ferrous gluconate) because they are born before the majority of their iron stores have crossed the placenta into the baby.

Fluoride is essential for the normal development of dental enamel and protects the child from subsequent dental decay. Fluoride in human milk varies with maternal ingestion but may be inadequate in some geographical areas. The dose is 0.1 mg/kg/day and is available as drops.

Breast feeding

Survival of the human species has until relatively recently been dependent, a least in part, on a close mother–infant dyad. The mother needed to be biologically capable of providing adequate volumes of milk formulated for the needs of her infant. Breast milk is almost perfectly adapted to the requirements of the infant and it has only been in the relatively recent past that in some parts of the world, safe alternatives to breast milk have become available.

The proportion of women breast feeding varies widely throughout the world. In 1981 the World Health Organization reported that in some countries all mothers breast fed for up to a year, but in others this figure was much smaller. In Britain over the last 10 years there has been an increase in the proportion of women who initially breast feed their infants. The DHSS report that in the early 1980s, 67% of mothers in England and Wales breast fed initially, and 40% were still breast feeding at 4 months. These figures are influenced by the socio-economic class of the family; 97% of women in the highest socio-economic group fed their first baby compared with a figure below 50% in a group of less advantaged women. The pattern in less developed countries is also mixed. In a group of women in rural Nigeria, 97% were still breast feeding at 1 year. Unfortunately the more economically advantaged women in Nigeria and other developing countries followed the Western pattern and stopped breast feeding after only a few months or weeks.

The factors that predict successful breast feeding are varied and include social class as mentioned above. The majority of women who planned to breast feed their baby while still pregnant had a much greater chance of this being successful than those who remained undecided during pregnancy and were encouraged to breast feed only after the birth of the baby. The attitude of the father and grandmother of the infant is also of great importance in determining whether a woman will breast feed her infant.

In developed countries the positive reasons to breast feed babies are mainly psychological rather than those of safety. Breast feeding is also free of cost which may be important in some parts of modern Britain. In developing countries the argument for breast milk being the safest way of feeding a baby is very strong. Formula feeds may be easily contaminated by polluted water used in making up the feed with the risk of fatal gastro-enteritis (p. 552).

Physiology of lactation

During pregnancy there is marked increase in the number of ducts and alveoli within the breast, in response to oestrogens, progesterone, placental lactogen and prolactin. The size of the nipple also increases. In the third trimester prolactin sensitizes the glandular tissue causing small amounts of colostrum to be secreted.

At birth, oestrogen levels fall rapidly while prolactin rises. This is stimulated further by the infant sucking at the breast. The prolactin secretion from the anterior pituitary maintains milk production from the breast alveoli. The volume of milk produced relates to the frequency, duration and intensity of sucking.

The flow of milk from the breast is under the control of the let-down reflex. The baby rooting at the nipple causes afferent impulses to pass to the posterior pituitary which secretes oxytocin. This passes, by the blood stream, to the breast where it acts on the smooth muscle fibres surrounding the alveoli so that milk is forced into the large ducts. Oxytocin also causes contraction of the smooth muscle of the uterus, thereby hastening involution. This is felt as 'after pains' and they may be severe for the first few days while breast feeding. As the baby takes less milk, the stimulus for prolactin production reduces, and lactation is inhibited. The hormonal maintenance of lactation is summarized in Fig. 6.1.

The let-down reflex is stimulated by contact with the baby including hearing the baby cry and handling him. Dripping of milk from the breast not being suckled is due to the reflex action; this diminishes after the first few weeks. Anxiety and embarassment suppress the reflex by action of the sympathetic nervous system. Every step possible should therefore be taken to put the mother at her ease and avoid unnecessary anxiety.

Variations in breast milk

Breast milk is a dynamic substance which changes its constituents with the post-natal age of the

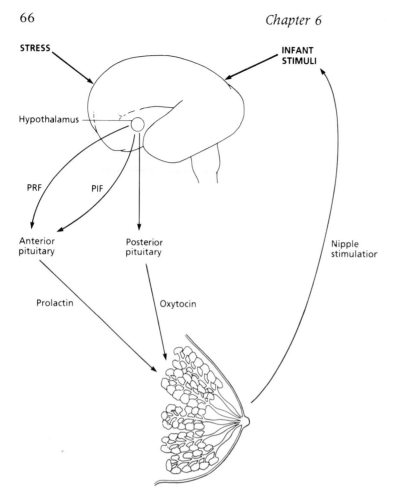

Fig. 6.1 The hormonal maintenance of lactation. PIF, prolactin inhibiting factor; PRF, prolactin releasing factor.

infant as well as showing consistent variations depending on the maturity at which the infant is born.

The newly born infant has a more immature physiology than babies of a few weeks or months of age. They are less able to conserve sodium by the kidney and may be less able to digest lactose and fat. Early breast milk is suited to the immature physiology and the milk contains more sodium (to account for renal wastage), less carbohydrate and less fat. Table 6.3 summarizes the changing constituents of human milk with post-natal age.

COLOSTRUM

The milk produced in the first few days after birth is called colostrum and is a thick, yellowish fluid. It is particularly valuable for the establishment of

lactobacilli in the bowel and contains less fat and energy, but more immunoglobulins and fat-soluble vitamins than later milk.

The constituents of milk do not reach their

Table 6.3 Composition of milk from women who are in the early stages of lactation (3 days after birth) and those who have been breast feeding for 1 month. All values are for 100 ml of milk.

	Days post-partum	
	3	28
Energy (kcal)	51	70
Protein (g)	3	2
Fat (g)	2	4
Carbohydrate (g)	6	7
Sodium (mmol)	3	1

mature proportions until about 10–14 days after birth and the secretion from the breast between colostrum and mature milk is referred to as transitional milk. The milk of mothers who deliver prematurely also varies in constituents compared to the milk of mothers delivering at full-term. Pre-term milk contains a higher protein and sodium content than term milk. Pre-term milk also contains considerably more IgA than term milk. The amount of lactose and fat (and consequently energy) may be less in pre-term milk and probably is associated with immaturity of the absorptive mechanisms of the pre-term infant.

Technique of breast feeding

The majority of the milk taken by a baby from the breast is consumed in the first 5 minutes of the feed. Much of the rest of the time is spent in non-nutritive sucking. The mother should be aware of the feeling of her breast being 'emptied' by her baby shortly after commencement of suckling, but the time spent at the breast following this is very important.

The mother should be encouraged to put the baby to the breast immediately after birth and the normal baby will attempt to suck. Little milk is produced, but the stimulation is important to establish lactation. The mother should be encouraged to put her baby to the breast on demand and she should also feed her baby during the first night if she is not too tired. The time the baby spends on the breast should be gradually increased so that the nipples become accustomed to the baby sucking.

Trauma to the nipple in the first few days after birth should be minimized. The baby exerts strong suction on the nipple and he should never be pulled off the breast. The mother should be shown how to release the baby by using her finger to depress the breast away from the corner of the baby's mouth. Every feed should be commenced on alternate breasts.

Babies are often given complement formula feeds in the early days of life by well-meaning staff in order to let the mother rest, but this is unnecessary. If the baby appears to be hungry and it is considered not appropriate to put him to the breast then he may be given a solution of dextrose and water.

INVERTED NIPPLES

Some women have abnormally inverted nipples and this should be detected during pregnancy. This condition is managed by wearing nipple shields under the bra for the last three months of pregnancy. The shield should also be worn after delivery.

CRACKED NIPPLES

This condition should be avoided by good breast feeding technique. If cracked nipples do occur, the first step in treatment is to alter the feeding position. Many mothers lose all pain if the baby is positioned with the body under the mother's armpit on the same side as the breast and the feet pointing backwards. If this fails a nipple shield should be used to protect the nipple during feeds. Between feeds, the nipples should be exposed to the air as much as possible and wearing a bra should be discouraged for a few days. The nipples must be kept dry. Gentle application of expressed breast milk directly to the cracked nipple has been recommended. Care should be taken to let the milk dry before replacing the breast in the bra.

Should these measures fail to relieve the pain, the baby must not be allowed to feed from the breast until the crack has healed. This usually takes 1–2 days if detected early. Milk is expressed either manually or by electric pump for feeding by bottle or spoon.

ENGORGEMENT

This occurs most commonly in primiparous women. Engorged breasts are full and painful, the overlying skin being red and oedematous. The baby should be allowed to feed generously from the breast at regular intervals to avoid milk engorgement. If the milk comes in so rapidly that it exceeds the baby's requirements in the early days, the breast can be expressed by hand or by an electric breast pump. Breast engorgement should not be confused with mastitis or early breast abscess.

BREAST ABSCESS

This is usually due to staphylococcal infection and is commonly a sequel to a cracked nipple. The first sign is either flushing of the skin over one area of the breast or a hard painful lump. This is due at first to retention of milk, but later it may become secondarily infected. At the first sign of infection, intramuscular flucloxacillin should be given and followed by oral medication. In early cases feeding from the affected breast should be continued, the breast being emptied of retained milk by expression. In late cases the breast should be firmly bandaged, feeding being permitted from the unaffected breast only. By this means lactation can be maintained in the normal breast but suppressed in the affected breast.

Advantages of breast feeding

The advantages of breast feeding can be summarized:
1 Perfect balance of milk constituents.
2 No risk of contamination with organisms.
3 Anti-infective properties.
4 Convenience.
5 No expense to purchase milk.
6 Psychological satisfaction.
7 Probably a reduced incidence of atopic illness.

Anti-infective properties

Breast-fed infants have a significantly lower risk of respiratory and gastrointestinal infections in the early months of life compared with formula-fed infants. Breast milk contains a number of important anti-infective properties:
1 Cells. Milk is teeming with white cells, mainly macrophages, polymorphs and both T and B lymphocytes.
2 Immunoglobulins. Secretory IgA is the predominant immunoglobulin found in breast milk. It is in particularly high concentration in the colostrum (early breast milk).

3 Lysozyme. This substance lyses bacterial cell walls.
4 Lactoferrin. Iron is necessary for the replication of some bacteria and lactoferrin binds the iron and inactivates it, thus depriving the organisms of this essential substance.
5 Interferon. This is found in low concentration in breast milk and has anti-viral properties.
6 Bifidus factor. The stool of breast-fed babies is more acid than that of artificially fed infants. This together with the carbohydrate bifidus factor encourages lactobacilli to flourish in the bowel. Lactobacilli inhibit the overgrowth of *Escherichia coli*. Unfortunately a single feed of formula milk is enough to disturb this delicate balance.

Contraindications to breast feeding

The contraindications to breast milk feeding can be considered as either maternal or neonatal. The latter group comprise contraindications to many forms of milk and not specifically human.

MATERNAL

1 Acute illness. This contraindication is relative and depends on the type and severity of the illness.
2 Neoplasm.
3 Psychosis, unless the mother can be very closely supervised.
4 Open tuberculosis (sputum positive to *Mycobacterium*).
5 Breast abscess (see above).
6 Drug ingestion (see above).

NEONATAL

1 Acute illness. Mothers should be encouraged to express milk whilst their baby is ill.
2 Severe cleft lip or palate. Feeding from the breast should be attempted but alternative methods of giving the baby breast milk may be necessary (p. 139).
3 Gastrointestinal abnormality. This includes congenital bowel obstruction and necrotising enterocolitis.

Table 6.4 A guide to the use of common drugs in breast feeding mothers.

Unsuitable for breast feeding mothers	Only use if mother and infant can be monitored	Safe to use in breast feeding mothers
Gold salts	Aminoglycosides	Codeine
Indomethacin	Co-trimoxazole	Non-steroidal
Phenylbutazone	Ethambutol	anti-inflammatories
Chloramphenicol,	Isoniazid	Paracetamol
Tetracyclines	Clonidine	Salicylates*
Phenindione	Diuretics	Cephalosporins
Lithium	Antidepressants	Erythromycin
Iodides	Carbamazepine	Metronidazole*
Oestrogens (high dose)	Phenytoin	Penicillins
Antimetabolites	Primidone	Rifampicin
Atropine	Carbimazole	Beta blockers
Ergotamine	Oral contraceptives	Digoxin
Opiates	Thiouracils	Heparin
	H_2 antagonists	Hydralazine
	Antihistamines	Methyldopa
	Theophylline	Warfarin
		Barbiturates*
		Benzodiazepines*
		Sodium valproate
		Corticosteroids*
		Progestogens
		Bulk laxatives
		Kaolin
		Inhaled bronchodilators

* Only if low dose regimes.

4 Metabolic problems. This includes galactosaemia, phenylketonuria and lactose intolerance.

Drugs in breast milk

Most drugs given to the mother are excreted to some degree in her breast milk but the exposure to the infant is usually so little that the risk is minimal. Table 6.4 lists the drugs that are definitely dangerous to the infant as well as those in which the risk can be minimized by careful monitoring.

Breast milk jaundice (see also Chapter 7)

An association between breast feeding and jaundice has been made and is due to a steroid compound in the milk which inhibits the conjugation of bilirubin. Hyperbilirubinaemia is never severe and breast feeding should not be withdrawn for this reason.

BREAST MILK BANK

There has been a fashion to give sick or premature babies the milk of well established breast feeding mothers of healthy babies. Many neonatal units ran a breast milk bank where the milk (either drip or expressed at the end of a feed) was delivered within 24 hours of collection to the bank and then frozen. The milk was then batched, pasteurized and refrozen until it was required by the baby.

Pasteurization refers to a precise method of heat treating the milk. It is rapidly heated to 62.5°C and held at that temperature for 30 minutes before being cooled and refrozen. Samples of the milk were taken for microbiological assessment prior to heat treatment (to exclude a toxin-producing organism) and immediately after pasteurization (to exclude pathogenic organisms in the milk surviving heat treatment).

Unfortunately, pasteurization destroys all the cells in the milk but it does conserve the majority of the immunoglobulin and other anti-infective proteins. Heating the milk to higher temperatures destroys the majority of these substances.

The role of the breast milk bank has diminished somewhat in recent years for two reasons. First, we now know that the milk of mothers who are established breast feeders is nutritionally inadequate for the needs of premature babies. Secondly, human immunodeficiency virus (HIV) may be spread in breast milk and all mothers donating milk must have their HIV antibody status known. This naturally discourages many of the donors in the community. It is not known for certain whether pasteurization destroys HIV.

It is not necessary to heat treat the milk of mothers who express milk for their own baby provided that this is done in a socially clean manner and the milk is frozen within 4 hours of expression.

Formula feeds

Safe alternative methods of feeding newborn infants are now available. These formula milks are based on cow's milk but are highly adapted to meet the basic nutritional requirements of grow-ing immature infants. A variety of components of cow's milk are utilized (Fig. 6.2). Skim milk is produced by removing the fat content, and the whey remains after removal of the curd (this is a step in the manufacture of cheese). The minerals are removed from the remaining whey and lactose by electrodialysis.

Formula feeds can then be assembled from these components together with other additives. Virtually all milks have added carbohydrate (Fig. 6.3a), usually lactose but sucrose and maltodextrins may also be used. Cow's milk fat is much less digestible than human milk fat and contains far less polyunsaturated fatty acids. Most milk manufacturers replace the cow's milk fat with a mixture of vegetable and animal fats (Fig. 6.3b). This alters the fatty acid profile to resemble more closely that of breast milk. A major difference between human and cow's milk is the protein fractions of curd (casein) and whey. Cow's milk contains mainly curd and to overcome this, modern formulas are based on demineralized whey. To this is added skim milk, more lactose and minerals. A mixture of fat, trace elements and vitamins (A, C and D) are than added (Fig 6.3c). Demineralized whey milks are amongst the most popular of modern formulas. Cow and Gate Premium, Ostermilk Complete Formula and SMA Gold Cap are of this type. Table 6.1 compares the major constituents of breast milk, raw cow's milk and a demineralized whey formula.

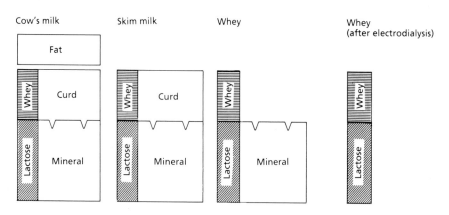

Fig. 6.2   Products of the dairy industry used in the manufacture of infant feeds. (Reproduced with permission from Wharton B.A., Berger H.M. *Br Med J* 1976.)

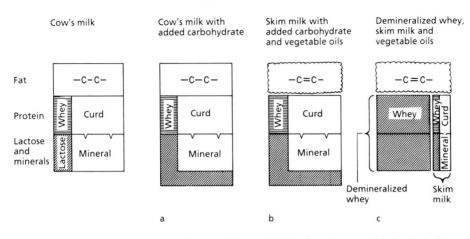

Fig. 6.3 Modifications of whole cow's milk in the manufacture of infant formulae. (a) added carbohydrate, (b) substituted fat, (c) demineralized whey. (Reproduced with permission from Wharton B.A., Berger H.M. *Br Med J* 1976.)

Preparation of feeds

Some mothers find it more convenient to make up the days supply of feeds at one time; this method being satisfactory provided they can be stored in a refrigerator. Mothers must be instructed to use a level measure of powder and not a heaped one which produces too concentrated a feed, especially in its electrolyte content. To obtain a level measure the excess powder is removed with the flat of a knife.

Scrupulous attention should be paid to sterility; bottles and teats being boiled between each feed. Sodium hypochlorite (Milton) is a useful disinfectant in which to store bottles and teats between feeds, but it is essential that the bottles are filled with the solution and the teats immersed. Immersion of the teats is achieved by placing them under glass covers, or in the bottle which is then laid on its side in a bowl containing Milton. This must be made up freshly every day.

Most mothers like to give the milk warm, although babies will take a cold feed just as well. To ensure that the feed is not too hot it should be tested by shaking out a little on to the back of the hand. The teat should not be touched or it will be contaminated. The hole in the teat should be of such size that when the bottle is inverted, milk comes out rapidly in drops but not a stream. To enlarge the hole a red-hot needle should be used.

Too large a hole causes the baby to choke on the feed and too small a hole leads to excessive air swallowing as a result of the baby vigorously sucking to obtain the milk.

Feeding the very premature infant

The nutritional requirements of very premature infants are significantly different to those of the full-term infant. There are two major reasons for this. First, the fetus at 28 weeks gestation is growing extremely rapidly and if delivered at this time probably requires more energy to grow than a mature infant. This increased demand is coupled with increased catabolism associated with premature delivery and the need for intensive care. The second reason is the very immature state of the absorptive mechanisms of the immature bowel. Malabsorption of fat and carbohydrate may easily occur if the gastrointestinal tract is overwhelmed by inappropriate nutrients.

It is now known that the milk of mothers delivering at full-term is nutritionally inadequate for the requirements of immature infants and they do not grow as well as if given the milk of their own mothers or other women delivering early. As mentioned above the milk of women delivering prematurely is of a different constitution to mature milk. At the present time, we believe that a very premature infant should be fed his own mothers milk and not mature breast milk.

Low birth weight formula

Low birth weight formulas have been developed by the milk manufacturers to mimic the milk of prematurely delivered mothers. These provide higher energy density with increased concentrations of protein and minerals, particularly sodium, calcium and phosphorus. Premature infants tolerate these milks well and grow adequately on them.

Premature breast milk does not, however, provide adequate mineral content for the needs of growing infants. Calcium and phosphorus content is inadequate and these infants are at risk of developing rickets of prematurity (p. 114). Supplementation of premature milk with extra phosphorus and vitamin D appears to be the best prophylaxis against this condition.

ROUTE OF FEEDING

Premature infants do not suckle as these reflexes are not yet developed. Alternative methods of feeding must be devised.

Nasogastirc tube

Milk can be delivered into the stomach by an indwelling tube passed through the nostril. The advantages of this method is that it is convenient, but aspiration of milk is the major disadvantage. This may be overcome by continuous infusion of milk through a pump.

Nasojejunal tube

This tube is made of fine silastic and is weighted at the end. It is passed into the stomach and the infant positioned on his right side to allow the tube to pass through the pylorus into the jejunum. This is a much more difficult technique but the advantage is that the pylorus prevents milk refluxing into the stomach with the risk of aspiration. Feeding milk directly into the jejunum is very unphysiological and this technique may be associated with necrotizing enterocolitis (p. 114). It is now not much used in routine practice.

Weaning

Healthy infants do not require weaning until 4−6 months of age. Breast or formula milk provide all their nutritional requirements in the early months. Some prematurely born infants do appear to require weaning relatively earlier than babies born at the right time and the relatively early introduction of mixed feeds may be necessary to satisfy them. Too early introduction of mixed feeding may be associated with obesity.

In developed countries there is a wide choice of weaning feeds. In Britain cereals and rusks are the favoured first solid food but package foods may also be used to which water is added. All modern cereals for babies are free of gluten and this may be associated with a reduction in. the incidence of coeliac disease (p. 196). The semi-solid food is given by spoon before offering the bottle or breast. Its timing should be whatever suits the mother. Alternative weaning foods are purées of protein such as fish or meat broth. These can be purchased in pre-prepared containers or be liquidized at home in a food blender.

In developing countries weaning is a vulnerable time in the child's development as protein–energy malnutrition may develop if an appropriate weaning diet is not available. In addition, vitamin deficiency syndromes (scurvy and rickets) as well as iron deficiency anaemia may develop and this is discussed in Chapter 29.

Babies are conservative individuals and dislike change. The earlier a new tasting food is introduced, the more likely it is to be accepted. Only one new feed at a time should be introduced and if disliked should be withdrawn for a few weeks and then tried again. When weaning the child, cup and spoon feeding should be introduced early in order to make the change easier and reduce the possibility of the baby refusing to give up the bottle.

As the child gets older his diet will become more like that of his parents and he will begin to try to

Table 6.5 Commercially available infant feeds for a variety of gastrointestinal or metabolic abnormalities.

Trade name	Protein	Fat	Carbohydrate	Indications
Comminuted Chicken*	Ground meat products	MCT oils	Nil	Carbohydrate intolerance Milk allergy
Formula S Soya Food	Soy protein	Vegetable oils	Glucose syrup	Lactose intolerance Galactosaemia Milk allergy
Galactomin 17*	Casein	Coconut and maize oils	Glucose syrup	Lactose intolerance Galactosaemia
Galactomin 19*	Casein	Coconut and maize oils	Fructose	Glucose–galactose intolerance
Minafen*	Low phenylalanine protein hydrolysate	Vegetable oils	Glucose	Phenylketonuria
Nutramigen	Hydrolysed casein	Corn oil	Sucrose and tapioca starch	Milk allergy Lactose intolerance Galactosaemia
Portagen	Casein	MCT and corn oil	Sucrose and corn syrup	Fat malabsorption
Pregestimil	Hydrolysed casein	MCT and corn oil Soy lecithin Soy oil	Glucose syrup Tapioca starch	Disaccharidase deficiency Milk allergy Fat malabsorption
Prosobee	Soy protein and methionine		Sucrose and corn solids	Milk allergy Lactose intolerance Galactosaemia

* Requires other dietary supplements.
MCT, medium chain triglycerides.

hold the spoon himself although he is likely to go through a stage of wanting to use his fingers only. Once the baby starts to chew his fingers and even before he has any teeth he can be a given a hard rusk or toast to chew on. At no time should the child be left alone whilst feeding for fear of choking.

By the age of 9 months, most babies are ready to eat at least one meal a day with the family. The food should be similar to the rest of the family group, but presented in an attractive and appropriate way, with meat cut up into small pieces and vegetables mashed. It will of course be necessary for the food to be given to the baby on a spoon or fork.

Babies can be given undiluted and unboiled, bottled cow's milk from 6 months of age. This can be served cold but as many infants are used to warm milk the child may initially reject it.

Specialized diets

There are a number of conditions which necessitate the infant being fed a specialized diet. These conditions may be either congenital or acquired and may provoke intolerance due to either the carbohydrate, protein or fat constituent of the milk.

Table 6.5 summarizes some of the special milk formulas that are commercially available for children with different forms of malabsorption.

Intolerance to carbohydrate

Lactose intolerance is due to deficiency of a particular disaccharidase, lactase, found on the brush border. It may be congenital or acquired following gastroenteritis (p. 200). Lactose-free milks are readily available.

Children with galactosaemia (p. 370) are intolerant of galactose which is predominantly derived from lactose. These children require a galactose free diet for life.

Intolerance to protein

There are a large number of inborn errors of protein metabolism which cause build up of certain amino acids in the blood which are toxic in high concentration. Phenylketonuria is the most common of these and is discussed in Chapter 22. Special diets and milks are available for children with these rare disorders.

Cow's milk protein intolerance is discussed on p. 198. Alternative milks that can be used in this condition include those containing protein hydrolysates of cow's milk, soy protein or goat's milk protein.

Intolerance to fat

Pancreatic lipase deficiency is common in cystic fibrosis (p. 199) and these children require dietary supplements to absorb fat. Bile salts are also essential for normal absorption of fat but medium chain triglycerides are absorbed directly through the bowel wall without the formation of micelles and are therefore useful in children with certain forms of fat malabsorption. A number of commercially available milks provide the fat in the form of medium chain triglycerides.

Feeding difficulties

Mucus vomiting

Vomiting in the first day or two of life is frequently associated with accumulation of mucus in the stomach. Gastric distension with swallowed maternal blood, or amniotic fluid may also cause the newborn infant to vomit. Babies born by caesarian section do not undergo abdominal and chest compression and consequently may have excess amniotic fluid in their stomach predisposing them to vomiting. It is routine practice to pass a nasogastric tube in all babies born by caesarian section to aspirate the stomach.

Babies with vomiting should have nasogastric suction with lavage and this may be repeated if mucus vomiting persists.

Vomiting is a symptom of a variety of important neonatal problems and should always be taken seriously. Bile-stained vomiting is always abnormal and suggests gastrointestinal obstruction. The causes of vomiting in the neonatal period are discussed in Chapter 7.

Aerophagy

Excessive air swallowing can occur in greedy feeders who gulp air with their first mouthfuls of milk. It may be due to faulty feeding technique including the use of a teat with too small a hole, or permitting the baby to suck air from the bottle because it is empty or not held fully inverted. Excessive air swallowing may also result from the hole in the teat being too large; this forces the baby to gulp in order to prevent drowning from the rapid flow of milk, and in so doing he also swallows a lot of air. Excessive crying, often due to underfeeding, will also lead to air swallowing.

Management is to assess the feeding technique and advise the mother how to avoid her infant swallowing air. If the infant is very greedy, the feed can be given initially by spoon to take the edge off the baby's hunger. Air swallowing is less of a problem if the infant is fed by spoon.

Evening colic

During the first 3 months of life it is common for babies to scream for long periods after the evening feed. This is frequently ascribed to colic, an unscientific label which in this situation is merely providing another name for screaming. It is usually related to the fact that this is the time when a mother's exhaustion is greatest and she is in a panic to try to get everything finished before her husband returns home. An explanation that a mother's haste and anxiety soon conveys itself to the baby may relieve the situation, particularly if she can delay the feed until after the return of her partner. This should make it possible for the baby to be played with after the feed instead of being put straight back into his cot.

Many babies with colic also have green stool. This simply indicates that the bowel transit time is increased and the bile has not been fully re-absorbed. Many parents accept that the baby cries because he is aware of the increased bowel motil-ity, but this is not painful. Antispasmodics are sometimes used for this condition, but this should be discouraged in most circumstances. Dicyclo-mine hydrochloride (Merbentyl, 2−5 ml 15 min-utes before a feed) has been used in the past but the manufacturers of this compound now recom-mend avoiding its use in infants under 6 months of age because of several reported cases of apnoea.

Regurgitation and rumination

Many babies bring up partially digested milk and spill it out of their mouths. This is termed reg-urgitation or possetting and is discussed in Chapter 3. This may lead to rumination where the milk is chewed over as a cow chews the cud. Rumination is a habit, the patients usually being bright babies who are bottle fed. The parents should be reas-sured that this is usually a benign condition but occasionally, babies will develop severe possetting and rumination and will fail to thrive. The term 'malignant ruminators' has been used to describe these infants and hospital admission with con-tinuous intragastric milk infusion of thickened feed may be successful by means of keeping the stomach empty.

Constipation

This is a term that should never be accepted with-out careful questioning of the parent as to pre-cisely what they mean by it. Many normal infants have infrequent stools and it is not abnormal for a baby who is breast fed to have his bowels open only twice a week. It simply means that there is a very low residue of the feed. Constipation, when applied to infants, is a term that should only be used if the stool is dry and hard or pellet-like.

Causes of true constipation include dehydration possibly due to the feeds being made up too con-centrated or an abnormality such as Hirschprung's disease. Constipation in older children is discussed in Chapter 12.

If an anatomical abnormality has been excluded the constipation can be treated with an alteration of the feeds. The use of extra water, and fruit or vegetable juice may be helpful. A time-honoured method is the use of sugar in the feed. This pro-duces an additional osmotic load with increased fluid volume of the stool. This method may cause obesity if used over a prolonged period and dental caries in infants with teeth. On the whole its use should be curtailed. A stool-wetting agent such as dioctyl sodium may be useful and milk of magnesia is a useful mild laxative. An infant with repeated episodes of constipation should be carefully evalu-ated by a paediatrician.

Diarrhoea

Diarrhoea is another potentially misleading term. The important feature is a watery stool as many healthy breast fed infants have frequent stools of the colour and consistency of mustard. Diarrhoea is considered in detail in Chapter 12. Treatment depends on the underlying cause but anti-diarrhoea medication is never indicated in infancy.

Parenteral nutrition

This refers to the intravenous infusion of a bal-anced nutritional regime when an infant is unable to tolerate a full enteral diet. The indications for total parenteral nutrition (TPN) are:

1 Gastrointestinal obstruction.
2 Post-gastrointestinal surgery.
3 Necrotizing enterocolitis.
4 Severe malabsorption where a special diet has failed.

5 An infant with severe respiratory problems in whom gastric feeding is unsafe.
6 The extremely premature infant.
7 Severe recurrent apnoea.

TPN includes the provision of carbohydrate, protein solution fat, minerals, vitamins and water in the corrrect proportions. A variety of solutions are available including a fat solution containing soya bean fat with glycerol and egg yolk lecithin (Intralipid) as well as solutions of synthetic amino acids. These solutions have been formulated for the needs of critically ill adult patients and not for children, but few serious adverse effects have been reported when they are used in paediatric practice.

The cocktail of solutions are infused either through a peripheral intravenous line or through a 'long line' directly into a central vein or the right atrium. There are a variety of methods to place the long line for prolonged periods but the major complication of these techniques is septicaemia. Close attention to aseptic technique and appropriate care of the lines will minimize this risk.

Complications

The major complications of TPN are:
1 Infection. The commonest causal organism is *Staphylococcus epidermidis*.
2 Tissue injury due to a peripheral drip leaking into the tissues. Most TPN solutions are highly acidic and cause major tissue necrosis with severe scarring.
3 Metabolic compromise due to overdosage of carbohydrate, fat or protein solution.
4 Inadequate supply of essential amino acids or fatty acids.
5 Cholestatic jaundice.
6 Metabolic acidosis.
7 Venous thrombosis.

Further reading

Lawrence RA. *Breast-feeding. A Guide for the Medical Profession.* C. V. Mosby, St Louis 1980.
McLaren DS, Burman D (Eds). *Texbook of Paediatric Nutrition,* 2nd Edn. Churchill Livingstone, Edinburgh 1982.

7

SPECIAL CARE OF THE
SICK NEWBORN INFANT

Approximately 10% of newborn infants will need medical attention for some reason. About 1% of infants are born with a major congenital malformation and these are discussed in Chapter 9. At one time all babies weighing under 2.5 kg were defined as 'premature'. This was unsatisfactory since there are two major causes of low birth weight; short gestation (i.e. pre-term) and growth retardation. Infants are now defined as being of *low birth weight* when the birth weight is under 2.5 kg, irrespective of the duration of pregnancy. The small baby may be either pre-term, small for gestational age or a combination of the two. Each infant must be carefully assessed to determine the reason for being small.

Small for gestational age infants

If the tenth centile is used to identify small for gestational age (SGA) infants, then theoretically the incidence of this condition should be 10% of the population. Babies who are small for pathological reasons will more likely be found in the lower centile groups, but being placed below the tenth centile does not prove the presence of an abnormality. If the infant is pathologically small then he has sustained intra-uterine growth retardation (IUGR) and has failed to reach his prenatal growth potential. The rate of prenatal growth is governed directly by maternal, placental and fetal factors. Table 7.1 lists causes of IUGR by these categories.

MATERNAL FACTORS

In world-wide terms, maternal malnutrition is probably the commonest cause of IUGR. Limited food supply, parasites and poverty are common in developing countries. Studies from South America have shown that calorie supplementation in pregnancy increases the average weight of a baby at

Table 7.1 Causes of intra-uterine growth retardation.

Maternal	Placental	Fetal
Maternal disease	Toxaemia of	Chromosomal
Toxins	pregnancy	Prenatal infection
Alcohol	Placental dysfunction	Rubella
Tobacco	Multiple pregnancy	CMV
Narcotics	Site of placental	Toxoplasmosis
Malnutrition	implantation	Dysmorphic syndromes
Short stature		(rare)
Poor socioeconomic status		
Maternal age		
Racial		
Previous small for		
gestational age baby		

term by 50 g for every 10 000 kcal (2500 kJ) consumed by the mother. Maternal short stature or low weight at booking puts the mother at greater risk of giving birth to a poorly grown infant. Poor weight gain during pregnancy (less than 5 kg) is also associated with diminished fetal growth. The socioeconomic status of the woman probably only acts on fetal size indirectly through the associated factors of nourishment, smoking, maternal size and ante-natal care. Very young (below 16 years) or older mothers (above 35 years) tend to have smaller babies. Maternal anaemia, alcohol consumption and smoking reduce fetal weight. Narcotic addiction is also associated with fetal growth retardation.

PLACENTAL FACTORS

Toxaemia of pregnancy and essential hypertension are the commonest causes of IUGR in developed countries. Placental abnormalities are usually present in these pregnancies and mainly affect the small blood vessels. This is probably due to reactive vasculitis in response to hypertension which consequently diminishes placental blood flow. Infarcts are often visible within the placenta. If the demands on placental function exceed its supply then growth failure occurs. This happens in multiple pregnancies but only from about 34 weeks onwards. Prior to this, growth of twin fetuses is usually normal.

FETAL FACTORS

Infants with chromosomal abnormalities are often born small. In trisomy 21 (Down's syndrome) gestation is often shortened, but growth retardation usually occurs despite this. Infants with trisomy 18 (p. 121) show severe growth restriction and in trisomy 13 there is also IUGR but less severe. The commonest fetal cause of IUGR is prenatal viral infection and the commonest agents to cause this are cytomegalovirus and rubella (p. 367). In addition, toxoplasmosis of prenatal origin may cause the infant to be SGA. Any process that interferes with early brain growth causes stunting

Table 7.2 Complications to which SGA and pre-term infants are particularly susceptible.

Small for gestational age	Pre-term
Hypoglycaemia	Respiratory distress syndrome
Asphyxia	Recurrent apnoea
Polycythaemia	Intraventricular haemorrhage
Pulmonary	Periventricular leukomalacia
haemorrhage	Patent ductus arteriosus
Meconium aspiration	Temperature instability
Temperature instability	Infection
Infection	Feeding problems
Hypocalcaemia	Necrotizing enterocolitis
	Retinopathy of prematurity

of somatic growth. Excessive radiation may cause this as may certain drugs such as steroids.

Problems of the SGA infant

The postnatal complications occurring in SGA babies are often quite different from those of normally grown infants. Table 7.2 lists the recognized complications occurring in SGA and pre-term infants. Several of these problems are common to both groups such as asphyxia, temperature instability and infection.

LONG-TERM OUTCOME

IUGR may permanently affect the child's physical and intellectual development but it is not possible to guess the outcome at birth in any particular infant.

Growth

In order for SGA infants to catch up in terms of growth they must be offered optimal nutrition and early feeds are essential. They should be fed to an expected weight. This is generally a point midway between their actual weight and their expected weight had they grown normally *in utero* (50th centile for gestational age). This should be recalculated every week and if they will tolerate more feed it should be offered liberally.

Despite these limitations it is possible to make

some general statements concerning the outlook for long-term growth in these infants:

1 On the whole the severity of IUGR does not seem to influence the growth potential strongly.

2 If catch up growth is going to occur it does so by 6 months. Catch up in head growth usually preceeds linear growth.

3 Full-term growth-retarded infants stand a good chance of catching up, particularly if growth retardation is due to maternal factors such as toxaemia.

4 Infants who are both severely growth retarded and premature are less likely to reach average size than infants of the same degree of prematurity but who are normally grown.

Developmental outcome

Probably the most important determining factor in how SGA infants will turn out depends on the environmental factors operating in the home. Those from deprived backgrounds are likely to do less well than those from caring and stimulating homes. The following statements can be made about the intellectual and neurological outcome of SGA infants:

1 Infants born SGA at term have more developmental, behavioural and learning difficulties, and males appear to be more vulnerable to this than females.

2 The severity of IUGR probably affects brain development but in some cases this does not relate to the severity of the neurological problems.

3 Effective catch up growth is associated with higher IQ scores than infants whose heads remain small.

Prematurity

An infant may be born premature (before 37 completed weeks of gestation) and/or SGA and accurate methods of assessing gestation may be necessary to distinguish the two (pp. 82–83). Over the last 15 years, neonatal intensive care has markedly improved and now most infants born at 26 weeks gestation and beyond survive, although they may require weeks of intensive care. Table 7.3 shows expected survival for various gestational age and

Table 7.3 Average survival figures for babies born prematurely and nursed in modern neonatal intensive care units. These figures exclude those infants born with major congenital abnormalities.

Gestational age (weeks)	Birth weight (g)	Survival percentage
<26	<750	20
26–28	750–1000	60
29–30	1000–1250	85
>30	>1250	90–95

birthweight groups in an average modern neonatal intensive care unit.

About 6% of all births are premature, and approximately 1% of infants weigh less than 1500 g at birth. The cause of premature labour is usually not apparent. Table 7.4 lists some recognized factors associated with prematurity. Cervical incompetance due to a previous surgical termination of pregnancy is the most important. Uterine distension due to twin pregnancy or polyhydramnios may also precipitate the onset of premature labour.

Obstetric care

In order to give a premature infant the best chance of intact survival, excellent obstetric care is necessary with careful management of labour. An attempt may be made to suppress premature labour with beta sympathomimetic drugs but this

Table 7.4 Factors associated with prematurity.

Previous termination of pregnancy
Multiple pregnancy
Cervical incompetence
Genital tract infection
Polyhydramnios
Maternal age <16 or >35 years
Previous premature birth
Premature rupture of membranes
Poor socioeconomic status
Pre-eclampsia
Short interval between pregnancies
Maternal disease
Antepartum haemorrhage

is often not successful for more than a few days. If the fetal membranes have ruptured then there is a risk of organisms ascending the birth canal and infecting the fetus; careful bacteriological surveillance is essential. Maternal or fetal infection is a contraindication to the suppression of labour. The obstetrician must pay careful attention to monitoring the fetus during labour and to protect the fetal head from too rapid delivery with consequent intracranial trauma.

The small pre-term head moves rapidly through the bony pelvis and vagina without being moulded, immediately impinging on the perineum which has not had time to stretch as in a full-term delivery. It is this collision between the soft unmoulded head and the hard perineum that may cause subdural haemorrhage due to shearing strains and tear of the tentorium or dura. It must therefore be routine for an episiotomy to be performed for the delivery of all pre-term babies. The additional measure of low forceps delivery to assist the head over the perineum is an added protection. The incidence of breech delivery is increased in pre-term babies and this increases the risks of intracranial injury. There is considerable debate as to the role of elective caesarian section in the delivery of very premature infant and this remains unresolved.

Assessment of gestation

Obstetric assessment

Accurate knowledge of the last menstrual period is essential in the assessment of gestation. Unfortunately this is not always available. An early clinical examination during the first trimester is helpful in assessing gestation, but the best method currently available is an early ultrasound scan. The diagnosis of IUGR is important in order to deliver a compromised infant from a hostile intra-uterine environment before severe growth retardation or even fetal death occurs.

Fetal well-being can be assessed by fetal heart rate patterns, biochemical assay (maternal oestriols or human placental lactogen) and serial ultrasound measurements of fetal growth. Radio-

graphic evidence of maturity from the appearance of the fetal epiphyseal centres of the knee and foot have been used but are unreliable. The centre for the lower end of the femur appears about the 34th week and that for the upper end of the tibia at about the 39th week. The absence of these centres has no significance in relation to maturity.

Clinical assessment of gestation

An attempt should be made to determine the gestational age of all infants at birth. Not only is this essential for small infants but also for larger ones whose maturity is in doubt. About half of all SGA babies will show loss of tissue mass and have a characteristic appearance (Fig. 7.1).

Brain growth is least affected by IUGR and continues to increase in size after the body has stopped growing. The liver and thymus are particularly small. The wasted SGA infant with a relatively large head is characteristic of these babies. Sometimes the head–body disproportion is so marked that hydrocephalus may be suspected. Lack of glycogen stores in the liver predispose to hypoglycaemia (p. 103). The uniformly growth-retarded infant who has a head in proportion to his body is more worrying since a congenital or chromosomal abnormality may have arrested total growth early in pregnancy.

The developing nervous system matures in an orderly and sequential manner throughout the course of gestation. It is possible to examine the infant at birth and accurately assess its gestation on the basis of both external and neurological criteria. The Dubowitz method of gestational assessment (Fig. 7.2) is the most widely used scheme. This method consists of 10 neurological items and 11 external criteria which are considered independently; at the end of the assessment the scores are added up and gestational age calculated.

Neurological items

These include mainly those of tone and were selected to be fairly independent of neonatal illness. The immature infant tends to be more floppy or hypotonic, the tone increasing with maturity.

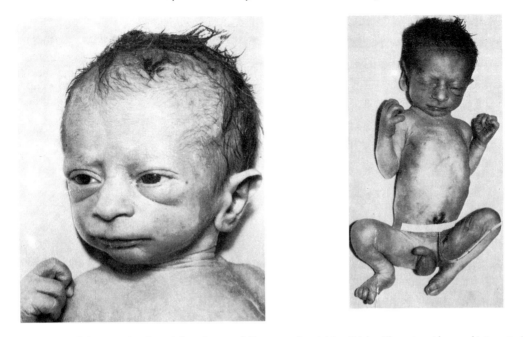

Fig. 7.1 Small for gestational age infant, born at full-term and weighing 2.1 kg. There is evidence of intra-uterine malnutrition with lack of subcutaneous fat and dry parchment-like skin.

At birth, immature infants adopt a more extended posture, but those born at term adopt the characteristic attitude of limb flexion. These changes are reflected in the baby's posture so that the limbs of the 28-week baby when supine are flat on the mattress. A baby born at term lies in a strongly flexed position and his trunk hardly touches the mattress (see Fig. 4.5). When held in ventral suspension, the very immature baby has a curved back and the limbs hang down in an extended posture. A full-term infant when held prone has flexed limbs.

Maturity can also be assessed by motor nerve conduction velocities which shorten in a predictable manner with increasing gestational age. This reflects progessive myelination of the immature nervous system.

External items

The more immature the baby the redder the skin. The colour is due to the thinness of the skin in which the capillaries appear more superficial.

Black babies are a light colour at birth, the most premature being the same red colour as those born to white parents. The genitalia is the first area to become pigmented.

Lanugo, the fine downy hair, is absent in the most immature infants and when it first develops is abundant and thick particularly over the back. It then begins to disappear 2 to 3 weeks before term.

The nails are soft and short, not reaching the tip of the finger or toe until term. Until 36 weeks the pinna is very soft and relatively shapeless. From then until full-term it becomes increasingly stiffened by cartilage which makes its folds stand out prominently. In very immature infants the ear can be folded with no recoil to its normal shape.

The size of the breast nodule is correlated with gestation. It cannot be felt until approximately 33 weeks, and by term measures 7 mm or more in diameter. The nipple size also grows in diameter in phase with breast nodule development.

Development of the skin creases on the sole of the foot is a reliable physical index of maturity. In immature infants there are no skin creases, and

Score (Neurological sign)

Neuro-logical sign	0	1	2	3	4	5
Posture						
Square window	90°	60°	45°	30°	0°	
Ankle dorsi-flexion	90°	75°	45°	20°	0°	
Arm recoil	180°	90–180°	<90°			
Leg recoil	180°	90–180°	<90°			
Popliteal angle	180°	160°	130°	110°	90°	<90°
Heel to ear						
Scarf sign						
Head lag						
Ventral suspension						

Score (External sign)

External sign	0	1	2	3	4
Oedema	Obvious oedema hands and feet, pitting over tibia	No obvious oedema hands and feet: pitting over tibia	No oedema		
Skin texture	Very thin, gelatinous	Thin and smooth	Smooth: medium thickness. Rash or superficial peeling	Slight thickening. Superficial cracking and peeling especially hands and feet	Thick and parchment-like, superficial or deep cracking
Skin colour (infant not crying)	Dark red	Uniformly pink	Pale pink: variable over body	Pale. Only pink over ears, lips, palms or soles	
Skin opacity (trunk)	Numerous veins and venules clearly seen, especially over abdomen	Veins and tributaries seen	A few large vessels clearly seen over abdomen	A few large vessels seen indistinctly over abdomen	No blood vessels seen
Lanugo (over back)	No lanugo	Abundant: long and thick over whole back	Hair thinning especially over lower back	Small amount of lanugo and bald areas	At least half of back devoid of lanugo
Plantar creases	No skin creases	Faint red marks over anterior half of sole	Definite red marks over more than anterior half: indentations over less than anterior third	Indentations over more than anterior third	Definite deep indentations over more than anterior third
Nipple formation	Nipple barely visible; no aerola	Nipple well defined; aerola smooth and flat; diameter <0.75 cm	Areola stippled, edge not raised: diameter <0.75 cm	Areola stippled, edge raised >0.75 cm	
Breast size	No breast tissue; palpable	Breast tissue on one or both sides <0.5 cm diameter	Breast tissue both sides; one or both 0.5–1.0 cm	Breast tissue both sides; one or both >1 cm	
Ear form	Pinna flat and shapeless. little or no incurving of edge	Incurving or part of edge of pinna	Partial incurving whole of upper pinna	Well-defined incurving whole of upper pinna	
Ear firmness	Pinna soft, easily folded, no recoil	Pinna soft, easily folded, slow recoil	Cartilage to edge of pinna, but soft in places, ready recoil	Pinna firm, cartilage to edge, instant recoil	
Genitalia: male; Females (with hips half abducted)	Neither testis in scrotum. Labia majora widely separated, labia minora protruding	At least one testis high in scrotum. Labia majora almost cover labia minora	At least one testis right down Labia majora completely cover labia minora		

Posture: Observed with infant quiet and in supine position. Score 0: Arms and legs extended; 1: beginning of flexion of hips and knees, arms extended; 2: stronger flexion of legs, arms extended; 3: arms slightly flexed, legs flexed and abducted; 4: full flexion of arms and legs.

Square window: The hand is flexed on the forearm between the thumb and index finger of the examiner. Enough pressure is applied to get as full a flexion as possible, and the angle between the hypothenar eminence and the ventral aspect of the forearm is measured and graded according to diagram. (Care is taken not to rotate the infant's wrist while doing this manoeuvre.)

Ankle dorsiflexion: The foot is dorsiflexed onto the anterior aspect of the leg, with the examiner's thumb on the sole of the foot and other fingers behind the leg. Enough pressure is applied to get as full a flexion as possible, and the angle between the dorsum of the foot and the anterior aspect of the leg is measured.

Arm recoil: With the infant in the supine position the forearms are first flexed for 5 seconds, then fully extended by pulling on the hands, and then released. The sign is fully positive if the arms return briskly to full flexion (Score 2). If the arms return to incomplete flexion or the response is sluggish it is graded as Score 1. If they remain extended or are only followed by random movements the score is 0.

Leg recoil: With the infant supine, the hips and knees are fully flexed for 5 seconds, then extended by traction on the feet, and released. A maximal response is one of full flexion of the hips and knees (Score 2). A partial flexion scores 1, and minimal or no movement scores 0.

Popliteal angle: With the infant supine and his pelvis flat on the examining couch, the thigh is held in the knee-chest position by the examiner's left index finger and thumb supporting the knee. The leg is then extended by gentle pressure from the examiner's right index finger behind the ankle and the popliteal angle is measured.

Heel to ear manoeuvre: With the baby supine, draw the baby's foot as near to the head as it will go without forcing it. Observe the distance between the foot and the head as well as the degree of extension at the knee. Grade according to diagram. Note that the knee is left free and may draw down alongside the abdomen.

Scarf sign: With the baby supine, take the infant's hand and try to put it around the neck and as far posteriorly as possible around the opposite shoulder. Assist this manoeuvre by lifting the elbow across the body. See how far the elbow will go across and grade according to illustrations. Score 0: Elbow reaches the opposite axillary line: 1: Elbow between midline and opposite axillary line: 2: Elbow reaches midline: 3: Elbow will not reach midline.

Head lag: With the baby lying supine, grasp the hands (or the arms if a very small infant) and pull him slowly towards the sitting position. Observe the position of the head in relation to the trunk and grade accordingly. In a small infant the head may initially be supported by one hand. Score 0: Complete lag: 1: Partial head control: 2: Able to maintain head in line with body: 3: Brings head anterior to body.

Ventral suspension: The infant is suspended in the prone position, with examiner's hand under the infant's chest (one hand in a small infant, two in a large infant). Observe the degree of extension of the back and the amount of flexion of the arms and legs. Also note the relation of the head to the trunk. Grade according to diagrams.

If the score for an individual criterion differs on the two sides of the baby, take the mean.

Fig. 7.2 The Dubowitz method for assessing gestation, with notes on techniques of assessment of neurological criteria. (Reproduced with permission from Dubowitz *et al. J Pediatr* 1970; **77**:1.)

they gradually develop initially over the anterior half of the sole. By 36 weeks there are one or two transverse creases. By 38 weeks more creases have appeared, but the heel is still smooth. At term the whole sole is covered with creases, some forming deep clefts.

The external genitalia vary with the degree of maturity. At 36 weeks the scrotum is small and its rugae are limited to the area of the median raphe. With advancing maturity the testicles may be seen in the groin (28 weeks), and in the scotum by 36 weeks. By term the scrotum should be covered with rugae. In the female at 36 weeks the labia majora are still poorly developed so that the clitoris and labia minora are easily visible. By term, growth of the labia majora has hidden these structures.

General principles of care

The survival rates of sick newborn infants are directly related to the skill of the nursing staff who should have received special training in their care. Weight by itself is not the deciding factor in where the infant is nursed but rather it is the condition of the baby. The modern trend is for fewer babies who are simply small, but otherwise well to be nursed in neonatal units and are best observed with their mothers on a transitional nursery. Infants who require respiratory support should be transferred to neonatal intensive care units where expertise and equipment are available to manage these critically ill infants. Intensive care implies the ability to monitor intensively these infants in order to detect abnormalities early and attempt to correct them before they become more serious.

Parents of ill infants find the neonatal intensive care unit a frightening place. There is much unfamiliar noise, activity, complicated equipment and in the centre their tiny infant. Parents' fears and anxieties must be anticipated and discussed frequently. They should also be encouraged to handle their baby and given an explanation of what the equipment does and what problems may develop. Expression of breast milk for her infant (even if the baby is not well enough to be given it

immediately) encourages the mother to feel that she is contributing to her baby's care. Unrestricted visiting is essential. It is best to be honest with the parents from the beginning and to give them a realistic chance of survival according to the survival figures in that hospital (see Table 7.3).

Infection

The premature infant is particularly prone to infection and prevention of cross-infection is of utmost importance. All staff must wash their hands with a bactericidal solution before and after handling each infant to avoid transmitting infection from one to another. All minor surgical procedures should be performed using aseptic techniques. Neonatal infection is considered in detail on p. 95.

Thermoregulation

Premature infants are less able to regulate their body heat at a constant level than full-term infants and care must be taken to avoid cold stress.

Babies try and conserve heat loss by a combination of the following methods:
1 Peripheral vasoconstriction.
2 Shivering. Premature infants cannot shiver.
3 Increased muscular activity but this is metabolically wasteful of energy.
4 Non-shivering thermogenesis. Mature infants are born with a layer of brown fat found mainly over the back. This can be rapidly metabolized to generate heat. Babies born prematurely have not laid down brown fat and are less able to protect themselves against a cool environment.

Heat is lost from the infant in one of the four methods shown in Figure 7.3. Careful attention must be paid to methods to minimize heat loss by each of these four ways.

EVAPORATION

Dry the infant immediately after birth. Very premature infants lose water continuously through their very thin skin. This is associated with heat

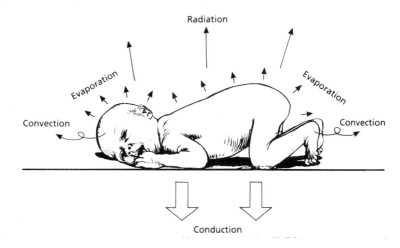

Fig. 7.3 The four ways in which an infant may lose body heat.

loss and can be minimized by nursing the infant in a humid atmosphere within the incubator.

RADIATION

Infants radiate heat through space to colder objects. Even within an incubator the infant will radiate heat to the colder walls of the incubator and thence to the colder room. Radiant heat loss can be minimized in three ways.
1 Maintain the nursery temperature as warm as is comfortable for the staff.
2 Double-lined incubator walls minimize radiant heat loss. This works in much the same way that double glazing conserves room heat.
3 Heat shield. This is a convenient and cheap method of providing a form of double glazing. A curved perspex shield is placed over the infant within the incubator. The temperature of the heat shield is higher than the walls of the incubator and therefore reduces radiant heat loss.

CONDUCTION

Avoid placing a warm baby on a cold surface. Pre-warm the cot or mattress upon which the infant is placed at birth.

CONVECTION

This can be minimized by avoiding draughts.

The thermoneutral environment

A healthy infant will maintain his core temperature despite being nursed in a variety of different ambient temperatures. If his environment is too hot he will vasodilate and sweat. If he is nursed in a cold environment he will vasoconstrict, move around more and utilize brown fat. He is using energy to maintain a constant body temperature. Neonatal care must be directed at conserving the infant's energy for growth and the infant should be nursed in an ambient temperature at which he expends the least amount of energy; this is referred to as the thermoneutral temperature. The optimal temperature depends on the postnatal age, on whether the infant is dressed or naked and on how much he weighs. A naked term infant at birth should be nursed in the first days of life in an incubator temperature of 32–34°C. An infant of 28 weeks gestation, nursed naked, requires an environmental temperature between 34°C and 35.5°C in the first week of life.

Respiratory distress

The four clinical features of respiratory distress in the neonate are:
1 Tachypnoea (respiratory rate over 60 breaths per minute).
2 Recession. This refers to indrawing of the

Table 7.5   Causes of neonatal respiratory distress.

Respiratory distress syndrome (hyaline membrane
  disease)
Pneumonia
Pneumothorax
Aspiration syndrome
  Meconium
  Milk
  Blood
  Amniotic squames
Congenital diaphragmatic hernia
Transient tachypnoea of the newborn
Tracheo-oesophageal fistula
Cardiac failure
Pulmonary hypoplasia
Persistent fetal circulation (primary pulmonary
  hypertension)
Bronchopulmonary dysplasia
Wilson–Mikity syndrome
Chronic pulmonary insufficiency of prematurity (CPIP)

sternum, or skin in the subcostal and intercostal
region.

3 Grunting.

4 Cyanosis.

These four symptoms may not all be present in
every case but the presence of two or more allows
the clinican to refer to the baby as having respiratory distress. This is a purely descriptive term and
does not imply a diagnosis. Although the respiratory distress syndrome may be the commonest
cause for respiratory distress the two terms are not
interchangable. Table 7.5 lists the causes of respiratory distress.

Respiratory distress syndrome (hyaline membrane disease)

Respiratory distress syndrome (RDS) is due to surfactant deficiency. Surfactant is a phospholipid
which lowers surface tension within the terminal
airway. Surfactant is secreted by the type II
pneumatocytes situated within the alveolar membrane. These cells are anatomically present by 20
weeks of gestation but usually do not become
functionally active until close to full-term. Various
stimuli can switch on surfactant production

including stress, premature rupture of the membranes and exogenous steroids given to the
mother. Maternal diabetes suppresses the development of surfactant and the infants of diabetic
mothers are more likely to develop RDS even if
born at full-term.

When the infant is born, fluid is squeezed out of
the lungs by compression of the chest wall. The
infant then takes his first breath and expands his
alveoli. If surfactant is present the alveoli remain
expanded, but if absent the alveoli collapse down
to their fetal state and the baby's next breath is
also a massive one to re-expand the terminal airways. Surfactant molecules form a monolayer on
the inside of the alveolar membrane. Due to their
chemical structure they are poorly compressable
and maintain the alveolus in an expanded state. In
RDS, each breath the baby takes is of similar
effort, the infant shows the clinical features of
respiratory distress, and soon gets tired.

INCIDENCE

RDS occurs in 1% of newborn infants but its incidence is closely related to immaturity. Approximately 60–70% of infants born at 28 weeks or
below will develop this condition and 20% of infants born at 34 weeks of gestation. Apart from prematurity, risk factors include being the infant of a
diabetic mother or a second twin, antepartum
haemorrhage, and shock. Male infants are more
susceptible to developing RDS than famale infants.

PATHOLOGY

The term hyaline membrane disease (HMD) which
is sometimes used synonomously with RDS refers
to the appearance of the terminal airway of
infants dying with this condition. Hyaline membranes are seen within the alveoli and represent part of the inflammatory response to this
condition.

CLINICAL FEATURES

The infants show signs of respiratory distress. This
is usually apparent very soon after birth but may

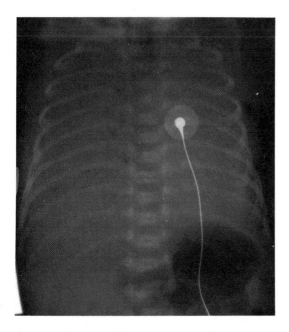

Fig. 7.4 Chest X-ray showing respiratory distress syndrome.

become progressively more obvious over the first day and may not reach its most severe form until the infant is 48 hours old or more. The infant is initially oliguric and often becomes oedematous. Diuresis often occurs just as the infant starts to improve clinically.

DIAGNOSIS

The diagnosis is made in the neonatal unit on the basis of a chest X-ray. The characteristic features are a 'ground glass' appearance reflecting airless alveoli together with an air bronchogram (Fig. 7.4). The severity of the clinical disease may not correlate very well with the degree of 'white out' seen on the X-ray.

The diagnosis may be anticipated by measuring directly or indirectly the amount of surfactant present in the amniotic fluid. Liquor may be collected if the membranes are ruptured or at amniocentesis. Gastric aspirate taken shortly after birth is largely made up of amniotic fluid and this can be examined. The lecithin : sphingomyelin (L : S) ratio reflects surfactant activity and a ratio of <1.5 predicts a high risk of RDS.

MANAGEMENT

As RDS is a self-limiting condition and the baby's lungs recover with the endogenous production of surfactant, management is directed towards supporting the infant whilst he has respiratory distress. These measures include:

Oxygen

Infants with mild disease require supplemental oxygen to maintain their arterial blood oxygen tension within the normal range (Pao_2 6.5–10.5 kPa) (50–80 mmHg). This can be achieved by placing the infant in a head box with careful monitoring of the fractional inspired oxygen (Fio_2). The inspired gases should be well humidified.

Continuous positive airway pressure (CPAP)

Infants with more severe disease in whom the blood gases are not maintained within the normal range by additional oxygen may be improved with CPAP. This form of treatment provides a constant positive pressure during expiration which limits the collapse of the alveoli. It may be provided by a tight-fitting face-mask, a nasopharyngeal prong or an endotracheal tube. It is often very effective treatment in more mature infants (those over 1500 g) but in very premature infants it may accelerate exhaustion with respiratory failure and is not recommended as the only form of respiratory support in this group.

Mechanical ventilation

The indications for ventilation are:
1 Hypoxia resistant to other measures when the Fio_2 exceeds 60% to maintain Po_2 >8 kPa (60 mmHg).
2 Hypercapnia. A rising Pco_2 which excees 8 kPa (60 mmHg) particularly if there is a falling pH (<7.25).
3 Apnoea.

Table 7.6 Complications of respiratory distress syndrome.

Pulmonary
Air leak
  Pneumothorax
  Pulmonary interstitial emphysema
Pneumonia
Atelectasis
Lobar collapse
Chronic lung disease

Extra-pulmonary
Patent ductus arteriosus
Intraventricular haemorrhage
Retinopathy of prematurity
Subglottic stenosis

General support

Careful attention should be paid to chest physiotherapy, particularly in mechanically ventilated infants, early treatment of infection, appropriate fluid intake, blood pressure monitoring and maintenance of the optimal environmental temperature.

Surfactant replacement therapy

Exogenous surfactant has been given to premature infants at birth or following birth if they show signs of RDS. This form of treatment is still being evaluated but does seem to reduce the severity of the disease in the majority of infants and is likely to become a standard method for managing these infants in the future.

COMPLICATIONS

These are listed in Table 7.6 and are discussed elsewhere.

PROGNOSIS

It is rare for an infant to die of RDS, and if death occurs it is usually related to a complication of the lung disease. The two most important causes of death in these infants are intraventricular haemor-

rhage (p. 101) and bronchopulmonary dysplasia (p. 94).

Pneumonia

Pneumonia may develop early (within 24 hours) as the result of intrapartum infection acquired during passage through the birth canal or later and usually affects infants with pre-existing lung disease.

EARLY ONSET PNEUMONIA

The most important organism is *Group B beta haemolytic Streptococcus*. This is present as a commensal organism in the genital tract of approximately 10% of pregnant women. A proportion of infants born through the colonized vagina may themselves become colonized with this organism, but only 1% of infants born to a mother carrying beta haemolytic streptococci will develop severe disease. This organism may cause pneumonia or meningitis.

The infant initially shows signs of respiratory distress. There may be an initial period of little or no symptoms and the baby may suddenly collapse with apnoea or severe respiratory compromise. The chest X-ray may be identical to that of RDS and *Group B beta haemolytic streptococci* should always be suspected in infants with early onset respiratory distress.

These infants are almost always septicaemic and may present with shock. They require intensive care and the prognosis for survival depends on how early antibiotics are started.

Other organisms that may cause early onset pneumonia include *Haemophilus influenzae* and the *Pneumococcus*.

Management

This includes respiratory support with supplemental oxygen and usually mechanical ventilation. Infection is usually assumed and antibiotics started on a best guess basis. Ampicillin (200 mg/kg) and gentamicin are the best combination to cover all the possible organisms and may be changed once the organism is detected and anti-biotic sensitivities are available.

LATE ONSET PNEUMONIA

These infants usually have damaged lungs and ventilated babies are particularly susceptible to secondary infection. The most common organisms are *Pseudomonas aeroginosa*, *Staphylococcus aureus*, *E. coli* and *Klebsiella*. Unusual opportunistic organisms such as candida or viruses may also cause serious pneumonia. The radiological appearance usually shows patchy involvement.

Treatment is with appropriate antibiotics together with vigorous chest physiotherapy.

CHLAMYDIA PNEUMONIA

This is an important perinatal pathogen and is contracted from passage through the birth canal. The infants often present initially with a purulent conjunctivitis and this is clinically indistinguishable from gonococcal ophthalmia. Specific culture techniques are necessary to isolate *Chlamydia trachomatis* from the conjunctiva.

Chlamydia pneumonitis usually develops 4–8 weeks after birth and may be preceded by conjunctivitis. The infants present with signs of respiratory distress and the X-ray shows diffuse infiltration through both lung fields.

Infants with chlamydial eye or lung disease must be treated with systemic erythromycin antibiotic as well as tetracycline eye ointment in the case of eye disease.

Pneumothorax

This is the most severe form of air leak from the alveoli. Air may escape into the lung interstitium causing a condition called pulmonary interstitial emphysema. The air tracks along the perivascular spaces and may rupture into the mediastinum (pneumomediastinum) or into the pleura causing a pneumothorax. Occasionally air may enter the pericardium (pneumopericardium) or track through the diaphragm into the peritoneum (pneumoperitoneum).

Pneumothorax may occur spontaneously at birth but is more likely to develop following resuscitation particularly if this is by bag-and-mask. Specific risk factors for the development of air leak include RDS, meconium aspiration and lung hypoplasia as occurs in conjunction with diaphragmatic hernia.

Up to 30% of infants who are mechanically ventilated develop pneumothorax and the method by which the infant is ventilated may modify the risk of this complication. If the baby is breathing spontaneously and actively expires against a positive pressure breath from the ventilator then air leaks may occur. This may be avoided by ventilating the baby at the same rate at which he is breathing or to give the baby a neuromuscular blocking agent (e.g. pancuronium) to produce muscle paralysis.

Diagnosis

Pneumothorax may be suspected clinically if there is a sudden deterioration in the infants condition. Breath sounds are diminished over the affected lung and a left-sided tension pneumothorax usually causes the heart to be displaced so that the heart sounds are best heard on the right.

Diagnosis is confirmed by chest X-ray (Fig. 7.5).

Management

A tension pneumothorax causes sudden and severe collapse and must be treated rapidly. Once the diagnosis has been made a plastic tube is inserted through the 2nd intercostal space in the mid-clavicular line into the pleura. The end of the tube is placed underwater (well below the level of the infant) to prevent air re-entering the pleura during expiration.

Pulmonary interstitial emphysema and pneumomediastinum are usually treated expectantly.

Meconium aspiration syndrome

During intrapartum asphyxia the fetus may pass meconium and in the presence of persistent asphyxia may start to gasp (see Chapter 5). This

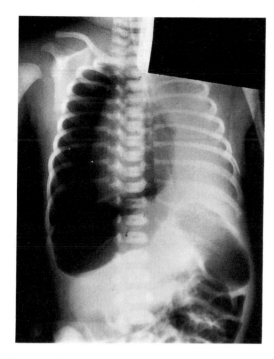

Fig. 7.5 Chest X-ray showing right-sided tension pneumothorax with displacement of the mediastinum and trachea to the left.

may result in meconium entering the smaller bronchi and when the infant is born and resuscitated the meconium is driven further down into the terminal airway. Meconium is an intensely irritant substance and causes a severe inflammatory reaction. Many infants have meconium present in their mouth and it may be seen below the vocal cords on resuscitation and yet they do not develop respiratory distress. It is the inflammatory effect of the meconium that causes the meconium aspiration syndrome.

Pathology

Meconium causes plugging of some airways with atelectasis distal to the block. A 'ball valve' effect may occur with hyperinflation of some parts of the lung and subsequent air leak. An intense inflammatory exudate develops and secondary infection may occur. Ventilation/perfusion inequality

develops causing the infant to become more hypoxic and in severe cases persistent pulmonary hypertension commonly develops (p. 93).

Diagnosis

The presence of meconium in the airway together with respiratory distress strongly suggests meconium aspiration syndrome. Diagnosis is made by chest X-ray which shows hyperinflation with diffuse patchy opacities throughout both lung fields.

Management

The respiratory distress is treated in the same manner as any infant with severe lung disease and most require mechanical ventilation. CPAP should be avoided and antibiotics are usually given.

Prophylaxis

Infants with meconium-stained liquor should be carefully evaluated at birth. The mouth is sucked out and the cords visualized with a laryngoscope. If there is meconium below the cords an endotracheal tube should be inserted to 'core out' the meconium and then withdrawn and this may need to be repeated on several occasions. The infant's trachea should then be washed out through the endotracheal tube with normal saline.

Milk aspiration

This occurs relatively commonly in small infants with gastro-oesophageal reflux. It is particularly common in infants who develop severe apnoea. Milk should not be fed directly into the stomach of infants who are at risk of aspirating and naso-jejunal feeding may be of value in this group.

Congenital diaphragmatic hernia

The incidence of this condition is approximately one in 2500 births. It is usually due to a defect in the posterolateral part of the diaphragm and occurs on the left side in 80% of cases. The significance of this condition depends on the size of the defect, the amount of the bowel in the chest and the timing of the herniation. Bowel in the chest may cause compression of the lungs with hypoplasia. If there is a large defect and the bowel has been present in the chest for much of the pregnancy then it is likely that both lungs will be severely hypoplastic, a condition incompatible with life (see below).

Clinical features

The infant presents with respiratory distress but the time of presentation depends on the size of the defect and the degree of lung hypoplasia. In severe cases the infant has marked symptoms from birth and in the others symptoms may be delayed for hours or days. The clinical signs suggestive of diaphragmatic hernia are a scaphoid (sunken) abdomen and apparent dextrocardia if the defect is left-sided as the mediastimum is pushed over to the right. Diagnosis is confirmed by chest X-ray (Fig. 7.6).

Management

The critical factor in the prognosis of this condition is the degree of lung hypoplasia. There is no advantage to be gained by immediate surgery and modern management concentrates on medical treatment to get the infant into the best possible condition before surgery. Operations may be delayed for hours or even days to achieve stability.

Medical management must concentrate on adequate ventilation, treating shock and persistent pulmonary hypertension which is a common complication of this condition.

Surgery involves pulling the bowel out of the chest and repairing the defect in the diaphragm.

Prognosis

This depends on the degree of pulmonary hypoplasia. Those infants presenting with symptoms after 6 hours have an excellent prognosis as their lungs are likely to be normally grown. Those presenting early (in the first 6 hours) may have a 60–70% mortality rate.

Transient tachypnoea of the newborn

This is a poorly understood condition and it is only possible to diagnose it in retrospect. It is benign and is probably related to delayed clearance of fluid from the lung in newborn, full-term infants. Those born by caesarian section are more likely to develop it presumably because lung fluid has not been squeezed out by passage through the vagina.

Clinical features

It should only be diagnosed in full-term or near-term infants. The infants show signs of respiratory distress but recover by 48 hours from birth. A chest X-ray may be helpful as it shows streakiness due to interstitial fluid and fluid in the horizontal fissure.

Management

These infants do not require respiratory support other than supplemental oxygen. If blood gases deteriorate and the infant requires mechanical ventilation, the diagnosis should be reviewed. The prognosis is excellent.

Pulmonary hypoplasia

Pulmonary hypoplasia is a relatively common condition and is due to three main groups of conditions as described in Table 7.7. For the lung to develop normally the fetus must be able to make breathing movements *in utero* and move a column of amniotic fluid up and down the major bronchi. Anything that interferes with this may cause the lung to fail to grow and these include:
1 A central nervous system problem with paralysis of respiratory activity will prevent chest wall movement.
2 Muscle disorder with weak respiratory muscles.
3 Compression of the lung with inhibition of expansion.
4 Lack of amniotic fluid. A considerable volume of amniotic fluid is produced as fetal urine. Any

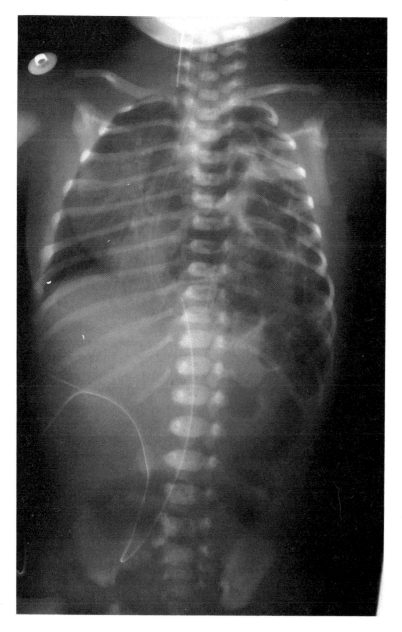

Fig. 7.6 Chest X-ray showing left-sided diaphragmatic hernia.

condition that inhibits fetal urine production is associated with lung hypoplasia (see Potter's syndrome, p. 250). Chronic loss of liquor as occurs in prolonged rupture of the membranes or early amniocentesis may also be associated with pulmonary hypoplasia.

Clinical features

The infant presents at birth with respiratory distress. Many of these infants will show features suggestive of the underlying pathology which has caused the lung hypoplasia. These include joint

Table 7.7 Causes of pulmonary hypoplasia.

Failure of fetal breathing
Brainstem abnormality
High spinal cord abnormality
Werdnig–Hoffman disease
Muscle disease

Inability to expand lungs
Diaphragmatic hernia
Chronic pleural effusions

Lack of amniotic fluid
Potter's syndrome
Leak of liquor

contractures (muscle disease or compression due to oligohydramnios), palpable renal masses in the abdomen or polyhydramnios (failure of the fetus to swallow as well as breathe).

Management

This is as for any cause of severe respiratory distress.

Prognosis

This depends on the severity of the lung hypoplasia. If it is severe the prognosis is hopeless, but if only moderate the lungs may grow postnatally if the infant can be kept in good condition.

Persistent fetal circulation

The fetus has a high pulmonary vascular resistance and blood is shunted away from the lungs through the ductus arteriosus and foramen ovale. At birth the communications close, the pulmonary vascular resistance falls and blood perfuses the lungs. In some infants pulmonary vasoconstriction does not resolve or may develop again in the presence of severe lung disease. This is known as persistent pulmonary hypertension.

Factors associated with pulmonary hypertension include:

1 RDS.
2 Meconium aspiration syndrome.

3 Diaphragmatic hernia.
4 Pneumothorax.
5 Hypoglycaemia.
6 Metabolic acidosis.
7 Polycythaemia.

Clinical features

The distinction between lung disease with persistent pulmonary hypertension and cyanotic congenital heart disease may be extremely difficult. The predominant feature is severe hypoxia without a reciprocally high arterial carbon dioxide tension.

Diagnosis

Identification of a recognized risk factor for this condition lends support to the diagnosis. Sometimes it may be necessary to perform cardiac ultrasonography to exclude a structural cardiac defect (see Chapter 13).

Management

Optimal ventilatory management is essential. Correction of hypoglycaemia, hypothermia and metabolic acidosis should be achieved before the use of specific drugs.

Pulmonary vascular resistance is lowered by hyperventilation producing respiratory alkalosis. If the infant remains hypoxic a pulmonary vasodilator may be used such as tolazoline or prostacyclin. Unfortunately neither of these drugs have specific action on the pulmonary arterioles and invariably cause the systemic blood pressure to fall. This should be anticipated and treated with inotropic agents.

Prognosis

This depends on the underlying pulmonary pathology.

Chronic lung disease

This is becoming an increasingly common problem now that methods of treating severe, acute lung

Table 7.8 Causes of chronic lung disease.

Bronchopulmonary dysplasia
Wilson–Mikity syndrome
Chronic pulmonary insufficiency of prematurity (CPIP)
Chronic aspiration of milk
Pneumonitis
　　Chlamydia
　　Viral
　　Pneumocystis carinii
　　Candida albicans
Neonatal rickets
Right-to-left shunt
　　Patent ductus arteriosus
　　Congenital cardiac anomaly

disease prevent early death. The definition of chronic lung disease is the sustained requirement of oxygen for more than 28 days. Table 7.8 lists the causes of chronic lung disease.

BRONCHOPULMONARY DYSPLASIA (BPD)

This condition occurs in 5–10% of VLBW infants. It is most likely in those who have required vigorous mechanical ventilation for severe RDS. It is probably due to the trauma of high pressure ventilation and may be exacerbated by infection, pulmonary interstitial emphysema and pulmonary oedema. The lung shows evidence of extensive scarring and the X-ray has a characteristic appearance. In the most severe form there is an irregular honey-comb appearance due to extensive cystic areas (Fig. 7.7).

There is some evidence that systemic corticosteroids (dexamethasone) may have a beneficial effect (albeit only transient) in the reduction of the inspired oxygen. Secondary infection is an almost invariable accompaniment of BPD and courses of antibiotics may be necessary. Steroids should not be used in the presence of infection.

The prognosis may be reasonably good. The lung has an impressive capacity for growth after birth and if the infant can be protected from further infection and damage he may eventually have functionally normal lungs. Some infants re-

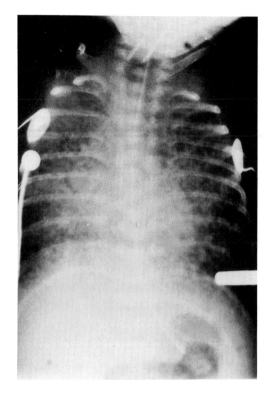

Fig. 7.7 Chest X-ray showing severe bronchopulmonary dysplasia.

quire additional oxygen for months or rarely years before they can be weaned into air.

An important complication of BPD is reactive pulmonary hypertension due to chronic hypoxia and this may cause *cor pulmonale* (p. 227). Careful monitoring of arterial haemoglobin saturation is essential to prevent this from happening. Infants who survive BPD can be shown to have increased airways resistance and are prone to recurrent episodes of wheeziness. The risk of cot death is considerably increased in these infants (see Chapter 28).

WILSON–MIKITY SYNDROME

The cause of this condition is unknown and usually occurs in premature infants who have never required mechanical ventilation. The onset is insidious, usually in the second or third week and progresses with increasing respiratory distress and persistent requirement for supplemental oxygen.

There is a characteristic X-ray appearance with uniform streaky infiltrates and small cystic areas throughout both lung fields.

The prognosis is good and there is no specific treatment. Similar appearances may be caused by infection, particularly with unusual organisms, recurrent aspiration of milk, or rickets and these must be excluded as far as possible.

CHRONIC PULMONARY INSUFFICIENCY OF PREMATURITY (CPIP)

This is a non-specific condition occurring in premature infants who have a uniformly hazy appearance on chest X-ray without evidence of specific abnormality to account for it. They have a persistent low grade oxygen requirement but appear to be well and thrive. It is probably due to non-compliant lungs perhaps due to relative surfactant deficiency which causes atelectasis and hypoxia. Treatment includes the use of methylxanthine drugs (p. 98) or occasionally CPAP (p. 87).

Infection

The newborn infant has incomplete development of the immune system so that infection is more frequent and may be more serious than in older children. Antibodies to infective agents are produced early in fetal life, but the major proportion of immunoglobulin is the IgG fraction which passes from the mother, across the placenta to the fetus largely in the third trimester. Infants born premature miss out on this transfer and are even more immunocompromised than the full-term newborn infant.

Infecting organisms

Distinction must be made between early (perinatal) infection which occurs in the first 48 hours of life and acquired infection usually as a result of cross-infection between parent, medical or nursing attendants and other babies. Early infection may be due to a vaginal organism acquired during passage through the birth canal, such as Group B beta haemolytic *Streptococcus* (GBS), *E. coli* and *Neissaria gonorrhoeae*. *Chlamydia trachomatis* is an organism which cannot survive outside cells and may cause early conjunctivitis and subsequent pneumonitis (p. 89). Herpes virus may be acquired perinatally and cause devastating infection. Of the organisms acquired later, *Staphylococcus epidermidis (albus)* is the most common pathogen. This bacterium like GBS, does not usually cause infection in adults and older children, but because of the immature state of the newborn immune system, opportunistic infections by these organisms are not uncommon. *E. coli*, *Pseudomonas aeruginosa* and *Staphylococcus aureus* may also occur but are becoming less common.

Clinical features

These are often non-specific when occurring in the newborn period and can be divided into general signs and symptoms and more specific ones.

General signs

These can be summarized as follows:
1 Poor feeding and lethargy.
2 Vomiting.
3 Unstable temperature. In small infants, a low temperature is as suggestive of infection as fever.
4 Apnoea.
5 Cyanotic attacks.
6 Irritability.
7 Hepatosplenomegaly.
8 Abdominal distension.

Specific signs

These point to infection at a particular site and may be similar to infection in older children. Specific signs are increasingly less frequently seen in the infants of lower gestational age.
1 Meningitis (p. 282). Convulsions, bulging fontanelle, hypertonia, irritability.
2 Pneumonia (p. 88). Respiratory distress, apnoea.

3 Septicaemia. The symptoms depend on the virulence of the organism. The infants with early onset infection often present with sudden and severe apnoea or shock with hypotension but in infants with *Staph. epidermidis* infection the symptoms and signs occur later and are usually much more general.

4 Osteomyelitis (p. 481). Pseudoparalysis (failure to move the affected limb), tenderness, swelling.

5 Urinary tract infection (p. 257). There are few specific signs and urine must always be cultured in any potentially infected infant.

Management

In view of the potential severity of any infection in the newborn period, prevention is the first line of management. This is effected by the avoidance of birth trauma and good nursing care, particularly an efficent barrier technique. The risk of *Pseudomonas* infection from equipment and from stagnant water used for humidification in incubators is great. For this reason equipment must never be washed in basins used for washing hands. The chance of cross-infection is much greater in hospital than in the home. It is always safer for the baby to be nursed with his mother, especially if they can be together in a single room, and for the baby to be breast fed. Scrupulous attention must be paid to the washing of hands before and after each baby is handled since this is the chief route by which infection, particularly *Pseudomonas*, is transferred from one patient to another.

Prophylactic antibiotics

This policy should be avoided as it increases the risk of multiply resistant organisms, but clinical staff should have a low tolerance for starting antibiotics in infants where there is a clinical suspician of infection. The policy of very early antibioitc treatment is recommended for infants with unexplained respiratory distress. They should be treated with broad spectrum antibiotics (ampicillin and gentamicin) in case the GBS organism is causing the early symptoms of infection.

ANTIBIOTIC TREATMENT IN THE NEWBORN

Antibiotics should be given at the earliest sign of infection without waiting for the results of bacterial investigations. A full infection screen, including lumbar puncture, should be initiated prior to starting antibiotics in all babies. In the absence of an exact knowledge of the infecting organism a combination of antibiotics should be used to be most effective against both Gram-positive and Gram-negative organisms. This combination will vary depending on the sensitivities of local organisms. For early infection a combination of ampicillin and gentamicin is effective and for late infections, gentamicin and flucloxacillin is recommended. If anaerobic organisms are suspected (most likely if there is the risk of faecal contamination) then metronidizole should also be included. These antibiotics are given intravenously for at least 7 days if organisms are cultured. If no organisms are grown and the infant recovers, a shorter course may be appropriate.

Tetracycline should not be used since it stains developing teeth yellow. Sulphonamides should be avoided since they increase the risk of displacing bilirubin from binding sites thereby predisposing to kernicterus.

Chloramphenicol can be used cautiously in the newborn where an alternative antibiotic is not available. In large doses it is toxic and causes the 'grey baby syndrome'. It is safe provided that the dose does not exceed 75 mg/kg/24 hours and serum levels are registered.

NON-SPECIFIC TREATMENT

In critically ill infants with infection, the following points should also be carefully considered:

1 Respiratory failure. Carefully monitor blood gases and ventilate if appropriate.

2 Shock. Monitor blood pressure and treat hypotension with plasma or inotropic agents (p. 244).

3 Convulsions should be treated with anticonvulsant medication.

4 Careful monitoring of fluid input, output and serum electrolytes in anticipation of renal compromise.

Congenital infection

The most important organisms causing congenital infection are toxoplasma, rubella and cytomegalovirus. Herpes, human immunodeficiency virus (HIV) and syphilis are also important. The term 'TORCH' infection is commonly used to describe this group: **T**, toxoplasma; **O**, other (syphilis, HIV); **R**, rubella; **C**, cytomegalovirus; **H**, herpes. These conditions are discussed in Chapter 21.

Apnoea

Apnoea is a common and very important symptom of newborn infants. Apnoea, in the neonatal period, is defined as a pause between breaths lasting for 20 seconds or more. Periods of apnoea lasting for less than 20 seconds may also be important if they are accompanied by change in colour.

In order for an infant to breath normally there must be normal integration between a number of organ systems. The respiratory centre within the brain stem sends messages via the spinal cord to intercostal muscles and the diaphragm which contract to produce negative intrathoracic pressure and air is sucked into the lungs. In addition, the airway must be unobstructed so air can flow freely. Apnoea can therefore be divided simply into central causes, muscle weakness and obstructive. These are summarized in Table 7.9.

Apnoea is a symptom and any infant with apnoeic episodes should be examined carefully and investigated to discover the cause. Apnoeic episodes are commonly associated with transient bradycardia in which the heart rate slows to 80 b.p.m. or less. These episodes may be self-limiting or require stimulation. They may also occur independently to apnoea.

Central apnoea

The most important condition which causes apnoea of sudden onset is infection. This is usually systemic (septicaemia) but may be the first symptom of meningitis, pneumonia, osteomyelitis or

Table 7.9 Causes of neonatal apnoea.

Central
Prematurity
Infection
Convulsions
Drugs (including maternal sedation)
Asphyxia
Hypoglycaemia
Intracranial haemorrhage
Polycythaemia
Necrotizing enterocolitis
Patent ductus arteriosus
High enviromental temperature
Reflex apnoea

Muscle weakness
Fatigue
Prematurity
Muscle disease

Obstructive
Choanal atresia
Pierre–Robin syndrome
Obstructed nares
Tracheomalacia
Milk aspiration

otitis media. All infants with sudden onset of apnoea should have a full infection screen including a lumbar puncture.

Drugs given to the mother (e.g. pethidine) may cause apnoea in the newborn infant in the first 6 hours of life. The maternal notes should be carefully examined for this possibility. Early onset apnoea should always be considered to be due to infection until proved otherwise.

A variety of neurological abnormalities may produce apnoea. These include convulsions, intraventricular haemorrhage, asphyxia, and cerebral anomalies. Apnoea may be the first symptom of necrotizing enterocolitis (p. 114).

There is evidence that a newborn baby's respiratory activity becomes less stable if he is nursed in too high an environmental temperature even though his body temperature is in the normal range (p. 84). Always check the incubator temperature in apnoeic infants.

'Apnoea of prematurity' is a diagnosis of

exclusion. It is thought that some infants are so premature that the respiratory centre has not fully developed and that this is the cause of the apnoea. It may be true that these infants have a reduced sensitivity to hypoxia and hypercapnia and therefore develop apnoea with less severe respiratory compromise than more mature infants, but the diagnosis of 'apnoea of prematurity' should only be made when other casues of apnoea have all been excluded.

Reflex apnoea occurs due to vagal stimulation and may be seen during resuscitation if a stiff suction catheter is blindly pushed down the baby's throat. Reflex apnoea may also occur during the passage of a nasogastric tube or at defaecation.

MUSCLE WEAKNESS

This is probably the commonest cause of apnoea in premature infants. The diaphragm is the main muscle of respiration in these infants and depends on a large proportion of non-fatiguable muscle fibres within it. Unfortunately these fibres do not develop until later in gestation and diaphragmatic fatigue occurs easily. The diaphragm works to better advantage when the infant is lying prone and this is the optimal position in which premature babies should be nursed.

OBSTRUCTIVE APNOEA

Babies are obligate nose breathers and if their nares become obstructed they may become apnoeic. More commonly, immature or sick babies may block their airway by milk, mucus or secretions. They continue to make vigorous respiratory efforts, but move no air in or out of their chest, become progressively cyanosed and then apnoeic. Apnoea monitors that register respiratory activity (as most do) will not detect airway obstruction in these infants until breathing eventually ceases.

Gastro-oesophageal reflux may be associated with obstructive apnoea and a trial of non-gastric feeds may help with discovering the cause of the apnoeic spells.

Investigations

The infant should be carefully examined and the following investigations carried out:
1 Full infection screen including lumbar puncture.
2 Blood glucose assessment.
3 Chest X-ray.
4 Full blood count.
5 Cranial ultrasound scan.
6 Serum electrolytes.
7 Arterial blood gases.

Observation of the infant during a period of apnoea may be helpful. If the infant goes blue prior to the apnoea this suggests that he may have an obstructive cause. Unusual movements such as sucking, blinking or twitching may suggest that the apnoeic spell is due to a fit and an EEG may give useful information.

Treatment

The infant should be carefully managed to avoid hypoxia or too high an environmental temperature which may predispose the infant to apnoea. Careful nursing with regular suction of secretions and placing the infant in the prone position is also helpful.

Figure 7.8 shows a form of action in infants in whom the apnoea monitor alarm starts. If the infant has a specific cause of apnoea such as infection or obstruction then this should be treated.

General methods

1 Nurse the infant prone.
2 Check environmental temperature and reduce if necessary.
3 Increase inspired oxygen by 5–10%.
4 Maintain venous haemoglobin above 12 g/dl.
5 Consider stopping gastric feeds.

Specific methods

1 Methyl xanthines. These drugs which include aminophylline, caffeine and theophylline have

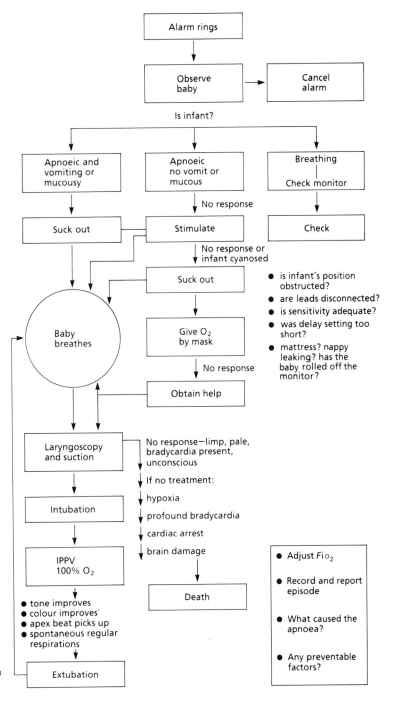

Fig. 7.8 Protocol for infants following an apnoea or bradycardia alarm.

multiple actions including an effect on the central control of breathing as well as a peripheral effect on muscle contraction.

2 CPAP. This may reduce apnoeic spells in some infants but is less effective in general terms than the methyl xanthines.

3 Doxapram. This drug is a central respiratory stimulant, but its use may be associated with unacceptable side-effects. It should only be used after a trial of methyl xanthines.

Neonatal convulsions

Convulsions in the neonatal period occur in approximately five infants per 1000. They are considerably more common in premature and sick infants than in healthy, full-term infants. Fits may be difficult to recognize or to distinguish from normal movements. Babies often show jittery behaviour which is not abnormal. They startle easily and may have rapid oscillatory movements particularly when crying or hungry. Convulsions may take the form of regular clonic movements which do not occur at a rate faster than 1–2 beats per second.

Clinical features

There is a wide diversity of seizure types in the newborn period. The premature infant with a less well developed central nervous system may show incomplete or subtle seizure patterns.

Subtle seizures. These may take the form of tonic or clonic eye movement, chewing or sucking movements, cycling type movements of the lower limbs or apnoea.

Tonic spasms. These are relatively common and may involve all four limbs. They are rarely benign. If the trunk is involved then the infant may adopt an opisthotonic posture.

Clonic seizures. These may be multifocal and transitory and may be benign. Focal clonic seizures are uncommon.

Myoclonic. Multiple myoclonic jerks are an ominous sign of severe cerebral dysfunction.

Aetiology

There are many causes of neonatal convulsions and these are listed in Table 7.10.

PERINATAL ASPHYXIA

This is the commonest cause of neonatal convulsions. Infants sustain hypoxic–ischaemic compromise during labour in 90% of cases. Ten percent of infants have a postnatal cause for their asphyxial insult. Asphyxiated infants show a consistent pattern of neurological abnormality which develops over the first day of life, remains constant for a day or more and then starts to resolve. The severity of the asphyxial insult can be determined by the degree of neurological abnormality following birth and can be divided into mild, moderate or severe categories (Table 7.11). These

Table 7.10 Causes of neonatal seizures.

Birth asphyxia
Intracranial haemorrhage
Infection
Developmental cerebral anomaly
Hypocalcaemia
Hypoglycaemia
Cerebral artery infarction
Drug withdrawal
'Fifth day fits'
Inborn errors of metabolism
Pyridoxine deficiency

Table 7.11 Classification of post-asphyxial encephalopathy.

Grade I (mild)	Grade II (moderate)	Grade III (severe)
Irritability	Lethargy	Coma
Hyperalert	Seizures	Prolonged seizures
Mild hypertonia	Differential tone	Severe hypotonia
Poor feeding	Requires tube feeds	Respiratory failure

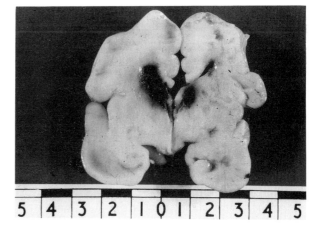

Fig. 7.9 Germinal matrix-intraventricular haemorrhage. Coronal section from a 28-week-gestation infant dying at 1 week of age. There is bilateral germinal matrix haemorrhage, with rupture on the right into the ventricle.

abnormalities are described as post-asphyxial encephalopathy (PAE). Only infants with moderate or severe encephalopathy develop fits and approximately two per 1000 full-term infants develop post-asphyxial fits.

INTRACRANIAL HAEMORRHAGE

There are a number of different types of intracranial haemorrhage which affect the newborn infant.

Subdural haemorrhage

This is now an uncommon condition and was due to obstetric trauma. In the era of modern obstetrics with carefully controlled delivery of the fetal head this condition is rarely seen.

Intraventricular haemorrhage (IVH)

This is a common condition in infants who are born prematurely. It affects approximately one-half of all infants with birthweight less than 1500 g. It is due to rupture of capillaries in the germinal matrix which is the site of production of glial cells located in the region of the caudate nucleus. Germinal matrix haemorrhage ruptures upwards into the lateral ventricle (Fig. 7.9) in the majority of cases, hence the term intraventricular haemorrhage. The term periventricular haemorrhage is

also used to describe this condition and strictly speaking this is more accurate.

IVH is due to changes in cerebral blood flow which are transmitted up to the capillaries of the germinal matrix and cause rupture. Bleeding into the ventricles may be extensive causing the ventricular system to be distended with blood and secondary intra-parenchymal extension may then occur with extensive cerebral injury (Fig. 7.10). In

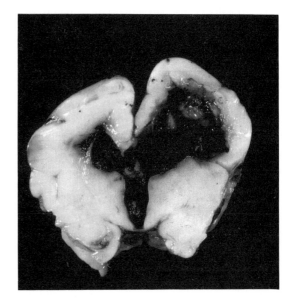

Fig. 7.10 Bilateral intraventricular haemorrhage with massive parenchymal involvement into the right hemisphere.

about 15% of cases of IVH, post-haemorrhagic hydrocephalus may develop (p. 146).

The prognosis in uncomplicated IVH (no parenchymal involvement nor hydrocephalus) is very good.

Subarachnoid haemorrhage (SAH)

This is also a common condition in the neonatal period and may cause convulsions. SAH is usually a benign condition and does not occur as the result of arterial rupture as is seen in older children and adults. Consequently the prognosis is good and the infant usually behaves quite normally between seizures.

HYPOCALCAEMIA

Today, hypocalcaemic fits are uncommon. Previously, hypocalcaemia occurred as the result of poorly modified milk feeds which had a high concentration of phosphate causing excretion of calcium. This form of hypocalcaemia occurred relatively late, usually after the first week of life and were either focal or multifocal.

Magnesium is also an important mineral for normal neuromuscular function and hypomagnesaemia may cause neonatal seizures.

INFECTION

Neonatal meningitis is usually associated with fits. The most common infecting organisms are *Group B beta haemolytic streptococci*, Gram-negative bacilli (*E. coli*) and prenatally acquired infections such as toxoplasmosis and cytomegalovirus.

'FIFTH DAY FITS'

This is a descriptive term referring to infants who are well but develop fits between the third and sixth day of life. They remain neurologically normal between fits. The convulsions are self-limiting and if short-lived probably require no specific anticonvulsant treatment. The cause of these fits is unknown and the prognosis is very good.

PERIVENTRICULAR LEUKOMALACIA (PVL)

This is a condition occurring in premature infants and is due to infarction of the periventricular white matter. If this is extensive then cavitation may occur (Fig. 7.11) and multiple cysts are associated with a very high risk of subsequent cerebral palsy (p. 320). PVL is due to ischaemia affecting a watershed region of the brain between two arterial sources. With advancing maturity, this watershed disappears due to effective anastomosis and the infant is no longer at risk of this form of cerebral pathology.

Diagnosis

Table 7.12 lists the investigations that should be performed in infants with neonatal seizures. These can be considered to be those that are necessary for all infants and those second-line investigations that are necessary when the first set of investigations have failed to find a cause for the seizures. If the infant remains neurologically abnormal and continues to have seizures then rare forms of metabolic disorders should be considered as discussed in Chapter 22.

Treatment

Treatment is directed towards the cause of the seizures. Causes such as hypoglycaemia and hypocalcaemia should be treated rapidly with the appropriate substance.

Table 7.12 Investigations to be performed in cases of neonatal convulsions.

Clinical history
  Evidence of asphyxia
  Family history of neonatal seizures
  Maternal drug ingestion
  Prenatal viral infection
Blood glucose (stick test)
Serum calcium and magnesium
Lumbar puncture
Serology for prenatal infection
Ultrasound brain scan
Urinary and serum amino acid profile
Urinary organic acid profile

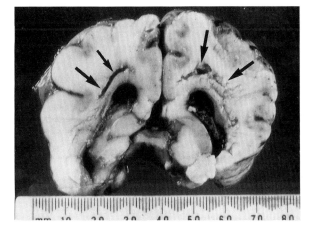

Fig. 7.11 Cavitating periventricular leukomalacia. Coronal section through the brain of a severely premature infant showing well-defined cavities (arrowed) in the periventricular white matter of both hemispheres.

Specific treatment of the fits should also be considered although this is not always essential. Seizures that last for 10 minutes or more and those that occur very frequently should be treated with an anticonvulsant. The main anticonvulsants used in the newborn period are:

1 Phenobarbitone. This is the first-line medication and should be given in a loading dose followed by maintenance. It is not effective for long-term use and should be changed after 6 months of age (p. 290).

2 Paraldehyde. This is a very short acting drug and is only useful to treat fits whilst waiting for the first-line drugs to have effect.

3 Phenytoin. This drug should not be used for maintenance therapy in the newborn but may be a useful drug given intravenously in a loading dosage. Oral or intramuscular absorption is very variable.

4 Clonazepam. This can be given intermittently if phenobarbitone fails to control the seizures or by continuous intravenous infusion. It should not be used in very premature infants.

Duration of anticonvulsant treatment

Anticonvulsants should be continued for as long as the infant remains neurologically abnormal. Many infants can have their medication stopped before discharge from the neonatal unit. Prolonged use of phenobarbitone is not recommended.

Prognosis

The prognosis depends on the underlying cause of the convulsions. Table 7.13 gives a guide to the risk of handicap depending on the aetiology of the seizures.

Hypoglycaemia

Glucose is a fundamental metabolic fuel which is burnt in the cell and in the presence of oxygen produces 38 molecules of high energy ATP. Hypoglycaemia is defined as a blood sugar below 2.2 mmol/l.

Table 7.13 Risk of severe handicap depending on cause of the neonatal seizures.

Aetiology of fits	Risk of severe handicap (%)
Asphyxia	50
Intracranial haemorrhage	25
Hypoglycaemia	50
Hypocalcaemia	10
Bacterial meningitis	50–80
Congenital cerebral anomaly	95
'Fifth day fits'	0
Unknown cause	25

Table 7.14 Common causes of neonatal hypoglycaemia.

Decrease in glucose availability
Intra-uterine growth retardation
Prematurity
Severe neonatal illness

Increase in glucose utilization
Hyperinsulinism
    Infants of diabetic mothers
    Rhesus iso-immunization
    Beckwith–Weideman syndrome
    Nesidioblastosis

Inborn errors of glucose metabolism
Glycogen storage disease
Galactosaemia
Aminoacidaemias

Aetiology

Table 7.14 lists the commoner causes of neonatal hypoglycaemia. These can be broadly divided into either a decrease in substrate availability or increased glucose utilization.

DECREASE IN GLUCOSE AVAILABILITY

This is most commonly seen in growth-retarded infants with depleted glycogen stores. Premature infants, particularly if sick, are also more likely to develop hypoglycaemia.

INCREASE IN GLUCOSE UTILIZATION

Insulin is necessary to drive the glucose into the cell and any cause of hyperinsulinaemia may cause neonatal hypoglyaemia. This is most commonly seen in the infant of a diabetic mother. These babies are exposed *in utero* to excess glucose due to the mother's hyperglycaemia. They secrete increased levels of insulin (i.e. they are hyperinsulinaemic) to maintain a normal blood sugar, but when the umbilical cord is cut they lose their continuous infusion of glucose and develop hypoglycaemia. Hyperinsulinism also occurs in infants with rhesus iso-immunization and very

rarely in those with hyperplasia of the pancreatic islet cells, a condition known as nesidioblastosis.

Clinical features

Many infants develop hypoglycaemia with no symptoms and this is referred to as asymptomatic hypoglycaemia.

If symptoms develop they are usually non-specific and include irritability, tremors, apathy, cyanotic spells, temperature instability, and apnoea. If the brain becomes hypoglycaemic the infant develops convulsions.

These symptoms are very similar to those that occur in infected infants and hypoglycaemia should be anticipated and checked in every unwell infant.

Investigations

Infants who are at risk of hypoglycaemia (particularly growth-retarded infants and those of diabetic mothers) should have a measure of blood glucose made very regularly. This is most conveniently performed by a heel-prick stick test (Dextrostix or BM stick). This should be done initially at 1 and 2 hours and thereafter 2-hourly after feeds until blood sugar levels have remained stable and normal for 8 hours. They should then be repeated 4- and then 8-hourly until the infant has been normoglycaemic for 48 hours.

Treatment

PREVENTION OF HYPOGLYCAEMIA

At-risk infants should be fed shortly after birth and then initially 2-hourly. If the blood sugar falls on regular testing a 10% solution of glucose water should be given in addition to the milk feeds.

ESTABLISHED HYPOGLYCAEMIA

If hypoglycaemia occurs despite regular feeds, an intravenous infusion of dextrose (glucose) should be set up. The concentration depends on the level of hypoglycaemia and its duration. Rapid infusion of highly concentrated dextrose (50%) should be avoided in hyperinsulinaemic infants as this may cause rebound hypoglycaemia.

In infants resistant to intravenous dextrose infusion, hydrocortisone, glucagon or diazoxide may be used. Partial pancreatectomy may be necessary to treat hypoglycaemia in nesidioblastosis successfully.

Prognosis

Convulsions due to hypoglycaemia are associated with severe mental retardation or cerebral palsy in 50% of cases. If the infants are symptomatic but do not develop fits then only 20% will be handicapped and is generally less severe in nature than those with fits. Asymptomatic hypoglycaemia is associated with an excellent prognosis.

Anaemia in the neonatal period

The newborn infant has a relatively high haemoglobin concentration compared with older children but this rapidly falls over the first weeks of life. The decline in haemoglobin concentration is referred to as physiological anaemia and these changes are summarized in Fig. 7.12. The fall is more marked in premature infants and reaches its lowest point about 6 weeks after birth in this group and at about 9 weeks in full-term infants.

The definition of anaemia at birth is a haemoglobin level below 14 g/dl. In premature infants anaemia is severe at a level below 8 g/dl.

Aetiology

There are a number of other important causes of anaemia.

ANAEMIA OF PREMATURITY

This refers to the exaggerated fall in haemoglobin seen in premature infants compared with the full-term infant. This is due to a number of factors:
1 Suppression of erythropoietin secretion.
2 A relative increase in the intravascular blood

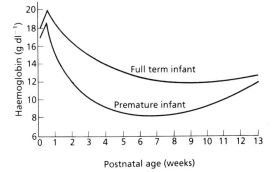

Fig. 7.12 Physiological anaemia. The two graphs show the normal fall in haemoglobin with postnatal age in mature and premature infants.

volume in the early months of life causing a dilutional effect.
3 Iron deficiency. A very premature infant is born with less than half the iron stores of a full-term infant.
4 Haemolysis. The immature erythrocyte is probably more prone to haemolysis.

HAEMORRHAGE

This may occur either during pregnancy or neonatal life.

Prenatal

Bleeding from the placenta is usually maternal in origin and therefore does not cause fetal anaemia. Occasionally bleeding may result from trauma to the umbilical cord producing fetal anaemia. The commonest cause of anaemia due to loss of fetal blood is either into the mother's circulation (fetomaternal) or into the twin fetus (fetofetal). Bleeding from the fetus into the maternal circulation may be severe and the mother usually shows no symptoms but fetal erythrocytes may be detected in the maternal circulation. Monozygotic twins share a placental circulation and there may be bleeding from one fetus into the twin causing one twin to be born anaemic and the other plethoric.

Table 7.15 Commoner causes of neonatal haemolysis.

Immune causes
Rhesus iso-immunization
ABO incompatability

Non-immune causes
Disseminated intravascular haemolysis
Prenatal infection
 Toxoplasmosis
 Cytomegalovirus
Red cell enzymes defects
 G6PD deficiency
 Others
Heriditary spherocytosis

Neonatal

Bleeding may be obvious or occult. Overt bleeding from the umbilical cord or into the subcutaneous tissues (e.g. cephalhaematoma) is usually fairly obvious. Bleeding may occur into the bowel, brain or lungs and not be obvious until specific investigations are performed.

HAEMOLYSIS

Haemolysis in the neonatal period is fairly common and can be divided broadly into immune and non-immune causes. Table 7.15 lists the commoner causes of neonatal haemolysis and these conditions are discussed in the section on neonatal jaundice (see below). Jaundice as well as anaemia is an important feature of haemolysis.

Clinical signs

The infant may look pale at birth or anaemia may be found on routine testing. Premature infants become most profoundly anaemic between 4 and 8 weeks after birth and may develop symptoms. The most important clinical feature is breathlessness particularly on feeding. Symptoms are unusual until the haemoglobin concentration falls below 8 g/dl. Some infants may develop apnoeic or bradycardic spells in response to severe anaemia.

Management

Symptomatic or severe anaemia should be treated by blood transfusion. Very sick infants with lung disease require a relatively higher haemoglobin concentration to provide adequate tissue oxygenation. Ventilated infants should have their haemoglobin maintained above 12 g/dl and infants breathing spontaneously but in oxygen should have their haemoglobin maintained between 10 and 12 g/dl. Supplemental iron is given by mouth to premature infants after 1 month of age.

Neonatal jaundice

Jaundice in the newborn period is a common symptom and is often completely benign. Bilirubin in high concentration is, however, severely neurotoxic and may cause permanent brain injury (kernicterus, p. 108) and all jaundiced babies require careful evaluation.

Bilirubin is produced in the unconjugated form as the result of red cell destruction in the reticulo-endothelial system. Unconjugated bilirubin is bound to albumin and then metabolized further in the liver to conjugated (water soluble) bilirubin by the action of the enzyme glucuronyl transferase. The conjugated bilirubin is excreted into the bile and into the small intestine. Some is metabolized further in the bowel back to the unconjugated form and reabsorbed. This is referred to as the enterohepatic circulation of bilirubin.

Aetiology

The causes of neonatal jaundice can be divided into unconjugated and conjugated (Table 7.16).

UNCONJUGATED HYPERBILIRUBINAEMIA

If severe or occurring on the first day of life, unconjugated hyperbilirubinaemia is usually due to haemolysis. Less severe jaundice, particularly when first apparent between days 2 and 5 is often referred to as physiological jaundice.

Table 7.16 Causes of neonatal jaundice.

Unconjugated
Haemolysis
 Rhesus incompatability
 ABO incompatability
 Hereditary spherocytosis
 G6PD deficiency
Prenatal infection
Septicaemia
Bruising and bleeding
Hypothyroidism
Polycythaemia
Breast milk jaundice
Crigler–Najjar syndrome

Conjugated
Neonatal hepatitis
 Prenatal infection
 Fructosaemia
 Tyrosinaemia
 Alpha-1 antitrypsin
Biliary atresia
Inspissated bile syndrome
Choledochal cyst
Cystic fibrosis
Rotor syndrome
Dubin–Johnson syndrome

Physiological jaundice

This is due to immaturity of liver metabolism, particularly the enzyme glucuronyl transferase. Physiological jaundice is a diagnosis of exclusion but if any of the following features are present, an alternative cause for the jaundice is very likely:
1 Clinically observed jaundice within 24 hours of life.
2 High levels of total bilirubin.
3 A conjugated level of bilirubin above 30 umol/l.
4 Persistent jaundice lasting more than 10 days in a full-term infant or 14 days in a premature infant.
5 An infant who is ill.

Breast milk jaundice

This is also a diagnosis of exclusion. Some mothers excrete a steroid in their milk which inhibits liver conjugation and the infant becomes jaundiced in the first week or two of life and remains jaundiced for several months although levels may decline before the infant is fully weaned from the breast. Hyperbilirubinaemia is never severe and the mother should be encouraged to continue to breast feed. The infants thrive despite mild to moderate jaundice.

Excessive haemolysis

Rhesus incompatability occurs in infants who are Rh-positive and are born to mothers who are Rh-negative. Approximately 15% of Caucasian women are Rh-negative but only 1% of Black women. The Rh-negative woman is sensitized by a small transfusion (as little as 0.25 ml) of blood from an Rh-positive individual and antibodies are produced. This most commonly occurs as a result of the fetus bleeding into the maternal circulation either at birth or at surgical termination of pregnancy. A previous uncrossmatched blood transfusion may also cause sensitization. Although sensitization may occur in the first pregnancy it is unlikely that sufficient antibodies have been produced to affect that fetus. In general rhesus haemolytic disease becomes more severe in successive affected pregnancies.

The rhesus factor is complex, comprising CDE/cde antigens. The commonest antigen is D and this accounts for 95% of cases. If the father is heterozygous for Rh-factor then some fetuses will be Rh-positive and others Rh-negative. This accounts for some siblings being affected and others escaping haemolysis in successive pregnancies.

Rh-negative women should be screened for rhesus antibodies at booking and again at 28, 32 and 36 weeks' gestation. If antibodies are present and if the titre in maternal serum is rising, amniocentesis should be performed. This should also be done if there is the history of a previously severely affected infant. Depending on the amount of bilirubin in the amniotic fluid a decision can be made to continue to manage the pregnancy with careful observation, or to give the fetus a blood transfusion. In the past this has been done by injecting blood under ultrasound control into the fetal peritoneum but more recently cordocentesis has been found to be very successful. In this procedure a needle is placed into a vessel at the base of the umbilical cord and blood injected directly into the fetal circulation.

Rhesus haemolytic disease can be prevented by giving anti-D gamma globulin (200 μg) to all Rh-negative women who deliver Rh-positive infants. Injection should be given within 72 hours of delivery. If antibodies are already present anti-D is not given. Anti-D should also be given following termination of pregancy, amniocentesis or any other procedure where a Rh-negative mother may be sensitized by a small transfusion of Rh-positive cells. Failure of anti-D to inactivate antibody occurs in women who produce non anti-D antibody (usually C).

Fetal disease depends on the severity and duration of the haemolysis. The fetus may be mildly affected and born with mild anaemia (10–12 g/dl) and moderate hepatosplenomegaly. The more severely affected infant is severely anaemic with massive hepatosplenomegaly. The most severe involvement causes high output cardiac failure with gross hydrops (oedema) and these fetuses often die *in utero* or shortly after delivery.

CONJUGATED HYPERBILIRUBINAEMIA

This is always significant and the infant should be investigated very carefully and rapidly. Neonatal hepatitis and biliary atresia must be distinguished as the latter condition can be cured surgically only if operated on very early in life. The causes of conjugated hyperbilirubinaemia are discussed in detail in Chapter 12.

Clinical features

Jaundice is clinically detectable then the level reaches about 100 μmol/l. Visible jaundice progresses in a centrifugal distribution from the head to the hands and feet. A rough idea of the approximate level of jaundice can be obtained by blanching the skin at different sites. This is done by pressing with a finger to drain the capillary blood and observing the yellow pigmentation be-

fore the capillaries refill. The approximate correlation between visible jaundice using this method and bilirubin levels are as follows:

Limited to head	100 μmol/l
Upper trunk	150 μmol/l
Lower trunk and thighs	200 μmol/l
Lower leg	250 μmol/l
Hands and feet	> 250 μmol/l

This technique does not apply if the infant has had phototherapy.

Clinical assessment of the infant should pay particular attention to the following points which suggest the infant should be carefully investigated:
1 Visible jaundice in the first 24 hours.
2 An unwell infant.
3 An infant with increasing jaundice.
4 Evidence of conjugated hyperbilirubinaemia (bilirubin in the urine).
5 Prolonged hyperbilirubinaemia.
6 Firm or enlarged liver.
7 Splenomegaly.

Attention should also be directed towards evidence of occult bleeding, anaemia, evidence of intra-uterine infection, neurological abnormality or abdominal distension.

Investigations

Investigating the jaundiced infant should be critical rather than haphazard. The first two factors to be elicited are whether there is a conjugated component to the hyperbilirubinaemia (presence of biliribin in the urine) and whether the jaundice is due to iso-immunization (Coombs' test positive). Infants with elevated bilirubin due only to insoluble unconjugated bilirubin do not have bilirubin in the urine. Once these two investigations have been performed further investigations are necessary to elucidate the precise cause. These investigations are summarized in Figure 7.13.

Complications

KERNICTERUS

This is the most important complication of hyperbilirubinaemia. Babies who die following a period

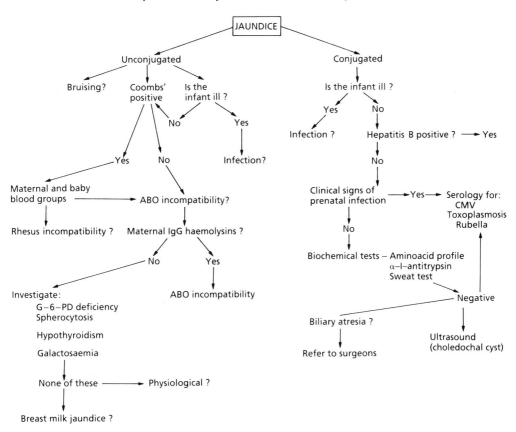

Fig. 7.13 A scheme for investigating neonatal jaundice.

of severe hyperbilirubinaemia show yellow staining of the basal ganglia and brain stem. This pathological appearance is described as kernicterus. Encephalopathy in the neonatal period may occur with very high levels of unconjugated bilirubin. These infants present with lethargy, stiffness and opisthotonus, high pitched cry and possibly convulsions. Survivors usually demonstrate major neurological sequelae including a choreo-athetoid form of cerebral palsy, high frequency hearing loss, paralysis of upward gaze and sometimes mental retardation. Abnormal findings may be less severe and the commonest isolated finding in infants with hyperbilirubinaemia is sensorineural deafness. Premature infants are more sensitive to hyperbilirubinaemia and may show fewer encephalopathic features than full-term infants.

The cause of the neurological sequelae is certainly due to hyperbilirubinaemia but the precise manner in which it damages the brain is unknown. It is often assumed that unconjugated bilirubin in the free (non-protein bound form) penetrates the brain and binds with sensitive neurones in the basal ganglia and elsewhere. There is, however, evidence that conjugated bilirubin may also be toxic and that opening of the blood–brain barrier by systemic compromise is the more likely explanation for bilirubin neurotoxicity.

Kernicterus as a clinical entity is preventable by careful management of severe hyperbilirubinaemia. Levels of total and unconjugated bilirubin must be carefully monitored and if they exceed preset levels phototherapy is instituted.

Management

Jaundice can be minimized by early feeding and keeping the infant adequately hydrated. If the level of bilirubin continues to rise to significant levels, phototherapy should be started. This treatment involves exposing the infant to light of 450 nm (the visible blue spectrum) which degrades bilirubin to non-toxic soluble products that are excreted in the urine. The infant's eyes should be protected from the light. If this is unsuccessful in controlling hyperbilirubinaemia, exchange transfusion is undertaken to bring down the bilirubin level and wash out some antibodies in the case of rhesus haemolytic disease.

The indications for exchange tranfusion depend on the infant's gestational age, postnatal age and general condition. The level at which bilirubin damages the brain is not known but bilirubin should not exceed 350 μmol/l in a full-term infant with haemolysis and 240 μmol/l in an infant less than 1500 g birthweight. Full-term infants with non-haemolytic forms of hyperbilirubinaemia may be allowed a level of unconjugated bilirubin of 400 μmol/l before exchange tranfusion is necessary.

Bleeding disorders in the newborn

Abnormal bleeding is a relatively common abnormality in newborn infants. It may present either as excessive bleeding into skin, bowel or urine or may become obvious if the infant oozes excessively from arterial or venepuncture sites.

Aetiology

Table 7.17 lists the most important causes of excessive or abnormal bleeding in the newborn period.

THROMBOCYTOPENIA

Iso-immune thrombocytopenia

In this condition the mother produces antibodies to fetal platelets in a similar manner to rhesus iso-immunization. Mother is platelet A1 antigen-

Table 7.17 Causes of excessive or abnormal bleeding in the neonatal period.

Thrombocytopenia
Iso-immune
Maternal idiopathic thrombocytopenia
Bacterial infection
Prenatal infection
Disseminated intravascular coagulation
Neonatal leukaemia

Haemorrhagic disease of the newborn

Clotting factor deficiency
Haemophilia
Christmas disease

negative and fetus is A1 antigen-positive. The mother produces IgG, in response to the fetal sensitization, which crosses the placenta and causes fetal thrombocytopenia. The maternal platelet numbers are normal. Although the neonatal thrombocytopenia may be severe initially it is a self-limiting condition which improves as the maternal IgG disappears from the newborn.

Maternal idiopathic thrombocytopenia (ITP)

Mothers with ITP produce an antibody which crosses the placenta and may cause her fetus to also develop thrombocytopenia. The lower the maternal platelets, the more severely affected the fetus is likely to be. Maternal platelet counts below 25 000 are almost always associated with severe neonatal involvement.

Disseminated intravascular coagulation (DIC)

DIC occurs as the result of a number of neonatal conditions including septicaemia, asphyxia and respiratory distress syndrome. Its aetiology, investigation and treatment are discussed in Chapter 24.

HAEMORRHAGIC DISEASE OF THE NEWBORN

This condition is due to vitamin K deficiency. Vitamin K is produced by the bacterial flora in the gastrointestinal tract but as the newborn infant has a sterile bowel at birth there is little production from this source in the first few weeks of life. All newborn infants should be given vitamin K1 at birth to prevent deficiency of the vitamin K-dependent clotting factors. It may be given intramuscularly or orally. It is particularly important to administer it to breast-fed infants.

INHERITED DISORDERS OF CLOTTING FACTORS

These are rare but important causes of neonatal coagulopathy. They are usually X-linked conditions and only affect male infants. They are becoming increasingly recognized as causes of prenatal intracranial haemorrhage.

Clinical features

The following features are suggestive of neonatal coagulopathy:

1 Oozing from venepuncture or arterial stab sites.
2 Generalized petechial or purpuric lesions. Traumatic petechial lesions are particularly common over the face of infants who have been exposed to a long second stage of labour. This does not suggest a bleeding disorder unless the lesions are generalized.
3 Intracranial haemorrhage in a full-term infant or fetus.

If coagulopathy is suspected, take a careful maternal history including family history of bleeding disorders, drug ingestion, ITP or viral infection in pregnancy. Examine the infant for the presence of congenital infection (hepatosplenomegaly or fundal abnormalities) and ensure that the infant does not have thrombocytopenia with absent radii syndrome (p. 436).

Investigations

Measure the following:
1 Platelets from a free-flowing venous sample.
2 Bleeding time.
3 Prothrombin time (PT).
4 Fibrinogen degradation products (FDPs).

Thrombocytopenia is the most common cause of neonatal coagulopathy. Bleeding does not occur spontaneously unless the platelets are less than $20\,000/mm^3$ and the infant may bruise easily to minor trauma at levels of $20\,000-50\,000/mm^3$.

Management

Severe thrombocytopenia ($<20\,000/mm^3$) is treated with platelet infusion and if severe bleeding has occurred the infant may need whole blood transfusion. Haemorrhagic disease of the newborn should be treated with intramuscular vitamin K1.

DIC is treated by appropriate management of the underlying cause. Specfic treatment is not indicated.

Birth injury

This may affect any organ and the commoner causes are shown in Table 7.18 related to organ systems. Premature infants are more likely to sustain birth trauma and vaginal breech deliveries are predisposed to brachial plexus injury.

Table 7.18 Common injuries associated with birth trauma.

Nervous system
Intracranial haemorrhage
Asphyxia
Overriding of the occipital bone with cerebellar trauma
Facial nerve palsy
Spinal cord lesion
Brachial plexus injury
  Erb's palsy
  Klumpke's palsy

Bone fractures
Skull fracture or depression
Clavicle, humerus, femur

Intra-abdominal
Viscus rupture (particularly liver)

Soft tissue
Cephalhaematoma
Bruising
Sternomastoid tumour

CEPHALHAEMATOMA

This is a common lesion and occurs in approximately 1% of newborn infants. It is discussed on p. 56.

SKULL FRACTURE

Linear fractures are usually benign. Depressed fractures should be carefully assessed and a brain scan performed. If cerebral contusion is present a neurosurgical opinion is indicated.

BRACHIAL PLEXUS INJURY

There are two forms: Erb's palsy and Klumpke's palsy.
1 Erb's palsy involves injury to the upper brachial plexus (5th and 6th cervical nerve roots). The arm is held in abduction with the elbow extended and the forearm pronated with the wrist flexed (Fig. 7.14).
2 Klumpke's palsy involves the lower brachial plexus (7th and 8th cervical and 1st thoracic segments). The infant shows wrist drop and paralysis of the hand with loss of the primitive grasp reflex.

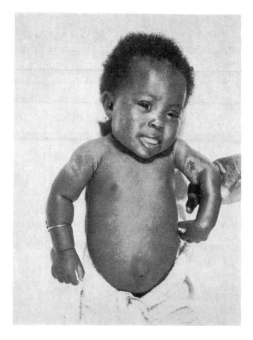

Fig. 7.14 Left-sided Erb's palsy showing the typical 'waiter's tip' position of the hand. In addition to the brachial plexus lesion the cervical sympathetic nerve supply has been damaged producing a Horner's syndrome on the same side, indicated by ptosis and enophthalmos.

FACIAL NERVE PALSY

This condition is detected by observation of the infant. He is unable to close the affected eye with lack of lower lip depression on crying (Fig. 7.15).

STERNOMASTOID TUMOUR

This is due to trauma to the sternomastoid muscle occurring at birth. Bleeding causes a firm swelling (tumour) which develops in the middle third of the muscle, but its appearance is often delayed for a number of days following birth (Fig. 7.16). Healing may be accompanied by shortening of the sternomastoid with limitation of neck turning.

Management

Prevention of joint contractures by passive physiotherapy is important in infants with brachial plexus injuries. Physiotherapy is also important in preventing contracture of the sternomastoid muscle following haematoma.

If the infant with a facial nerve palsy cannot close his eye spontaneously, artificial tears should be applied regularly and the eye may need patching to prevent corneal injury.

Fractures of the long bones should be discussed with an orthopaedic surgeon experienced in the care of children. Often no specific treatment is necessary.

Retinopathy of prematurity (ROP)

This is an important condition which is confined to the newborn period. It was previously referred to as retrolental fibroplasia (RLF) but the modern terminology is more accurate. In Britain the incidence of this condition in very premature infants

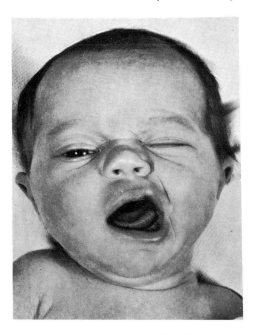

Fig. 7.15 Right facial nerve palsy. The right eye cannot be closed and the mouth is drawn to the left side.

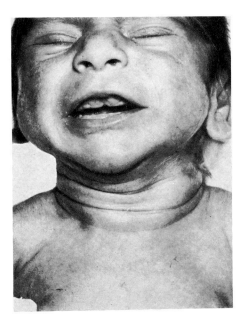

Fig. 7.16 Sternomastoid tumour with a visible lump on the left side of the neck.

(32 weeks gestation and below) is about 50% and its incidence increases with reducing gestational age. Although it is a common condition it is rarely severe. Most cases of acute ROP undergo spontaneous resolution, and in those in whom regression does not occur scarring may develop with visual impairement. This occurs in only 1% of premature infants.

Aetiology

When ROP was first recognized in the 1950s it was a condition seen in relatively mature infants and was due to hyperoxia. This probably caused spasm of the retinal vessels with resultant retinal ischaemia, scarring and blindness. Today ROP should never be seen in mature infants and remains a problem only in more immature infants. Its cause in these infants is unknown. Although hyperoxia may have an aetiological role it is only one of many factors; the most important one being the severity of illness the infant is suffering from. There is some evidence that vitamin E supplements may limit the severity of this condition but this is as yet unproven.

Clinical features

This condition can only be diagnosed in the actue stages by using an indirect ophthalmoscope following pupil dilatation with 0.5% cyclopentolate eye drops, and therefore the infants must be seen by an ophthalmologist with an interest in this condition. Infants with the severe scarring form of this condition may show a white reflex on shining a light into their eye (see Chapter 5).

Management

Although oxygen is not the only important risk factor it is important to monitor arterial levels of oxygen tension carefully to avoid a Pao_2 above 10–12 kPa depending on the gestational age of the infant. The majority of infants with signs of acute ROP spontaneously resolve. Severe scarring may be limited by the use of cryotherapy to the retina.

Neonatal rickets

The extremely low birth weight infant is particularly at risk of poor bone mineralization; a condition referred to as neonatal rickets. These infants have a relatively high vitamin D requirement (1000 units/day) but the cause of neonatal rickets is inadequate mineral intake. Breast milk is poor in phosphorus and is inadequate for the requirements of very tiny babies (those less than 1000 g birth weight). These infants should be supplemented with extra phosphorus and calcium if breast fed, or given a low birth weight formula (p. 72).

Full-term babies may be born with rickets if their mothers are deficient in vitamin D. The baby may present with hypocalcaemic tetany and X-rays show the characteristic metaphyseal changes. The alkaline phosphatase level is usually markedly elevated.

Diagnosis

This is made radiologically. The bone looks porotic, but the main feature is broadening and cupping of the metaphyses. In severe cases fractures may be seen. Many babies with radiological features of neonatal rickets have a very high alkaline phosphatase value (> 1000 KA units) but this is not essential to make the diagnosis.

Necrotizing enterocolitis (NEC)

This is an inflammatory disorder of the bowel occurring usually in the newborn period. It most commonly affects the terminal ileum or sigmoid colon and the bowel is inflamed, ulcerated and may perforate. Organisms invade the mucosa and produce gas within the bowel wall and this gives the characteristic radiological appearance on abdominal X-ray.

Its precise cause is unknown but risk factors include asphyxia with bowel ischaemia, impaired bowel blood flow (secondary to an umbilical venous catheter, patent ductus arteriosus or polycythaemia), hypoxia (it is commoner in cyanotic

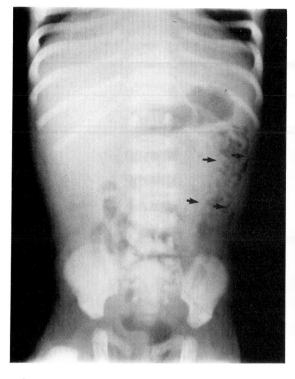

Fig. 7.17 Necrotizing enterocolitis. Abdominal X-ray showing intramural gas (arrowed) in the wall of the descending colon.

heart disease), infection and an osmotic load on the bowel as may occur in early feeding.

Infection is commonly present in infants with NEC, and *Clostridium difficile* is sometimes isolated from the stool. There is little evidence that infection is the primary cause in the majority of cases and probably represents a secondary occurrence. NEC is also seen later in the first year of life in infants with Hirschprung's disease.

Clinical features

The first signs of NEC are usually insidious with apnoea, lethargy, bile-stained aspirates from the stomach and failure to maintain body temperature. Established cases usually show marked abdominal distension, blood in the stool and cardiovascular collapse with shock.

Investigations

Abdominal X-ray usually shows intramural gas (pneumatosis coli) (Fig. 7.17). There may also be distended loops of bowel and free gas in the peritoneum which indicates perforation has occurred. Rarely gas may be seen in the portal vein.

Faeces and blood should be cultured for bacterial and viral pathogens.

Management

In infants in whom NEC is suspected, gastric feeds should be withdrawn for 2 weeks. Broad spectrum antibiotics are indicated in all cases for at least 5 days. These should include metronidizole to cover the possibility of anaerobic organisms.

The indications for surgery include perforation or failure to respond to medical treatment. At laparotomy the peritoneum should be drained and an ileostomy fashioned from normal-looking bowel. Massive resection of bowel is to be avoided in the acute stage of the illness.

Most infants with NEC have a temporary lactase deficiency and when started back onto feeds they should be given a lactose-free milk.

Complications

1 Lactase deficiency.
2 Stricture occurs in approximately 15% of infants following NEC and usually affects the splenic flexure and descending colon.

8

INHERITED DISORDERS AND GENETIC COUNSELLING

Although there is little to suggest that inherited disorders are becoming more common, two factors have prompted awareness of their increasing relative contribution to childhood morbidity and mortality. First, there is a greater understanding and appreciation of the role of genetic factors in the cause of many disorders of childhood, particularly the common malformations and multiple congenital anomaly syndromes. Secondly, as a consequence of major advances in medicine and public health, sweeping progress has been achieved in the management of formerly common environmental disorders, leaving a large residue of conditions, often severe and untreatable, which are largely or entirely genetic in origin.

Given that approximately one in 40 of all babies has a congenital malformation, which is likely to be at least partly genetic in origin, and that inherited disorders account for up to 30% of all childhood deaths and hospital admissions, it is clearly important that doctors working with children should be familiar with the basic principles of human inheritance. Consideration of the nature of genes and chromosomes provides a useful starting point.

Structure of genes

Until recently it was conventional to regard the gene as a simple unit made up of DNA comprising two chains of nucleotides coiled around each other in a double helix, with each set of three nucleotide bases coding for an amino acid. The chromosome was seen as consisting of a long series of sequential genes, each producing a particular protein.

Whilst this can still be accepted as a reasonable overview, the structure of the human genome is now known to be much more complex. The total length of the haploid human genome is approximately 3 million kilobases (3000 million base pairs). Yet each of the estimated 50 000 human structural genes (i.e. genes coding for a protein product such as an enzyme or cell receptor) is likely to be no greater in length than 10–15 kilobases, so that well over 50% of the total DNA must be non-functional or 'redundant' as far as final protein product is concerned.

It emerges that a large proportion of the human genome consists of repetitive or highly repetitive DNA, most of which is not transcribed. Curiously, some forms of this show striking variation in length from person to person, a factor of no obvious clinical significance, but analysis of which can be elegantly exploited in the technique known as genetic finger-printing. This involves the study of hypervariable mini-satellite DNA, a particular type of repetitive DNA which is widely scattered throughout the genome and which shows marked variation from person to person to the extent that no two individuals, with the exception of monozygotic twins, will have absolutely identical patterns.

This abundance of non-transcribed DNA is found not only between the genes but also within them. Recent studies have revealed that most genes are much longer in their genomic structure than would be expected on the basis of analysis of the final protein product. For example, the locus for the Duchenne muscular dystrophy gene occupies approximately 2000 kilobases of the short arm of the X-chromosome. Yet only 0.7% of this (14 kilobases) codes for 'dystrophin', the protein product now believed to play a crucial role in muscle contractility and survival.

This discrepancy in length between the genomic sequences and those of the transcribed DNA can be accounted for by (a) regulatory sequences which appear to play a critical role in control of protein synthesis, and (b) the presence of non-protein coding segments known as introns, which intervene between those parts of the gene which are expressed and which are known as exons. The degree of complexity of these systems, the functions of which are far from clear, is illustrated by the meagre size of the 14 kilobase Duchenne muscular dystrophy gene transcript which is formed by 60 exons scattered amongst 2000 kilobases of genomic DNA.

Chromosome structure and function

The fundamental unit of inheritance is the gene. Genes are tightly packaged in chromosomes and are present in all nucleated cells. The precise nature of this packaging is complex and poorly understood. Under the electron microscope chromosomes can be seen to be made up of nucleoprotein fibres known as chromatin. This is composed of histone proteins, rich in basic amino acids and constant in structure throughout the animal kingdom, around which the DNA is coiled. In some curious and totally mysterious way this complex packaging process must have evolved to facilitate cell division, permitting chromosome replication in somatic cell division (mitosis), and halving of the normal diploid number in spermatogenesis and oogenesis (meiosis).

Normal karyotype

To analyse an individual's chromosome constitution or karyotype, it is necessary to obtain nuclei from cultured dividing cells. This is achieved in the laboratory by arresting cell division during metaphase, the stage of maximum chromosome condensation. The cell nuclei are then swollen using a hypotonic solution thus separating the individual chromosomes and rendering them readily visible under the light microscope. The resulting metaphase spread can be analysed by staining the chromosomes with particular dyes. Normally it requires a minimum of 3 days for the production and analysis of a karyotype from peripheral blood lymphocytes.

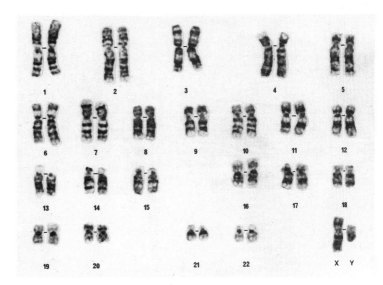

Fig. 8.1 A normal human male karyotype showing the banding pattern obtained using Giemsa stain.

Certain stains, such as Giemsa, are taken up preferentially in different parts of a chromosome producing an effect known as banding. Alternating light and dark bands produce, with very few exceptions, a consistent and recognizable pattern in the chromosomes of all individuals. Careful analysis of these banding patterns permits confident identification of chromosome abnormalities.

A typical G-banded karyotype from a normal male is shown in Fig. 8.1. Each chromosome consists of two parallel strands joined at a constriction point known as the centromere. The strands are known as chromatids. The normal human karyotype consists of 23 pairs of chromosomes arranged in decreasing order of size. The pairs numbered 1 to 22 are the autosomes, with the remaining pair of sex chromosomes consisting of two X-chromosomes in the female and one X and one Y in the male. The short and long arms of each chromosome are labelled p and q respectively.

The introduction of chromosome-banding techniques, which are rapidly becoming more sophisticated, has led to the identification of a plethora of chromosome syndromes resulting from loss or gain of even a tiny amount of visible chromosome material. It is perfectly possible that submicroscopic chromosome abnormalities may account for a large proportion of children with unexplained mental retardation or dysmorphic syndromes. Hopefully the future application of molecular genetic technology shall radically augment the definitive power of existing diagnostic chromosome analytical techniques.

Inheritance of disease

Disorders in which genetic factors are implicated can be considered under the following three headings.

Chromosomal

The normal human has 46 chromosomes, made up of 22 pairs of autosomes and a single pair of sex chromosomes, XX in the female and XY in the male. During meiosis each pair divides so that each gamete receives a single or haploid set. Fertilization results in restoration of the diploid chromosome constitution.

Any aberration of the autosomes resulting in loss or gain of chromosome material is likely to result in mental retardation and physical anomalies. Alterations in the sex chromosome constitution are generally less deleterious.

Most chromosome abnormalities occur as *de novo* events in a family, resulting from an error in gametogenesis in one of the parents. However, some chromosome rearrangements may exist in a balanced form in one of the parents, in which case there may be a previous history of similar problems in the family.

The implications of this for genetic counselling and family evaluation are discussed in the section on Down's syndrome.

Single gene (Mendelian)

Over 4000 conditions or traits showing probable single gene inheritance have been identified. A condition which is manifest in the heterozygote, who by definition has only one copy of the abnormal gene, is said to be dominant. A recessive disorder is expressed only in the homozygote, who has two copies of the abnormal gene having inherited one from each parent. If the abnormal gene is situated on an autosome, then the resulting condition is said to show autosomal dominant or recessive inheritance: if it is on the X-chromosome then the term sex-linkage is applied.

Polygenic or multifactorial

Many common conditions, including malformations such as spina bifida and disorders of adult life such as schizophrenia show a clear familial tendency which does not conform to any recognized mode of single gene inheritance. It is postulated that these disorders result from the interaction of an underlying familial predisposition, controlled by many genes at different loci (polygenic), with adverse environmental factors which are often poorly understood. It may well be that many different mechanisms contribute to the pathogenesis of multifactorial disorders.

Chromosome abnormalities

It is extremely difficult to gauge the incidence of chromosome abnormalities at conception since many have such a devastating effect on cell division and morphogenesis that implantation or subsequent establishment of pregnancy is not achieved. For example, trisomy of chromosome number 1 has never been observed in a naturally conceived human conceptus. Up to 50% of first trimester spontaneous abortions are chromosomally abnormal, with triploidy, monosomy X and various autosomal trisomies, particularly trisomy 16, featuring prominently. At least 90% of Turner's syndrome embryos and 60% of Down's syndrome embryos are spontaneously miscarried in early pregnancy.

By term the incidence of chromosome abnormalities has fallen to one in 200. Many of these babies die shortly before or after birth, accounting for 3–4% of total perinatal mortality in England and Wales. Others, particularly those with sex chromosome anomalies, may not present until adult life. Finally, there are undoubtedly many individuals with balanced rearrangements or insignificant abnormalities, such as 47,XXX, who never come to medical attention, other than by chance or, in the case of a balanced rearrangement by malsegregation resulting many years later in the birth of an abnormal child.

It is also worth noting that somatic acquired chromosome aberrations probably occur regularly in all humans and may, on rare occasions, be associated with the genesis of malignancy by altering the function of genes controlling cell division. It is postulated that the loci of these 'oncogenes' or their adjacent regulatory control genes are disrupted in some way by the chromosome rearrangement.

Down's syndrome (trisomy 21)

This condition derives its name from Dr Langdon Down who first described it in the Clinical Lecture

Reports of the London Hospital in 1866. However, children with Down's syndrome have probably been recognized since antiquity as several ancient paintings and carvings depicting the typical facial characteristics have been identified.

The incidence of Down's syndrome has been found to be approximately one in 650 to one in 750 in all ethnic communities in which it has been studied. At the chromosomal level this disorder is well understood, but the primary factors responsible for generating the chromosome abnormalities are largely unknown. Clues are provided by the well documented association with advanced maternal age and a tentative suggestion that a history of maternal exposure to diagnositc radiation may be relevant.

Table 8.1   Common abnormalities in Down's syndrome.

Neonatal
Hypotonia, lax joints and absent Moro reflex
Excess nuchal skin and 'well behaved'

Craniofacial
Brachycephaly and epicanthic folds
Upward slanting palpebral fissures
Brushfield spots in iris
Small ears and protruding tongue

Limbs
Small middle phalanx of fifth finger
Single palmar crease
High incidence of ulnar loops on fingers
Wide gap and plantar crease between first and second toes

Cardiac
Common atrioventricular canal
Atrial septal defect and ventricular septal defect
Patent ductus arteriosus
Tetralogy of Fallot

Other
Short stature and strabismus
Duodenal atresia and anal atresia
Increased incidence of leukaemia and thyroid disorders

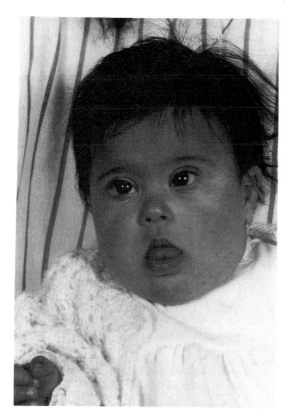

Fig. 8.2   A female infant with Down's syndrome.

CLINICAL FEATURES

The diagnosis of Down's syndrome is usually readily apparent at the first neonatal examination, but very small babies or those hidden by the paraphernalia of intensive care may present diagnostic difficulties. The characteristic features in the neonate are listed in Table 8.1. In infancy, muscle tone slowly improves as the familiar physical features become more obvious (Fig. 8.2). Cardiac anomalies account for the death of 15–20% of all Down's syndrome babies.

Down's syndrome children show a broad spectrum of intellectual ability with IQ scores ranging from 25 to 60. Social skills tend to be better developed than those parameters measured by IQ tests, and many Down's syndrome children are happy, friendly and thoroughly lovable.

Recently attention has focused on the intriguing observation that most adults with Down's syn-

drome develop pre-senile dementia in their fourth decade. The pathological findings in the brain are identical to those seen in Alzheimer's disease. In this relatively common disorder there is deposition of fibrillary amyloid proteins both within and outside cerebral neurones and blood vessels. The major protein subunit of this amyloid fibril is coded for by a gene on chromosome 21. Thus it appears that the pre-senile dementia commonly seen in Down's syndrome is a direct consequence of a primary gene dosage effect.

GENETIC ASPECTS

The chromosome findings in Down's syndrome are listed in Table 8.2. The additional number 21 chromosome in children with trisomy 21 is derived from the mother in 80% of cases. Presumably this relates in some way to the fundamental

Table 8.2 Chromosome abnormalities in Down's syndrome.

Trisomy 21 (e.g. 47,XY,+21)	95%
Mosaicism (e.g. 46,XY,/47,XY,+21)	2%
Translocation (e.g. 46,XY,−14,+t(14q21q)*	3%

*Karyotypes are described using a complex nomenclature system. In this example the child will be a male with Down's syndrome resulting from an unbalanced Robertsonian translocation involving the long arms of chromosomes number 14 and 21.

Table 8.3 Risk of Down's syndrome in relation to maternal age.*

Maternal age at delivery (years)	Incidence of Down's syndrome in liveborn infants
30	1 in 700
35	1 in 450
36	1 in 400
37	1 in 250
38	1 in 200
39	1 in 150
40	1 in 100
41	1 in 80
42	1 in 60
43	1 in 50
44	1 in 40
45	1 in 30

*The maternal age-specific risk of Down's syndrome tends to be higher in chorion villus biopsy and amniocentesis studies. Presumably this reflects preferential spontaneous loss of Down's syndrome conceptions throughout pregnancy.

differences in gametogenesis between the sexes and the well established maternal age effect. Risks for specific maternal age have been derived and are indicated in Table 8.3. Parents under age 35 years who have a baby with trisomy 21 can be quoted a recurrence risk for chromosome abnormality of approximately 1%. Over 35 years the maternal age specific risk is appropriate, although some authorities suggest that this should be increased by 1%. Advanced paternal age is of little or no significance.

About 2% of children with Down's syndrome show mosaicism for trisomy 21. In these indi-viduals cytogenetic studies reveal the existence of two cell lines, one normal and the other trisomy 21. These children tend to show clinical features intermediate in severity between normality and the classical trisomy 21 phenotype. The risk to future children for a couple who have a baby with mosaic trisomy 21 is probably comparable to that for a couple who have a child with full-blown trisomy 21.

Cytogenetic studies in the small remaining number of children with Down's syndrome show a translocation. This is usually of a particular type, known as Robertsonian, involving fusion at the centromeres of the long arms of one number 21 chromosome and one of the other acrocentric chromosomes (numbers 13, 14, 15, 21, 22). It is absolutely essential that parental chromosome studies are undertaken when a Down's syndrome child is found to have a translocation, since in about 25% of cases one of the parents will be found to carry the rearrangement in a balanced form. In the remaining 75% of cases the translocation will have arisen as a *de novo* event in gametogenesis and risks for future children will be as already outlined for trisomy 21.

Recurrence risks have been derived for the in-herited translocations and tend to be of the order of 2% if the father is the balanced carrier and 10% if it is the mother. In the very rare situation when one of the parents has a balanced 21 : 21 Robertso-nian translocation, the risk of Down's syndrome in liveborn offspring will be 100%. This is one of the very few occasions in genetic counselling when risks to offspring exceed 50%. Others include un-treated maternal phenylketonuria and marriages in which both partners have an autosomal domi-nant disease.

Trisomy 18 (Edwards' syndrome)

This disorder was first identified in 1960, shortly after it became possible to study human chromo-somes and 1 year after the chromosome abnor-mality in Down's syndrome was first identified. Trisomy 18 affects approximately one in 3000 newborn children and is more common in females than males. The prognosis is universally gloomy.

CLINICAL FEATURES

Frequently this disorder first presents during pregnancy when the baby is noted to be small for gestational age. An increased incidence of delivery by caesarean section has been noted. These babies tend to be scrawny at birth with reduced activity and a feeble cry.

Numerous abnormalities have been observed in trisomy 18, the most common of which are listed in Table 8.4. The diagnosis can usually be suspected by inspection of the face and hands (Fig. 8.3), which are invariably clenched with overlapping fingers and small fifth fingernails. This hand appearance is not pathognomonic for trisomy 18 and is also seen in certain forms of arthrogryposis. Cardiac abnormalities occur in 90% of cases and contribute to poor survival. Over 50% of these babies die within the first week of life and well over 90% have perished by the age of 1 year. Long-term survivors show very severe mental handicap.

GENETIC ASPECTS

In cases with typical clinical features chromosome studies almost always reveal straightforward trisomy 18. Very rarely there may be a translocation, or occasionally mosaicism may be found in less severely affected children. The mean maternal age at birth for these babies is increased when compared with the figures for all births (26 years in England and Wales). The recurrence risk for serious chromosome abnormality is 1%. For older mothers a risk figure of maternal age specific risk (see Table 8.3) plus 1% would be appropriate.

Trisomy 13 (Patau's syndrome)

Trisomy 13 shares many features in common with trisomy 18. It was first delineated in 1960, has an incidence of approximately one in 5000, and conveys an equally gloomy prognosis.

CLINICAL FEATURES

Babies with trisomy 13 are usually grossly abnormal. The more common features are listed in Table

Table 8.4 Clinical features of trisomy 18.

Craniofacial
Prominent occiput
Low set dysplastic ears
Narrow short palpebral fissures
Small mouth and micrognathia

Limbs
Clenched hands and overlapping fingers
Hypoplastic nails
Rocker bottom feet and talipes
Short dorsiflexed big toes

Cardiac
Ventricular and atrial septal defects
Patent ductus arteriosus
Coarctation of aorta
Bicuspid aortic valve

Other
Hypoplastic radii
Tracheo-oesophageal fistula
Oesophageal atresia
Short sternum
Cryptorchidism
Renal anomalies
Spina bifida

Table 8.5 Common clinical findings in trisomy 13.

Craniofacial
Microcephaly
Facies type I, holoprosencephaly and hypotelorism
Cyclops, absent philtrum and nares
Facies type II, microphthalmia and large bulbous nose
Cleft lip and palate
Small auricles, often low set
Occipital scalp defects

Limbs
Single palmar crease
Post-axial polydactyly
Hyperconvex nails

Cardiac
Atrial and ventricular septal defects
Patent ductus arteriosus and dextrocardia

Other
Single umbilical artery
Cryptorchidism
Exomphalos
Polycystic kidneys

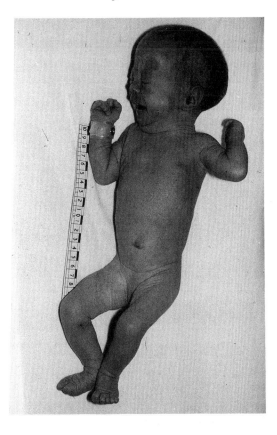

Fig. 8.3 A female infant with trisomy 18. Note the characteristic prominent occiput and clenched overlapping fingers.

8.5. Some babies show the typical facial appearance associated with holoprosencephaly in which there is hypotelorism, or even a single eye (cyclops), and agenesis of the premaxilla resulting in absence of nostrils and philtrum. Others show bilateral microphthalmos with bilateral cleft lip and palate and a large bulbous nose (Fig. 8.4). Scalp defects localized in the occipital region (Fig. 8.5) and post-axial polydactyly are characteristic, to the extent that a combination of these findings and a typical facies is strongly suggestive of the diagnosis.

Cardiac abnormalities occur in 80% of babies with trisomy 13 and neurological dysfunction, including convulsions, severe hypertonia and apnoeic spells, is common. At least 50% of babies with trisomy 13 die in the first month of life and survival beyond 1 year is very unusual. As with trisomy 18, long-term survival is associated with very severe mental retardation.

GENETIC ASPECTS

Chromosome studies show trisomy 13 in 80% of cases. The mothers of these children tend to be older than average and the recurrence risk is likely to be of the order of 1%. The remaining 20% show an unbalanced Robertsonian translocation most commonly involving the long arms of one number 13 and one number 14 chromosome (i.e. 46,XY,−14,+t(13q14q)). In these families parental chromosome studies are mandatory. A small number of children with mosaic trisomy 13 (46,XY/47,XY,+13) have been identified. These are usually much less severely affected than in the full-blown syndrome.

Turner's syndrome (45, X)

Dr Turner documented the classic clinical features of this condition in 1938. The absence of a Barr

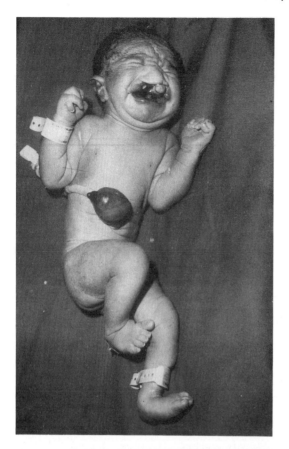

Fig. 8.4 A baby with trisomy 13. Obvious external abnormalities include bilateral cleft lip and palate, polydactyly and exomphalos.

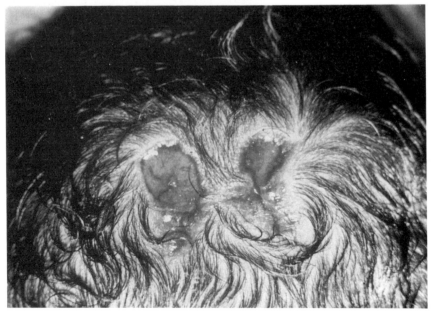

Fig. 8.5 Characteristic butterfly shaped occipital scalp defects often found in trisomy 13.

body, suggesting the presence of only one X-chromosome, was noted in 1954 and cytogenetic confirmation of this was forthcoming in 1959. This disorder is common after conception, but spontaneous pregnacy loss of approximately 97% of Turner's syndrome conceptions results in a live-born incidence of one in 5000 females.

Semantic confusion has arisen over use of the term 'male' Turner's syndrome. This is more correctly known as Noonan's syndrome, which shows autosomal dominant inheritance and affects both males and females.

CLINICAL FEATURES

Presentation may be in (a) pregnancy, (b) the newborn period, (c) childhood, or (d) adolescence.

Routine ultrasonography during the second trimester of pregnancy may show fetal oedema limited to the nuchal region or generalized. Thus Turner's syndrome features in the differential diagnosis of fetal hydrops, which includes Rhesus disease, α thalassaemia, congenital infection and severe cardiac failure. At birth, babies with Turner's syndrome may manifest the residue of this oedema with neck webbing, puffy hands and feet, and narrow hyperconvex nails (Fig. 8.6). Short stature may prompt investigation in childhood when other clinical stigmata may be apparent (Table 8.6). Finally, some patients do not present until adolescence with delayed puberty.

In the absence of a severe life-threatening cardiac malformation, which occurs only rarely, life expectancy in Turner's syndrome is normal.

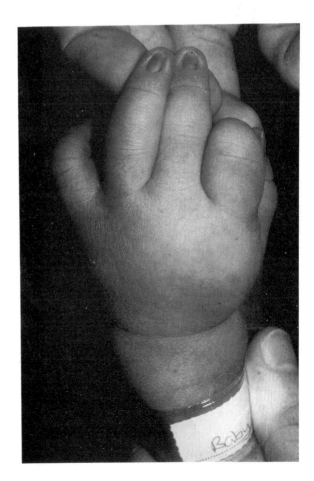

Fig. 8.6 Hand of a newborn baby with Turner's syndrome showing oedema and narrow hyperconvex nails.

Chapter 8

Table 8.6 Clinical features of Turner's syndrome.

Hallmarks
Short stature and ovarian dysgenesis

Craniofacial
Prominent ears
Neck webbing
Low posterior hairline
Ptosis

Limbs
Cubitus valgus
Short fourth metacarpal
Puffy hands and feet
Hyperconvex nails

Other
Coarctation of aorta
Horseshoe kidney
Shield chest
Madelung deformity
Conductive deafness (mild)

Intelligence is also normal contrary to inaccurate statements which have appeared in the past. Several women with Turner's syndrome have led very distinguished academic careers.

GENETIC ASPECTS

A 45,X karyotype is found in 50% of patients. The remaining 50% may show a variety of chromosome anomalies including mosaicism (e.g. 45,X/ 46,XX), a deletion of the short arm of one X-chromosome (46,X, del (Xp)) and an isochromosome of the long arm of one X-chromosome (46,X, i(Xq)). In 75% of 45,X cases the error has occurred in paternal gametogenesis, i.e. the X-chromosome which is present is maternal in origin. No formal studies of recurrence risk have been undertaken; for cases of 45,X this is likely to be very low.

Klinefelter's syndrome (47,XXY)

Dr Klinefelter and colleagues reported this condition in 1942. The presence of an additional X-chromosome was first demonstrated in 1959. The incidence in surveys of newborns is 1.5 per 1000 males, but it is quite probable that many cases never come to medical attention.

CLINICAL FEATURES

Boys with Klinefelter's syndrome show no dysmorphic features. Intellectual skills, particularly speech and reading, are mildly impaired and mean IQ is reduced by 15–20 points when compared with unaffected siblings.

Usually the diagnosis is first suspected during investigation of infertility. Gynaecomastia may be present and the testes are usually small and soft. Adult males are usually above average in height with a low upper to lower segment ratio. Other occasional findings include scoliosis, diabetes mellitus and lower leg skin ulcers. Treatment with testosterone is beneficial for development of secondary sexual characteristics and prevention of osteoporosis.

GENETIC ASPECTS

In 80% of cases, chromosome studies show a 47, XXY karyotype. The additional X-chromosome is maternally derived in 60% of cases and, as in the autosomal trisomies, there is a maternal age effect. The recurrence risk is low and certainly no greater than 1%.

The remaining 20% of cases show either mosaicism (e.g. 46,XY/47,XXY) or the presence of two or more additional X-chromosomes (e.g. 48,XXXY). This latter group of patients show marked hypogonadism and moderate to severe mental retardation.

Fragile X syndrome

For many years it has been recognized that severe mental retardation is more common in males than in females. Several studies have indicated that this is due to the existence of at least one form of sex-linked recessive mental retardation. Recently, it has emerged that in at least one-third of these families there is a strong association between the presence of retardation and a constriction or fragile site at the end of the long arm of one X-chromosome.

The fragile X-syndrome is now believed to be the second most common genetic cause, after Down's syndrome, of severe mental retardation, affecting one per 1000 newborn males.

CLINICAL FEATURES

Older boys and adult males have a recognizable facial appearance with high forehead, large ears, long face and prominent jaw. The irides are often a striking shade of pale blue. After puberty macro-orchidism is characteristic. Mild connective tissue weakness and skin striae have also been observed.

Mental retardation is usually moderate with a mean IQ of 50, although values lower than 30 have been recorded. Speech tends to be halting and repetitive. A history of convulsions is common and autistic behaviour may occur.

GENETIC ASPECTS

Although this condition shows a clear association with the fragile site on the X-chromosome, the mode of inheritance is not that of simple recessive sex-linkage. One-third of female heterozygotes show mild intellectual impairment, whereas some males who must have transmitted the causative agent to a daughter, are of normal intelligence. One theory postulates that the fragile X-gene, or genes, may exist in a pre-mutated unstable state, which only causes mental retardation when it changes to the abnormal form following recombination with another X-chromosome during meiosis in females. Much remains to be learned about the genesis of this curious but very important disorder.

Investigation of a family is complicated further by the difficulties which arise in demonstrating the fragile site in karyotypes derived from cultured lymphocytes. Affected males rarely show the abnormality in more than 40% of cells, and in some obligatory carrier females no abnormality whatever can be demonstrated. Thus genetic counselling involves very careful painstaking evaluation of each family.

Autosomal dominant disorders

Well over 1000 conditions showing autosomal dominant inheritance have been described. These may present at birth, and thus justify the label congenital, or they may not be manifest until late adult life. The effects may be limited to a single organ or body system, or may involve several different systems, a phenomenon known as pleiotropy. Some of the more common autosomal dominant disorders are listed in Table 8.7

Figure 8.7 shows a pedigree in which the typical features of autosomal dominant inheritance are apparent. Males and females are affected in equal numbers and each may transmit the condition to sons or daughters. Thus the condition is said to show 'vertical' inheritance affecting members of each generation.

When an affected individual has children, then there is a 50% chance that each child, male or female, will inherit the abnormal gene. Thus on average 50% of offspring will be affected, although by the laws of chance, some sibships will have more than 50% of members affected, others less. The situation is analogous to that of tossing a coin.

Occasionally two people with the same autosomal dominant condition marry and wish to know of possible risks to children. These are as indicated in Figure 8.8. Often, as in achondroplasia, a baby receiving a double dose of the abnormal gene will be so severely affected that long-term survival is very unlikely. For many autosomal dominant conditions the homozygous state is probably lethal, resulting in early pregnancy loss.

Sometimes an autosomal dominant disorder may appear to skip a generation. If examination of the obligatory gene 'carrier' shows no abnormality, then the disorder is said to show reduced penetrance. For example, only 80% of individuals with the gene for the autosomal dominant form of retinoblastoma, an embryonic tumour of the retina, actually develop the tumour (p. 470). Thus penetrance equals 0.8, so that any child of someone with the inherited form of retinoblastoma runs a risk of 40% (50% × 0.8) for developing this tumour.

Table 8.7 Examples of autosomal dominant disorders (many of which are discussed in detail elsewhere in this book).

System	Principal clinical features
Skeletal and connective tissue	
Achondroplasia	Large head, short stature and short limbs
Marfan's syndrome	Tall stature, lens dislocation and aortic aneurysm
Osteogenesis imperfecta	Brittle bones, blue sclerae and deafness
Malformations	
Apert's syndrome	Craniosynostosis and syndactyly
Holt–Oram syndrome	Atrial septal defect and thumb abnormality
Noonan's syndrome	Pulmonary stenosis, ptosis and neck webbing
Phakomatosis	
Neurofibromatosis	Cafe-aù-lait patches and neurofibromata
Tuberose sclerosis	Adenoma sebaceum and depigmented naevi
Neurological	
Huntington's chorea	Adult onset chorea and dementia
Myotonic dystrophy	Myotonia, muscle weakness and wasting
Peroneal muscular atrophy	Distal muscle weakness and wasting
Gastrointestinal	
Peutz–Jeghers syndrome	Oral freckling and intestinal polyps
Polyposis coli	Intestinal polyps, and high risk of malignancy
Haematological and metabolic	
Familial hypercholesterolaemia	Xanthomata and coronary artery disease
Spherocytosis	Mild haemolysis
Von Willebrand's disease	Haemorrhage and factor VIII deficiency
Renal	
Adult polycystic kidney disease	Renal cysts and renal failure
Alport's syndrome (some forms)	Nephritis and deafness

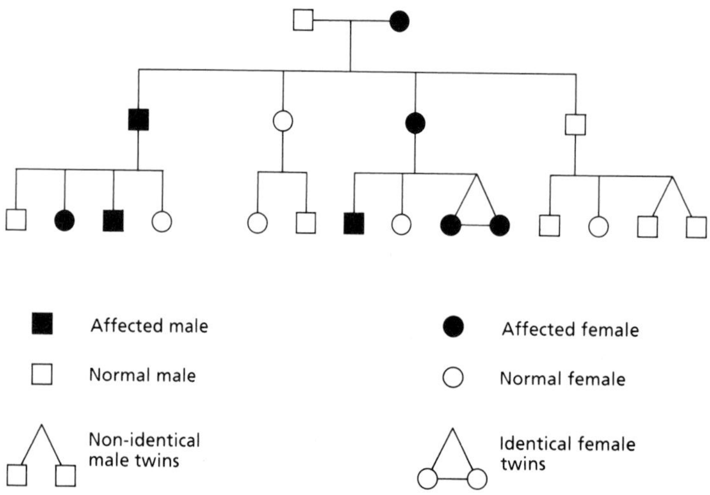

■	Affected male	● Affected female
□	Normal male	○ Normal female
Non-identical male twins		Identical female twins

Fig. 8.7 A pedigree illustrating autosomal dominant inheritance.

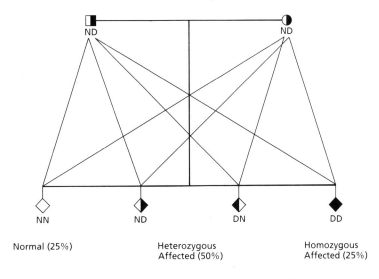

Fig. 8.8 Risks for the offspring of two individuals who have the same autosomal dominant disorder. On average one child in four will be normal (NN), two in four will be affected (ND and DN) and the remaining one in four will be homozygously affected (DD), a condition which is often incompatible with survival.

For many autosomal dominant conditions, the degree of severity varies from person to person even within a family. This phenomenon of variable expression or expressivity is epitomized by tuberose sclerosis which may cause severe mental retardation in some individuals and only minor skin anomalies in others. This emphasizes the importance of careful examination of all relevant family members in genetic counselling.

All autosomal dominant conditions have to start somewhere. The individual in whom the condition first occurs is referred to as representing the new mutation. The risk to each child of this person will be 50%. The precise causes of mutations are unknown, but one clue is provided by an association with advanced paternal age. Thus in several autosomal dominant disorders, such as achondroplasia and Apert's syndrome, the mean paternal age at birth of children representing new mutations will be slightly but significantly greater than the mean paternal age in the general population (approximately 29 years in England and Wales). Overall, however, the risk of a new mutation in the offspring of an older father is much smaller than the risk of chromosome abnormality in older mothers, and for genetic counselling purposes a figure of 0.5% is appropriate for a 50-year-old man planning to have a child.

Autosomal recessive disorders

Autosomal recessive inheritance has been established beyond all doubt for approximately 600 disorders. As with diseases showing autosomal dominant inheritance, all systems of the body may be affected, but in contrast to autosomal dominant disorders, which tend to present as major structural anomalies, autosomal recessive conditions

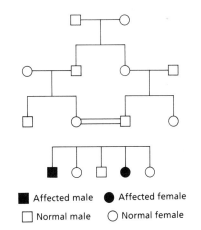

Fig 8.9 A pedigree showing autosomal recessive inheritance. In this family the parents of the affected children are first cousins. There is an increased incidence of consanguinity amongst the parents of children with rare autosomal recessive disorders.

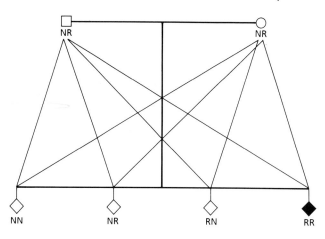

Fig. 8.10 Autosomal recessive inheritance. Two out of three healthy siblings are hererozygous for the abnormal allele (R).

often result in enzyme deficiencies. Most inborn errors of metabolism show autosomal recessive inheritance.

A typical autosomal recessive pedigree is portrayed in Fig. 8.9. Generally equal numbers of males and females are affected. Individuals with autosomal recessive conditions are usually limited to a single sibship within a family, i.e. 'horizontal' inheritance as opposed to the 'vertical' pattern seen in autosomal dominant inheritance.

The mechanism underlying autosomal recessive inheritance is illustrated in Fig. 8.10. When two carriers have children, on average one in four of their offspring will be homozygous normal (NN), two in four will be heterozygous like their parents (NR and RN) and the remaining one in four will be homozygous for the abnormal gene (RR) and will be affected. Thus since two out of three healthy siblings will be heterozygous, the likelihood that the healthy sibling of someone with an autosomal recessive disorder will be a carrier equals two in three.

This information can be utilized in determining risks to various family members for having an affected child. Consider the healthy sister of someone with cystic fibrosis. There is a two in three probability that this lady is a carrier. The likelihood that her healthy and unrelated spouse, who has no family history of cystic fibrosis, is a carrier will be the incidence of carriers in the general population from which these individuals are

drawn. This can be calculated using Hardy–Weinberg equilibrium by multiplying the square root of the incidence of the disease by two. Thus if the general population incidence is $1:1600$, the carrier incidence will be $2 \times 1:40$ which equals $1:20$. Thus it can be concluded that the risk of cystic fibrosis in the first child of this couple will be $2:3 \times 1:20 \times 1:4$ which equals $1:120$.

Most individuals in the general population carry at least one recessive gene. Thus if close blood relatives marry they may both carry the same deleterious recessive gene by descent from a common ancestor. This explains why rare recessive disorders occur more commonly in the offspring of consanguineous parents. Very rarely, in highly inbred communities a phenomenon known as pseudodominance may be observed. This occurs when an affected homozygote marries a carrier and they then have an affected child, thus simulating the vertical inheritance pattern seen in autosomal dominant disorders.

Several autosomal recessive conditions are known to have a high incidence in particular ethnic communities. Common examples are given in Table 8.8. Possible reasons for this include (a) a founder effect, (b) social, geographical and hence genetic isolation of a sub-group, and (c) heterozygote advantage implying that carriers have a biological and hence reproductive advantage over non-carriers. When carrier detection tests are available, as is the case for Tay Sach's disease and

Table 8.8 Autosomal recessive disorders showing high incidence in particular ethnic groups.

Ethnic group	Disorder
Afro-Caribbeans	Sickle cell disease
Ashkenazi Jews	Familial dysautonomia
	Tay Sach's disease
Caucasians	Cystic fibrosis
Eskimos	Congenital adrenal hyperplasia
Finns	Congenital nephrosis
Greek-Cypriots	β thalassaemia
Norwegians	α_1-antitrypsin deficiency

the haemoglobinopathies, screening of the relevant population can be offered aimed at alerting heterozygotes to their carrier status. Programmes of this nature have been initiated for thalassaemia in the Greek-Cypriot community with considerable success.

Sex-linked disorders

Sex-linkage, or more precisely X-linkage, has been confirmed beyond all doubt for approximately 140 disorders. These range in severity from entirely trivial problems such as red–green colour blindness which affects one in 10 males, to very much more serious and fortunately much rarer conditions such as haemophilia and Duchenne muscular dystrophy. Some of the more common X-linked disorders which present in childhood are listed in Table 8.9.

The mechanism of inheritance is illustrated in Fig. 8.11. The abnormal gene is located on the X-chromosome. The heterozygous or 'carrier' female is protected from the effects of a recessive gene on one X-chromosome by the normal allele on her other X-chromosome. However, the hemizygous male will be at the mercy of any recessive mutation on his X-chromosome since the Y chromosome, with very few exceptions, is not homologous to the X.

A typical X-linked recessive pedigree is shown in Fig. 8.12. On average a heterozygous female will transmit the abnormal gene to half her daughters, who will thus be carriers, and to half her sons who will be affected. A male will transmit the abnormal gene to all his daughters, who will therefore be obligatory carriers, and to none of his sons. Thus male to male transmission cannot occur in X-linked inheritance. This pattern of transmission has been likened to that of the 'knight's move' in chess.

Rarely a female may manifest an X-linked recessive disorder. This may be due to:
1 Homozygosity due to inheritance of two abnormal alleles, one from her carrier mother and one from her affected father.
2 Turner's syndrome, in which only one X-chromosome is present.

Table 8.9 Clinical features and examples of X-linked disorders.

Recessive	
Red–green colour blindness	Mildly impaired colour vision
Glucose-6-phosphate dehydrogenase deficiency	Drug-induced haemolysis
Haemophilia A	Haemorrhage, factor VIII deficiency
Haemophilia B (Christmas disease)	Haemorrhage, factor IX deficiency
Bruton's agammaglobulinaemia	Recurrent bacterial infection
Duchenne muscular dystrophy	Progressive muscle weakness, pseudohypertrophy.
Lesch–Nyhan syndrome	Neurodegeneration, self-mutilation
Dominant	
Pseudohypoparathyroidism	Short stature, obesity, cataracts
Vitamin D-resistant rickets	Rickets, low serum phosphate
Dominant	
Incontinentia pigmenti	Abnormalities of teeth, eyes and skin pigmentation; lethal in males

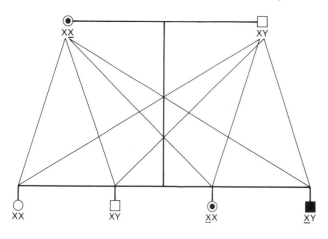

Fig. 8.11 Sex-linked recessive inheritance. The chromosome with the abnormal gene is underlined, i.e. X̲. Carrier females are denoted as ◉.

3 A skewed pattern of lyonization in a heterozygote, in which by chance the X-chromosome bearing the normal allele is inactivated in well over 50% of cells.

Carrier detection of X-linked recessive disorders in females can be extremely difficult for several reasons. For example, it may be that cells in which the X-chromosome bearing the normal allele is active have an enormous advantage over cells in which the X-chromosome bearing the abnormal gene is active; thus the majority of cells in the carrier female will be normal. Alternatively, cells in which the X-chromosome bearing the normal allele is active may be able to correct the biochemical error in cells in which the other X-chromosome is active, so that study of tissue

biochemistry *in vitro* will be unhelpful. Some of these difficulties have been bypassed using new molecular genetic techniques which rely on direct analysis of the genes rather than their products or secondary effects.

A few conditions, such as vitamin D-resistant rickets and pseudohypoparathyroidism, show X-linked dominant inheritance, in which the effects of the mutation on the X-chromosome are manifest in the female, albeit usually to a lesser degree than in the male. Some X-linked dominant conditions, such as incontinentia pigmenti, appear to be lethal in the male, so that the disorder is seen only in females.

The Y-chromosome appears to carry only a few expressed genes consisting chiefly of a testis deter-

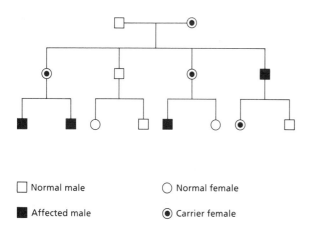

☐ Normal male

■ Affected male

○ Normal female

◉ Carrier female

Fig. 8.12 A pedigree showing sex-linked recessive inheritance. All of the daughters of an affected male will be obligatory carriers.

Table 8.10 Empiric recurrence risks for common multifactorial malformations.

Disorder	Incidence	Recurrence risk for siblings (%)
Neural tube defects	1:300	5
Cleft lip ± cleft palate	1:500	2–6*
Pyloric stenosis	1:300	2–10*
Congenital dislocation of the hip	1:200	1–10*
Congenital heart disease:		
Ventricular septal defect	1:400	4
Atrial septal defect	1:1000	3
Patent ductus arteriosus	1:1000	3

*Recurrence risk varies depending on degree of severity or sex of index case (see text).

mining factor. Holandric (Y-linked) inheritance has not been confirmed for any human disorders, with the possible exception of the male family surname!

Polygenic or multifactorial disorders

Multifactorial inheritance, implying the interaction of adverse environmental factors on an underlying polygenic predisposition, has been postulated for many of the more common malformations. Complex mathematical models have been derived to calculate recurrence risks for various relatives based on the proportion of genes shared with the affected individual and the incidence of the disorder in the general population.

For most of the presumed multifactorial conditions listed in Table 8.10, the calculated risks for first degree relatives (siblings and offspring) tend to correspond closely with figures obtained from large family studies. These are known as 'empiric' risks and are widely used in genetic counselling.

According to the multifactorial model, risks to relatives will be greater if:

1 More than one close family member is affected. For example, for neural tube defects, the risk to the sibling of one affected child is 5%, but rises to 12% if there are two affected children in the sibship.

2 The index case is very severely affected. Thus the risk of facial clefting for the sibling of someone with isolated cleft lip is 2% but a figure of 6% is quoted if the index case has bilateral cleft lip and palate.

3 The index case belongs to the sex which is only rarely affected. This suggests that he or she must have more 'bad' genes than affected individuals of the opposite sex. Thus for pyloric stenosis, which shows a male to female ratio of 5:1, a much higher risk is quoted for the sibling of an affected girl (10%) than for the sibling of an affected boy (2%).

Much remains to be learned about the precise mechanisms underlying multifactorial inheritance. Already the molecular biologists are exploring ways of identifying particular genes or patterns of genes (haplotypes) which may confer susceptibility. This strategy is likely to have considerable implications for the prevention of late onset multifactorial conditions such as hypertension and diabetes mellitus if individuals at high risk can be identified.

Meanwhile it seems more appropriate to pursue environmental factors which may be implicated, an approach which has already proved fruitful for neural tube defects. Provisional results from several UK centres suggest that the recurrence risk of neural tube defects can be reduced substantially if 'at risk' mothers take particular vitamin supplements before and during early pregnancy. The results of these studies remain somewhat controversial and await confirmation, but they do point the way to a universally acceptable means of true or primary prevention.

Genetic counselling

Essentially genetic counselling is concerned with the provision of information. It can be seen as a non-judgemental communication process by which patients and/or relatives are alerted to (a) the nature of the disorder for which their children may be at risk; (b) the probability of developing or transmitting it; and (c) the approaches which can be employed for prevention or amelioration.

There are several important steps involved in the genetic counselling process. First, and by far the most important is establishing the diagnosis. Many inherited disorders show genetic heterogeneity so that the same clinical picture (phenotype) can result from different genetic errors (genotype). Thus lengthy investigations and family studies are often necessary if correct conclusions are to be reached. Without the correct diagnosis, wrong information may be imparted with tragic consequences.

Secondly, the imparting of information in a sympathetic and comprehensible fashion. This requires time and a relaxed informal atmosphere. If parents are going to make fundamental decisions about future children they are entitled to more than a few minutes discussion in a busy clinic.

Consideration of possible options for reducing or avoiding risks is essential so that patients may be fully informed about possible carrier tests or prenatal diagnosis. This is obviously an area which has to be handled with tact and sensitivity. There

has been very rapid progress in prenatal diagnostic techniques to the extent that some means of attempting this can now be offered for most disorders.

It cannot be overstressed that no attempt should be made to be directive. The counsellor's role is to provide information about risks, implications and options, rather than to indicate to patients what they should do. Paternalistic directive counselling may be well intended, but it is the patient, not the doctor, who has to live with the consequences. Thus the entire process is orientated towards ensuring that patients may reach their own informed decisions about future childbearing fully equipped with all of the relevant facts.

The potential complexity of this lengthy process is amply illustrated by the family shown in Fig. 8.13. in which three males have, or have had, Duchenne muscular dystrophy. Individual III-2 wishes to know if she is a carrier of this X-linked recessive disorder, and if so whether prenatal diagnostic tests can be carried out in early pregnancy.

Having reviewed the family history and confirmed the diagnosis, it can be concluded that individual III-2 commenced life with a 50% chance of being a carrier. Until recently the only carrier test of any possible value was assay of serum creatine kinase, an enzyme which leaks out of dystrophic muscle. All affected males show very high levels of creatine kinase activity, whereas mildly elevated

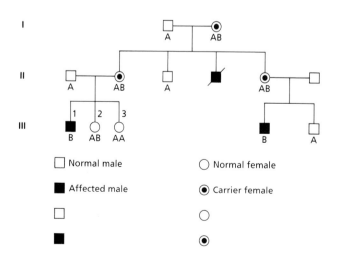

Fig. 8.13 Pedigree of a family in which Duchenne muscular dystrophy is segregating. The letters A and B indicate polymorphic marker alleles at a locus very closely linked to the disease locus. Inspection of the pedigree indicates that it is the grand-maternal B allele which is on the same chromosome as the disease gene. Thus III-2 is very likely to be a carrier and any of her male offspring with the B allele will be affected.

levels are noted in approximately 65% of carriers.

Over the last few years a new approach to carrier detection and prenatal diagnosis has evolved using molecular genetic techniques. The ability to analyse DNA using (a) restriction enzymes, which cleave DNA at specific sequences, and (b) gene probes derived from different parts of the X-chromosome, has resulted in the detection of polymorphic (showing normal variation) X-chromosome loci, closely linked to the Duchenne locus. By tracking the co-segregation of the disease and closely adjacent 'linked' polymorphic markers, it is now often possible to predict with precision whether or not a woman such as III-2 in Fig. 8.13 is or is not a carrier.

Thus for the family in Fig. 8.13, it is apparent that the Duchenne gene is co-segregating with marker B. If linkage between this marker locus and the Duchenne gene is known to be tight, i.e. the loci are so close together that recombination in meiosis is very unlikely, then it is highly probable that III-2 is a carrier and equally probable that III-3 is not. Prenatal diagnosis could be offered by analysis of material obtained by chorion biopsy during the first trimester. This is a considerable advance on the non-selective termination of a male pregnancy which was all that could be offered until very recently.

The investigation and evaluation of a family such as this is a lengthy and complex process, which should be undertaken well in advance of a planned pregnancy. The introduction of these novel techniques for the study of conditions such as the haemoglobinopathies, cystic fibrosis and Duchenne muscular dystrophy has enabled many couples who would otherwise have had no further children, to embark upon subsequent pregnancies secure in the knowledge that their future baby stands as good a chance as any other child of being perfectly healthy.

Further reading

Connor JM, Ferguson-Smith MA. *Essential Medical Genetics*, 3rd Edn. Blackwell Scientific Publications, Oxford 1990.

Emery AEH, Mueller RF. *Elements of Medical Genetics*, 7th Edn. Churchill-Livingstone, Edinburgh 1988.

Harper PS. *Practical Genetic Counselling*, 3rd Edn. John Wright & Sons Ltd, Bristol 1988.

McKusick VA. *Mendelian Inheritance in Man*, 8th Edn. Johns Hopkins University Press, Baltimore 1988.

9
CONGENITAL ABNORMALITIES APPARENT AT BIRTH

Approximately 2% of all infants born in the UK have a congenital malformation and Table 9.1 lists the incidence of some of the commoner congenital abnormalities. Some of these lesions are obvious at birth and others become apparent with the passage of time.

A congenital abnormality may be due to either a malformation, a deformation or a disruption.

1 *Malformation* refers to abnormal development of a tissue or organ.

2 *Deformation* refers to a tissue which has developed normally but has been adversely affected by external forces. Talipes is an example of this type of abnormality.

3 *Disruption* refers to a tissue which has developed normally to begin with but is then injured by

Table 9.1 Frequency and expected incidence of congenital malformations (diagnosed in the first week of life) in the UK for 1982 (OPCS).

	Rate/ 1000 births	Expected incidence
Total malformations	21.1	1:30
Central nervous system	1.6	1:300
Eye	0.2	1:3000
Ear	1.0	1:600
Cleft lip and/or cleft palate	1.4	1:500
Intestinal	0.7	1:900
Cardiovascular system	1.4	1:400
External genitalia	1.4	1:300
Limbs	8.0	1:75
Chromosomal	1.0	1:600

Table 9.2 Some teratogenic factors associated with congenital malformations or deformations.

Drugs
Thalidomide
Anti-neoplastic agents
Sex hormones (progestogen, oestrogen)

Toxins
Alcohol
Heroin
Cocaine
?Tobacco smoking

Infection
Rubella
Cytomegalovirus
Toxoplasmosis

Maternal disease
Diabetes
Phenylketonuria
Hyperthyroidism

Irradiation
X-rays
Nuclear power station accidents
Radio-iodine

Fever
Maternal infection
Sauna

Compression
Oligohydramnios
Abnormal uterus

some process which causes it to break down. Common causes of disruption are infection (cytomegalovirus) or vascular abnormality (infarction).

The aetiology of congenital malformations is often multifactorial but genetic factors are a major contributor, as discussed in Chapter 8. The incidence of some of the common malformations is shown in Table 8.10. The interaction of a genetic predisposition with environmental factors is particularly important. A teratogen is a factor which causes malformation or deformation and some of the better recognized teratogenic agents are listed in Table 9.2.

This chapter is not a comprehensive review of all congenital abnormalities but discusses some common conditions obvious at, or shortly after, birth. Many congenital abnormalities are discussed in the appropriate chapter dealing with the relevant organ system.

Syndromes

A syndrome is a constellation of abnormalities which together represent a recognizable developmental defect. They may be genetic or secondary to the action of external agents such as drugs. Approximately 30% of syndromes are due to a chromosomal or genetic anomaly. Table 9.3 lists some of the common syndromes based on a chromosomal defect. Table 9.4 summarizes some of the commoner non-chromosomal syndromes and indicates whether they show a distinctive pattern of inheritance. Some of these conditions are described in more detail elsewhere.

Table 9.3 Commoner syndromes due to a chromosomal abnormality.

Down's syndrome (trisomy 21)	see p. 119
Edward's syndrome (trisomy 18)	see p. 121
Patau's syndrome (trisomy 13)	see p. 122
Turner's syndrome (45,X)	see p. 123
Klinefelter's syndrome (47,XXY)	see p. 126
Fragile X syndrome	see p. 126

Gastrointestinal malformations

These may involve structures from mouth to anus.

Table 9.4 Some inherited syndromes apparent at, or shortly, after birth.

	Description	Mental retardation	Inheritance
Beckwith–Wiedemann	Large tongue Exompholos Pancreatic islet cell hyperplasia with hypoglycaemia	No	Sporadic
Crouzon	Proptosis Craniosynostosis of facial bones and abnormal facies	No	Dominant with variable expression
Apert	Craniosynostosis Abnormal facies Abnormalities of the hand	Unusual	Dominant many cases are new mutations)
Laurence–Moon–Biedl	Obesity Polydactyly Retinal pigmentation Genital hypoplasia	Yes	Autosomal recessive
Pierre Robin	See p. 138	No	Sporadic

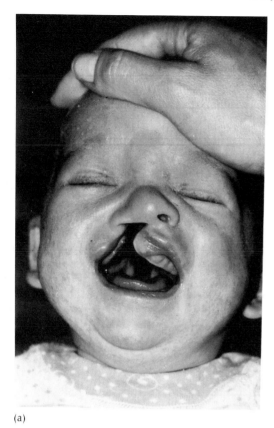
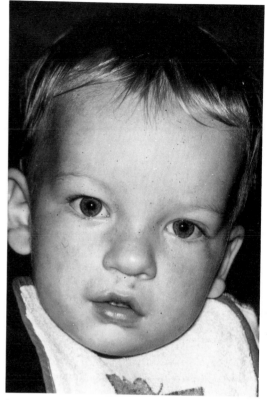

(a)   (b)

Fig. 9.1 Cleft lip and palate. (a) At birth the infant has a right-sided cleft lip and palate. (b) The same infant following surgical repair.

Cleft lip and palate

Cleft lip generally occurs to one side of the midline (Fig. 9.1), may be single or bilateral and may exist alone or in association with a cleft palate. It occurs in 1:1000 births and has a polygenic form of inheritance. A median cleft lip and palate is very rare and is usually associated with cranial abnormalities and/or trisomy 13.

Cleft palate is a common condition with an incidence of 1:400. In its mildest form it exists as a cleft of the uvula and progressively more severe forms are represented by cleft of the soft palate and cleft of both the hard and soft palate. Bony clefting with intact mucosa or palatal musculature defect may occur and this is referred to as the submucous cleft. It may be difficult to diagnose at birth. A lateral cleft palate is usually associated

with cleft lip but a midline cleft palate is rarely associated with lip involvement.

PIERRE ROBIN SYNDROME

In this condition there is severe under-development of the lower jaw, referred to as micrognathia (Fig. 9.2), and is often associated with a cleft palate. The main problem associated with Pierre Robin syndrome, other than the cosmetic appearance, is the tendency for the tongue to fall back into the throat (glossoptosis) causing respiratory obstruction with cyanotic spells. These infants should be nursed prone and a special frame may be necessary. This problem is usually self-limiting as catch-up growth of the lower jaw often occurs over the first 6 months of life when the problem of respiratory obstruction recedes.

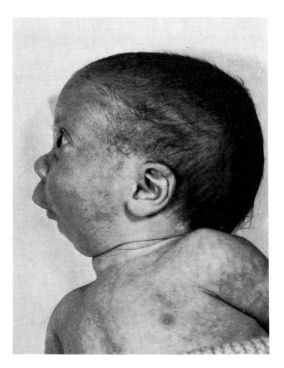

Fig. 9.2 Pierre Robin syndrome showing micrognathia. This infant also had a median cleft palate.

Treatment

Cleft lip is an unsightly condition which causes much parental distress. Both parents must be seen as soon after birth as possible and it is helpful to show them photographs taken before and after surgery to show the excellent outcome following surgery (see Fig. 9.1). Serious feeding problems rarely occur with cleft lip alone although there is often dribbling of milk from the mouth. The lip is usually closed surgically at about 6–12 weeks.

Cleft palate is commonly associated with severe feeding problems. Although some babies do feed well from the breast or teat, in many, a specially long (lamb's) teat or flanged (Great Ormond Street) teat is used. An acrylic obturator may be helpful where feeding remains a problem. These are made by a dental technician and when *in situ* produce an artifical palate. This oral appliance may stimulate the growth of the underdeveloped maxilla. Surgical closure of the palate is usually undertaken at about 9 months of age and well before the acquisition of speech.

Prognosis

The child with a cleft palate is particularly at risk of a number of important complications.
1 Unclear speech. Particular attention must be paid to speech as nasal escape and poor articulation are anticipated. The parents should be introduced to a speech therapist after the birth who is experienced in the care of these children.
2 Hearing impairment. These children are particularly prone to development of recurrent otitis media and conductive deafness. Regular hearing assessment and ENT supervision are essential.
3 Dental development. Cleft palate often involves the gum and close orthodontic supervision should be maintained throughout childhood.

Oesophageal atresia and tracheo-oesophageal fistula (TOF)

This is a common congenital abnormality with a frequency of approximately 1 : 2500 births. Oesophageal atresia is associated with tracheo-oesophageal fistula in 95% of cases. In 85%, the fistula occurs at the lower end of the trachea and communicates with the lower oesphageal pouch. The varieties of this condition are shown in Fig. 9.3. TOF is associated with other major congenital abnormalities in about 30% of cases. These involve the heart, kidneys, vertebrae, limbs and anus.

Clinical features

The pregnancy is often complicated by polyhydramnios because the fetus cannot swallow amniotic fluid. At birth the baby is 'bubbly' due to an inability to swallow secretions. If this is ignored the infant will become acutely ill at the first feed due to aspiration of milk into the lungs.

The rare form of an H-type fistula may not present immediately and is often suspected in infants with episodes of recurrent aspiration of milk.

Investigations

Confirmation of the diagnosis of the oesophageal atresia is made by passing a stiff (size 10 FG)

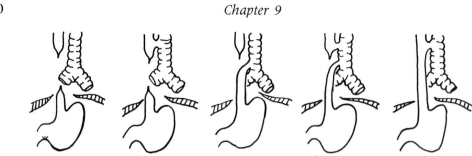

Fig. 9.3 Five variants of tracheo-oesophageal fistula, with or without oesophageal atresia. Type c accounts for over 85% of all cases.

radio-opaque nasogastric feeding tube into the oesophagus and determining the level at which it obstructs. A plain X-ray is helpful to confirm the level of obstruction. In the presence of oesophageal atresia, gas in the stomach confirms that there must be a tracheo-oesophageal fistula.

Diagnosis of an H-type fistula may be much more difficult and may require contrast studies or cine swallow radiography.

Management

Once the diagnosis has been made the infant should be nursed in a head-up position to avoid reflux of gastric secretions through the fistula into the lungs resulting in a chemical pneumonitis. In addition, secretions collecting in the upper pouch should be continuously drained by means of a Replogle catheter and suction pump.

The definitive treatment is surgical and involves tying off the fistula and anastamosing the two ends of the oesophagus. If this is not possible initially, an oesophagostomy is performed with subsequent further surgical treatment.

Prognosis

A number of major problems may develop in these infants. These include stenosis at the site of the anastomosis with dysphagia, gastro-oesophageal reflux and tracheomalacia or bronchomalacia. These infants often develop an unpleasant barking cough which is distressing.

Table 9.5 Causes of gastrointestinal obstruction presenting in the neonatal period.

Anatomical	Functional
Oesophageal atresia	Pyloric stenosis
Duodenal atresia	Hirschsprung's disease
Jejunal atresia	Meconium plug syndrome
Volvulus due to malrotation	Meconium ileus
Colon atresia	
Stricture secondary to necrotizing enterocolitis	

Congenital intestinal obstruction

Intestinal obstruction, presenting shortly after birth, can be divided into anatomical and functional causes (Table 9.5). It is a common condition and occurs in 1 : 1000 births.

There are four major features of intestinal obstruction:
1 Bile-stained vomiting.
2 Failure to pass meconium.
3 Abdominal distension.
4 Visible peristalsis.

If the obstruction is high in the gastrointestinal tract then abdominal distension may not be seen and the infant may pass copious amounts of meconium from below the obstruction. The stool, however, does not show a change from meconium to products of milk digestion.

Bile-stained vomiting is always abnormal and strongly suggests obstruction. In the rare case of early pyloric stenosis, the vomitus does not contain bile.

Table 9.6 Causes of abdominal distension presenting in the neonatal period.

Gastrointestinal obstruction
Ascites
Massive hepatomegaly
Hydronephrosis
Distended bladder
   Urethral valves
   Denervation (spina bifida)
Pneumoperitoneum
Tumour (rare)

Abdominal distension in the neonatal period suggests intestinal obstruction but the other causes must be considered and these are listed in Table 9.6.

Investigations

In all infants with obstruction, dehydration must be carefully considered. Vomiting for only a short time in a newly born baby may cause major electrolyte disturbances. Measurements of electrolytes and urea should be made regularly. An erect and supine abdominal radiograph is the most useful diagnostic test. These will demonstrate dilated loops of bowel and fluid levels. It is not possible in many cases to diagnose the level of obstruction based on the radiological appearances, with the exception of duodenal atresia. In this condition the classical 'double bubble' is seen on the erect film (Fig. 9.4). If the obstructed bowel is ischaemic, perforation may occur, leading to free air in the peritoneal cavity which is usually visible on the X-ray film. Contrast studies may be helpful to delineate the site of obstruction, particularly if Hirschprung's disease or meconium ileus is suspected.

Management

Careful fluid management is mandatory. The child should be rehydrated and the electrolyte imbalance corrected. Any bile-stained aspirate should be replaced with intravenous normal saline, volume for volume, in addition to the child's normal fluid requirements.

Once the diagnosis of intestinal obstruction has been made, the opinion of a paediatric surgeon should be urgently obtained. Provided that the infant is well hydrated and in good condition,

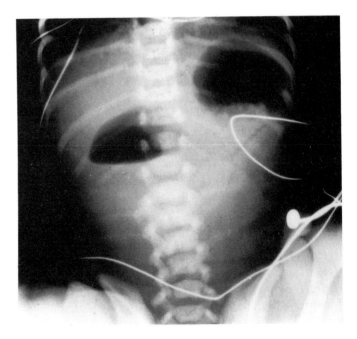

Fig. 9.4 Erect abdominal X-ray showing the 'double bubble' sign characteristic of duodenal atresia.

nothing will be gained by a period of conservative treatment in infants with anatomical obstruction. In some infants with functional obstruction, a decision may be made to observe the child to see if spontaneous resolution occurs. If this is done the child must be regularly reassessed by an experienced paediatrician every 4–6 hours.

The management of intestinal obstruction is usually surgical. An end-to-end anastomosis is usually performed for simple atretic segment provided the bowel looks healthy. In the presence of an unhealthy bowel or where it is unsafe to rely on an anastomosis, an ileostomy or colostomy should be fashioned in healthy bowel proximal to the site of obstruction.

Duodenal atresia

This may be either due to atresia or extrinsic obstruction by means of Ladd's peritoneal bands. It occurs relatively commonly in association with Down's syndrome. Rarely an annular pancreas may constrict the duodenum.

Small bowel atresia

Jejunal atresia is a relatively common isolated abnormality, although multiple atretic sites may occur. Evidence suggests that some cases may be due to compromise of the bowel blood supply *in utero*. This is often a disruption rather than a malformation.

Malrotation

During the course of bowel development, the gut is temporarily outside the abdomen, which then rotates and is withdrawn back into the abdominal cavity. Malrotation, as the name implies, refers to the situation where the bowel has not rotated normally prior to its return into the abdominal cavity and is not fixed to the posterior abdominal wall in the usual anatomical position. The caecum remains undescended in the right hypochondrium. This is a potentially dangerous state because the bowel may twist on its mesentry and impair the blood supply causing volvulus. It is

essential to make the diagnosis rapidly to avoid the bowel becoming necrotic.

Anal atresia

This defect should be found at routine newborn examination. Treatment depends on whether the atretic segment is long or short. Sometimes the anus is covered by a membrane which can be cut back exposing normal anatomy and the child will have normal anal function. High lesions, above the puborectalis muscle, require more extensive surgery.

Anal atresia is commonly associated with a fistula through which the meconium emerges. In males it is often a rectovesical fistula and in females a rectovaginal fistula.

Elucidation of the height of the lesion may be aided by an X-ray with the child in an upside down position and a radio-opaqe marker on the anal dimple. The distance between the marker and the air in the rectum gives an idea of the length of the atretic section.

Management

High lesions require a defunctioning colostomy on the first day of life. Subsequent surgery is necessary to produce normal functioning. Approximately one-third will eventually be continent, one-third continent with soiling and one-third incontinent of faeces.

Meckel's diverticulum

This structure is a finger-like protrusion from the lower ileum and is due to the persistence of a portion of the omphalomesentric duct. It may never cause symptoms but can give rise to a number of complications. It frequently contains aberrant gastric mucosa which may cause ulceration and perforation. It is also a cause of rectal bleeding.

The omphalomesentric duct may remain patent, causing a discharge from the umbilicus, or it may form a vestigial band and lead to intestinal obstruction. A Meckel's diverticulum may form the apex of an intussusception.

Exomphalus

In this condition the child is born with bowel extruding through the umbilical cord due to failure of the bowel to spontaneously withdraw into the abdomen. The exomphalus may be small with just one loop of small bowel involved or be massive with the entire bowel and liver in the sac. Exomphalus may be associated with Beckwith–Weidemann syndrome (p. 137).

Gastroschisis

In this condition there is a full thickness defect in the anterior abdominal wall through which the abdominal contents protrude. It is often separated from the umbilicus by a bridge of skin to the right of the umbilicus.

Management

The treatment of both conditions is relatively urgent. The bowel should be placed in a sterile plastic bag prior to surgery as the water and heat loss through the exposed bowel is massive. The surgeon replaces the bowel and closes the abdominal wall defect. Occasionally the defect is so large that primary closure may be impossible.

Inguinal hernia

In children this is an indirect hernia due to failure of closure of the processus vaginalis. It is much more common in boys and may be associated with an undescended testicle on the same side. It occurs in about 25% of very premature infants.

The child presents with a bulge in his groin which may be intermittent. It is usually reducible by milking it up the inguinal canal. A child with an incarcerated (irreducible) hernia should be admitted to hospital because of the risk of strangulation of the bowel within the hernial sac.

All children with an inguinal hernia should have the lesion surgically closed early in life. Chil-dren who present with an incarcerated hernia should be put in gallows traction in an effort to reduce the hernia prior to surgical closure.

Malformations of the nervous system

Malformations of the central nervous system are the commonest of all major congenital abnormalities and often the most devastating. The largest group of malformations are those referred to as neural tube defects.

Neural tube defects (NTD)

The neural tube starts to develop in the fourth week of embryonic life. The tube elongates at the cranial end to develop into the brain and the caudal end forms the spinal cord. The primitive neural tube submerges and becomes covered with tissue which later develops to form spine and skin. It is failure of the neural tube and its contiguous structures to close that cause the spectrum of neural tube disorders. This ranges from anencephaly at the most severe to asymptomatic vertebral arch defects at the mildest end. Spina bifida is the term used to describe failure of development of any part of the midline structures over the back.

The incidence of the NTD disorders have fallen in recent years and spina bifida occurs now with a frequency of about 1 : 2000 births. There is some evidence that folate deficiency may be an important factor in the causation of the NTDs. Screening programmes for open NTD disorders are widely used in some parts of the world where this is a common condition. Alpha fetoprotein (AFP) is derived from central nervous tissue and in the presence of an open spina bifida lesion or anencephaly, excess AFP is found in the maternal blood. Blood is routinely taken from the mother at 14–18 weeks and those with high levels should have a careful ultrasound assessment. Conditions other than open NTD which may cause high AFP levels include twin pregnancy and gastroschisis. In some centres, amniotic fluid AFP is also assayed. Only 10% of women with abnormally high serum AFP measurements actually have a fetus with a significant NTD. AFP screening will not detect closed lesions.

Anencephaly

The anencephalic child is usually born with no recognizable structures above the brain stem. Anencephaly occurs more commonly in females then in males and polyhydramnios, due to impaired fetal swallowing, affects the majority of these pregnancies. Although these children may breathe at birth the prognosis is obviously hopeless and they die soon afterwards.

Encephalocele

In this condition there is a failure of closure of the occipital bone and a skin-covered sac is present (Fig. 9.5). This may contain fluid only, but in severe cases much of the brain may be contained within the sac. Neurosurgical treatment is necessary to amputate the sac and close the bony defect. Prognosis depends on the amount of brain removed in the sac.

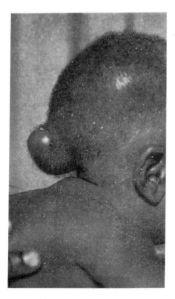

Fig. 9.5 Occipital encephalocele.

Spina bifida

Spina bifida can be subdivided into different categories (Fig. 9.6)

SPINA BIFIDA CYSTICA

In this condition, there is absence of the vertebral arches and failure of closure of the overlying skin. It can be further subdivided into:
1 Meningocele. The spinal cord is normally formed but a thin sac of meninges is exposed which contains CSF.
2 Myelomeningocele. In this condition the child is born with a meningocele which often ruptures at birth and the underlying cord is abnormally formed (Fig. 9.7). This condition accounts for 80% of the cases of spina bifida cystica.

SPINA BIFIDA OCCULTA

This implies that the skin over the lesion is intact and the condition may be benign. In other cases serious neurological deficits develop and great care must be taken in the management of the child. It can be subdivided into:
1 Dermal sinus. This is a tract that runs from the sacrum, dorsal spine (or rarely scalp) to terminate at a deeper level. It is often associated with a tuft of hair or midline naevus over the abnormal vertebrae. In the most severe form, the sinus communicates with the dura and the child may develop meningitis from this route.
2 Lipomyelomeningocele. This refers to a pad of fat over the spine with a stalk passing into the cord. As the child grows he may develop signs of neurological deficit in the lower limbs or sphincter disturbance. A midline fatty swelling over the spine should always be referred to a neurosurgeon as a matter of some urgency.
3 Diastematomyelia. In this condition the spinal cord is split by a bony or cartilaginous spur. Neurological signs do not usually develop until 3–4 years and the diagnosis is made by a myelogram. The child should be urgently referred to a neurosurgeon.

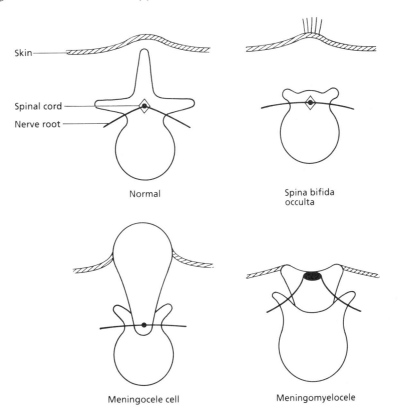

Skin

Spinal cord

Nerve root

Normal

Spina bifida occulta

Meningocele cell

Meningomyelocele

Fig. 9.6 Varieties of neural tube defects.

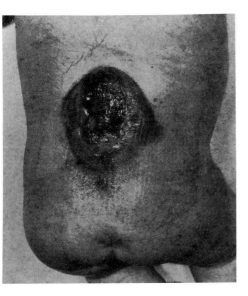

Fig. 9.7 Open myelomeningocele involving the lumbosacral region. Note the patulous anus.

Assessment

The child must be carefully assessed to establish the extent of neurological deficit. Spina bifida cystica is usually associated with sensory and motor deficit depending on the level of the lesion. The level of paralysis should be documented by observation and assessment of muscle power. The sensory level can also be relatively accurately assessed at birth. The anal sphincter is observed and is patulous if paralysed. The bladder should be carefully palpated to establish whether it is distended and neurogenic. Two additional investigations are essential in evaluating the child with spina bifida. Ultrasound examination of the head will detect early hydrocephalus (this occurs in about 90% of children with spina bifida cystica) and ultrasound examination of the kidneys will establish whether hydronephrosis has developed secondary to bladder paralysis.

Management

It is difficult to give a clear statement as to the management of spina bifida. It is now clear that aggressive early surgical treatment leaves the child very severely disabled but every child should be carefully assessed, preferably by a paediatrician and a neurosurgeon. Signs at birth which are used to indicate a poor prognosis include a large thoracolumbar lesion, scoliosis or kyphosis present at birth, gross hydrocephalus and other severe congenital abnormalities. Children in this group are usually not benefitted by surgical treatment and this is usually not advised.

Children managed surgically should have the back lesion closed within 24 hours of birth and the majority will also need a ventriculoperitoneal shunt for the treatment of progressive hydrocephalus. Careful management of bladder and renal function is also essential for many years and a number of orthopaedic procedures may also be necessary. Multi-speciality follow-up into adult life is essential in all these cases.

Hydrocephalus

Hydrocephalus is due to an obstruction to the free flow of cerebrospinal fluid (CSF) which is produced at the choroid plexus within the brain. It flows out of the intracerebral compartment at the level of the fourth ventricle to be absorbed over the surface of the brain at the arachnoid granulations. Pressure increases as a result of fluid obstruction and the child may show symptoms of raised intracranial pressure.

Hydrocephalus is a descriptive term and is not helpful as a diagnosis. In addition the infant born with a large head may not have hydrocephalus. Table 9.7 lists the causes of a large head at birth.

Table 9.7 Causes of a large head at birth.

Hydrocephalus
  Communicating
  Non-communicating
Benign external hydrocephalus
Hydranencephaly
Megalencephaly

Congenital hydrocephalus is a relatively common malformation present at birth. The finding of fetal hydrocephalus on prenatal ultrasound examination is also common as many women are examined routinely during pregnancy. Fetal hydrocephalus must alert the obstetrician to examine the fetus carefully for associated lesions such as spina bifida. The prognosis for fetuses found to have hydrocephalus is bad.

The single most important investigation is real-time ultrasound. This will determine whether there is excess fluid within the ventricles and will usually delineate the level of obstruction.

Arnold–Chiari malformation

This condition is seen in almost every baby with spina bifida. There is herniation of part of the cerebellum thorough the foramen magnum, together with deformity of the brain stem. Abnormalities of the skull bones are also seen on radiological examination. Hydrocephalus usually occurs with the Arnold–Chiari malformation and is due to blockage of CSF circulation at the level of the abnormal fourth ventricle.

Communicating hydrocephalus

This refers to hydrocephalus due to blockage of CSF absorption at a site beyond the fourth ventricle. This means that CSF flows freely into the lumbar subarachnoid space and a specimen can be obtained at lumbar puncture. The two commonest causes of communicating hydrocephalus are seen following intraventricular haemorrhage in newborn infants (p. 101) and meningitis. It is due to fibrosis or inflammatory obstruction at the level of either the exit from the fourth ventricle or the arachnoid granulations. Very rarely a tumour of the choroid plexus causes communicating hydrocephalus.

Non-communicating hydrocephalus

This occurs less commonly than communicating and is more likely to be due to a developmental abnormality. The commonest malformation is stenosis of the aqueduct of Sylvius and this is often a genetically determined disorder. Obstruction at the outlet of the fourth ventricle may occur following intraventricular haemorrhage or meningitis, but this is less common than when obstruction occurs over the surface of the brain.

External hydrocephalus

This is not strictly speaking a form of hydrocephalus but rather complete replacement of the intracranial contents, above the level of the mid-presents in the first year of life with an increasing head circumference, crossing centile lines in an upward direction. Brain scanning usually shows an excess of CSF over the surface of the brain but, with normal or only minimally dilated ventricles. There is almost always a close family member with an abnormally large head. Providing the child's developmental milestones are normal and he shows no signs of intracranial hypertension, the parents should be strongly reassured. Treatment is rarely indicated.

Hydranencephlay

This is not strictly speaking a form of hydrocephalus but rather complete replacement of the intracranial contents, above the level of the midbrain, with fluid. This is due to a devastating event in the first trimester of pregnancy; usually bilateral infarction of the internal carotid arteries. The infant may have a normal or enlarged head at birth but the prognosis for development is hopeless.

Clinical features

If hydrocephalus presents in infancy the child often has an abnormally large head. This may be accompanied by downward deviation of the eyes ('setting sun' sign), lethargy and vomiting. The symptoms of raised intracranial pressure are discussed in Chapter 17.

Treatment

In very immature infants who may be too small or sick for immediate surgery, temporary measures to relieve intracranial hypertension may be used. These include regular lumbar puncture or drug (isosorbide, acetazolamide) treatment. Definitive treatment is insertion of a ventriculoperitoneal shunt to drain CSF continuously from the lateral ventricles to the peritoneal cavity.

Developmental anomalies

Microcephaly

The size of the head is dependent on the growth of the brain, therefore, except for craniosynostosis (see below) all cases of microcephaly result from failure of brain growth. This may be affected by influences during pregnancy, during labour or in the first 2–3 years of life after which time brain growth is almost complete.

Microcephaly may be due to a developmental defect (primary microcephaly) or an insult which affects the developing brain (secondary microcephaly). The most important causes of secondary microcephaly apparent at birth are prenatal infection (toxoplasmosis, cytomegalovirus and rubella). A rare primary form of microcephaly is inherited as an autosomal recessive or less commonly, dominant form.

Secondary microcephaly may be due to events occuring at or after birth and these include severe birth asphyxia, meningitis or metabolic encephalopathy.

Children with secondary microcephaly are all very severely mentally handicapped and usually also have severe cerebral palsy. Children with primary microcephaly due to genetic causes may not be severely retarded although they usually have impaired intelligence. Cerebral palsy does not develop in this group.

Craniosynostosis

In this condition there is premature fusion of one or a number of the cranial sutures. The shape of the head is altered depending on which sutures are involved. Sagittal suture synostosis occurs most commonly and causes a long narrow head referred to as scaphocephaly. Coronal suture synostosis causes a flattened head with a high forehead and flat occiput. This is referred to as brachycephaly. Premature fusion of a single coronal suture causes plagiocephaly (see below).

Although this condition causes cosmetic problems it only restricts the head growth very rarely when there is fusion of all the sutures.

Treatment

This should be undertaken early when the diagnosis is first made. The synostoses are excised and material placed between the bones to prevent premature refusion. The cosmetic results with early treatment are usually excellent.

Plagiocephaly

In this condition the head is asymmetrical. Rarely it is a congenital condition when associated with unilateral synostosis of a coronal suture, but is more commonly due to compression after birth. It may be due to limitation of head movement from the shortening of a sternomastoid muscle and the infant always lies in the same position when supine thereby flattening the head in an asymmetrical manner.

Sternomastoid shortening, if present, must be treated with stretching exercises. In other cases the parents should be reassured that there is no abnormal pressure on the brain and that the condition is harmless. As the child gets older the asymmetry becomes less obvious as well as being obscured by the growth of hair.

Malformations of the genito-urinary tract

Renal agenesis

Bilateral renal agenesis is a relatively common malformation and is incompatible with life, although infants often live for several hours after birth. The pregnancy is associated with oligohydramnios because the fetus produces no urine, a major constituent of the amniotic fluid volume. Bilateral renal agenesis is associated with a charac-

teristic phenotype, including typical squashed facial features and prominent epicanthic folds (see Fig. 15.3). The infants always have lung hypoplasia and this is the cause of death.

Other major congenital malformations of the renal tract are also associated with Potter's facies. This includes renal obstruction and congenital urethral valves (see Chapter 15)

Unilateral renal agenesis is quite common. The normal kidney is slightly hypertrophied at birth and may be palpable. The child shows no clinical abnormality and this condition is entirely compatable with normal existence.

Hypospadias

This is a common malformation in which the urethral opening is on the ventral surface of the glans or shaft of the penis. In glandular hypospadias the abnormal opening may be missed because it is small but the prepuce is always abnormal. Instead of encircling the glans, it is gathered as a hood on the dorsal surface (Fig. 9.8). Some degree of chordee is usually present causing the penis to be curved. Epispadias refers to the urethra opening on the dorsal surface of the penis.

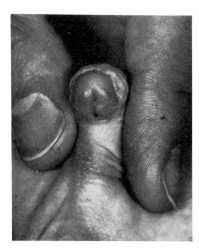

Fig. 9.8 Glandular hypospadias. The opening of the urethra can be seen below the blind pit. The prepuce is 'hooded' instead of encircling the glans. A moderate degree of chordee is present.

If the testicles are undescended, or if the degree of hypospadias is severe then the child's chromosomes should be examined to exclude an intersex state (p. 418).

Treatment

Hypospadias, if mild, can be repaired as a one stage procedure at about 6 months. If severe, several operations may be necessary but these should be complete well before the age that the child starts school. Circumcision must not be permitted as the prepuce is required for repair.

Deformations of the joints

Congenital orthopaedic abnormalities are almost always due to compression rather than a malformation in the development of the structures. As a group they form a very common cause of congenital abnormality apparent at birth. In all children with severe deformities of the lower limbs, the spine must be examined and the nerve supply to the legs, anus and bladder carefully assessed in order to exclude spina bifida as the cause of intra-uterine limb immobility.

Talipes (club foot)

Talipes is subdivided according to whether the foot is held in a toe down or a heel down position.
1 Talipes equinovarus. This occurs in 1 : 1000 infants (Fig. 9.9). If severe it may be associated with wasting of the muscles in the lower leg.
2 Talipes calcaneovalgus. In its severe form this is 5–10 times less common that the equinovarus disorder.

Treatment

The range of movements of the ankle joint should be carefully assessed. If the ankle can be moved to the extremes of their normal range then no treatment is necessary other than physiotherapy. If there is a fixed deformity, then serial splinting is

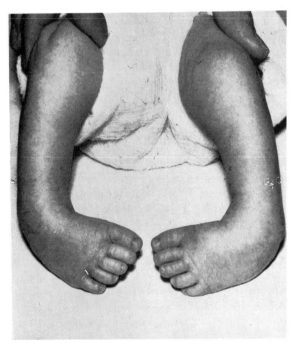

(a)

Fig. 9.9 Bilateral talipes equinovarus.

carried out and some cases may require subsequent corrective surgery.

Children with metatarsus varus require no specific treatment other than observation. When the child starts to walk there is often spontaneous resolution.

Congenital dislocation of the hip

This condition shows a female preponderance of about 7 : 1 and has an incidence at birth of 5–10 per 1000. The left hip is dislocated four times more commonly than the right. There are a number of associated factors:
1 Polygenic. There is often a family history.
2 Joint laxity. This is probably the reason that more girls than boys are affected.
3 Presentation. It is 10 times more common in infants born by the breech.
4 Neuromuscular factors. Muscle or spinal abnormalities are important predisposing factors.

Diagnosis

Congenital dislocation of the hip should be routinely diagnosed in the newborn period as every newborn baby must have a careful examination of the hips. Two tests are performed: (a) the Ortolani's (reduction) test (Fig. 5.7), and (b) the Barlow test (Fig. 5.8). Routine examination of the hips is described in Chapter 5.

Abnormalities of the hip can be described on the basis of these tests as:
1 Dislocated. The hip is out of joint and cannot be abducted.
2 Dislocatable. The hip is in joint but can be dislocated by Barlow's test.
3 The clicky hip. This is due to a ligamentous laxity and is not a sign of abnormality. These babies should be re-examined at about 6 weeks.

LATE DISLOCATION OF THE HIP

It is now well recognized that some infants found to have dislocated hips during late infancy had an entirely normal hip examination at birth. All babies when seen for any reason should have their hips examined for the maximum degree of abduction. A dislocated hip will not abduct normally.

Investigation

A hip X-ray in the neonatal period is not very helpful because the hip joint at birth is poorly ossified. Ultrasound examination is much more helpful to establish normality of the acetabulum. Some infants show an abnormally shallow acetabulum and these infants probably require treatment.

Treatment

The dislocated and dislocatable hip requires immediate treatment by splinting. The principle of treatment is to immobilize the hip in an abducted position for a period of 2–3 months. If the hip is clinically stable the child should be reassessed radiologically at regular intervals to ensure normal bone development. Surgery is indicated when the dislocated hip cannot be reduced or there has been a failure of splinting.

The prognosis for dislocated hip diagnosed in the neonatal period is excellent if appropriate management is instituted.

Arthrogryposis multiplex

In this condition two or more joints are contracted and have severely diminished movement. The joints in severe cases may be entirely fused as a result of replacement with fibrous tissue. The joints are usually extended or more rarely flexed and a degree of talipes is often present.

There are a number of underlying conditions which cause arthrogryposis multiplex:
1 Neurogenic causes such as spinal muscular atrophy (p. 300).
2 Myogenic causes such as congenital muscular dystrophy (p. 301).
3 Compression as occurs in severe oligohydramnios or bicornuate uterus.

Treatment

Physiotherapy and orthopaedic surgery may produce vast improvement in some, particularly if due to compression alone. Children with congenital neuromuscular disorders may be improved little even after years of treatment.

Further reading

Levene MI, Tudehope D, Thearle J. *Essentials of Neonatal Medicine*. Blackwell Scientific Publications, Oxford 1987.

Smith DW. Recognizable patterns of human malformation. In: *Major Problems in Clinical Pediatrics*, Vol VII, 3rd Edn. WB Saunders, Philadelphia 1982.

10

DISORDERS OF THE EAR, NOSE AND THROAT

The ear

Disorders affecting the ears are probably the most common reason for parents to seek medical advice about their child. This section will deal with diseases of the outer and middle ear and hearing impairment is discussed in Chapter 18.

The pinna, external auditory canal and middle ear structures develop from the first two branchial arches during the embryonic period. At birth, the mastoid process contains no air cells and they do not start to develop until well after birth.

Examination of the ear

The outer ear, or pinna, shows great variation in shape and these patterns often run in families. Preauricular ear tags and pits are common and may require cosmetic surgery. Congenital atresia of the external auditory meatus occurs rarely. Low set ears together with downward sloping palpebral fissures are a feature of the Treacher Collins syndrome, an autosomal dominant condition.

Every doctor involved in the care of children should be able to examine the ear competently. Examination of the ears is traditionally left to the end as it is most likely to upset the young child. The child should be held by the mother on her lap with the child's head against her chest. If the child is likely to struggle the mother's other hand should restrain his arms, and his legs can be gripped gently between the mother's legs (Fig. 10.1).

The examiner should hold the auriscope be-

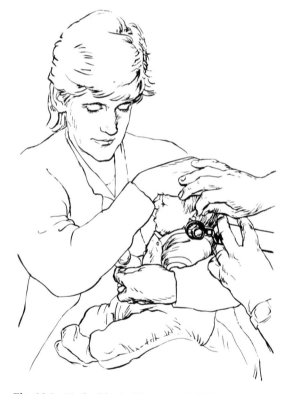

Fig. 10.1 Method for holding a small child during ear examination.

tween fingers and thumb, resting his hand against the child's temple so that the instrument will move with the child. The top of the pinna is grasped by the examiner's other hand and pulled up to straighten out the external auditory meatus.

152

The largest possible speculum is chosen which will comfortably enter the meatus and is not advanced more than 0.5 cm in infants and 1 cm in older children. If wax is present, an attempt should be made to remove it gently.

The drum should be carefully visualized and the normal appearance is shown in Figure 10.2a. The tympanic membrane is normally white in colour and translucent, with a light reflex at its lower pole. Some middle ear structures can be observed through the membrane including the manubrium and the umbo. The normal drum lies in a neutral position. If there is increased pressure in the middle ear as occurs in otitis media the drum bulges forward and is inflamed (Fig. 10.2b). If the drum is retracted, as occurs in some cases of glue ear, the light reflex is lost, the drum is dull and both the manubrium and malleus are very obvious (Fig. 10.2c). In some cases, a fluid level can be seen through the membrane and air bubbles may also be present. Assessment of drum mobility is helpful but this requires specialized equipment and skill. Air is pumped through the auroscope speculum which forms a tight seal with the meatus and

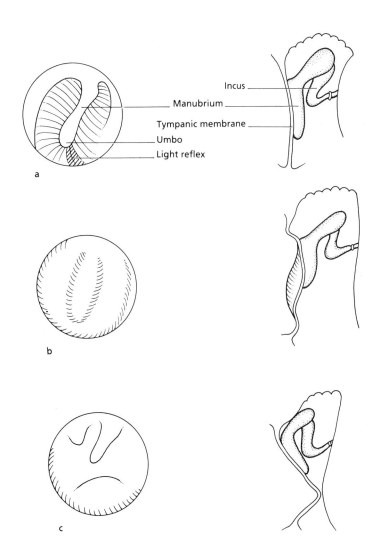

Fig. 10.2 Appearances of the tympanic membrane with a profile view on the right. (a) Normal tympanic membrane; (b) bulging tympanic membrane (acute otitis media); and (c) retracted tympanic membrane (glue ear).

movement of the tympanic membrane can be assessed.

Otitis externa

This refers to inflammation of the external auditory meatus with discharge. Discharge from the meatus may be primary or secondary to perforation of the tympanic membrane. Otitis media may be due to the presence of a foreign body, local trauma or infection. *Candida* or *Staphylococcus* are the most commonly seen infectious agents. Infection may be acquired from infected water in swimming pools.

Clinical features

The ear is extremely painful, this being exacerbated by movement of the pinna, or lying on the affected side. The external auditory meatus is red, soggy and swollen and may be almost closed. The discharge is often scanty but smells offensive. A painful enlarged lymph node may be palpable in front of, below or behind the pinna.

Treatment

The insertion of a gauze wick which has been soaked previously in glycerine with 10% ichthammol gives relief. Local antibiotic cream should only be used if infection has been shown to be present on microbiological culture.

Otitis media

This is an extremely common childhood disorder and occurs most frequently in the first 3 years of life. It is also seen commonly between the ages of 5 and 7 years and may occur in the newborn period particularly during the course of tracheal intubation.

Otitis media occurs due to Eustachian tube dysfunction which may be due to either obstructive or functional factors.

1 Obstruction is due in most cases to adenoidal hypertrophy and very rarely associated with a tumour.

2 Functional disorders are due to the Eustachian tube being patulous and failing to maintain its patency. This commonly occurs in very young children. Infected material is more likely to be aspirated into the patulous tube from the nasopharynx which then infects the middle ear. Cleft palate is an important cause of a functionally abnormal Eustachian tube and children with this condition are much more prone to recurrent otitis media. Very young children and those with Down's syndrome have facial anatomy more likely to predispose to Eustachian tube dysfunction and are also more likely to develop otitis media.

The infecting organisms are most likely to be *Streptococcus pneumoniae* and *Haemophilus influenzae*. More rarely a beta haemolytic *Streptococcus* or a virus may be the cause.

Clinical features

The children present with fever, painful ear and hearing loss. It is usually preceded by an upper respiratory tract infection. In younger children, anorexia, vomiting and diarrhoea may be the presenting features and there may be no obvious symptoms pointing to the ear as the source of infection. For this reason routine aural examination should be performed on all unwell children. Examination of the ear reveals the tympanic membrane to be inflamed and bulging, with loss of the light reflex (Fig. 10.2b).

Management

Ampicillin is the antibiotic of choice. Nasal drops containing ephedrine 0.5% in saline may be of value in the acute phase to maintain drainage through the Eustachian tube. Myringotomy is rarely required but should be performed if there is still pain and a bulging drum 48 hours after the start of treatment.

The children should be re-evaluated 2 weeks after starting treatment. If the ear is abnormal at that time, further examination should be under-

Table 10.1 Complications of acute otitis media.

Serous otitis media
Conductive deafness
Mastoiditis
Perforation of the tympanic membrane
Chronic otitis media
Cholesteatoma
Facial palsy

taken 4 weeks later. Persistent abnormality may indicate serous otitis media (see below).

Complications

These are shown in Table 10.1 and are discussed elsewhere.

SEROUS OTITIS MEDIA (GLUE EAR)

This condition, also known as catarrhal otitis media, occurs as a result of failure of resolution of acute otitis media. The two main factors determining whether a child will develop this condition are the degree of inflammatory exudate associated with the acute infection and the degree of drainage through the Eustachian tube. Inflammatory exudate develops as the result of acute infection which is partially resorbed to leave thick serous or mucoid fluid within the middle ear and is referred to as 'glue'.

Clinical features

The presenting complaint is usually deafness, although this may be unrecognized until the child is screened for hearing impairment. Glue ear is the commonest form of hearing impairment seen in children. The child may also complain of earache. Glue ear may be found in children presenting with any upper respiratory tract infection.

Examination of the tympanic membrane reveals a dull, opaque retracted drum (Fig. 10.2c). The light reflex is absent. A horizontal fluid level or air bubbles are often seen through the drum. The tympanic membrane is immobile on pneumatic

testing. Hearing impairment often shows a conductive impairment but this rarely exceeds 40 dB.

Management

There is considerable controversy as to the best management of this condition. The natural history of glue ear is spontaneous resolution with improvement in hearing and any treatment must be compared with the tendency for the child to recover naturally. Treatment with Actifed (triprolidine hydrochloride and pseudoephedrine hydrochloride) or Sudafed (pseudoephedrine hydrochloride) for 4–6 weeks is sometimes effective but if hearing impairment is present a surgical opinion should be sought.

As the condition is related to failure of the middle ear secretions to drain, therapy is directed towards establishing adequate drainage. Small plastic drainage tubes (grommets) have for many years been inserted through the tympanic membrane to allow equalization of pressure and aeration with resolution of the 'glue'. These appear to cause rapid improvement in the child's hearing but may require replacement every 6 months to maintain continued drainage. After grommets are inserted, normal activities including swimming should be encouraged, but diving is forbidden.

Another approach to treatment is surgical adenoidectomy. This permits drainage to occur over a much longer period of time but resolution of the hearing impairment is slower. A practical method to treat these children is to perform adenoidectomy and place a grommet in the worst affected ear thereby gaining rapid improvement in hearing with more prolonged drainage.

Mastoiditis

This is now a very rare condition and results from inadequate or inappropriate treatment of otitis media. The mastoid process becomes tender and inflamed; the pinna may be pushed forwards. X-rays show clouding of the mastoid air cells. Most cases respond to intravenous antibiotic therapy; surgery rarely being required.

Table 10.2 Causes of earache.

Acute otitis media
Upper respiratory tract infection
Otitis externa
Mumps
Serous otitis media
Referred pain to the ear
   Tonsillitis
   Teething
   Temporomandibular joint
   Dental caries

Earache

This is a common symptom in children. Very young children are irritable and may pull at their ear. The child should be examined carefully as pain in the ear may be referred from a lesion in the throat such as tonsillitis. Earache may also be felt in association with mumps. The ear itself must be carefully examined before considering that the pain is referred from another site. Table 10.2 lists the commoner causes of earache.

Symptomatic relief for the pain can be obtained from a hot water-bottle or a pad of warm cotton wool bandaged over the ear.

Nose

The nasal compartment separates from the mouth early in development. Initially the posterior nares are separated from the nasopharynx by the bucconasal membrane which disappears at about 5 weeks of development. Failure of this membrane to degenerate causes choanal atresia (see below). The nasal sinuses are present at birth in a rudimentary form, but the frontal sinus does not start to develop until about 6 months after birth. Sinus development continues into adult life.

Choanal atresia

This is due to failure of the bucconasal membrane to degenerate early in fetal development. Bilateral choanal atresia is rare, but unilateral atresia is considerably more common and usually does not present until later in childhood.

Clinical features

Infants are obligate nose breathers and complete nasal obstruction will cause a dramatic picture of cyanosis and vigorous efforts to inspire with no air movement (obstructive apnoea). Bilateral choanal atresia presents shortly after birth with severe respiratory obstruction. Crying often results in some improvement as air can be aspirated through the open mouth.

Unilateral atresia may cause few symptoms but classically there is a persistent white discharge from the affected nostril which is so stringy it can be drawn out with forceps.

Investigations

Diagnosis is made by the inability to pass a firm catheter through the posterior nares into the pharynx. If the diagnosis is in doubt a small volume of radio-opaque dye is instilled into the nares and a lateral X-ray with the neck extended will show the extent of the blockage.

Management

Emergency treatment of bilateral choanal atresia involves the passage of a plastic oral (Guedel) airway to allow the infant to breath. Subsequent surgery is required to establish patency but this may require a number of surgical procedures and bilateral choanal atresia may be associated with considerable morbidity.

Table 10.3 Causes of epistaxis.

Trauma
Nose picking
Coryza
Foreign bodies
Upper respiratory tract infection
Hypertension
Bleeding disorders
Leukaemia

Epistaxis

Nose bleeding is a common symptom in childhood. In most cases it is due to a local cause but it can result from generalized disease. Table 10.3 lists the important causes of epistaxis.

Bleeding usually occurs within Little's area on the anterior portion of the nasal septum where there is a plentiful supply of blood vessels. Nose picking is particularly likely to traumatize this area.

Management

First aid treatment involves sitting the child upright and leaning forward with the soft part of the nose compressed continuously between finger and thumb for up to 10 minutes. Most nose bleeds will stop spontaneously within this time.

Prophylactic treatment of repeated epistaxis involves regular application of vaseline on the tip of the little finger to the mucosa of the nasal septum. Cauterization of the offending vessel is undertaken in some cases.

Severe life-threatening epistaxis occurs rarely. Treatment involves packing of the nose with ribbon gauze by an experienced surgeon.

Rhinitis

Rhinitis refers to nasal discharge which may be clear or purulent and which may be persistent or episodic. There are a number of important causes of this very common symptom and these are listed in Table 10.4.

COMMON COLD (CORYZA)

This is due to a viral infection. Children are especially susceptible when they start playgroup or

Table 10.4 Causes of rhinitis.

Coryza
Upper respiratory tract infection
Allergy
Foreign body
Unilateral choanal atresia

school and mix with large numbers of people in confined spaces. On average each child develops five colds per year. Viruses implicated in causing the common cold include rhinoviruses, respiratory syncitial virus, parainfluenza, influenza and coronaviruses. Over 100 antigenically distinct forms of rhinovirus alone exist and it is not surprising that repeated infections occur.

The symptoms of cold include sneezing, rhinitis, nasal congestion, cough and fever. It should be distinguished from upper respiratory tract infection (URTI) by lack of lymphadenopathy. In addition URTI is usually associated with pharyngitis and red tympanic membranes. Coryza in young babies is particularly distressing because nasal congestion may cause severe respiratory embarrassment.

Treatment is symptomatic. Decongestants (pseudoephedrine) reduce the degree of nasal congestion. Antibiotics should not be given and vitamin C is ineffective.

ALLERGIC RHINITIS

This occurs rarely in young children below the age of 5 years but is common in adolescence. There is usually an atopic family history and it is necessary for the child to be sensitized previously by an allergen. These commonly include grass pollens and moulds. It is often seasonal (when it is called hay fever) but may also be perennial.

The episode starts with sneezing, followed by profuse clear rhinorrhoea. Intense irritation of the nasal mucosa and eyes usually accompanies the other acute symptoms. Examination of the nose reveals red, congested mucosa.

The condition is due to a local type I hypersensitivity reaction mediated by IgE antibodies. Treatment is directed towards avoiding the precipitating allergens, together with antihistamines. Pseudoephedrine may be helpful in treating the nasal congestion. Ephedrine nasal drops may be of some value for relief of snuffliness but must not be used for more than a few days, otherwise reactive vasodilatation may occur. Severe symptoms may be relieved by beclomethasone nasal spray or insufflation of sodium cromoglycate into the nose.

Sinusitis

In young children the paranasal sinuses are relatively underdeveloped and their drainage ostia are large. This makes acute sinusitis uncommon as retention of infected material within the sinuses is the underlying cause of this condition. Infection causes swelling of the mucosa with inflammatory exudate which may block the ostia; further build up of exudate causes pressure and pain. The commonest organisms causing acute sinusitis are *Haemophilus influenzae*, *Streptococcus pneumoniae* and less commonly viruses.

Clinical features

The maxillary sinus is most commonly affected. The child usually presents with fever and facial pain (usually infra-orbital) during the course of, or immediately following, upper respiratory tract infection. Swelling around the eye or cheek may occur and headache is common. Purulent nasal discharge and cough may be the main features in younger children.

Acute ethmoiditis

This is a rare but dangerous form of sinusitis occurring in young children. It is usually due to *H. influenzae*. The child becomes acutely ill with proptosis and periorbital oedema of the affected side. An orbital abscess may develop.

Investigations

The diagnosis is confirmed radiologically or by ultrasound examination. Opaque sinuses on X-ray indicate the presence of fluid or pus. Thickening of the mucosa is a particularly common finding in children with maxillary sinusitis.

Treatment

Treatment is with antibiotics (ampicillin or amoxycillin) and 0.5% ephedine nasal drops. Sinus puncture is very rarely indicated if appropriate antibiotic treatment is carried out.

Complications

1 Osteomyelitis of the facial bones.
2 Cavernous sinus thrombosis.
3 Subdural empyema.
4 Cerebral abscess.
5 Chronic sinusitis.

Adenoidal hypertrophy

The adenoids are an aggregation of lymphoid tissue situated in the midline at the junction of the roof and posterior wall of the nasopharynx. They enlarge during childhood, reaching maximum size between the ages of 5 and 25 years.

Clinical features

Children with enlarged adenoids have a characteristic appearance. They stand with their mouth open and sniff constantly. Catarrhal fluid often appears on the upper lip which they sniff up or wipe with the back of their hand or sleeve.

Adenoidal hypertrophy causes two major clinical problems:
1 Otitis media with glue ear due to obstruction to the drainage of the Eustachian tube and this is discussed in detail above.
2 Obstructed breathing. In milder cases the children present as mouth breathers. They have noisy breathing particularly at night and spend much of their time with the mouth open due to their posterior nasal obstruction. They have hyponasality of speech.

More severe cases may develop sleep apnoea due to prolapse of the adenoidal tissue during sleep. These children show marked episodic desaturation of their haemoglobin which can be monitored non-invasively during sleep. They are at risk of cor pulmonale due to unrecognized chronic hypoxia.

Investigations

The adenoids can only be seen by means of posterior rhinoscopy but a good idea of their size can be obtained from the appearance of the nasopharynx. A large pad of adenoidal tissue pushes the uvula forwards and upwards thereby increasing the depth of the pharynx.

Management

The indications for adenoidectomy are:
1 Repeated episodes of otitis media with conductive hearing loss.
2 Stertorous breathing with sleep apnoea.
3 Chronic hypoxia during sleep.

Adenoidectomy must not be performed on children with cleft palate or submucous cleft as this will exacerbate nasal escape on vocalization.

Throat

The structures destined to form the larynx and trachea separate from the oesophageal structures in the fourth week of development. The neonate is born with a proportionately small larynx and it remains small until puberty. The subglottis is the narrowest part of the upper airway at birth and during early childhood. The epiglottis and larynx are relatively softer in early life until mature cartilaginization occurs.

Stridor

This refers to an audible inspiratory noise which may be present at birth or develop subsequently. The degree of stridor usually depends on the inspiratory breath. A stridulous noise is usually louder when the child cries and is softer during sleep. Table 10.5 lists the causes of congenital and acquired stridor.

LARYNGOMALACIA

This is the commonest cause of congenital stridor. It is due to an excessively soft immature larynx which is sucked towards the glottis at each inspiratory breath. Although it is usually present at birth its onset may be delayed for some weeks. It tends to improve spontaneously with time.

It is not possible to confirm the diagnosis of laryngomalacia unless direct laryngoscopy is performed and this is not necessary in mild cases. Other more serious causes of congenital stridor must always be considered and laryngoscopy undertaken if there is doubt as to the diagnosis or if the child becomes worse, or if there is not resolution within 6 months.

CONGENITAL LARYNGEAL OBSTRUCTION

Rarely the infant is born with a laryngeal web or cyst which causes stridor in about 5% of congenital cases. Laryngeal cleft may also present with stridor. A subglottic haemangioma may cause stridor and this is often not present at birth and develops as the haemangioma grows.

These diagnoses can only be made at laryngoscopy performed under a general anaesthetic. Tracheostomy may be required if obstruction is feared.

ACUTE LARYNGOTRACHEOBRONCHITIS (CROUP)

This is an infectious disease usually due to parainfluenza virus 1 or 2. It occurs most commonly in young children of 6 months to 2 years. The infection starts with an upper respiratory tract illness which proceeds rapidly to fever, a barking cough and stridor. The stridor may be intermittent due to laryngeal spasm. Further progression down the respiratory tract may cause wheezing and tachypnoea. The infection is often mild but in some children it may rapidly progress to become extremely severe and life threatening. The child may be

Table 10.5 Causes of stridor.

Congenital	Acquired
Laryngomalacia	Acute laryngotracheobronchitis
Laryngeal web	Acute epiglottis
Laryngeal cleft	Subglottic stenosis
Haemangioma	Allergic laryngeal oedema
Bilateral vocal cord palsy	Diphtheria
Subglottic stenosis*	Foreign body
	Laryngeal papilloma

* Although the lesion may be congenital, stridor often develops late.

cyanosed and toxic and in the most severe form the stridor may appear to improve as the respiratory effort deteriorates. Acute epiglottitis (see below) must always be considered in cases of severe croup.

Management

The child should be placed in a well humidified environment. In mild cases the child can be left at home providing the parents are warned about the signs of deterioration. A closed bathroom with all the hot taps on will soon produce a misty humid environment. If there is any doubt as to the parents ability to cope, the child should be admitted to hospital for observation. A steam tent (croupette) is placed over the cot and the child carefully observed. This is often frightening for the child and the mother should be encouraged to get into the steam tent with him. Adequate fluids are essential to avoid dehydration with crusting of the upper airway mucosa. The condition. is self-limiting and acute laryngotracheobronchitis does not require antibiotics. Severe cases with threatened airway obstruction should be intubated by an experienced doctor. Tracheostomy should not be necessary.

ACUTE EPIGLOTTITIS

This is a most feared and life threatening condition. It usually occurs in the winter months and affects slightly older children (2−4 years) than croup. It is due to *H. influenzae* and many of these children are also septicaemic.

Clinical features

They present as extremely toxic, feverish and often drool from the mouth as they are unable to swallow. They sit up and lean forward with their chin jutting out. They are not hoarse and rarely cough.

If this condition is suspected, examination of the mouth must not be attempted outside hospital as acute airway obstruction may occur. The child should only be examined with an experienced

anaesthetist or throat surgeon standing by. The epiglottis is bright red and oedematous and resembles a cherry.

Management

Intubation is the emergency treatment of choice but requires an experienced clinician in view of the difficulties created by the swollen epiglottis. For this reason, tracheostomy may be an alternative but less good form of treatment. In some parts of the world many strains of haemophilus are resistant to ampicillin and intravenous chloramphenicol is the best drug to use until the sensitivities are known. Blood cultures should always be taken from these children before treatment is started. Extubation is usually possible within 48 hours of admission.

SUBGLOTTIC STENOSIS

This is becoming an increasingly common problem probably because many more ill neonates are ventilated with endotracheal tubes for long periods of time. Rarely it is due to congenital narrowing in the subglottic region.

In premature babies who have been ventilated, stridor may not be apparent for days, weeks or even months following extubation. Many go home apparently well and then return with severe stridor and upper airway obstruction associated with upper respiratory tract infection.

Management

Children with severe subglottic stenosis will require tracheostomy and later reconstructive surgery to the subglottis.

Infection of the throat

During the first year of life the tonsils are always small. Infection of the throat during this period affects the whole pharynx rather than the tonsils alone as in older children, so that it is more correct to refer to acute pharyngitis in babies.

ACUTE PHARYNGITIS

This is a very common infection and is seen in conjunction with viral upper respiratory infection. The pharynx, soft palate and tonsillar fauces are inflamed and swollen. There is usually associated lymphadenopathy of the neck. Specific infections which cause acute pharyngitis include:

1 Measles. Examine for Koplik's spots (p. 357).
2 Infectious mononucleosis (p. 360).
3 Vincent's angina. This is a particularly severe form of pharyngitis due to infection simultaneously by two organisms; a spirochaete and a Gram-negative bacillus. There is redness and swelling of the mouth and a characteristic grey membrane on the gums which bleeds easily when scraped. Treatment is with penicillin.
4 Diphtheria (p. 362).
5 *Candida*. This is due to *Candida albicans* infection and is common in babies but may also be seen in immunosuppressed patients. White plaques are seen on the buccal mucosa and occasionally the pharynx. They cannot be removed by scraping. They respond to nystatin drops or miconazole (Daktarin) oral gel.

ACUTE TONSILLITIS

In acute tonsillitis the tonsils become enlarged and inflamed, often with a white exudate on the external surface of the gland when the term acute follicular tonsillitis is used. This white exudate·must be differentiated from the creamy material which may be visible in the tonsillar crypts and does not necessarily indicate infection.

Tonsillitis is usually due to viral infection, particularly in young children. The commonest organism causing tonsillitis between the ages of 5 and 17 years is the haemolytic *Streptococcus*. Exudate on the tonsil must make the clinician consider other infection particularly infectious mononucleosis (p. 360) and diphtheria (p. 362).

Clinical features

The child is feverish and may complain of sore throat. In younger children, pain may not be local-ized to the throat but they may complain of abdominal pain probably due to mesenteric adenitis. This emphasizes the need for the throat to be examined in all children with stomach pain. Lymphadenopathy is seen in all children with bacterial tonsillitis. The jugulo-digastric nodes, palpated just below the angle of the jaw, are enlarged and painful.

Treatment

Symptomatic relief in older children may be obtained with salt water gargles. Pyrexia in younger children responds to paracetamol elixir. Most cases of tonsillitis do not require antibiotics. Antibiotics may be helpful in children with more systemic symptoms and those with exudate. A throat swab should be taken in all cases. Streptococcal tonsillitis should be treated with benzyl penicillin for 10 days.

Complications

These include:
1 Otitis media.
2 Chronic tonsillitis.
3 Peritonsillar abscess (quinsy). This is seen more commonly in older children. There is acute pain and swelling around the affected tonsil with pyrexia and malaise. The lymph nodes are swollen and the child often complains of dysphagia. Intramuscular penicillin should be used if the diagnosis is made early but later incision of the abscess will be necessary. This must be done under general anaesthetic and with great care to avoid aspiration of infection material.
4 Post-streptococcal allergic disorders. The two most important are acute nephritic syndrome (p. 260) and rheumatic fever (p. 476).

CHRONIC TONSILLITIS

This condition results from repeated attacks of tonsillitis. Here the doctor should be more influenced by the history of recurrent attacks than by the appearance of the tonsils. Enlargement of the tonsils is no indication that they are unhealthy, as they grow, in common with lymphoid tissue elsewhere in the body, throughout childhood. Tuberculosis of the tonsil is now a very rare cause of chronic tonsillitis in developed countries (p. 561).

Clinical features

The children are often listless and pale. Examination may reveal either large or small tonsils. The most important features are the presence of pus in the crypts and persistent enlargement of the jugulo-digastric lymph nodes, palpated just below the angle of the jaw. Large tonsils alone do not indicate chronic tonsillitis and are usually benign. Airway obstruction and dysphagia rarely occur due to gross tonsillar hypertrophy but hypoxia, hypercapnia and cor pulmonale may result from obstruction.

Treatment

Tonsillectomy is one of the commonest operations performed on children but the indications for it are poorly understood. The usually accepted indications for tonsillectomy are:
1 Recurrent infection. More than five attacks of tonsillitis per year for 2 years or more.
2 Airway obstruction with sleep apnoea, hypoxia and/or hypercapnia.
3 Following peritonsillar abscess (quinsy).

Hoarseness

This may occur acutely and is usually due to laryngitis. Occasionally in children it is chronic and other causes must be considered. All children with hoarseness lasting for more than 3 weeks should be investigated and have direct laryngoscopy. The commoner causes of hoarseness in children follow.

ACUTE LARYNGITIS

This is usually preceded by upper respiratory tract infection, tonsillitis or croup. The child is usually pyrexial and unwell when hoarseness develops usually with cough and sometimes stridor. It is usually due to a viral infection. The condition is self-limiting and the voice improves in a short period of time.

CHRONIC LARYNGITIS

This is uncommon in children and may be associated with infection or misuse of the voice; excessive screaming or shouting is a major factor. Laryngoscopy should be performed and speech therapy is often helpful.

VOCAL CORD PARALYSIS

This may be congenital or acquired. It is unilateral in the majority of cases and if bilateral may cause severe respiratory obstruction. Trauma to the cords by intubation is an important factor. Rarely recurrent laryngeal nerve palsy occurs following cardiac surgery.

In congenital paralysis the cry is usually hoarse or weak. Stridor may also be present. Diagnosis is confirmed by direct laryngoscopy.

PAPILLOMATA OF THE LARYNX

Multiple benign papillomata are the commonest tumour to affect the larynx in children. They are liable to recur after treatment.

Neck swelling

Swelling in the neck is a common finding and may cause the parents great concern. There are a large number of causes of such swelling and meticulous history with careful examination is necessary in all cases. The presence of a swelling at birth reduces the differential diagnosis. Localization of the swelling to either the anterior or posterior triangle of the neck (Fig. 10.3) also helps to narrow the differential diagnosis. Lymphadenopathy is a common cause of neck swelling and the child should be carefully examined for sites of local infection as well as the presence of generalized lymphadenopathy or splenomegaly. The swelling

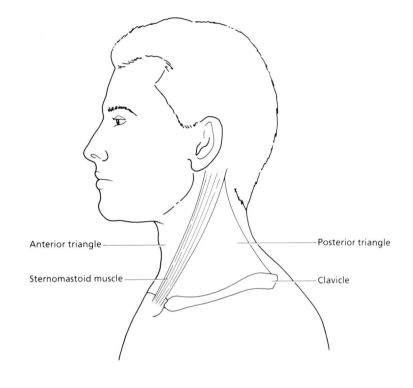

Fig. 10.3   The anterior and
posterior triangles of the neck.

should be assessed as to its nature (solid or fluctuant), whether it moves on swallowing or is transilluminable and whether it is mobile or fixed to deeper structures. Table 10.6 lists the causes of neck swelling, many of which are discussed elsewhere.

BRANCHIAL CLEFT CYSTS

These arise from remnants of the second branchial cleft and may be present at birth. More commonly they are first detected at about 5 years of age. They lie in the anterior triangle of the neck opposite the middle third of the sternomastoid muscle. They do not transilluminate.

Together with the cyst, or separate from it, there may be a branchial sinus just anterior to the mid-portion of the sternomastoid muscle. In some cases this may connect to the tonsil through a fistulous connection.

Treatment is surgical excision of the cyst. If a fistula is present this should also be excised. Its

Table 10.6   Causes of neck swelling.

Branchial cleft cyst
Cystic hygroma
Thyroglossal duct cyst
Lymphadenopathy
Goitre
Thyroid nodule
Lymphoma
Sternomastoid tumour
Mumps
Rhabdomyosarcoma
Neurofibrosarcoma
Neuroblastoma

path lies between the internal and external carotid arteries and surgery may be hazardous.

CYSTIC HYGROMA

This is a mass of lymphatic tissue that causes a swelling in the posterior triangle of the neck, often present at birth (Fig. 10.4). The mass is soft and trans-illuminates brilliantly. Although some

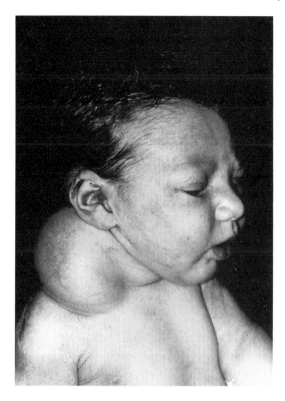

Fig. 10.4 Cystic hygroma.

form anywhere in its tract, but usually lies below the hyoid bone. It is always midline and rarely present at birth. It is best seen when the child slightly hyperextends his neck. It moves with protrusion of the tongue and swallowing. The lump should be surgically excised if large enough to be prominent.

Midline tumours such as a thyroglossal duct cyst must be distinguished from other lumps in the midline of the neck, including ectopic thyroid nodules (which may be malignant) and dermoid cysts. The latter are always attached to the skin.

LYMPHADENOPATHY

Enlarged lymph nodes in the neck may be solitary or multiple and may be part of a generalized lymphadenopathy which is discussed in detail on p. 440. A lymph node abscess is relatively common in children. It presents as a painful lump, usually in the neck, which is tender on palpation, red and may be pointing. Surgical incision of the node is indicated if it is pointing, otherwise a course of antibiotics may resolve the lump.

regression in size may occur with time, the best treatment is complete surgical excision.

THYROGLOSSAL DUCT CYSTS

The thyroglossal duct potentially lies in the line of the embryonic thyroid migration. A cyst may

LYMPHOMAS

These are discussed in detail in Chapter 25. Hodgkin's disease and lymphosarcoma are the two most common lymphomata to present with swelling in the neck.

11
RESPIRATORY DISORDERS

Respiratory complaints make up the single largest group of disorders about which family doctors are consulted and also account for 30% of acute medical paediatric admissions to hospital. The contribution of acute and chronic respiratory symptoms towards school absenteeism and family disruption is very great but difficult to quantify. Pre-school children have up to nine respiratory infections per year and approximately 3% of all young children are admitted to hospital with such infections. In addition, 12% of school children have clear symptoms of asthma and in some, medical help has not been sought or incorrect diagnosis or management has occurred. Probably one in five pre-school children wheeze at some time. The frequency, age profile and severity of respiratory symptoms and infections is obviously greatly affected by many environmental and social factors such as parental (and possibly child) smoking, age of starting playgroup or school, number and age of siblings, immunization status, ethnic background and overcrowding. Hence respiratory disease forms a major part of any paediatric practice.

Lung development

The lungs develop as an outgrowth from the foregut and by 16 weeks gestation the bronchial tree has its full complement of generations. Thereafter the vascular supply continues to develop and the number of bronchioles increase. Alveoli are not present at term, but develop rapidly in the first few months after birth although the normal adult number is not reached until near to the end of the first decade. The sequence and timing of lung growth and development has implications for the type and severity of lung disease, as well as the possibility for recovery from insults occurring at different stages in lung development. Thus a diaphragmatic hernia present from the first trimester will cause a reduced number of bronchial divisions which cannot change even if the abnormality is successfully dealt with after birth. A diaphragmatic hernia occurring much later in gestation will not alter bronchial divisions but will still interfere with saccule and early alveolar development. Successful surgical repair may allow some natural improvement in these abnormalities to occur. It is this situation which has resulted in diaphragmatic hernia being one of the conditions in which prenatal surgery has been contemplated in order to allow normal lung development from before birth. Severe acquired lung disease after birth, for example in association with prematurity, has potential for continued repair of damage over many years if the patient can be supported through what may be a period of years of compromised lung function.

Anatomy and function

The air passages are usually divided somewhat arbitrarily into three levels: upper, middle and lower (Table 11.1). Pathology affecting the respiratory tract does not abruptly change at those divisions but symptoms and signs vary such that careful consideration of these often allows the major site of the problem to be ascertained by clinical means. Division of lungs into lobes and, within

Conducting zone	Respiratory zone	**Table 11.1** Simplified division of the respiratory tract.
Extra thoracic		
Upper airway		
Nose		
Pharynx		
Sinuses		
Middle airway		
Larynx		
Upper trachea		
Intra-thoracic		
Lower airway	Respiratory bronchioles	
Lower trachea	Alveolar ducts	Intra-thoracic
Bronchi	Alveolar sacs	
Terminal bronchioles		

lobes, into bronchopulmonary segments is of clinical importance both in the anatomical localization of abnormalities detected on examination and in the interpretation of chest X-rays. Lung function can be assessed clinically in terms of exercise tolerance, by lung function testing and by blood gas values, some of which can be obtained with some accuracy non-invasively (oxygen saturation and to a lesser extent oxygen and carbon dioxide tensions).

Standard lung volumes are illustrated in Figure 11.1 and can be measured with a spirometer which school-age children are usually able to cope with if not too nervous or too breathless. A simpler and more convenient tool is the peak flow meter which is helpful in assessing and monitoring children with obstructive airway disease, particularly asthma. If taught over a period of time when they are not acutely ill, some children as young as 4 years can use peak flow meters which can then be issued for home use in selected cases.

Arterial blood gas analysis in childhood is rarely warranted outside an intensive care setting because of the pain and distress caused by the procedure. Capillary samples from a prewarmed toe or heel may be justified to monitor hypercapnia or acidosis in infants with acute respiratory disease,

for example bronchiolitis, but requires some skill to get satisfactory samples. Acid–base problems are discussed in Chapter 16.

Symptoms of respiratory disease

Cough

This is the single most common symptom about which parents consult GPs and is a feature of a wide range of diseases. In taking the history of the cough it is important, and usually possible, to differentiate it from simple clearing of the throat which is common and may be a feature of postnasal drip. Opportunity to hear the child's cough should be taken, as the nature of it may be very helpful in making a diagnosis. Cough is essentially a symptom of disease at or below the larynx although a foreign body in the ear may cause cough in some people due to reflex stimulation. An anatomically arranged list of causes of cough is given in Table 11.2.

Lower respiratory tract disease can usually be recognized by other features in the history and on examination. It should be realized that infants and young children do not expectorate but that sputum may be seen and described in vomitus.

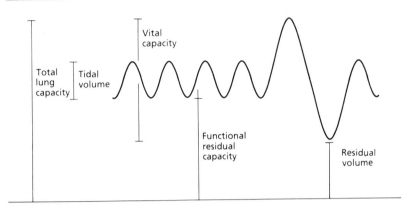

Fig. 11.1 Standard lung volumes.

Table 11.2 Anatomical classification for the causes of chronic cough.

Upper airway
Post-nasal drip
Foreign body in ear

Middle airway
Laryngeal foreign body
Compression
  Hilar nodes and/or other masses
  Aberrant blood vessels
Tracheomalacia

Lower airway
Asthma
Foreign body
Pertussis

Pulmonary
Consolidation
Collapse
Bronchiectasis

Cardiac
Pulmonary venous congestion
Pulmonary oedema

Psychogenic

Table 11.3 Causes of haemoptysis in children.

Common
Pneumonia
Inhaled foreign body
Laryngo-tracheitis

Uncommon
Cystic fibrosis
Arteriovenous malformation
  Airway
  Pulmonary
Complex cyanotic congenital heart disease
Tuberculosis
Haemosiderosis
Tumour

Exclude
Nasal, pharyngeal, oral bleeding
Haematemasis

Clearly a description of sputum can be helpful and although small amounts of blood in sputum are not uncommon in children with acute infections of their middle airways, large or repeated haemoptysis requires careful evaluation beginning with confirmation of the observation and exclusion of haematemesis and bleeding from nose and throat. Causes of haemoptysis are given in Table 11.3.

Airway disease frequently causes cough and it may be the initial or only manifestation of bronchial hyper-reactivity without the other classic features of asthma. Thus to include exercise, excitement, allergens, cold air as well as respiratory infections in the list of precipitants enquired about is important. Sometimes peak flow measurements before and after exercise will be required to demonstrate that cough is a feature of bronchial lability or a trial with a bronchodilator (e.g. salbutamol) or prophylactic agent (e.g. sodium cromoglycate) may be needed. The cough of acute or chronic laryngeal disease has a croupy, hoarse or barking nature and is usually accompanied by hoarseness and inspiratory stridor. Children with tracheo-malacia have a characteristic low pitched bovine cough which is more marked with intercurrent infections. Tracheomalacia is frequently seen in association with a previous history of oesophageal atresia and tracheo-oesophageal fistula repaired in the neonatal period. During exacerbations, they often have predominantly expiratory stridor which is a sign of intrathoracic middle airway collapse or narrowing and is otherwise uncommon. Stridor is discussed in Chapter 10.

PSYCHOGENIC COUGH

Cough of psychogenic origin is one that persists after an initial clear physical cause for the cough is likely to have resolved. It disappears in sleep (many causes for cough are worse at night, when lying or when exposed to house dust mite or other allergens in the bedroom) and is commonest in adolescents. It is frequently described as honk-ing like a goose. Often secondary gain from the symptom can be identified and it normally, but not always, responds to sympathetic talking through the problem with the child and family. Antitussives are rarely, if ever, indicated in paediatrics; attempts to find specific treatments for the cough in pertussis have not been particularly successful.

Dyspnoea

Dyspnoea means shortness of breath. Young children and infants cannot complain of shortness of breath and even some school-age children will find it hard to express themselves. Parents' reports of 'breathing difficulty' need to be enquired into more closely to see if they mean noisy respiration, fast breathing, reduced exercise tolerance or difficult and uncomfortable looking respiration. In babies, breathlessness most commonly shows itself as difficulty in taking or completing feeds hence this complaint requires, amongst other things, detailed consideration of the respiratory history. Table 11.4 lists the possible causes. Stridor and

Table 11.4 Classification of the commoner causes of dyspnoea.

	Examples
Airway obstruction	
Congenital abnormality	Laryngomalacia
Compression	Hilar lymphadenopathy
Foreign body	
Asthma	
Pulmonary	
Collapse/consolidation	Infection, foreign body
Over inflation	Congenital lobar emphysema, foreign body
Cardiac	
Severe hypoxaemia	Cyanotic congenital heart disease
Pulmonary plethora	Large ventricular septal defect
Pulmonary venous obstruction	Heart failure
Metabolic	
Metabolic acidosis	Diabetic ketoacidosis
Neurological	
Cerebral irritation	Meningitis

nasal obstruction should be distinguished from true dyspnoea. Neonatal causes of respiratory distress are dealt with in Chapter 7.

Wheeze

This refers to an almost musical noise predominantly expiratory in timing coming from intrathoracic airways. Lay people may describe a number of respiratory noises as wheeze and it is necessary to clarify what type of noise they are describing in their child. Many parents will have a good idea as to whether a noise is originating in the throat, neck or chest. Having established that wheeze is the problem, the doctor then tries to find out what precipitating factors are suspected, whether the noise is constant or variable, whether there is predictable diurnal or seasonal variation and to what extent the child is ill or breathless with the symptom. Family history may also be helpful, not only of wheeze, but of other respiratory problems and of atopic or allergic illnesses.

As previously stated, one child in five will wheeze at some time in the first 5 years of life and in many of these the symptom will be mild, causing very little disturbance. The challenge is to detect those children with asthma who will benefit from treatment. Particular features that indicate the need for investigation are onset at a very young age, asymmetry of rhonchi heard on auscultation, absence of intercurrent viral infection as a precipitant in young children, constant wheeze, asymmetry of chest movement, persisting chest X-ray abnormalities or failure to thrive, with or without, diarrhoea. Foreign travel, contact with possible tuberculosis and sudden onset leading to suspicion of foreign body inhalation are also indications to consider diagnoses other than simple wheeze-associated respiratory infection. Table 11.5 gives causes of wheeze at different ages.

It should be emphasized that most wheezy infants and pre-school children do not need investigation if the episodes are short lived in association with viral infections, recovery is complete and general health, growth and development are normal.

Table 11.5 Causes of wheeze in childhood classified by age.

Infancy
Acute
  Bronchiolitis
  Other viral infections
  Pertussis
  Tuberculosis
  Cardiac failure
  Foreign body

Chronic or recurrent
  Cystic fibrosis
  Cardiac failure
  Recurrent aspiration
  Bronchial or lower tracheal obstruction
    Compression—aberrant vessels, nodes, masses
    Foreign body
    Tracheomalacia, bronchomalacia
  Obliterative bronchiolitis

Older children
Acute
  Viral infections
  Mycoplasma infection
  Foreign body

Chronic or recurrent
  Asthma
  Cystic fibrosis
  Bronchiectasis
  α_1 antitrypsin deficiency

Hyperventilation

The entity of chronic hyperventilation causing multiple symptoms and not being readily apparent on talking to, or examining, the patient is a controversial one and relates mainly to adults. In children acute hyperventilation is relatively common and is perceived by child and parents as a respiratory problem in some cases, although in others the presentation may be of funny turns or strange sensations in hands or feet. When a child presents with fast breathing the possibility of an underlying respiratory problem, for example asthma, or of metabolic acidosis must be considered and can usually fairly easily be confirmed or refuted. Confusion can arise when the child also suffers from a chronic illness such as asthma, cardiac disease or diabetes mellitus which may cause similar breathing problems and produce the background anxieties often present in over-breathing problems. Furthermore, hyperventilation may induce bronchospasm in some people.

The problem of primary hyperventilation is one of older children with the exception of the very rare Joubert's syndrome in which periods of very fast respiration in association with major brain malformation (particularly absence of cerebellum) are present from the newborn period.

A history of paraesthesiae of fingers and toes and sometimes of carpopedal spasm due to respiratory alkalosis suggest hyperventilation. If presentation is in the form of fainting turns a change in respiratory pattern and sensation as well as the presence of paraesthesiae must be specifically asked after. Observers may have noted strange respiration preceding the neurological episode. A classic history particularly if a spontaneous attack is witnessed or one can be induced allows a positive diagnosis to be made with certainty. Sometimes a capillary blood gas sample and a peak flow reading during an episode are helpful. If other diagnoses need to be ruled out this is better done at initial presentation so that appropriate reassurance and instructions for prevention can be given with confidence. Causes of stress and anxiety are often easily identified and recognition of the problem may allow simple measures such as deliberately breathing slowly and rebreathing into a paper bag. If there are major psychosocial or emotional problems referral to a child psychiatrist may be helpful but in many cases this is not necessary.

Respiratory failure

This is said to exist when gaseous exchange through the lungs is inadequate to maintain arterial blood gas tensions of oxygen and carbon dioxide within the normal range.

Aetiology

A list of causes of respiratory failure in childhood is given in Table 11.6. Some of these conditions

Table 11.6 Causes of respiratory failure.

Neurological
Head injury
Meningitis
Encephalitis
Drugs
Spinal muscular atrophy

Muscular
Muscular dystrophies

Skeletal
Injury to chest
Scoliosis
Asphyxiating thoracic dystrophy

Cardiological
Severe heart failure
Obstructed pulmonary venous return

Obstructed airway
Inhaled foreign body
Laryngeal web
Laryngo-tracheobronchitis
Epiglottitis
Bronchial stenosis
Congenital lobar emphysema
Asthma
Cystic fibrosis

Reduced lung volume
Pulmonary agenesis/hypoplasia
Pulmonary collapse/consolidation
Cystic fibrosis
Pleural effusions

will be immediately recognizable or have specific treatment (e.g. foreign body inhalation, asthma, epiglottitis) but the general approach remains the same.

Clinical features

These are listed in Table 11.7 and will be influenced by the underlying cause. Certain signs are particularly valuable and at times allow diagnosis to be made and management to be begun without distressing the child further with blood gas analyses. Arterial blood samples can be difficult and are painful for the children.

Table 11.7 Features of progressing respiratory failure.

Clinical
Worsening cyanosis, increased oxygen requirement
Rising pulse rate
Increased pulse volume with hypercapnia
Increasing respiratory rate
Flaring nostrils
Increasing recession
Restlessness
Reduced conscious state

Investigations
Falling arterial oxygen tension
Rising carbon dioxide tension
Falling pH
Falling transcutaneous oxygen tension
Rising transcutaneous carbon dioxide tension
Falling oxygen saturation on oximetry

Arterialized capillary samples will give information on pH and carbon dioxide tensions but decisions to relieve airway obstruction or mechanically ventilate are usually based on clinical assessment. Rate, effort and pattern of respiration are all important as well as the presence of respiratory noise. Cyanosis, tachycardia and confusion or altered conscious state are serious signs, warm peripheries with bounding pulses signify hypercapnia.

Investigations

Some features of respiratory compromise may be well tolerated and the respiratory acidosis induced by hypercapnia may become well compensated (by maintaining a high plasma bicarbonate) if the time scale is long enough for this form of compensation to occur. Hypoxaemia without carbon dioxide retention may occur if hyperventilation accompanies the disease (for example in acute asthma or acute pneumonia) and can be a feature of non-respiratory disease, particularly cyanotic congenital heart disease. Severe hypoxaemia may result in metabolic acidosis, particularly if poor tissue perfusion (ischaemia) also occurs. It is the combination of hypoxaemia and ischaemia that is especially damaging to brain and other vital structures. Hypoxaemia due to respiratory disease without concomitant hypercapnia will usually be improved by increasing inspired oxygen concentration. The presence of hypercapnia as well as hypoxaemia requires assisted ventilation unless the cause can be rapidly, effectively and safely dealt with.

Management

Giving oxygen is important, the risks of suppressing respiratory drive in chronically hypercapnic children by doing this is small and in any case such patients are going to be observed closely and looked after in a unit where tracheal intubation could be immediately performed if necessary. Trends in all clinical parameters are important and a short period of careful and close monitoring with application of any specific treatments usually allows assessment of need for more aggressive care to be made. Controlled intubation by an experienced operator with sedative and neuromuscular blocking agents being used is preferable to crisis intubation when respiratory arrest occurs. Management of respiratory failure is simply outlined in Table 11.8.

Abnormalities of the chest wall

Children with chronic or recurrent respiratory difficulties may develop abnormally shaped chests, similarly those with unusually soft bones (e.g. rickets) will do so in response to normal or mildly increased respiratory effort. Pre-term babies therefore may have chest deformity persisting some years after their respiratory problems have resolved. Table 11.9 lists types of chest wall deformity.

Table 11.8 Simplified approach to respiratory failure.

1 Ensure good airway:
    Deal with secretions and bronchospasm
    Intubate if necessary
2 Give increased inspired oxygen
3 Check for respiratory acidosis:
    (Arterial blood gas)
    Ventilate if necessary
4 Treat underlying cause

Table 11.9 Types of chest wall deformity seen in children.

Harrison's sulcus
Pectus excavatum (funnel chest)
Pectus carinatum (pigeon chest)
Congenital absence of one or more ribs
Scoliosis

HARRISON'S SULCI

These represent the attachment of diaphragm to the inner aspect of the rib cage (Plate 1) and their presence should alert the clinician to a history of airway obstruction (for example, by massive tonsillar enlargement) or recurrent chest problems of some sort, such as asthma or cystic fibrosis. Abnormally pliable bones as are seen in rickets would be a very uncommon cause in developed countries and other features should also be present including swollen epiphyses of wrist and ankle, as well as the 'rickety rosary'. Minor degrees of Harrison's sulci are seen in some normal children.

PECTUS EXCAVATUM

Pectus excavatum, also called funnel chest, is an abnormality which is usually apparent to some degree at birth; it may progress or regress thereafter. Not infrequently there is a family history. It is a matter of debate as to whether the abnormality causes any symptoms. Various respiratory complaints have been attributed to it but its chief importance is two-fold; first, the cosmetic aspect, and secondly, it may be associated with Marfan's syndrome (p. 485) and related disorders which have major implications for the child and his family. Isolated pectus excavatum, without scoliosis or other skeletal abnormalities, can result in the cardiac apex appearing to be displaced laterally with an unusual cardiac contour on X-ray together with unusual electrocardiographic findings. These must not cause the diagnosis of a non-existent cardiac problem to be made. Indication for surgical correction of isolated pectus excavatum is cosmetic and rarely appropriate.

PECTUS CARINATUM

Pectus carinatum (pigeon chest) is a rarer congenital abnormality which is usually only of cosmetic importance. Some children with chronic obstructive lung disease or congenital heart disease have a very prominent sternum sometimes similar to pectus carinatum but history, examination, chest X-ray and electrocardiogram will differentiate these conditions.

Congenital abnormalities of the lower respiratory tract

Structural congenital abnormalities of upper and middle airways have been dealt with in Chapter 10.

Tracheal abnormalities

Tracheal agenesis is clearly incompatible with extra-uterine life. Tracheal stenosis will cause stridor and respiratory difficulties from birth and tracheostomy is likely to be needed as the initial form of management. Acquired tracheal or sub-glottic stenosis is much commoner, being seen in those children who had had prolonged or repeated tracheal intubation for respiratory disease as neonates or infants. Tracheomalacia has already been discussed in the section on cough.

Tracheo-oesophageal fistula was discussed in Chapter 9 and usually accompanies oesophageal atresia. It rarely occurs as an isolated abnormality in which case the child usually presents with choking on feeds and recurrent pneumonia. Considerable delay often occurs in making the diagnosis which is best demonstrated by contrast swallow or endoscopy.

Bronchial abnormalities

Bronchial stenosis may be congenital or acquired and will cause varying degrees of collapse, consolidation or over-inflation of lung distal to the stenotic segment. Other causes of extrinsic compression to the lower airway includes aberrant or

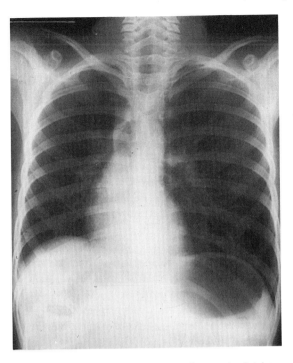

Fig. 11.2   Radiograph showing partial agenesis of right lung producing mediastinal shift to the right.

enlarged blood vessels, massive cardiomegaly, mediastinal tumours and hilar lymphadenopathy. Bronchogenic cysts are a rare cause of such compression which may be detected coincidentally when a chest X-ray is performed for some unrelated reason.

Pulmonary abnormalities

Hypoplasia, aplasia or agenesis of a lobe or whole lung (Fig. 11.2) may occur either alone or in conjunction with other congenital abnormalities, for example, cardiac malformations. Respiratory difficulty ranges from none to severe depending on the amount of lung missing, the degree of mediastinal shift and the presence and type of other abnormalities. Thus a cardiac lesion with a large left to right shunt or a stenosed proximal airway will greatly exacerbate problems encountered with absence of a lobe or lung. Babies with congenital diaphragmatic hernia have hypoplastic lungs on both sides, although, more gross on the herniated side. Survival after surgery is basically determined by the degree of lung hypoplasia.

CONGENITAL LOBAR EMPHYSEMA

Congenital softening or absence of bronchial cartilage in one or more lobes may allow the affected areas to become over-inflated thereby producing congenital lobar emphysema. Symptoms are often progressive and may be absent at birth. Feeding difficulty, tachypnoea, indrawing, asymmetry of chest movement with unilateral over-inflation are increasingly apparent over the first few months of life. Chest X-ray shows over-inflation of one or more lobes with compression of adjacent ones and mediastinal shift (Fig. 11.3). Left upper, right middle and right upper lobes are most commonly affected. Associated cardiac and other anomalies must be sought, and external compression or intrinsic acquired obstruction of affected bronchi has to be considered. Spontaneous resolution is recognized but many cases need lobectomy to relieve symptoms and to allow collapsed lobes to re-expand.

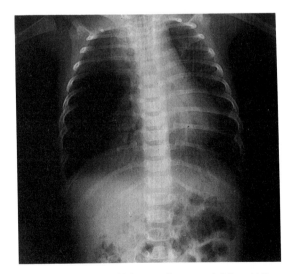

Fig. 11.3   Congenital lobar emphysema of right middle lobe. The X-ray shows compression of the right upper and lower lobes.

SEQUESTRATED LOBE

Occasionally a lobe of lung derives its arterial supply from branches off the aorta and drains venous blood into the right atrium usually indirectly via the inferior vena cava or azygos vein. Such lobes are abnormally formed and do not connect normally to the bronchial tree if at all. They are termed sequestrated, are more common in males and may be asymptomatic. They may produce a characteristic curve (scimitar) on chest X-ray because of abnormal vasculature draining from them. The haemodynamic effects caused by a sequestrated lobe are usually insignificant but they provide a nidus for sepsis which may be recurrent and may develop into lung abscess. It is for these reasons that removal is indicated.

Extremely rare lung malformations include cystic adenomatous malformation, pulmonary lymphagiectasia and pulmonary arterio-venous malformations. The reader is directed to larger works for details of these (see Further Reading at the end of the chapter.

Disorders of the pleura

Many pleural diseases are infective in origin and as such are often associated with underlying pulmonary infection and merely represent secondary extension of primary lung pathology. Primary infection of the pleura and special aspects of pleural infection will be dealt with here, the overall approach to infections of the lower respiratory tract is covered in the section on pneumonia.

Pleurisy

This is usually due to infection. The degree of systemic disturbance, pyrexia and elevation of white cell count depends on the causative organism, but primary and predominantly pleural infection is usually viral, relatively mild and self-limiting.

Clinical features

Pleuritic pain is typically sharp and stabbing in nature being made worse by coughing or deep inspiration. If diaphragmatic pleura is involved,

pain may be referred to the shoulder tip. Pain of this nature is very characteristic when a child can describe it. In younger children the splinting of part of the chest wall and rapid shallow respirations may provide the clue. Peritonitis and pericarditis can give very similar pictures; underlying pneumonia may be responsible. Diminished breath sounds over the affected area and a pleural rub are not necessarily detected; signs of consolidation or effusion may be found. Chest X-ray can be normal or may show pneumonic changes or an effusion, which is usually small.

Management

Simple analgesia is all that is required providing the diagnosis is not seriously in doubt; such cases are rarely seen in hospital and many probably do not even come to the family doctor's attention. The differential diagnosis of viral pleurisy includes Bornholm disease.

BORNHOLM DISEASE (EPIDEMIC MYALGIA)

This is sometimes called pleurodynia, is caused by Coxsackie B viruses and is associated with spasms of severe pain. These spasms may also affect the abdominal wall musculature when differentiation from intra-abdominal pathology may be difficult.

Pleural effusion

This may be unilateral or bilateral and may be due to pulmonary, pleural or systemic disease. A list of causes is given in Table 11.10. Clinical features include reduced chest expansion, dull percussion note, reduced breath sounds (sometimes with bronchial breathing at the upper border) and mediastinal shift away from the affected side in very large unilateral lesions. There are two indications for tapping or draining an effusion; for diagnosis and far less commonly for the relief of respiratory compromise in very large effusions. Diagnostic tests on pleural fluid are given in Table 11.11. Investigations vary according to the suspected aetiology and treatment is that of the underlying disorder. Grossly purulent effusion is

Table 11.10   Causes of pleural effusion in childhood.

Infection
Acute pyogenic pneumonia
Tuberculosis

Cardiac
Heart failure

Hypoalbuminaemia
Nephrotic syndrome
Protein losing enteropathy

Collagen vascular disease
Rheumatoid arthritis
Systemic lupus erythematosus

Chylous effusion
Idiopathic
Post surgical

Malignant
Lymphoma
Leukaemia
Ewing's tumour

Table 11.11   Diagnostic tests on pleural fluid.

Microscopy
White blood cells, number, type
Other cells (cytology)
Fat globules

Gram stain
Organisms

Ziehl–Neelsen stain

Biochemistry
Protein
Glucose
Triglycerides

Immunological tests
Rheumatoid factor
Antinuclear factor

Culture

termed empyema and is secondary to pyogenic pneumonia. Pus should be removed for bacteriological diagnosis and to prevent a septic focus persisting. Open surgical drainage may be necessary if repeated aspirations are required or percutaneous insertion of a chest drain fails to release pus.

Pneumothorax

Outside the spectrum of neonatal lung disease, pneumothorax is infrequent in children (Fig. 11.4). The commonest cause is trauma and haemothorax may also occur. Pulmonary air leak may occur in any respiratory illness which is severe enough to require assisted ventilation and is a well recognized, albeit rare, complication of asthma, cystic fibrosis, lung abscess and congenital emphysema.

In acute asthma, pulmonary air leak is quite common if small amounts of mediastinal or subcutaneous air are looked for on X-ray. Subcutaneous emphysema in the suprasternal and supraclavicular regions is occasionally found and indicates the need for chest X-ray to detect

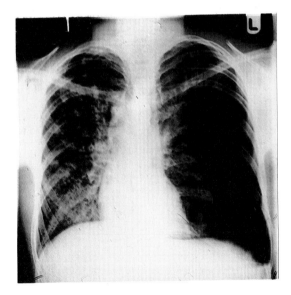

Fig. 11.4   Left-sided pneumothorax in a child with cystic fibrosis.

pneumothorax which may be hard to detect clinically and requires urgent drainage. In cystic fibrosis, pneumothorax may be recurrent and the risk of bronchopleural fistula and emphysema are real.

Management can be difficult both in terms of

Table 11.12 Causative organisms of pneumonia in a normal host.

Streptococcus pneumoniae
Mycoplasma pneumoniae
Haemophilus influenzae
Staphylococcus aureus
Chlamydia trachomatis
Virus
Respiratory syncytial virus
Influenza
Parainfluenza viruses
Adenoviruses
Coxsackie viruses
Rhinoviruses

resolution of an acute episode and in preventing relapse. The introduction of sclerosing agents into the pleural cavity to obliterate it is probably preferable to surgical removal of the parietal pleura.

Respiratory infections

Infections of upper and middle respiratory tract are dealt with in Chapter 10 and will only be referred to here in so far as they often co-exist or predispose to lower respiratory infections.

Pneumonia

This is caused by a wide range of micro-organisms in otherwise healthy individuals (Table 11.12). Any of those aetiological agents can also affect immunocompromised hosts but other micro-organisms occur particularly or exclusively in those with impaired immune responses. Indeed, the detection of an unusual organism should alert the clinician to the possibility of an underlying immune defect. Congenital abnormality of the bronchi or lung parenchyma, previously inhaled foreign body, prolonged pulmonary collapse and acute or chronic aspiration may predispose to lung infection. Babies and children with plethoric lungs due to a large left to right shunt have frequent respiratory symptoms, but it is not clear whether they are at greatly increased risk of pneumonia. Children unable to clear secretions efficiently for

any reason are at increased risk. Chronic sinusitis is associated with chronic or recurrent lower respiratory infection, classically bronchiectasis. The common entity of the child with repeated or constant coryza and cough is probably in the vast majority of cases not truly a problem of significant lower respiratory infection and will be discussed later.

Lung consolidation may be focal and limited by segments or lobes (Fig. 11.5) or it can be diffuse and patchy causing bronchopneumonia (Fig. 11.6). The precise pattern depends on many factors including the infecting organism (e.g. *Pneumococcus* usually causes lobar pneumonia) and what predisposing factors, if any, exist. Ineffective clearance of secretions favours the development of bronchopneumonia.

Clinical features

Acute pneumonia presents with a short history of systemic disturbance and often pleuritic pain. Cough is not a marked feature. Signs include a flushed miserable and pyrexial child. There may be laboured respiration with grunting or more subtle flaring of the nostrils and tachypnoea with intercostal recession. Signs of consolidation should be detected in older children, but in infants they are often hard to define. Meningism may be present and shoulder tip or abdominal pain can also divert attention from the correct diagnosis.

Investigations

Streptococcus pneumoniae is still a common cause of this clinical picture although *Mycoplasma pneumoniae*, *Haemophilus influenzae*, *Staphylococcus aureus* and several viruses can also produce it. Gram stain and culture of the sputum are helpful if a sample can be obtained and blood culture may be positive. In the UK, many febrile children will have received doses of oral antibiotic prior to attending hospital and culture results therefore can be misleading. White cell counts are seldom of practical value in differentiating aetiology. In a classic presentation it is reasonable to treat as if pneumococcal

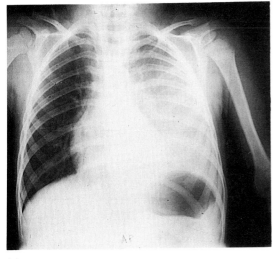

(a)

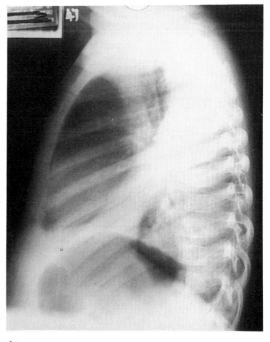

(b)

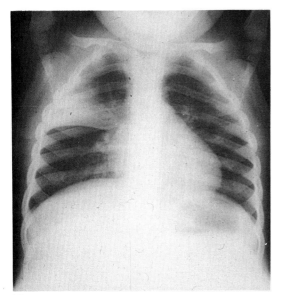

(c)

Fig. 11.5 Radiographic appearances of consolidation. (a) Postero-anterior (PA) view; (b) lateral view of left lower lobe consolidation; and (c) right upper lobe (anterior segment) consolidation.

pneumonia is the infecting organism; blood and sputum cultures having been obtained prior to treatment with antibiotics.

Serum for cold agglutinins (in *Mycoplasma* infections) and viral serology should be obtained if there is not a dramatic improvement within 24 hours of starting treatment. Alternative infective agents should be considered and antibiotic spectrum broadened if the child is very ill, several lobes are involved, previous antibiotic therapy has

been properly given and failed, or the history is more than a few days (Table 11.13). In infants *Streptococcus pneumoniae* may cause bronchopneumonia with correspondingly less localized and specific signs and patchy not focal changes on X-ray. Most causative agents for acute pneumonia can cause similar clinical features. Bronchopneumonia is more likely in infancy and certain clinical association can point to particular diagnoses (Table 11.14).

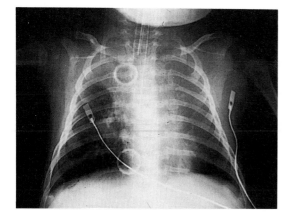

Fig. 11.6 Radiographic appearance of diffuse pneumonic changes. There is also collapse of the right upper lobe.

Table 11.14   Clinical correlations with pneumonia.

Feature	Probable organism
Acute lobar consolidation	*Streptococcus pneumoniae*
Infant, with gradual onset, and previous history of sticky eyes	*Chlamydia*
Infant, with associated meningitis or epiglottitis	*Haemophilus influenzae*
Widespread X-ray changes, toxic	*Staphylococcus aureus*
Scchool-age child with bullous myringitis, arthralgia, headache	*Mycoplasma pneumoniae*
Previously debilitated infant or child	Gram-negative bacilli

Management

Seldom can clinical signs or simple immediate investigations diagnose viral pneumonia with certainty. Thus antibiotics are appropriate. Route of administration depends on how ill the child is, what the suspected aetiology is and what antibiotic is to be used. Attention should be paid to fluid and electrolyte balance as severely ill children with pneumonia may retain fluid excessively or may become dehydrated through tachypnoea and fever. Analgesia and antipyretics may be needed. Physiotherapy has little or no role in the acute stages. Oxygen should be given to those with marked respiratory distress who usually have extensive changes on X-ray. Occasionally ventilatory support is needed.

Complications

Complications of acute pneumonia are listed in Table 11.15. Any organism can cause lung abscess, although this is a particular feature of *Staph. aureus* infections. This organism along with some Gram-negative ones is particularly prone to causing empyema, but any organism can be associated with serous sympathetic pleural effusions. Distant

Table 11.13   Antibiotic treatment of pneumonia.

Acute lobar pneumonia	Parenteral penicillin, *or* oral amoxycillin, *or* if allergy, erythromycin
If severely ill	Ampicillin and flucloxacillin
If widespread pneumonic changes	Parenteral antibiotics initially
If suspicion of either *Mycoplasma* or *Chlamydia*	Erythromycin
In debilitated patients, if severely ill	Start with ampicillin, flucloxacillin and gentamicin; change antibiotics in light of cultures/response Also consider pneumocystis

Table 11.15 Complications of pneumonia.

Acute	Chronic
Dehydration	Persisting lobar collapse
Hyponatraemia	Bronchiectasis
Respiratory failure	Recurrent pneumonia
Lung abscess	
Empyema, pleural effusion	
Pyogenic foci	
Brain	
Pericardium	
Endocardium	
Bone	
Skin	
Kidney	
Pneumothorax	

Table 11.16 Some unusual causes of pneumonia.

Pneumocystis carinii	Acute lymphoblastic leukaemia
	HIV-infected infants
Cytomegalovirus	Immunodeficiency states, congenital, acquired including post-transplantation
Measles virus	Humoral immunodeficiency states
Fungi (*Candida, Aspergillus*)	Cellular immunodeficiency
	Prolonged exposure to antibiotic and tracheal intubation
Legionella pneumophilia	Exposure to contaminated air-conditioning system

(haematogenous) spread to pericardium or bone is rare in pneumoccal disease but common in staphylococcal sepsis. Local spread to the pericardium is also possible. *Haemophilus influenzae* may cause epiglottitis or meningitis in the same patient. Pneumococcal meningitis and pneumonia rarely coexist. Long term sequelae are rare in developed countries. Chickenpox pneumonitis can leave diffuse calcified lesions on X-ray without clinical problem. Adenovirus pneumonia can cause pulmonary fibrosis and broncholitis obliterans in a significant number of cases. Bronchiectasis is a very rare occurrence in previously healthy children, although measles and pertussis are predisposing factors in some cases.

PNEUMONIA IN IMMUNOCOMPROMISED HOSTS

Certain organisms are unlikely to infect previously healthy children. After the newborn period infection by unusual organisms may present in unusual ways and point to an underlying predisposition. When a child is already known to be at risk of such infections, diagnosis should not be delayed. Table 11.16 lists the more unusual micro-organisms likely to be encountered in immuno-incompetent patients together with the likely underlying conditions predisposing to infection. Clinical features of such infections may be subtle or non-specific and may not even point particularly to the respiratory system, thus a high index of suspicion is required. Chest X-ray may give diagnostic clues but may also be unhelpful. The pathogen may be identified from blood and/or sputum cultures relatively quickly. Virus cultures from upper respiratory tract secretions and serological tests take longer and pneumocystis, at present, can only be reliably diagnosed by open lung biopsy.

Specific treatment should be used where possible, but broad spectrum 'blind' therapy aiming at likely pathogens is often necessary in ill patients. Supportive measures and clarification of underlying predisposition are of course important. In children with acute leukaemia on cytotoxic treatment, regular co-trimoxazole is an effective prophylaxis against pneumocystis pneumonia (see Chapter 25).

Bronchiolitis

This is an acute viral lower respiratory tract infection occurring in epidemics in the winter months in temperate climates. It affects children under 18 months of age and respiratory syncytial virus (RSV) is responsible for the majority of cases although parainfluenza viruses and adenoviruses are sometimes identified.

Clinical features

Classically, an infant develops coryza, a characteristic cough, tachypnoea and feeding difficulty over a period of 3–5 days. Wheeze may be a feature but even without it the chest is over-inflated. Scattered crepitations on auscultation are characteristic. Mild cases will not reach hospital but apnoeic episodes, marked respiratory distress, feeding difficulty or cyanosis warrant admission.

Investigations

Chest X-ray shows over-inflation, sometimes peribronchial infiltrates and lobar collapse or consolidation may develop in some cases. RSV can be rapidly identified in the nasopharynx by immunofluorescent antibody techniques and this allows positive diagnosis which may influence decisions about isolation in hospital and withholding antibiotics.

Management

Physiotherapy is not indicated unless pulmonary collapse or consolidation develop; bronchodilators and steroids have no role. Added oxygen, tube feeding or intravenous fluids are indicated for more severe cases. Mechanical ventilation for either recurrent severe apnoea or respiratory failure is needed in 5–10% of those admitted to hospital. Recently the antiviral agent Ribavirin has been found to have some influence on the course of RSV bronchiolitis. This is not dramatic and experience is limited. If used at all it should be for those known to be at very high risk of dying from the disease such as babies with congenital heart disease and pulmonary hypertension, or those with chronic lung disease following neonatal respiratory problems. Complete recovery from uncomplicated bronchiolitis may take 2 or 3 weeks although hospital admission is usually much shorter than this.

Complications

The relationship between bronchiolitis in infancy and subsequent recurrent chestiness including asthma is complex, certainly those who wheeze with their first RSV infection are more likely to develop asthma subsequently but cause and effect cannot be differentiated. Obliterative bronchiolitis is a chronic pulmonary complication which may result in a unilateral small, but radiologically hyperlucent lung (McLeod's syndrome). Alternatively the child may have bilateral over-inflated lungs, but in either case, recurrent lower respiratory infections occur. This destructive process in lung tissue with ensuing fibrosis is a sequelae of adenovirus bronchiolitis rather than RSV infection. Older children and adults get repeated RSV infections as immunity is short lived but the clinical picture is generally different and milder than that seen in infancy, although a remarkably similar picture has been described in old age.

Pertussis (whooping cough)

Recent experience in the UK has shown that when immunization rates fell on account of exaggerated fears about vaccine toxicity, the number of cases of pertussis rose dramatically. This condition is discussed in the section on infectious diseases (p. 363).

Bronchitis

This term is often used to describe a variety of clinical conditions including viral laryngo-tracheo-bronchitis with short lived stridor, barking cough and hoarseness as well as the rare and usually more severe bacterial membranous tracheitis. A single acute feverish illness with productive cough, a few crepitations or rhonchi in the chest without evidence of pneumonia may be attributed to bronchitis. If such illnesses become recurrent or are associated with marked wheeze, with or without tachypnoea, then bronchitis is probably not a good description and wheeze-associated respiratory infection or asthma are more likely diagnoses. This is important if widespread use of antibiotics is to be avoided in viral illnesses; bronchodilators and asthma prophylaxis are more appropriate. If recurrent episodes are also associated with atopy and/or chronic nasal congestion, then the diagnosis of asthma with rhinitis is even more likely. Underlying bronchiectasis with chronic sinusitis must be excluded under these circumstances. This is usually fairly simple by means of history and examination with a chest X-ray if necessary. Childhood chronic bronchitis is a diagnosis very rarely made by paediatricians in the UK.

Tuberculosis

World-wide, this is a major problem and enters into the differential diagnosis of every respiratory symptom and sign encountered in childhood. It is not rare in Britain, but because it is more frequently seen in the developing world it is discussed in detail in Chapter 29.

Bronchiectasis

This is a condition in which bronchial damage or persistent pulmonary collapse results in dilatation of bronchi and bronchioles which become chronically infected. Underlying causes are detailed in Table 11.17 and may result in bronchiectasis either localized to one lobe or generalized throughout the lung. In some cases an underlying cause is not apparent, but these cases are becoming rare in communities with good nutrition, without extreme social deprivation and with good access to medical services. Not all cases show progression and, clinically if not radiologically, some actually improve with time.

Clinical features

The condition is characterized by chronic, productive cough with purulent sputum together with haemoptysis in some cases. Poor growth and chest deformity may be apparent, clubbing is present in some. Crepitations and rhonchi are heard in the chest. Progression to evidence of pulmonary hypertension and right heart failure are very uncommon in childhood. Chest X-ray can be normal or may show local or generalized tramline and ring shadows outlining thickened and dilated bronchi with small areas of consolidation. Its precise nature and extent can be demonstrated by bronchography but this is not indicated unless surgery is being considered (Fig. 11.7).

Investigations

Appropriate investigations to reveal any underlying cause should be performed. This should now include tests of cilia structure and function as some cases will be a manifestation of the immotile or dysmotile cilia syndrome. Lung function tests may help in assessing need for and response to bronchodilators.

Management

Management should include specific treatment for any underlying cause, prompt and relevant antibiotic treatment for exacerbations (sputum culture should be performed regularly), regular postural drainage and physiotherapy and attention to nutritional state. Prophylactic antibiotics (with cotrimoxazole, amoxycillin or a cephalosporin) may help some patients in winter months and influenza immunization is recommended for those over 4

Table 11.17 Predisposing factors in bronchiectasis.

Localized	Generalized
Inhaled foreign body	Severe pertussis or measles
Persisting lobar collapse	Immune deficiency, hypogammaglobulinaemia
Congenital bronchial stenosis	Cystic fibrosis
Tuberculosis	Immotile cilia syndrome

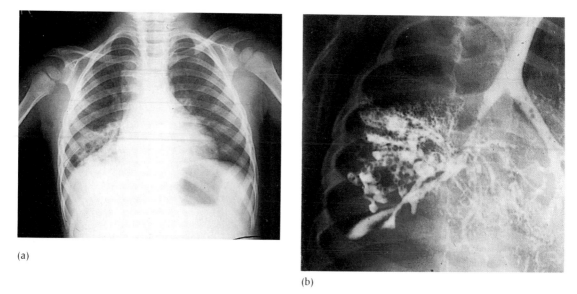

(a)

(b)

Fig. 11.7   Bronchiectasis. (a) Chest x-ray; and (b) bronchogram showing invovement of the right lower lobe.

years old. Smoking, active or passive, should be discouraged very strongly. Some patients will need prophylactic and therapeutic regimes for their accompanying sinusitis and chronic dental sepsis.

Removal of an affected lobe is only rarely indicated, even if the rest of the lung seems disease free and medical management is not controlling symptoms. In those with a suspected or confirmed underlying predisposition to generalized bronchiectasis, disease may still show itself in other parts of the lung after removal of an apparently isolated affected lobe. For this reason surgery should be even more cautiously embarked on in such patients.

Immotile cilia syndrome

Disorders of ciliary ultrastructure and function are being increasingly recognized. There is no doubt that structurally normal respiratory ciliated mucosal cells temporarily function abnormally and inadequately in response to a variety of noxious stimuli including viral infections and cigarette smoke. There is, however, a group of patients in whom abnormalities of ciliary structure detected

by electron microscopy are associated with permanent abnormalities of function noted by dissecting microscopic examination of ciliated epithelium.

Clinical features

Clinical spectrum in such individuals is from normality through recurrent chestiness and sinusitis to full-blown Kartagener's syndrome with dextrocardia, bronchiectasis and chronic sinusitis. Some forms of this condition show autosomal recessive inheritance, with affected males having reduced fertility because spermatozoal motility is also adversely affected.

Investigations

Diagnosis is made by clinical suspicion and confirmed by obtaining nasal or bronchial ciliated mucosa for conventional and electron microscopy. Facilities for obtaining satisfactory nasal brush samples of mucosa are not widespread in the UK and bronchial biopsy is only done if bronchoscopy with or without bronchography are indicated. Practical implications of making the diagnosis are probably not dramatic although in mild cases without established bronchiectasis a more vigorous approach to episodes of chestiness may be advised. Natural history in those mildly affected in terms of respiratory morbidity and the value of more aggressive diagnostic and management strategies are unclear. Genetic implications for parents and possible future subfertility in affected male children also raise difficult issues at the present time.

Asthma

Asthma is defined clinically as episodic reversible intrathoracic airways obstruction; the reversibility being either spontaneous or in response to treatment. Pathophysiologically, airway secretions, mucosal swelling and bronchial smooth muscle constriction all contribute to airway obstruction. Such pathological changes will occur in anyone in response to certain noxious stimuli (for example sulphur dioxide) but only in some people in response to intercurrent infection, allergens, exercise and changes of air temperature. Such persons are said to have hyper-reactive airways. This condition may be only temporary after infections such as pertussis and mycoplasma. In others, the tendency to bronchial hyper-reactivity or lability persists longer although clinical problems may not always occur. Thus one of the parents of an asthmatic child may have abnormal bronchial lability demonstrable on lung function testing but deny any lower respiratory symptoms at all. In addition, there may or may not be a parental history of childhood cough and wheeze or of present symptoms of another atopic or allergic condition.

Much dispute surrounds the issue of whether infants with recurrent cough and wheeze have asthma. They do not consistently show a clinical response to bronchodilators and not all of them develop typical asthma as older children. Conversely, many asthmatic children do have symptoms dating back to the first year or two of life even if they were mild or were not recognized for many years as manifestation of bronchial hyper-reactivity. In asthmatic children and their families there is a high incidence of other atopic illnesses such as hay fever, rhinitis, eczema, urticaria and food or drug intolerance due to allergy producing gastrointestinal or dermatological symptoms. The relationship between such allergies and behaviour problems is much less clear.

Clinical features

Asthma classically shows itself by recurrent episodes of cough, wheeze and breathlessness. One of these symptoms may predominate to the extent that others are only admitted to after careful questioning. Severe cases will still show periodicity in severity but may not become entirely asymptomatic. Precipitants include intercurrent viral infections especially in younger children, running, being tickled, getting excited, changes in temperature or humidity, and allergens. Sometimes more than one precipitating or exacerbating factor needs to be present for bronchospasm to occur, thus running may be tolerated unless it is very cold or the grass has just been cut. A curious relationship to drinking cola style drinks and developing wheeze some hours later is recognized.

History taking will give clues to the particular precipitating factors. Features to note include seasonal variation (alternaria mould spores in autumn, viral infections in winter), diurnal variation (symptoms from house dust mite allergy are likely to be worse at night), recent move of house or cavity wall insulation installation and intermittent or regular contact with animal hair or fur. This last point is emotive in many households. Daily contact with animal dander directly or via contaminated carpets and furniture may keep bronchi especially labile without symptoms being particularly brought on by handling the pet. Removal of the animal from the home for short trial periods will not remove its dander from the house and no improvement may be seen. Complete separation of the patient from the contaminated environment may produce improvement.

History taking must include details of how disruptive to life asthma is in terms of exercise tolerance, activities curtailed or avoided, school time missed, nights disturbed and medication usage. Features in the history which undermine the diagnosis of asthma should be thought about carefully, these include no periodicity, presence of symptoms from birth, no family or personal history of atopic illnesses and no response at all to properly administered asthma treatments in children over 18 months of age. In an acute attack details of suspected precipitant, frequency of and response to bronchodilator administration, degree to which walking or talking are impaired and the presence of blue lips at any time must be sought.

Physical examination of a mild asthmatic between episodes may be normal, but some clues such as mild Harrison's sulci or the production of prolonged expiration or expiratory rhonchi when the child is asked to breathe out fast and hard through an open mouth may be elicited. Evidence for other atopic illnesses should be looked for, such as eczema, rhinitis with a transverse crease across the nose from much rubbing, shiny smooth nails from scratching itchy, but not overtly eczematous skin, and creases under the eyes. Growth should always be plotted. More severe cases may have evidence of Harrison's sulci and even when claiming to be well there may be over-inflation of the chest with audible wheeze or expiratory rhonchi on auscultation. Growth delay and marked chest deformity are only rarely seen.

Abnormalities on cardiovascular examination other than tachycardia, evidence of tracheal deviation, asymmetry of any chest signs and the presence of clubbing are not features of asthma and cast major doubt on the diagnosis. Clinical features in acute episodes are listed in Table 11.18.

Investigations

Investigations of mild cases can be minimal; a chest X-ray when well should be normal. Lung function tests, either using a peak flow meter or spirometer, to confirm diagnosis or assess response to drugs may be helpful. If there is initially no evidence of airway obstruction this may be demonstrated after exercise in a high proportion of cases. This is rarely necessary, but if symptoms are not typical it may save much anxiety and time. Peak flow meters can be issued for use at home in selected cases where there are diagnostic or therapeutic problems. Demonstrating eosinophilia or elevated total IgE levels is not particularly helpful. Specific IgE levels or allergen skin-prick testing are greatly used by some and they reveal allergic children, but in terms of advice to families a detailed history is usually sufficient as house dust mite and grass sensitivity can be suspected on this basis and other allergens producing positive skin or IgE results may not be the cause of symptoms.

Management

Treatment of asthma requires attention to a number of aspects in addition to drug therapy. Precipitant avoidance is theoretically pleasing but practically limited in value. Viral infections cannot be avoided, exercise should not be avoided and allergens may not be identifiable. Cut grass or an offending animal not living with the family can probably be largely avoided. The family pet can be kept from the bedroom and certain families can be advised against getting furry or hairy pets. House dust mite reduction in the bedroom is worth a vigorous 4 or 6 weeks trial in those with predominantly nocturnal symptoms and should only be continued in those convinced of benefit. Desensitization is dangerous and ineffective. Physiotherapy and breathing exercises have little role. Encouraging a frightened child with mild asthma to relax and breathe more calmly in an attack by education when well sometimes helps.

An essential part of all asthma management in

Table 11.18 Clinical features of acute asthma.

	Mild	Severe
Speech	Normal	Impossible
Pulse rate	Normal	Marked tachycardia
Character	Normal	Paradoxical
Colour	Pink	Cyanosed
Respiratory rate	Normal	Increased
Indrawing	Absent	Marked
Posture	Normal	Marked over-inflation
		Hands on hips or head
Wheeze	Variable	Absent
Mental state	Normal	Very anxious
		Restless
		Drowsy

childhood is two-way communication between professionals and both child and family, this should result in proper understanding of the illness, proper use of all treatments including hospital admission, and hopefully minimum interference with daily life most of the time. Encouraging physical activity is especially important, swimming is very popular with asthmatics as many are less troubled by symptoms whilst swimming than by other forms of exercise.

Drug therapy

Drug treatment is a major part of the management of asthma. Details of regimes for different degrees of asthma and for acute severe asthma are given in Table 11.19 and Figure 11.8. Treatment for acute asthma is indicated when increasing the use of a bronchodilator in its regularly used form has not kept symptoms under control. The drugs used to treat asthma can be divided into a number of groups with specific actions:

Betamimetics. These drugs can be used for either prophylaxis or in established attacks. Salbutamol and terbutaline are both selective β_2 adrenoceptor stimulants that are widely used in paediatric practice. They may be given orally, intravenously and by inhalation. The latter route is associated with fewer side-effects and has a more rapid action. There are a wide variety of dispensers commercially available for these drugs. These drugs have little effect in the first year of life.

Xanthine derivitives. Aminophylline and theophylline are useful drugs in the treatment of asthma. They may have some synergistic action with the betamimetics. They are particularly useful as sustained-release preparations often used in nocturnal asthma. Aminophylline is a valuable intravenous preparation for the management of a severe acute asthmatic attack, but the dose used must take into account whether the child is already on maintenance theophylline or not.

Sodium cromoglycate. This is a drug used in the prophylaxis of asthma and can only be given by inhalation. Its action is to stabilize the mast cells and is particularly useful in the management of allergy and exercise-provoked asthma. It must be

Table 11.19 Drug therapy of asthma.

Symptoms	Bronchodilator (e.g. salbutamol, terbutaline)	Prevention
Mild intermittent	As needed, inhaled if possible; oral if too young to inhale	None
Mild, but frequent	As needed	Inhaled cromoglycate *or* oral theophylline if too young for Spinhaler. Nebulized cromoglycate if oral theophylline not working
Severe, frequent	Regular 6–8-hourly, increase to 3–4-hourly if needed; may need home nebulizer	Inhaled corticosteroid (beclomethasone, budesonide) Oral steroids, alternate mornings, rarely needed
Provoked by exercise		Inhaled β_2 agonist 5 min before, cromoglycate 20 minutes before

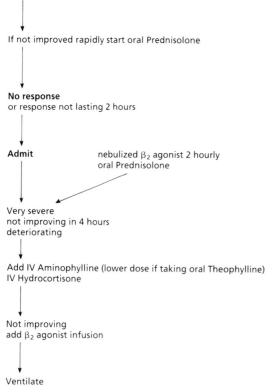

Inhaled β₂ agonist (may need delivery device or nebulizer)
3 hourly

↓

If not improved rapidly start oral Prednisolone

↓

No response
or response not lasting 2 hours

↓

Admit   nebulized β₂ agonist 2 hourly
                             oral Prednisolone

↓

Very severe
not improving in 4 hours
deteriorating

↓

Add IV Aminophylline (lower dose if taking oral Theophylline)
IV Hydrocortisone

↓

Not improving
add β₂ agonist infusion

↓

Ventilate

Fig. 11.8   Treatment of acute severe asthma.

taken regularly, 3–4 times per day and should be used for at least 3 months before deciding it is of no benefit.

Steroids. Inhaled steroids are of great value in the prophylactic management of moderately severe asthma. The most commonly used topical steroids are beclomethasone and budesonide. There is very little risk of clinically significant adrenal supression unless the inhalers are used very frequently; their main side-effect being oral thrush.

Systemic steroids (prednisolone) are used in cases of severe acute asthma, not responsive to betamimetic agents. Oral prednisolone given early in an attack may avoid the need for hospitalization in children with severe asthma. Adrenal supression is an important consideration with this form of therapy.

Complications

These include lobar collapse, particularly of the right middle lobe which responds to aggressive bronchodilator usage and physiotherapy. Pneumothorax is rare but must be considered during a severe episode that is unresponsive to treatment. Poor growth is a feature of severe chronic asthma, but ought not to be a side-effect of administered corticosteroids even in those receiving regular systemic treatment. Family disruption and schooling problems must be listed as complications, but careful attention to communication about the disease should avoid this. In addition, professional contact with school where necessary can be very helpful. Deaths from asthma in childhood do occur and are not declining, this is in spite of increasing hospital admissions and greater awareness of the disease. This indicates the scope and necessity for much more basic and applied research into the condition and its treatment.

ASPERGILLOSIS

A few chronic childhood asthmatics have allergic bronchopulmonary aspergillosis in which colonization of the respiratory tract with *Aspergillus fumigatus* results in episodic fever, productive cough, night sweats and weight loss in addition to symptoms of chronic asthma. Lung function testing may show restrictive and obstructive features. There is peripheral blood eosinophilia and *Aspergillus* can be identified in sputum. Specific IgE and IgG are elevated and both immediate and delayed skin hypersensitivity is present. *Aspergillosis clavatus* can cause extrinsic alveolitis and patients with

Table 11.20   Some allergens in extrinsic alveolitis.

Cow's milk	Ingested or possibly aspiration
Actinomyces	Humidifier systems
Bacillus subtilis	Humidifier systems
Bird protein	Pigeon, parrot, chicken droppings
Pig pancreatic protein	Inhalation of pig pancreas extract
Micropolyspora, Thermactinomyces	Mouldy hay

pulmonary cavities from any cause can develop an aspergilloma. Debilitated immunocompromised patients may develop disseminated aspergillosis. These conditions due to *Aspergillus* species are different clinical entities. Asthmatics with allergic bronchopulmonary aspergillosis may need systemic corticosteroids for long periods to control symptoms. Antifungal agents do not work in this condition.

Alveolitis

Extrinsic allergic alveolitis

In addition to asthma there are a number of lung diseases in which allergy appears to play an important part, these diseases are rare in childhood and can be grouped together as extrinsic allergic alveolitis. Some recognized allergens are given in Table 11.20. The sufferers may or may not be atopic and the chief symptoms are cough and breathlessness. This can occur 6–10 hours after exposure to antigen and resolve within a day or be a more chronic process. Tachypnoea and crepitations with or without cyanosis are the chief findings on examination, poor growth or even weight loss may be noted. In acute cases fever is common. Diffuse reticulonodular densities are characteristic when seen on X-ray and lung function tests show a restrictive pattern. Recognition of a particular antigen is made by clinical history and detection of serum IgG precipitations to the offending antigen. Treatment is by removal of antigen wherever possible, steroids may be needed in severe acute attacks or chronic disease when antigen removal is not possible.

Idiopathic fibrosing alveolitis

This has some clinical similarities with extrinsic allergic alveolitis, but onset is usually insidious and clubbing is more common. Chest X-ray abnormalities are more likely to be confined to lower zones and of course evidence for an external precipitant is lacking. The condition may be associated with a number of systemic diseases including rheumatoid arthritis, histiocytic disorders (p. 472), and lung

irradiation. Diagnosis is ultimately by lung biopsy when precipitating and associated factors have been excluded.

Chronic lung disorders

Cystic fibrosis

This is the commonest autosomal recessive inherited condition affecting Caucasians, with an incidence of 1 : 2500. It is also seen in non-white races but is considerably less common. The severity of cystic fibrosis varies greatly from patient to patient, but it is a chronic, usually fatal disease with a tendency to affect many organs. The lethal nature of cystic fibrosis is most commonly due to respiratory involvement, but symptoms are also often seen in the gastrointestinal system and these are discussed in Chapter 12.

The underlying cause of cystic fibrosis is not known, but it is a generalized disease affecting many organs including:

1 Lungs.
2 Heart. Cor pulmonale develops secondary to chronic lung disease.
3 Sweat glands. There is a high concentration of salt in the secretions (p. 188).
4 Liver. Cirrhosis and liver failure occurs in some patients.
5 Pancreas. Fat malabsorption is very common. Rarely diabetes mellitus develops in older patients.
6 Bowel. The meconium is abnormal with a high albumin level. Meconium ileus is the presenting feature in 10% of cases. Rectal prolapse is seen with increased frequency in toddlers with cystic fibrosis.
7 Genital abnormality. Sterility is almost invariable in males. Females are fertile.
8 Sinuses. Chronic sinus infections are not very common. Multiple nasal polypi are seen in 10% of those suffering from the disease.

PRESENTING FEATURES

The earliest presentation is in those infants with meconium ileus (p. 199). The commonest presenting symptoms are directly related to gastrointestinal or respiratory symptoms or failure to thrive. Failure to thrive is associated with steatorrhoea and recurrent respiratory infections.

The major underlying factors in lung involvement are thick tenacious sputum plugging the medium-sized bronchioles together with chronic infection. This leads to a vicious cycle which may evolve to extensive bronchiectasis, respiratory failure, cor pulmonale and death.

Symptoms relate to the progression of the disease. Initially, the child develops repeated lower respiratory tract infections. Cough is a prominent symptom and is particularly persistent and paroxysmal. Small stature, low weight, finger clubbing and an over-inflated chest are seen in varying degrees. Crepitations and rhonchi are heard in the chest.

Diagnosis

Sweat test. The definitive diagnosis of cystic fibrosis is made on the sweat test. Normal sweat contains not more than 50 mmol/l of both sodium and chloride. Levels of sweat sodium above 70 mmol/l are found in patients with cystic fibrosis. Sweat is collected by various different techniques, the most widely used being pilocarpine iontophoresis in which sweat is collected on a pre-weighed filter paper. Falsely elevated sodium results may be obtained if less than 100 mg of sweat is collected.

Screening tests. In cystic fibrosis pancreatic tryptic activity is reduced and trypsin is elevated in the serum. This is present in newborn infants affected by the disease and immunoreactive trypsin can be measured on a dried blood spot. This is the best method for screening the newborn population for the presence of this condition. It is to be hoped, but is not yet proven, that early detection by screening improves outlook.

Treatment

There is no cure for cystic fibrosis and treatment is essentially palliative. A number of heart–lung transplant operations have been carried out for end-stage cystic fibrosis and it is of interest that the transplanted lung is not prone to the retention of secretions. Unfortunately, this operation is never likely to offer significant hope to the majority of sufferers. Porta-caval anastomosis for complications of portal hypertension is sometimes performed.

The keystones of management are aggressive respiratory care and attention to absorption and nutrition.

Physiotherapy. Adequate drainage of secretions by vigorous postural physiotherapy is essential and this can be performed at home by the mother under the supervision of an experienced physiotherapist. Mucolytic agents may be helpful when secretions are particularly viscous and difficult to drain by physiotherapy.

Antibiotics. Infection is the most destructive process in cystic fibrosis. If the diagnosis is made in infancy, particularly if there is an affected sibling, prophylactic antibiotics are used by many from the time of diagnosis for the first 2 years of life. An effective anti-staphylococcal agent such as flucloxacillin is used. Once the child develops infection, vigorous and appropriate antibiotic management should be introduced. *Pseudomonas* is the most important organism in older children, and the antibiotics should be given intravenously during the course of infection and may also be given by nebulized solution, as may bronchodilators.

Nutrition. Optimal nutrition is essential together with pancreatic enzyme replacement. This is discussed in Chapter 12.

Prognosis

Over 70% of children with cystic fibrosis survive to 16 years, but females have a worse prognosis than males. Girls appear to develop more severe respiratory disease which is the most important factor in predicting risk of early death. Other adverse prognostic features are poor weight gain and an abnormal chest X-ray in the first year following presentation. Some children have remarkably mild disease and their prognosis may be excellent.

ALPHA-1 ANTITRYPSIN DEFICIENCY

This is an autosomal recessive disorder which may present as neonatal hepatitis. In adults it can cause generalized emphysema, a very rare condition in childhood. The major childhood implication of this deficiency in relation to respiratory disease is that those known to be homozygous (by virtue of having had neonatal hepatitis), or suspected as being heterozygotes, ought to be encouraged as strongly as possible not to smoke as to do so makes respiratory manifestations in adult life virtually certain. Children with obstructive airways disease not definitely asthma warrant serum α_1 antitrypsin assay.

PULMONARY HAEMOSIDEROSIS

This is a very rare condition in which chronic bleeding into alveoli occurs. It can be primary or secondary to cardiac disease (mitral stenosis for example), collagenoses or haemorrhagic diseases. Primary disease is less rare in childhood and may be associated with cow's milk protein sensitivity. Children present with either chronic refractory iron deficient anaemia or with haemoptysis, cough or wheeze. Nephritis may also be present (Goodpasture's syndrome) so that haematuria may be reported. Chest X-ray features are variable and sometimes transient. Mild diffuse infiltrates, focal collapse or consolidation and hilar adenopathy all may be seen. Lung function tests show obstructive changes and gastric juice will contain iron-laden macrophages. Lung biopsy is diagnostic but not always necessary. Treatment with transfusion and respiratory support may be needed. Cow's milk should be excluded if serological evidence of sensitivity is found; steroids and other immunosuppressives have their advocates. Associated or predisposing diseases should be treated appropriately.

Lung masses

Primary and secondary tumours involving the lung are extremely rare in childhood (see Chapter 25). Congenital cysts of lung, bronchus, gastrointestinal tract or pericardium present as lung or mediastinal masses either by compressive infective symptoms or as coincidental findings on X-ray. Anterior thoracic myeloceles and neural crest tumours cause posterior mediastinal masses. Thymus tumours are exceedingly rare in children.

Diaphragmatic abnormalities

Congenital diaphragmatic hernia is dealt with elsewhere (Chapter 9). Eventration of the diaphragm due to underdevelopment of diaphragmatic muscle is usually asymptomatic and detected as an elevation of part of one hemidiaphragm. X-ray or ultrasound screening of diaphragmatic movement may show it to be paradoxical. Paralysis of one hemidiaphragm due to phrenic nerve injury, for example at cardiac surgery, causes a similar picture and rarely causes a major respiratory problem. Bilateral phrenic nerve palsy is much more serious and causes severe respiratory failure.

Preventative aspects of paediatric respiratory diseases

Many respiratory symptoms are more frequent when overcrowding, social deprivation and passive smoking are present. Therefore improvement in these aspects of the environment are important. Children should be very strongly discouraged from smoking, not only for their health in early years but also to reduce the heavy toll on health that smoking takes in adult life. Breast feeding probably has some slight preventative effect on acute respiratory infections during the period that breast feeding continues. Immunization against pertussis is valuable in reducing risk of contracting the disease and in reducing its severity. BCG immunization at birth for high-risk groups is widely practised in the UK (p. 355). This is specifically with a view to reducing risk of miliary tuberculosis with meningitis in childhood. Immunization of teenagers and of childhood contacts of open cases against tuberculosis is still considered of value in preventing respiratory tuberculosis. Measles immunization is very effective in preventing severe disease, thereby reducing both acute and chronic respiratory effects. Many of these preventative measures are even more important world-wide when malnutrition makes any respiratory infection more dangerous, thus immunization and adequate nutrition are high priorities in developing countries (see Chapter 29).

Acknowledgement

I am indebted to Dr David Lindsell, Consultant Paediatric Radiologist, John Radcliffe Hospital, Oxford, for many of the radiographs used in this chapter.

Further reading

Godfrey S, Baum JD (Eds.) *Clinical Paediatric Physiology.* Blackwell Scientific Publications, Oxford 1979.

Kendig EL, Chernick V (Eds) *Disorders of the Respiratory Tract in Children,* 4th Edn. WB Saunders, Philadelphia 1983.

Phelan PD, Landau LI, Olinsky A (Eds) *Respiratory Illness in Children,* 2nd Edn. Blackwell Scientific Publications, Oxford 1982.

West JB. *Respiratory Physiology — The Essentials,* 2nd Edn. Williams and Wilkins, Baltimore 1979.

12
DISORDERS OF THE GASTROINTESTINAL SYSTEM

The major role of the gastrointestinal tract is to digest food and absorb nutrition to enable the child to achieve his optimal growth and development. The gut is embryologically derived from endoderm and is morphologically well developed by the twelfth week of gestation, so that even very pre-term babies are able to sustain nutrition by the enteral route, although some enzymes, such as pancreatic amylase, may only reach full adult levels 6−9 months after birth.

Disease processes affecting the alimentary tract may present with symptoms of disordered function, such as diarrhoea, and subsequent malabsorption, or more insidiously with evidence of failure to thrive and poor linear growth.

Dysphagia

Difficulty in swallowing or feeding, is an important symptom in children. Discoordinate oesophageal motility may be related to cerebral palsy and this, if accompanied by extensor spasms and thrusting of the tongue, creates major feeding difficulties. A modified barium swallow examination, using video recording, has proved to be very useful in the diagnosis of this abnormal form of contraction. Desensitization of hypersensitive areas of the face by firm stroking may help to reduce the tongue thrusting and this type of manoeuvre coupled with the help of a speech therapist may often alleviate these difficulties. Feeding in a high back chair so that the pharynx is not occluded during the extensor spasms may also prevent the child choking, and hence make feed

times much less of the battle that they may become without such assistance.

Obstruction of the oesophagus may also result in dysphagia. If this is due to external compression, as a result of vascular anomalies such as a double aortic arch, there may also be associated stridor due to pressure on the trachea. The diagnosis is confirmed by barium swallow, which demonstrates the oesophageal compression. Treatment is by surgical correction of the anomaly.

Intrinsic obstruction rarely occurs due to congenital abnormalities such as a web, which again may be demonstrated by means of a barium swallow. More commonly, oesophageal strictures may result either from the accidental ingestion of corrosives, or from oesophagitis, as a consequence of severe reflux. The degree of obstruction can be assessed by oesophagoscopy, and the stricture dilated at the same time by the use of increasing diameter bougies.

Vomiting

Vomiting, to a greater or lesser degree, is a common symptom in infancy; indeed, it is almost the norm, but it is often very distressing for parents. Many children are simply possetting, or regurgitating small amounts of feed. This is entirely benign and is not associated with failure to thrive. The only treatment required is reassurance, but it is wise to check the volume of feed that is being given, as overfeeding can also result in vomiting. An unwell child who is vomiting may have a systemic disease not associated with the gastro-

Table 12.1 Causes of acute vomiting.

Infectious gastroenteritis
Intestinal obstruction
Infection from a non-intestinal site
  Otitis media
  Urinary tract infection
  Meningitis
Ingestion of toxic substances
Increased intracranial pressure (p. 296)
Encephalopathy
Pancreatitis
Self-induced

intestinal tract, such as infection, particularly of the meninges and urinary tract or an abnormality of amino acid or organic acid metabolism. A thorough examination and investigation is mandatory in all vomiting babies. Bile-stained vomiting is always pathological and indicates intestinal obstruction, although occasionally an obstruction above the level of the ampulla of Varter will not produce bile staining. Table 12.1 lists the common causes of vomiting.

Gastro-oesophageal reflux

Some babies may present with vomiting in the first weeks after birth, sometimes with failure to thrive, and the vomitus may be blood stained. If the reflux is severe, then recurrent episodes of aspiration will lead to the symptoms of repeated chest infections. The reflux of milk from the stomach to the lower oesophagus is common because of the normal immature development of the cardia.

Investigations

The diagnosis is confirmed by barium swallow, during which a coexistent hiatus hernia is often found. It is now apparent that episodes of reflux may not always be evident on X-ray, and the use of a pH probe placed at the lower oesophagus may be more accurate in detecting this condition. The technique of gastroscopy enables direct vision of

the oesophagus and easily demonstrates the presence of oesophagitis.

Management

The treatment of reflux consists of positioning the infant after feeding in an upright position. Nursing the baby prone in a slight head up position (30 degrees) has also been shown to be helpful. Thickening of the milk with cornstarch or carob seed (Nestargel or Carobel) is often required and is usually beneficial. The use of agents that also contain an antacid, such as Gaviscon, have also been used before feeds but caution is needed because of their high sodium content. Drugs that alter gastric emptying, such as Maxolon and domperidone, have also been used, but they should only be resorted to in extreme cases. Only very rarely are these measures ineffective but occasionally the failure to thrive continues, with the possible development of an oesophageal stricture. This necessitates a surgical repair such as a Nissen fundoplication. *In toto*, 95% of patients cease to vomit as they assume a more upright position and consume a more solid diet, usually at about 1 year of age. The presence of a hiatus hernia does not alter this good prognosis.

Pyloric stenosis

The onset of projectile vomiting at 6 weeks of age suggests pyloric stenosis, although other causes must be considered. The condition has an incidence of approximately 1 in 3000 in the UK and is commoner in first born male infants. The strongest linkage, however, is in those infants born to a mother who also had pyloric stenosis. Recent studies, using ultrasound, have shown that the muscular thickening of the pylorus is not present at birth, but develops during the first month of life.

Clinical features

The vomiting occurs immediately after a feed and characteristically the baby is ravenously hungry, and often has a worried appearance. Examination of the baby is directed to assess the degree of dehydration, and palpation of the tumour during a test feed. The infant is nursed on his mother's lap and given a milk feed, during which the abdomen is observed for the presence of visible peristalsis. If right handed, the examiner places his left hand on the infant's abdomen to palpate the tumour.

The pylorus is felt in the right hypochondrium, and when enlarged has the consistency and size of an olive. In difficult cases the thickened pyloric muscle can be readily visualized by abdominal ultrasound.

Management

The prolonged vomiting may result in profound electrolyte abnormalities specifically hyponatraemia, hypokalaemia, and a metabolic alkalosis. It is essential that these, along with the dehydration, are corrected prior to surgery. The alkalosis is not treated specifically but responds to the administration of sodium chloride. The operative repair is by means of a Ramsted procedure during which the muscle is divided down to the mucosa, through a transverse incision. The use of atropinic agents, even in the very minor degrees of obstruction, is contraindicated in view of the excellent results achieved by surgery.

Abdominal distension

The average normal toddler has the appearance of a 'pot-belly' due to the relatively small size of the pelvis. Distension is usually noticed by parents, and is best visualized by standing the child sideways. The factors responsible may be intraluminal, where malabsorption results in excess gas formation, ascitic fluid, or tumours, the most common being nephroblastoma and neuroblastoma. The causes of abdominal distension are listed in Table 12.2.

Aerophagy, or compulsive air swallowing, often results in gross abdominal distension in an otherwise well child. The abdomen is tympanitic to percussion. The habit can normally be broken by

Table 12.2 Causes of abdominal distension.

Intestinal causes
  Gas in the bowel
  Coeliac disease
  Cow's milk protein intolerance
  Carbohydrate intolerance
  Cystic fibrosis
  Protein losing enteropathy
  Constipation
  Hirschsprung's disease
  Metabolic disturbances (e.g. hypokalaemia)

Ascites
  Nephrotic syndrome
  Cirrhosis
  Hepatic failure

Intra-abdominal mass
  Hydronephrosis
  Polycystic kidney
  Wilm's tumour
  Neuroblastoma
  Hepatosplenomegaly

simple explanation to both the child and parents, but where there is associated discomfort, the use of charcoal biscuits can result in considerable relief.

Acute diarrhoea

Infective gastroenteritis

Despite the rigorous measures instituted by the World Health Organization (WHO) to improve sanitation and to promote breast feeding, gastroenteritis remains one of the leading causes of infant death in the developing world, particularly in those infants less than 6 months of age. This is discussed fully in Chapter 29. Breast feeding affords some protection, not only by avoiding the risk of preparing bottle feeds with contaminated water, but also by specific factors such as IgA, lactoferrin, antiviral factors, and the promotion of the growth of lactobacillus in the colon, which suppresses the growth of potential pathogens (p. 68).

Table 12.3 The commoner infective causes of
gastroenteritis.

Viruses
  Rotavirus
  Parvovirus
  Astrovirus
  Calicivirus
  Adenovirus

Bacterial
  Campylobacter jejuni
  Shigella
  Salmonella
  E. coli
  Yersinia enterocolitica
  Cholera
  Staphylococcus
  Bacillus cereus

Parasites
  Entamoeba histolytica
  Giardia
  Cryptosporidium

AETIOLOGY

The pathogens causing gastroenteritis are listed in
Table 12.3. In the UK, rotavirus, which was first
identified in the late 1960s, is the commonest
single pathogen in infancy and accounts for up to
75% of episodes of gastroenteritis with seasonal
peaks throughout the winter months. The virus
was named because of the radial spokes observed
with the aid of electron microscopy. Other viruses
may also be isolated, although less commonly, and
these include: parvovirus, adenovirus, and small
round viruses such as astrovirus and calicivirus.
The production of diarrhoea in viral infections is
believed to be due to invasion of the crypt enterocyte by viral particles, which results in functionally
immature enterocytes present at the villous tip,
thereby disrupting normal absorption. The diarrhoea is often preceded by a period of vomiting,
particularly in rotavirus infections.

Campylobacter has emerged as the leading
bacterial cause over the last 10 years. This apparent increase is related to the improved culture of
the organism, which is micro-aerophilic, and re-

quires special techniques for detection. Bacteria
produce diarrhoea in a number of ways:

1 They may invade the mucosa (*Campylobacter*,
Shigella and *Salmonella*).
2 Produce an enterotoxin (cholera and certain
serotypes of *E. coli*).
3 Adhere to the enterocyte (serotypes of *E. coli*).

The clinical symptoms give a clue to the underlying organism. The presence of blood and mucus
suggest the presence of an invasive organism,
whereas the so-called rice water stools indicates
the presence of enterotoxin production. Abdominal pain is uncommon, except for *Campylobacter*
infections, when combined with blood in the
stool, a surgical condition is often suspected.

Clinical features

A careful clinical examination of the child with
gastroenteritis is critical to good management, as
therapy is primarily directed to the correction of
dehydration. The clinical features of dehydration
are listed in Table 12.4. It is also essential, particularly in the small child, to exclude causes of secondary diarrhoea due to overwhelming infections,
for example meningitis. It is relatively easy to
underestimate the severity of the stool losses because the fluid stool pools within the gut, and the
stool which is passed may often be mistaken for
urine in the nappy. In those children with severe
to moderate dehydration it is also essential to
measure the serum sodium to exclude hypernatraemic dehydration (serum sodium concentration
greater than 150 mmol/l) because in this clinical
situation the skin has a doughy feel which may

Table 12.4 Clinical assessment of dehydration.

Degree (% body weight)	Signs
<5	Thirst, dry mucous membranes
5–10	Sunken eyes, sunken fontanelle, reduced tissue elasticity, oliguria
10–15	Circulatory failure, hypotension, tachycardia

lead to an underestimation of the degree of dehydration (see also Chapter 16). Investigations should also include stool culture for both bacterial and viral pathogens, with blood and CSF cultures if septicaemia is suspected.

Management

The treatment of gastroenteritis has been greatly altered over the last decade with the advent of oral dehydration solutions containing sodium and glucose (p. 552). Water absorption is coupled to sodium absorption, with glucose to aid co-transport. Solutions containing less sodium than the WHO recommended oral rehydration solution (35–45 mmol/l of sodium) are more commonly used in Britain and are adequate due to the lesser incidence of endotoxin-mediated diarrhoea. The solution is provided as a dry powder and made to 200 ml with sterile or boiled water. Oral rehydration solution (ORS) is given to provide 150 ml/kg/24 hours maintenance fluid; additional volume is required to replace the losses due to dehydration and the ongoing stool losses. If the baby is breast fed then the losses are replaced by ORS and the maintenance fluids are given as breast milk. If the baby is unable to tolerate the large volumes of solution, due to vomiting, then the frequency of the feeds may be increased and consequently the volume of each feed reduced.

In Europe and the USA, moderate dehydration is usually managed by intravenous rehydration, but even this degree of fluid loss has been successfully managed by ORS in the developing world. Severe dehydration, greater than 15% fluid loss, will require the urgent re-establishment of circulatory volume with 20 ml/kg of plasma.

In hypernatraemic dehydration, the replacement of fluid should be carried out slowly to avoid the sudden osmotic changes and resultant rapid fluid shifts that lead to cerebral injury and cerebral venous thrombosis. ORS is preferable and the losses should be replaced over a period of 12 hours. If intravenous fluids are required they should initially be given as half strength dextrose saline, and again rehydration should proceed slowly. Fortu-

nately this complication has become much less common over the last decade, and is probably due to the production of 'humanized' formula milks, as well as better education regarding the preparation of infant feeds.

The use of antibiotics should be discouraged, as these do not appear to alter the course of the disease and may lead to the development of resistant organisms. Two possible exceptions to this rule are *Campylobacter*, where erythromycin may alleviate the abdominal pain, and the use of Septrin in *Shigella* septicaemia. Drugs such as opiates and binding agents such as kaolin are not used because they do not significantly reduce fluid losses. They may result in respiratory depression and can delay clearing of the organism further by reducing peristalsis.

Regrading

When rehydration has been established, and ongoing losses hve ceased, usually after 24 hours, the patient is regraded back on to normal feed. Traditionally this has involved the gradual, step-wise introduction of increasing concentrations of milk over several days, but recently it has been suggested that this is unnecessary, particularly in infants greater than 6 months of age, and they can be regraded directly on to full strength milk. This is particularly important in those countries where malnutrition is common. Babies under the age of 6 months should still be regarded conventionally to avoid complications.

Recovery from the initial episode may be delayed due to the development of lactase deficiency, which will result in the continuation of diarrhoea associated with the presence of reducing substances in the stool. This condition is temporary and responds to a lactose-free milk. If more than three attempts at regrading fail then cow's milk protein intolerance must be considered.

Chronic diarrhoea

The persistence of an increased stool volume for longer than 2 weeks is considered to indicate

Dietary intolerance	Coeliac disease
	Cow's milk protein intolerance
	Carbohydrate intolerance
Inborn errors	Chloridorrhoea
	Acrodermatitis enteropathica
	Abetalipoproteinaemia (p. 372)
Surgical	Malrotation
	Blind loop syndrome
	Stenosis
Pancreatic insufficiency	Cystic fibrosis
	Shwachman's syndrome
Immunodeficiency	Severe combined immunodeficiency
	Hypogammaglobulinaemia
	Opsinization defect
	HIV infections (AIDS)
Tumours	Ganglioneuroma
	Lymphoma
Others	Intestinal lymphangiectasia
	Addison's disease
	Auto-immune enteropathy
	Congenital microvillus atrophy

Table 12.5 Causes of chronic diarrhoea in children.

chronic diarrhoea. This must be differentiated from the normal stool of the breast-fed infant which are often water, and the overflow incontinence of fluid stool that is frequently seen in chronic constipation. The child should be examined carefully for signs of muscle wasting, particularly of the limb girdles, both shoulder and pelvic, which suggest malabsorption. The differential diagnosis of chronic diarrhoea is shown in Table 12.5.

Toddler diarrhoea

Although a benign disorder, toddler diarrhoea or 'peas and carrots syndrome' after the appearance of vegetable matter in the stool, is a cause of great anxiety to parents and is a common reason for seeking medical advice. The incidence is greatest in boys and usually occurs between the ages of 6 months and 2 years, although the symptoms can persist for as long as 5 years. The aetiology remains unsure, but recent studies indicate that there is a decreased gut transit time, which may be related to abnormalities of prostaglandin synthesis and metabolism, which have been demonstrated in this condition.

The cardinal features of toddler diarrhoea are the very frequent passage of watery stools containing particles of vegetable matter and the fact that the child continues to thrive.

Treatment is mainly to reassure the parents that the diarrhoea will improve and the child is not suffering from a serious bowel disorder. Moderate restriction of fibre and 'squash' type drinks may alleviate the symptoms. In those children with excessive diarrhoea loperamide may prove helpful.

Coeliac disease

Coeliac disease has long been recognized as a cause of failure to thrive during childhood. Samuel Gee, in 1888, gave what is now a classic description of the disease, but it was not realized that gluten was the causative agent until 1953. This protein is found predominantly in the cereals wheat, rye and the possibly barley and oats. It is composed of many subunits and it is now established that the alpha gliadin fraction of gluten is responsible for the changes observed. The incidence of coeliac disease shows great variability with a frequency ranging from 1 : 300 on the western coast of Ireland to 1 : 6000 in the UK. The disease is most common in Caucasian races and with the advent of genotyping it is now appreciated that there is a strong association with the HLA B8 DRW3 histocompatibility antigen, but an environmental trigger appears to be required for full expression of the disease. A risk factor of 20% has been quoted for the first degree relatives of patients with coeliac disease. Over the last 5 years it is becoming clear that its incidence is declining, possibly due to changes in infant feeding practices, specifically the later introduction of cereals.

PATHOLOGY

The pathological lesion of coeliac disease is total and uniform villous atrophy of the proximal small intestine and this can be seen on examination of biopsy tissue under a dissecting microscope (Plate 2). The epithelium is infiltrated with lymphocytes and there are an increased number of plasma cells in the lamina propria (Plate 3). The thickness of the mucosa is actually increased due to hypertrophy of the crypt region.

Clinical features

The clinical features usually develop a couple of months after the introduction of weaning cereals. The classical symptoms are failure to thrive, diarrhoea and abdominal distension, although constipation, vomiting and short stature may also occur. The child is extremely miserable and an improvement in mood is often the first response to treatment. It is important to examine the patient standing sideways, when the buttock wasting and abdominal distension are more apparent (Fig. 12.1). The associated malabsorption results in low levels of protein, particularly albumin, but only in extreme cases is oedema present. The haemoglobin is typically low, due to iron deficiency, as a result of both microhaemorrhages and malabsorption. A megaloblastic picture has been described due to folate deficiency, but it is very rare. Reduced red blood cell folate levels are usually present.

Diagnosis

The diagnosis is made by jejunal biospsy, at the level of the duodeno-jejunal flexure, using a modification of the Crosby capsule. This contains a spring-loaded knife blade, and is positioned using X-ray screening. Suction on an attached syringe 'fires' the capsule. The diagnosis can sometimes be made by examining the tissue under a dissecting microscope. Detailed histological examination should always be carried out in addition to this. There are no adequate alternatives to biopsy for diagnosis, alpha gliadin antibodies have been suggested and indeed they may be helpful for screening purposes and monitoring progress, but many normal people also possess such antibodies and so the test lacks specificity. Alteration of the diet without a tissue diagnosis should be discouraged as treatment is required for life and it is essential that an accurate diagnosis is made early.

Management

Treatment involves the total exclusion of gluten from the diet. It is important that the diet is reviewed by a dietician, and much practical advice can be obtained by the patient joining the Coeliac Society. On such a regime the jejunal lesion heals completely and such children can lead an absolutely normal life, but the diet must be maintained for life. There is an increased risk of developing small bowel lymphomas and adenocarcinoma, although the preventative role of strict dietary adherence has yet to be demonstrated.

The recognition of the rare syndrome of transient gluten intolerance has meant that the patients are normally challenged a couple of years after diagnosis. A biopsy on gluten-free diet shows a normal mucosa, a gluten-containing diet is then given, and a repeat biopsy performed after approximately 3 months, at which stage the mucosa, in those patients with coeliac disease will have become flat. If a normal biopsy is obtained at 3 months, then they are repeated at regular intervals

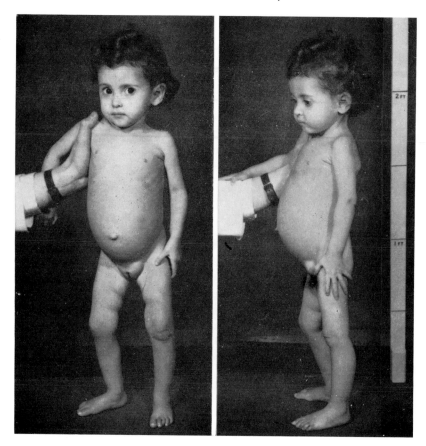

Fig. 12.1 Coeliac disease in a child of 18 months. The abdomen is distended; there is wasting of the limbs and buttocks.

for 2 years to allow for the possibility of a delayed response.

Cow's milk protein intolerance

Cow's milk allergy may present with eczema, wheezing, or vomiting. There are, however, two cow's milk protein syndromes that involve the alimentary tract; cow's milk protein intolerance (CMPI) which affects the small bowel, and cow's milk colitis resulting from inflammation of the colon. The principle allergen is beta lactoglobulin, but lactalbumin may also contribute to the effect. Breast feeding is obviously protective, but some cow's milk protein allergen ingested by the mother has been shown to enter human breast milk and sensitize the infant.

Clinical features

CMPI presents as chronic diarrhoea, usually following an acute infective gastroenteritis, and is always associated with some degree of failure to thrive. Children under the age of 6 months seem to be particularly prone to this complication and research from the developing world suggests that it may be an important cause of malnutrition following gastroenteritis. There are no specific diagnostic tests, but skin testing to cow's milk and the detection of specific IgE antibodies, demonstrate an atopic tendency. A jejunal biopsy demonstrates a patchy enteropathy with eosinophilic infiltration of the mucosa (Plate 4), the specimen is usually thin compared to the uniform change and thick biopsy specimen found in coeliac disease.

Management

The withdrawal of milk from the diet, results in healing of the mucosal changes and improvement of growth, but it is also important that milk solids are removed. The use of several milk substitutes have been well described, particularly those based on soy protein, but it should be remembered that allergy to this protein occurs in approximately 20–30% of patients, and so a milk based on hydrolysed cow's milk protein may be preferable. Goat's milk should not be used because it is very low in folic acid, and the strict bacteriological control found in the dairy industry does not apply to goat's milk. The syndrome is transient and commonly resolves at 1 year of age, when a cow's milk challenge is performed. This should be undertaken in hospital because of the risk of anaphylaxis. Milk is first applied to the lips and if no reaction is seen then increasing volumes are given orally starting at 1 ml.

COW'S MILK COLITIS

The colitic form of the syndrome presents shortly after birth, with blood-stained diarrhoea. It is important to consider bleeding and infective disorders, which produce the same symptoms. The diagnosis is confirmed by colonoscopy, which shows ulceration and eosinophilic infiltration of the colonic mucosa, but where no such facilities are readily available, withdrawal of cow's milk is often both diagnostic and curative. The prognosis is good with most cases becoming tolerant to milk again at 1 year of age. Follow-up of a group of such patients at Great Ormond Street Hospital has suggested that further allergies may develop later. Allergy to other foods, such as fish, rice, chicken and egg have all been described but with the exception of egg they are rare.

Cystic fibrosis (see also p. 187)

Although the major impact of this disease is upon the respiratory tract, cystic fibrosis must enter into the differential diagnosis of the child with chronic diarrhoea and failure to thrive, particularly if this is associated with recurrent chest infections. Cystic fibrosis as it relates to the respiratory system is discussed in Chapter 11. The absence of pancreatic enzymes result in gross malabsorption of fat and leads to steatorrhoea. The replacement of these enzymes with pancreatic extract, particularly the newer longer acting preparations, has resulted not only in the resolution of diarrhoea, but also in a generally improved nutritional state. These children should receive 150% of the total recommended dietary allowance of nutrients including fat. High dose vitamins are also provided to prevent deficiency syndromes. Vitamin E deficiency is a particularly important condition which may cause a peripheral neuropathy.

Ten per cent of patients with cystic fibrosis present in the neonatal period with meconium ileus and intestinal obstruction. X-rays show the 'bubble'-like appearance of meconium at the terminal ileum. The treatment of meconium ileus is normally surgical, although a diagnostic gastrograffin enema may occasionally result in resolution of the obstruction.

Giardia

This protozoan is found world-wide, but appears to have areas of increased incidence such as Leningrad. The infection is produced by ingestion of the cyst from contaminated water supplies. Many people remain asymptomatic, but in a few it results in chronic diarrhoea and malabsorption. Patients with immunodeficiency are at risk, but children with a normal immune system may also acquire the infection.

Stool examination may reveal the cystic form of the organism, but the best method for diagnosis is to perform a jejunal biopsy and examine the duodenal aspirate where the organisms can be clearly identified. *Giardia* associated with the condition of chronic diarrhoea will also result in a flat biopsy, but the differentiation from coeliac disease is usually easy because of the visible parasites. Electron microscopy has shown that *Giardia* produce their clinical effect by adhering to the enterocyte. A 10-day course of metronidazole, results in complete eradication.

Carbohydrate intolerance

Lactose intolerance is either a primary autosomal recessive condition, presenting with diarrhoea at birth, or secondary to mucosal damage accompanying such conditions as gastroenteritis and coeliac disease. Lactase levels normally decline with age, particularly in Negro and Asian children.

Sucrose-isomaltase deficiency is also inherited as an autosomal recessive condition and is more common than primary lactase deficiency. The infant is asymptomatic until sucrose or dietary starches are introduced into the diet at the time of weaning, when diarrhoea and failure to thrive may become apparent. There is, however, a broad spectrum of involvement from severe diarrhoea to mild discomfort.

Glucose-galactose malabsorption results in diarrhoea from birth, and if not recognized early often results in death. Fortunately, it is rare, and the treatment is the substitution of fructose as the major carbohydrate in the diet.

Investigations

The diagnosis of these brush border enzyme deficiencies is confirmed by jejunal biopsy and direct enzyme assay. However, the hydrogen breath test provides an indirect measurement and has the advantage of being less invasive. This procedure relies on the fact that unabsorbed sugars are metabolized by colonic bacteria to produce hydrogen, which is absorbed and excreted in the breath. Antibiotics may disrupt the colonic microflora and give rise to a false negative result. This may be excluded by the administration of a non-absorbed sugar, such as Lactulose, which will produce hydrogen even in the normal subject.

Chloridorrhoea

With the advent of improved methods of investigation, rare causes of chronic diarrhoea are being increasingly recognized, so reducing the number of patients with the so-called idiopathic label. Abnormalities of electrolyte absorption will result in diarrhoea from birth, the best recognized condition being chloridorrhoea, where an increased loss of chloride in the stool can be measured. This is present ante-natally and result in gross polyhydramnios.

Intestinal lymphangiectasia

This condition produces diarrhoea as a result of protein loss in the small intestine, due to 'leakage' from dilated lymphatics. The loss of albumin may be so great that oedema and ascites may occur. The diagnosis may be suspected from the peripheral blood which shows a depletion of lymphocytes. Shrinkage of the lymphatics is obtained by a diet high in medium chain triglycerides. Breast feeding is contraindicated because of the high long chain fat content of breast milk.

Congenital microvillous atrophy

This condition causes diarrhoea from birth. This is believed to be due to an enterocyte cytoskeletal abnormality and the diagnosis is made on electron microscopy where the microvilli can be seen to be disrupted and contained in intracellular vesicles. At present no satisfactory treatment is available other than long-term total parenteral nutrition.

Constipation

This symptom is a major cause of maternal anxiety, although the child is only rarely seriously unwell. There is also much confusion amongst both parents and medical staff concerning the definition of constipation. Not all babies pass stools on a daily basis and an interval of up to 1 week is not unusual. It should also be remembered that babies who are fed with a formula milk will normally have firmer stools than those who are breast fed.

The commonest cause in the UK is functional constipation, but it is imperative to consider other causes including hypothyroidism, electrolyte disturbance, such as that found in renal tubular acidosis, and neurological lesions such as cerebral palsy and lesions involving the lower spinal cord.

The pattern of stool withholding may start early in life with excessive parental concern in potty training, or may be triggered by an event which results in pain on defaecation, for example an anal fissure. This encourages the child to avoid the passage of stool which becomes hard and a vicious cycle of stool withholding develops (p. 30). In the older child, factors surrounding the embarrassment about using outside toilets at school or uncomfortable toilets at home will aggravate the situation.

Clinical features

Examination of the abdomen will demonstrate the degree of faecal loading, and rectal examination will reveal hard stools. There may also be associated soiling. The presence of an anal fissure will be evident upon examination of the anal margin and in this situation a rectal examination should not be performed as it will result in undue pain for the child.

Management

The essence of treatment is primarily to reassure both the parents and the child that there is no serious abnormality and to relax the all too frequent excessive parental concern over bowel actions. The normal response of the internal anal sphincter is to relax with distension of the rectum, and with faecal loading this response is blunted. It is important therefore to re-establish normal rectal diameters. Laxatives, including Lactulose, a bulking agent and Senokot, a bowel stimulant, should be given in large doses to establish a normal bowel pattern, and so avoid the need for enemas and suppositories which are so often distressing for the patient and hospital staff, although these will be required if there is no response to laxatives. The use of star charts may greatly improve motivation and reduce the incidence of soiling. Intense support of the child and family is required with regular, and initially, frequent outpatient visits to assess the response. It is often helpful to enquire about the diet as the intake of fibre-containing foods are frequently reduced, especially if a lot of 'junk food' is consumed. Medication should be

withdrawn slowly over a period of 3–4 months after the bowel actions have been normal for 3 months.

Encopresis

This term refers to the passage of a normal stool but in abnormal situations. It is usually associated with behavioural abnormalities, and such children need psychological assessment and therapy. This is fully discussed in Chapter 20.

Hirschsprung's disease

This is due to an absence of ganglion cells in the intramuscular and submucous plexuses of the large bowel and involves a variable length of intestine from the anus extending proximally. This causes functional intestinal obstruction.

Clinical features

Hirschsprung's disease most commonly presents in the neonatal period with a delay in the passage of meconium beyond 24 hours. This is usually associated with gross abdominal distension and the later onset of vomiting. A later presentation, with history of chronic constipation may be due to an ultra-short segment of involvement. Diagnostic delay in the neonatal period is associated with an increased mortality due to the development of necrotising enterocolitis. Rectal examination in this condition reveals an empty rectum and dilation of the constricted region with the examining finger results in the explosive passage of stool.

Investigations

The diagnosis is confirmed by suction biopsy of the rectal mucosa which shows the absence of ganglion cells and an increase in positive cholinesterase staining due to the increased number of nerve fibres present. Ano-rectal manometry will demonstrate a failure of the normal relaxation of the internal anal sphincter with rectal distension, it is occasionally used as a diagnostic tool but is less reliable than a biopsy.

Management

The treatment of Hirschsprung's disease is surgical, and in the neonatal period this consists of a defunctioning colostomy. The definitive repair is undertaken at about 1 year of age. Following complete repair, there is often faecal incontinence, but full continence is eventually acquired in 70–90% of cases.

Inflammatory bowel disease

The advent of endoscopy in paediatrics has resulted in the earlier diagnosis of inflammatory bowel disease. Both Crohn's disease and ulcerative colitis occur in childhood, and although comparatively rare, their incidence appears to be increasing.

Crohn's disease

Crohn's disease involves the whole length of the intestine from the mouth to the anus, and the changes are not uniform, resulting in the skip lesions which were originally described on barium X-rays. The most frequently affected areas are the distal ileum and the proximal colon. The histological features are those of granulomatous change and affect the full thickness of the bowel wall, which will result in the adherence of bowel leading to the formation of fistulae, which may occasionally include the bladder.

Clinical features

The symptoms of this condition are many and often rather vague, which means that there is often a long delay between the onset of symptoms and diagnosis of the disease. In one study the interval was as long as 2 years. The common gastrointestinal symptoms are abdominal pain, diarrhoea which may be blood stained, mouth ulceration, and both anal fissures and fistulae. The systemic features are anorexia, arthritis and finger clubbing. Delayed puberty and poor growth are very common and are found in approximately 30% of affected children.

Investigations

The investigation of these children will show anaemia and elevation of acute phase reactants such as the ESR and C-reactive protein levels. Protein loss leads to low serum albumin levels. The mainstay of diagnosis is colonoscopy to the level of the terminal ileum, which will also provide biopsy material for histological examination. A small bowel barium meal is also necessary to demonstrate possible involvement of the ileum.

Management

The aim of treatment is to induce a remission and prednisolone is used in a dose of 2 mg/kg/day for a period of 2 weeks. Sulphasalazine may have a steroid sparing effect, and is very effective in Crohn's colitis, but it has no prophylactic role. Many patients can thereafter be maintained on alternate daily steroids. Bowel rest with total parenteral nutrition seems to have a beneficial effect in those patients with severe disease although the mechanism of action is unknown. Recently it has been shown that the use of an enteral diet is almost as effective in the induction of a remission as the use of steroids, but again the mechanism is unknown. The growth failure so often seen in these children may result from both the usage of steroids and the disease itself. If only localized lesions are present, then surgical intervention may be warranted to gain a period of good growth, but should be used cautiously because of the risk of fistula formation postoperatively. The nutritional monitoring of these patients is crucial because the anorexia coupled with malabsorption may lead to marked malnutrition.

Prognosis

The overall prognosis is guarded, the mortality is low (2.4%), but multiple relapses are common well into adult life. Colonic disease tends to have more extra-intestinal symptoms and a poorer prognosis.

Ulcerative colitis

This is less common than Crohn's disease in children, and unlike Crohn's there is an increased risk in siblings of 5–10%. The inflammatory lesion is superficial and restricted to the colon, and tends to progress from the distal bowel proximally.

Clinical features

The onset is again insidious with the passage of blood and mucus which is initially worse at night. Tenesmus and abdominal pain may also be features. Uveitis and pauciarticular arthritis may occur and other systemic symptoms such as fever, erythema nodosum and disordered liver function may be present.

Investigations

A barium enema will show a loss of haustrations and an abnormal mucosal pattern with crypt abscess, but the cornerstone of the diagnosis is again colonoscopy. Investigation of the stools for infective agents is mandatory and amoebic dysentery should be excluded by serology.

Management

The treatment of ulcerative colitis is similar to Crohn's disease with steroids, but sulphasalazine may have a prophylactic role. In localized proctitis topical steroids given as enemas are effective. Colectomy is curative, but is not usually performed in childhood unless there are frequent relapses, or severe extra-intestinal problems. The major acute complication is toxic megacolon, which is often precipitated by the use of opiates or anticholinergic drugs. The treatment of this requires a period of complete bowel rest with parenteral nutrition and steroids. Ulcerative colitis also carries an increased risk of malignant changes; 3% in the first decade, and 20% per decade for patients with active disease irrespective of the age of onset. It is for this reason that all patients should have regular colonoscopic examinations.

Rectal bleeding

The passage of fresh blood from the rectum can be extremely frightening for both the child and his parents. A carefully taken history can be helpful in the diagnosis and in directing further investigations. Pain on defaecation associated with fresh blood on the outside of the stool is suggestive of an anal fissure, particularly when constipation is present. The fissure is normally easily visible on inspection. The use of stool softeners, for example Lactulose, will ease the pain by preventing straining at stool and allows healing to take place. The application of a topical anaesthetic agent has been suggested but it is often difficult to apply in active toddlers.

Fresh blood, often fairly profuse, at the end of defaecation, which is painless and not associated with an alteration of bowel habit, suggests the presence of a rectal polyp. These can occasionally be palpated on rectal examination, but colonoscopy is required because although commonly single, they can be multiple. The polyps can be removed by a snare during the same procedure. Juvenile polyps of the colon are hamartomatous, with no tendency to malignant change, but a family history suggests familial adenomatous polyposis coli, which has an autosomal dominant mode of inheritance. This is an important diagnosis as these lesions are premalignant and colectomy is the treatment of choice. Peutz Jegher syndrome has the same inheritance, but the polyps are benign hamartomata and occur throughout both the colon and small intestine. In this latter condition there may be associated pigmented lesions on the

Table 12.6 Causes of rectal bleeding in the neonate.

Anal fissure
Necrotizing enterocolitis (p. 114)
Cow's milk colitis
Haemorrhagic disease of the newborn
Other bleeding disorder
Meckel's diverticulum
Intussusception
Idiopathic

lips, face and fingers. The treatment is conservative although if symptomatic the polyps can be removed by colonoscopy.

Rectal bleeding in the newborn should always be carefully evaluated. Table 12.6 lists important causes for this.

Rectal prolapse

Rectal prolapse may present with rectal bleeding, but more commonly the parents notice the protruding rectal mucosa. The association between this and cystic fibrosis is well described, but any chronic diarrhoea, such as that coincident upon a heavy parasite load or straining at stool may produce a prolapse. The mucosa can normally be replaced digitally, and the concomitant use of stool softeners obviates the need for straining. In cystic fibrosis the prolapse responds to the addition of pancreatic supplements. If the prolapse recurs immediately after being replaced, strapping the buttocks reduces the frequency, and maintains the rectum in place, only very rarely is surgery required.

Intussusception

Intussusception is an important cause of abdominal pain and bleeding in the child aged 3 months to 2 years. It commonly affects previously healthy children, but a recent history of respiratory or gastrointestinal infection is not uncommon.

Clinical features

The symptoms results from invagination of one segment of bowel into another. The commonest site is the terminal ileum into the caecum. Classically the child presents with pain which is episodic and severe with associated screaming and drawing up of the legs. The so-called 'redcurrant jelly' stools consisting of blood and mucus is passed in approximately 75% of cases. A detailed examination will often demonstrate a sausage-shaped mass in the right side of the abdomen, and a rectal examination will occasionally reveal the convex mass of the intussusception but this is a late sign.

Investigations

A plain X-ray of the abdomen shows signs of obstruction with the typical cresenteric shadow of the lesion in the right hypochondrium (Fig. 12.2).

Management

In those patients with a history of less than 24 hours and no evidence of peritonism or shock, a barium enema may be used to reduce the bowel but high pressures should not be used because of the risk of perforation. The mortality rate is still 1% and this is usually related to a delay in diagnosis. The cause is unknown in most cases and commonly no precipitating factor is found, but there is a recurrence rate of approximately 5% and very occasionally a polyp is found to be the lead of the intussusception.

Abdominal pain

Chronic abdominal pain of childhood is an extremely common condition and readers are referred to the excellent monograph written by the late Dr Apley. The aphorism that the further away from the umbilicus the pain is sited, the more likely the cause is organic holds true. The child with recurrent abdominal pain commonly points to the umbilicus, although obviously this must be treated with some degree of caution. A thorough examination is both reassuring to the parents and important in the exclusion of other causes. Investigations should not be excessive, but it is usual to measure the haemoglobin and ESR to rule out Crohn's disease, and to culture the urine. Recently, abdominal ultrasound has proven to be of benefit to examine the pancreas for signs of chronic pancreatitis as well as the liver and kidneys. The management of abdominal pain is largely reassurance.

Peptic ulceration

Abdominal pain that wakes the child at night is not usually benign. There is increasing evidence that suggests that peptic ulceration is a relatively

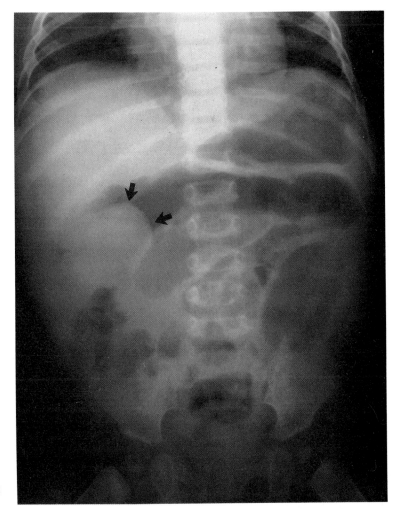

Fig. 12.2 Plain abdominal X-ray showing intussusception. Note the leading edge of the intussuscepting bowel arrowed.

common occurrence. Duodenal ulceration is more common that gastric and in such cases there is frequently a positive family history. The diagnosis is made by gastroscopy, as barium studies rarely reveal the presence of ulcers. Massive bleeding is uncommon, but occasional coffee ground vomits are described. Cimetidine and the use of antacids bring about symptomatic relief and healing of the ulcer. Therapy is continued for 12 months to reduce the incidence of relapse but this still occurs in 10–25% of cases. Recent evidence suggests that infection with the bacteria helicobacter pyloriditis may be one causative agent, but much further work is required before its true role is known for certain.

Acute appendicitis

This is one of the commonest abdominal childhood emergencies, but the diagnosis and the mortality can be high especially in the very young.

Clinical features

The clinical features are central abdominal pain and anorexia. The child who continues to have a healthy appetite does not have appendicitis. The pain may not move to the right iliac fossa, but classically this occurs a few hours after onset. The abdomen is tender with guarding. There may also be rebound tenderness, which is elicited by the presence of maximum discomfort on suddenly removing the palpating hand. Vomiting is a constant feature with a low grade fever and leucocytosis. Constipation is common but diarrhoea may also occur. Rectal examination is often extremely tender particularly in the case of retrocaecal appendix. The bases of the lung must be auscultated as basal pneumonia is occasionally mistaken for appendicitis.

The differential diagnosis should also include mesenteric adenitis and it is this condition that commonly results in the removal of a normal appendix. This is normally secondary to an acute upper airways infection, commonly tonsillitis. There may be a history of a few days malaise before the acute onset, and a history of sore throat may be elicited. The pain is colicky in nature, and the temperature commonly high. The enlarged abdominal glands are not palpable and a period of observation is often required to establish the di-

agnosis and exclude appendicitis. The symptoms usually resolve in a few days.

Henoch–Schönlein purpura (p. 261) may also present as acute abdominal pain, but other features such as the classic rash and arthralgia, should suggest the diagnosis. Gastrointestinal bleeding occurs due to the presence of the purpuric lesions within the bowel mucosa.

MECKEL'S DIVERTICULUM

This is a remnant of the omphalo-mesenteric duct. It may remain asymptomatic, but it frequently contains gastric mucosa which can ulcerate and give rise to abdominal pain and intestinal haemorrhage. Very occasionally the lumen can obstruct mimicking appendicitis. The diagnosis may be confirmed by a technetium scan which demonstrates the ectopic gastric tissue as a hot spot.

Hepatic disease

Jaundice is the accumulation and retention of bilirubin in the skin and other tissues. It may be an important symptom of liver disease or

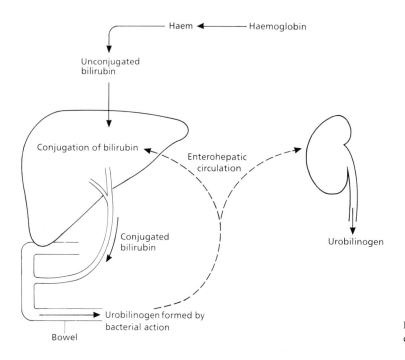

Fig. 12.3 Production and excretion of bilirubin.

Table 12.7   Causes of jaundice due to hyperbilirubinaemia. See also neonatal jaundice p. 106

Predominately unconjugated		Predominately conjugated	
Haemolysis	Hepatic	Hepatic	Obstructive
See p. 430	Drugs Gilbert's syndrome Criggler–Najjar syndrome	Hepatitis Metabolic diseases Cirrhosis Drugs Wilson's disease α_1-antitrypsin deficiency Cystic fibrosis Dubin–Johnson syndrome Rotor syndrome	Hepatitis Biliary atresia Gallstones Choledochal cyst

haemolysis. Bilirubin levels must exceed 190 µmol/l (2.5 mg/dl) before it is visible in the skin. Bilirubin is produced by the breakdown of haem from haemoglobin which is initially insoluble until metabolized in the liver to a soluble conjugated form. Soluble bilirubin is then excreted into the bowel via the hepatic and bile ducts. Figure 12.3 illustrates the major components of bilirubin metabolism.

Jaundice results from excessive haemolysis, hepatic cell dysfunction or failure to excrete bilirubin through the biliary tree. Jaundice may therefore be considered to originate from either prehepatic, hepatic or posthepatic causes. This classification may become confusing as prehepatic jaundice may induce cholestasis with posthepatic abnormalities as well. Unconjugated hyperbilirubinaemia is particularly common during the neonatal period and is discussed in Chapter 7.

Causes of jaundice can be conveniently divided into either those which cause predominately unconjugated (insoluble) hyperbilirubinaemia or predominately conjugated jaundice. Conjugated hyperbilirubinaemia can be further subdivided into either cholestatic (obstructive) or non-cholestatic in nature. Table 12.7 lists the causes of jaundice in children categorized in this manner.

Clinical evaluation

A careful history together with clinical examination will often allow the doctor to narrow the differential diagnosis to a relatively small group of conditions. Acute anaemia in the presence of sudden onset of jaundice strongly suggests haemolysis. Acholuric (normal-coloured urine) jaundice indicates an unconjugated cause, also suggestive of haemolysis. Dark, tea-coloured urine means that soluble bilirubin is present and in this case the stools are pale. This is strongly suggestive of a cholestatic or obstructive form of the disease. Bilirubin in the skin causes intense itching and extensive scratch marks may be seen.

Liver size is variable and is not particularly helpful in making a diagnosis. Massive hepatomegaly with jaundice suggests long-standing haemolysis or infestation such as malaria (p. 572). Steatorrhoea occurs in the majority of children with long-standing chronic liver disease due to the absence of bile salts in the bowel. The stools smell very offensive and usually float in the toilet pan. Fat-soluble vitamin deficiency states may also be apparent on examination.

Management

Specific treatment depends on the cause of the jaundice and careful investigation must be undertaken in every case. Non-specific management may be helpful, particularly in cholestatic causes of jaundice.

Dietary supplements. Malabsorption is due to lack of bile salts and this may cause malnutrition. A diet high in medium chain fatty acids, which do not require bile salts for their absorption, is an important dietary supplement.

Vitamin supplementation. Fat-soluble vitamins will be malabsorbed. Particular clinical problems include vitamin A deficiency (p. 546), vitamin E deficiency, metabolic bone disease (vitamin D deficiency) and hypoprothrombinaemia due to vitamin K deficiency. This vitamin must be given regularly, either parenterally or as a water-soluble preparation.

Pruritis. Intense itching is a feature of cholestatic jaundice due to accumulation of bile salts and cholesterol in the skin. Cholestyramine is particularly helpful in reducing the irritation.

Liver transplantation. This is now undertaken in some centres for end-stage liver failure and may become a valuable therapeutic option in the future.

Prolonged neonatal jaundice

A full discussion of the causes of neonatal jaundice is found in Chapter 7, but jaundice that persists for longer than 2 weeks in the neonatal period is by definition prolonged. It is predominantly due to retention of conjugated bilirubin, although this is not always the case. This results in the clinical picture of pale stools and dark urine due to the respective lack of bile pigment and increased urinary excretion. Two major clinical entities must be considered, neonatal hepatitis and extra hepatic biliary atresia. The diagnosis must be made as soon as possible, as a delay beyond 1 month in biliary atresia may seriously jeopardize the prognosis.

Neonatal hepatitis

The incidence of neonatal hepatitis is approximately 1 : 3000 live births, however, in only 40% of cases can a cause be defined. The onset may be from birth, when it is confused with physiological jaundice, but the presence of acholuric stools should arouse suspicion. The causes can broadly

Table 12.8 Causes of the neonatal hepatitis syndrome.

Metabolic
  Galactosaemia
  Fructosaemia
  Tyrosinosis
  Niemann–Pick syndrome
  Gaucher's disease
  Wolman's syndrome
  Zellweger's syndrome
  Rotor syndrome
  Parenteral nutrition

Hormonal
  Hypothyroidism
  Hypopituitarism

Infective
  Hepatitis A and B
  'TORCH' infections
  Coxsackie virus

Genetic
  α_1-antitrypsin deficiency

be divided into metabolic, hormonal, infective and genetic (Table 12.8). The full investigation of the neonate must be undertaken quickly to identify those aetiologies which are potentially treatable such as galactosaemia, fructose intolerance, hypothyroidism, hypopituitarism, and infective agents including urinary tract infections, toxoplasmosis, and syphilis. It is also essential to monitor liver function, especially clotting studies as morbidity may be increased by bleeding.

Of the genetic causes, by far the most common is α_1-antitrypsin deficiency. The disease is inherited as an autosomal recessive disorder, with the PiZZ (protease inhibitor) electrophoretic pattern being associated with cholestasis. One-half of neonates born with the PiZZ genotype will have an asymptomatic rise in transaminase levels only, but 11% will develop cirrhosis which carries a grave prognosis. Associated disorders of the respiratory tract are rare in childhood.

The pathology of the neonatal hepatitis syndrome, seen on biopsy of the liver, shows inflammatory cell infiltration of the portal system, with the presence of characteristic giant cells.

These changes are non-specific and do not give any indication as to the aetiology. The liver in α_1-antitrypsin deficiency can be characterized by the presence of PAS-positive material in the hepatocytes.

Treatment is very much dependent upon the aetiology, but in those cases where no treatable cause is identified, bile flow may be stimulated by the use of phenobarbitone and cholestyramine.

Extrahepatic biliary atresia

The importance of this syndrome lies in the fact that an early differentiation from neonatal hepatitis is essential, as a delay longer than 60 days has been clearly shown to adversely affect the prognosis. Clinical examination alone is not a useful discriminator, as both syndromes may be associated with pale stools and dark urine. Liver function tests may be helpful in certain cases, and the use of certain biochemical markers, such as gamma glutamyl peptidase and lipoprotein X in atresia have been used but are not reliable enough to be used alone. The presence of a cause of hepatitis should be actively sought which may be helpful to exclude biliary atresia. The use of radioisotopes that are selectively excreted by bile, such as the rose bengal iodine test, and the newer technetium-labelled DISIDA scans are helpful in many cases but a grey area often exists between the two syndromes. The use of phenobarbitone coupled with radioisotope scans may be helpful in those cases of hepatitis with a severe obstructive element. Ultrasound imaging is important as it may easily demonstrate a choledochal cyst, which may also obstruct the biliary tree, although the resolution is not good enough to define atretic ducts. The demonstration of an absent gall bladder suggests biliary atresia.

The diagnosis is usually confirmed by liver biopsy in which the characteristic proliferation of the intrahepatic bile ducts may be seen. The pathogenesis of the atresia is still unknown, but an infective agent, such as reovirus type 3 is a likely candidate, and would account for the cases that have been documented to occur postnatally.

Management

The treatment of biliary atresia is surgical, using a Roux-en-Y loop to establish bile drainage. The best known procedure is that first described by Dr Kasai from Japan, a country with a high incidence of this condition. The prognosis is reliant upon the diameter of the ducts at the portahepatis found at the time of operation.

Atresia of the intrahepatic ducts is also well described, but this is normally part of a syndrome and the diagnosis can often be inferred by careful examination of the child. Of these, Alagille's syndrome is probably the most common and comprises a characteristic facies, vertebral anomalies and the presence of peripheral pulmonary stenosis.

Hepatitis A

Infection with this virus is the commonest cause of hepatitis in childhood, although cytomegalovirus and Epstein–Barr virus infections may produce a similar clinical picture. The disease is spread by faecal contamination of food and drinking water, and so is far commoner in areas of poor sanitation. The highest incidence is in those children aged between 5 and 15 years. The incubation period of hepatitis A is approximately 1 month.

Clinical features

The onset is often insidious associated with anorexia, nausea and malaise for 4–5 days before the onset of jaundice. The urine becomes dark due to bilirubin, and the levels of the serum transaminases are usually raised, often before the onset of jaundice. On examination there are no signs of chronic liver disease, such as clubbing, spider naevae or ascites, but the liver is normally tender on palpation. The diagnosis can now be confirmed by serology.

Management

There is no specific treatment required, and the child feels much improved with the onset of jaundice. Strict bed rest was often advocated in the past, but this is no longer thought to be necessary. Although the child with hepatitis is usually nursed in an isolation cubicle, by the time of the onset of jaundice the patient is no longer shedding the virus, and so this may not be required. Few children with hepatitis A require admission to hospital.

Hepatitis B

Infections with this agent are much less frequent than hepatitis A. The incubation period is much longer, between 50 and 180 days. The epidemiology is also very different and rarely affects healthy children. One of the major routes of contamination used to be blood products, but donors are now routinely screened for infection. More common in the paediatric population is vertical transmission from an infected mother, but saliva can also contain viral particles, as can semen.

Clinical features

The clinical features are similar to hepatitis A, but the incidence of systemic symptoms, such as urticaria and arthralgia are more frequent. The clinical course is benign in the majority of cases, but the progression to chronic hepatitis is more frequent than in hepatitis A infections. Chronic carriers have a higher incidence of hepatocellular carcinoma in later life.

Investigations

The serology of this infection is now well described. The Australia or surface antigen (HBsAg) is positive, the core antigen (HBeAg) and corresponding antibody correlates with the duration of the infection, and is of particular use during pregnancy. A mother who is HBeAg positive is highly infectious. If she also has antibody to HBe (HBeAb positive) there is little risk of her infecting her baby. The incidence of the carrier state is increased in those patients infected during the neonatal period, and this risk is strongly correlated with an 'e' antigen-positive mother. It is for this reason

Table 12.9 Causes of chronic liver disease.

Chronic active hepatitis
Chronic persistent hepatitis
Wilson's disease
α_1-antitrypsin deficiency
Recurrent cholangitis (following biliary atresia)
Neonatal hepatitis
Drugs
Inflammatory bowel disease

that pregnant women in many centres are now screened and those infants found to be at risk are immunized with hepatitis B vaccine at birth and again at 1 month and 1 year of age. Immunoglobulin is also given at birth to afford some protection until the baby seroconverts from the vaccine.

Chronic liver disease

This is uncommon in children and Table 12.9 lists the most important causes.

Chronic hepatitis

Two syndromes are recognized as being associated with chronic hepatitis, chronic persistent hepatitis and chronic active hepatitis. Of these two, chronic persistent hepatitis carries the better prognosis.

CHRONIC PERSISTENT HEPATITIS

It is usually diagnosed following the detection of raised serum transaminase levels, subsequent to an episode of acute hepatitis, and 80% are found to be surface antigen (HBeAg) positive. The confirmation of the diagnosis is made by liver biopsy, no treatment is required and the disease spontaneously resolves in about 1–4 years.

CHRONIC ACTIVE HEPATITIS

This condition arises acutely with hepatitis and is most common in young girls over the age of 10 years. A subacute presentation with anorexia, weight loss and hepatomegaly may also occur. In chronic active hepatitis, liver function is greatly disturbed with signs of bleeding disorders with hypoproteinaemia and ascites. There may also be signs of other auto-immune phenomena such as glomerulonephritis, thyroiditis, fibrosing alveolitis, ulcerative colitis and pericarditis. Again the diagnosis is made on a liver biopsy, taking care to check the child's clotting status prior to undertaking this procedure.

Management

The treatment is initially that of acute hepatic failure, correcting clotting by means of plasma, and increasing the low plasma albumin levels, taking care not to give diuretics. A course of steroids in high dosage is given to induce a remission, and then maintenance steroids are prescribed for approximately 1 year. In adults this treatment has resulted in a 10-year survival in 60% of patients, the outlook for children is probably better than this. Before steroid treatment was introduced, 90% of cases developed cirrhosis.

Bacterial infections

In general, bacterial infections of the liver are rare and commonly produce their effects by means of abscess formation. Diagnosis can be made by ultrasound scan of the liver. If jaundice develops then this denotes a bad prognosis.

Parasitic infection of the liver in global terms is more frequent; the type of organism is dependent on the particular endemic area. Amoebiasis and leishmaniasis are perhaps the most common, but in areas of sheep farming hydatid disease of the liver also affects children. These infections rarely present with jaundice.

Reye's syndrome

Typically, Reye's syndrome (pronounced ryes) affects young children and is associated with a dramatic deterioration in a child thought to be recovering from a viral infection. The liver is enlarged and on biopsy is infiltrated with fat. Electron microscopy demonstrates disruption of the

mitochondria. Liver failure may result in disordered clotting, the transaminases are raised and the serum ammonia is greatly elevated. There is usually marked hypoglycaemia. Cerebral oedema develops rapidly with progressive deterioration in conscious level, proceeding to coma.

The management of these children is best undertaken in an intensive care unit with facilities for the measurement and treatment for raised intracranial pressure. This may be reduced by the infusion of mannitol and by hyperventilation to maintain the carbon dioxide tension at 3.5 kPa (26 mmHg). There is a high mortality associated with Reye's syndrome, and as yet the aetiology is unknown, although there appears to be a relationship with viral infections, principally chicken pox and influenza. Recently salicylates have been implicated, and it is for this reason that the use of aspirin in children is no longer sanctioned. There has been a dramatic reduction in the prevalence of Reye's syndrome in the last few years, possibly related to the publicity about aspirin.

Cirrhosis

In children, cirrhosis is frequently the end-point of either a metabolic disease process, such as galactosaemia or α_1-antitrypsin deficiency, the end-stage of an uncorrectable extrahepatic biliary atresia, or the result of a congenital condition such as familial childhood cirrhosis. The signs of chronic liver failure are, however, normally present.

Clinical features

The liver is initially firm and increased in size, there may be clubbing of the nails, with palmar erythema and spider naevi, accompanied by ascites. Liver failure may not be suspected until the child presents with a bleeding episode, or steatorrhoea.

Management

The management of these children requires specialist expertise and involves attempting to prevent progression to hepatic coma. In severe cases, the intake of sodium is restricted to 1 mmol/kg, as well as total fluids to 60% of the normal maintenance volume which help to compensate for the hyperaldosteronism which is usually present. The diet must be high in energy but low in protein and so for practical purposes consists of a high carbohydrate intake. In those patients in incipient hepatic failure, the monitoring and treatment of raised intracranial pressure is also essential. In addition the breakdown products of the bowel microflora is reduced by oral neomycin coupled with magnesium sulphate for its laxative effect. Because of the associated fat malabsorption these children also need high replacement levels of the fat-soluble vitamins. With the advent of transplantation techniques and improved methods of controlling rejection episodes, more children in end-stage liver disease are being offered transplants but, as yet, the numbers are small and carried out in only a few centres.

Wilson's disease

Although rare (approximately five cases per million population), this autosomal recessive disease is of great importance because it is a potentially treatable cause of liver failure. The disease process is the abnormal deposition of copper within the basal ganglia of the brain and within the liver. The levels of copper are high and those of caeruloplasmin are characteristically low. Abnormal deposition with the eye gives rise to the characteristic Kayser–Fleischer ring. Both the liver disease and central nervous system signs eventually develop usually late in the first decade of life, although initially liver disease may be the sole feature. The predominant symptom is often choreoathetosis (p. 323). The excess of copper is removed by the regular use of the chelating agent penicillamine.

Portal hypertension

There may be very little warning that a child has portal hypertension until a massive haemorrhage from ruptured oesophageal varices has taken place. This is one of the commonest causes of major haematemesis or melaena in childhood.

Aetiology

The causes can be divided into the site of obstruction, i.e. prehepatic, hepatic and posthepatic. Of these the prehepatic type is the most common, and is usually the result of umbilical sepsis in the neonatal period, although it can occur following umbilical venous cannulation, which should therefore be used with caution in neonates. Hepatic causes are the result of those disease processes that progress to cirrhosis. Cystic fibrosis is also emerging as an important aetiological factor and patients with this condition should be examined for the presence of splenomegaly.

BUDD–CHIARI SYNDROME

This is the best example of a posthepatic lesion and is a result of thrombosis of the hepatic vein, an unusual cause is the consumption of bush tea containing senna alkaloids which is consumed in Jamaica.

Clinical features

An initial evaluation of the patient should determine the presence of splenomegaly (this may not be palpable immediately following a bleed) and for signs suggestive of chronic liver disease. In the case of portal venous obstruction, there may be a caput medusae (dilation of veins flowing from the umbilicus). Hepatic vein thrombosis will result in ascites and dilated veins in the distribution of the inferior vena cava flowing to that of the superior vena cava.

Management

The majority of bleeding episodes cease with conservative management, but balloon compression of the oesophageal varices with a Sengstaken tube may occasionally be needed, combined with a pitressin infusion. There is no place for emergency shunt procedures in childhood. Further investigation after the acute phase with endoscopy will demonstrate varices, and indeed they may be sclerosed directly at endoscopy. Of the various

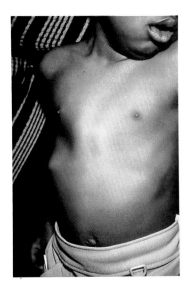

Plate 1 Harrison's sulci and prominent sternum secondary to chronic severe upper airway obstruction.

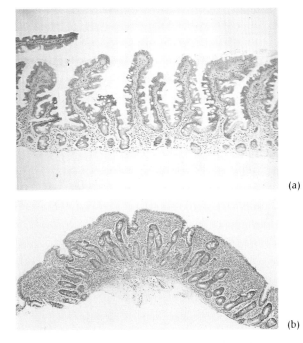

(a)

(b)

Plate 3 Small bowel histology in (a) a normal child, and (b) a child with coeliac disease.

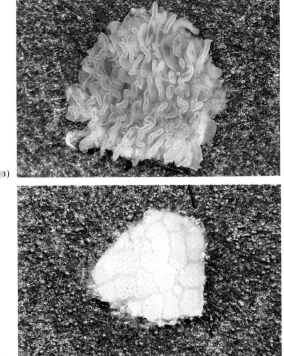

(a)

(b)

Plate 2 Appearances of a jejunal biopsy under the dissecting microscope. (a) Normal, and (b) coeliac disease. Note the completely flat appearance compared with normal.

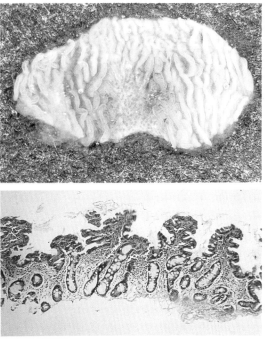

(a)

(b)

Plate 4 Small bowel biopsy in a child with cow's milk protein intolerance. (a) Dissecting microscope showing patchy atrophy, and (b) histological appearance.

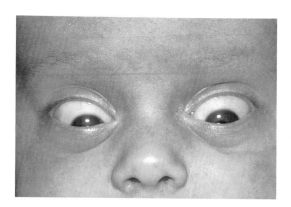

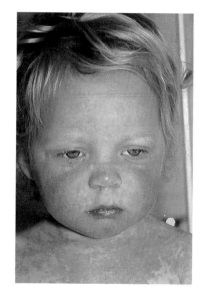

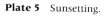

Plate 5 Sunsetting.

Plate 6 Typical rash of measles. Note that the child looks miserable and has conjunctivitis.

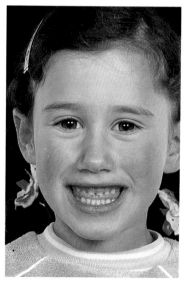

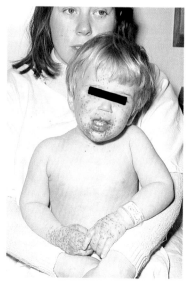

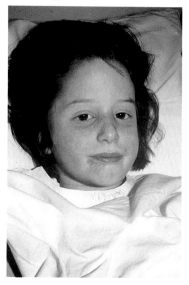

Plate 7 The erythematous 'slapped cheeks' of Fifth disease.

Plate 8 Eczema herpeticum. The areas of skin previously eczematous are affected with vesiculation.

Plate 9 The typical facial rash of scarlet fever. Note the circumoral pallor.

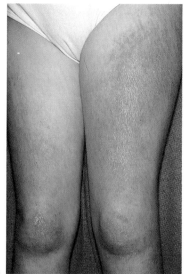

(a)

Plate 10a   Skin lesions of dermatomyositis. Heliotrope rash on thighs.

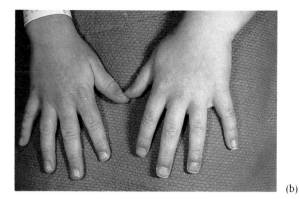

(b)

Plate 10b   Skin lesions of dermatomyositis. Violaceous rash on the extensor surfaces of the fingers.

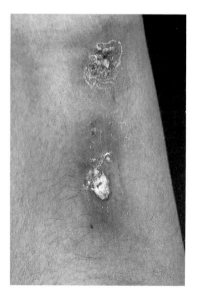

Plate 11   Dermatomyositis showing calcification extruding through the skin.

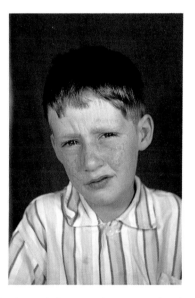

Plate 12   Systemic lupus erythematosus showing the characteristic rash in the butterfly distribution of the face.

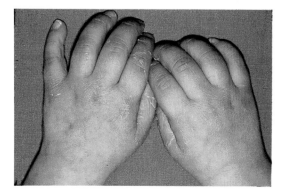

Plate 13   The hands of a child with Kawasaki's disease.

options regarding contrast radiology, coeliac axis arteriograms with a film taken in the venous phase appears to be the most advantageous. The long-term management is as conservative as possible; children with hepatic causes tolerate a shunt procedure poorly. Of those that do require such a procedure, a mesocaval shunt where the superior mesenteric artery is anastomosed to the inferior vena cava is preferred. This can normally be delayed until after 10 years of age as it is commonly unsuccessful below this age and the frequency of bleeding episodes naturally decline with increasing age.

Acknowledgment

The photomicrographs are reproduced with the kind permission of Mr A. Philips of the Queen Elizabeth Hospital for Children, Hackney, London.

Further reading

Anderson CM, Burke V & Gracy M. *Paediatric Gastroenterology*. Blackwell Scientific Publications, Oxford 1978.

Apley J. *The Child with Abdominal Pains*. Blackwell Scientific Publications, Oxford 1978.

Walker-Smith J. *Diseases of the Small Intestine in Childhood*. Pitman Medical, London 1989.

13

DISORDERS OF THE
CARDIOVASCULAR SYSTEM

The study of cardiac anatomy can become extremely complex, but in order to understand the clinical implications in the majority of cases of structural cardiac disease only a fairly superficial knowledge of anatomy is required. More complex lesions can at least be partly understood if certain basic facts of nomenclature are grasped. Systemic venous return to the heart is usually via the inferior vena cava and a right-sided superior vena cava to a morphologically right atrium. When the

right atrium drains through a tricuspid valve to a morphologically right ventricle and the left atrium opens via a mitral valve to a morphologically left ventricle, atrioventricular concordance is said to be present. If the right ventricle gives rise to a pulmonary artery and the left to an aorta then ventriculo-arterial concordance exists.

These descriptions all relate to the morphological characteristics of the cardiac structures concerned and do not necessarily describe spatial

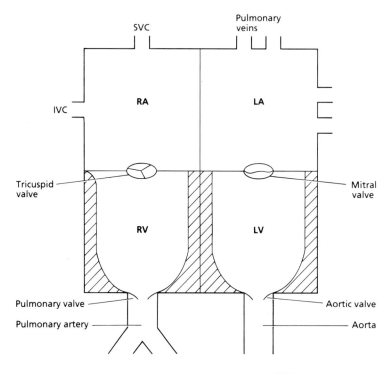

Fig. 13.1 Schematic diagram showing normal cardiac relationships. IVC, inferior vena cava; LA, left atrium; LV, left ventricle; RA, right atrium; RV, right ventricle; SVC, superior vena cava.

relationships within the chest. Pulmonary veins normally drain into the morphologically left atrium. The usual arrangement is that the heart is mainly in the left hemithorax (laevocardia) with the apex pointing to the left and the morphological left atrium is on the left. This atrial arrangement is termed atrial situs solitus or usual atrial arrangement. The normal cardiac configuration is illustrated in Figure 13.1.

Cardiac disease in childhood can be either congenital or acquired and although the former is the commoner in developed countries, acquired heart disease still occurs and enters the differential diagnosis of many conditions. World-wide, acquired paediatric heart disease is still a major prob-

Table 13.1 Causes of acquired heart disease in developed countries.

Pericarditis
Viral myocarditis
Infective endocarditis
Rheumatic fever, acute and chronic effects
Cardiomyopathy
Kawasaki disease
Cardiac involvement in collagen vascular diseases

lem. Acquired heart diseases encountered in children in developed countries are listed in Table 13.1 and will be discussed later. Congenital heart disease occurs in the region of 8 per 1000 live births in the UK. Up to 30% of these congenital

Table 13.2 Aetiology of congenital heart disease.

Cause or association	Detail or example
Clear genetic association Autosomal dominant	Rare families with ASD
Part of genetic syndrome Autosomal dominant	Holt–Oram syndrome (upper limb abnormalities and ASD) Noonan's syndrome (Turner-like phenotype and pulmonary stenosis)
Autosomal recessive	Ellis-van Creveld (polydactyly, short limbs, dysplastic nails and AV septal defect)
Part of sporadic syndrome VACTERL association	Vertebral, ano-rectal, oesophageal abnormalities and tetralogy of Fallot
Associated with chromosomal abnormality Down's syndrome (trisomy 21) Edwards' syndrome (trisomy 18) Patau syndrome (trisomy 13) Turner's syndrome (46XO)	AV septal defect, VSD, PDA ASD, VSD Complex lesions Coarctation
Intra-uterine infection Rubella embryopathy	Cerebral, eye, ear abnormalities and PDA, VSD, coarctation
Maternal diabetes	VSD, cardiac hypertrophy
Drugs in pregnancy Phenytoin	ASD, PDA (microcephaly, facial abnormality, nail hypoplasia)
Alcohol	ASD, VSD (typical facies, mental retardation, small stature)

ASD, Atrial septal defect; AV, atrioventricular; PDA, patent ductus arteriosus; and VSD, ventricular septal defect.

cardiac abnormalities will cause symptoms in the neonatal period or early infancy.

The aetiology of congenital cardiac defects·is usually multifactorial, i.e. polygenic and environmental. Once a couple have had an affected child for which no cause was found, their risk of having another affected child increases to around 3% depending on the particular lesion. There are a number of recognized causes and these should always be considered when congenital heart disease is identified. A list of common and important causes or associations is given in Table 13.2.

Investigative techniques

Heart disease, or suspected heart· disease, can be investigated in a number of ways, but careful history taking and thorough physical examination should always be the starting point. These may be all that is needed to give accurate information on the nature and severity of the lesion.

Electrocardiography

This gives information about heart rhythm and conduction, chamber size, dominance and hypertrophy. The normal electrocardiogram changes throughout childhood and when any doubt exists, reference must always be made to a table of normal values. Systematic analysis of an electrocardiogram will make mistakes less likely and a simple scheme for this is shown in Table 13.3. Table 13.4 gives normal values for certain parameters and Table 13.5 gives some important markers of abnormality seen on electrocardiograms.

Table 13.3 Systematic electrocardiographic analysis.

Rate	
Rhythm	
P wave	Axis, height, duration, configuration
PR interval	
QRS	Axis, duration, configuration, voltages, progression across chest leads
ST segment	Elevated or depressed
T wave	Flat, peaked or inverted

Table 13.4   Some normal ECG values.

P wave

Height <2.5 mm	At any age
Duration <0.12 sec	

PR interval

0.06−0.12 sec	Neonate
0.08−0.14 sec	1 month−3 years
0.10−0.18 sec	3−12 years
0.12−0.21 sec	Adult

Frontal QRS axis

60° to 180°	1 day
20° to 120°	1 month
0° to 100°	1−5 years
−20° to 100°	5−16 years

Table 13.5   ECG features of abnormality.

P wave

Height 3 mm or more, right atrial enlargement
Width 0.12 sec or more, left atrial enlargement

Right ventricular hypertrophy

QRS right axis deviation
   R wave V_1 beyond upper limit
   S wave V_6 beyond upper limit
   Upright T in V_1 when R dominant after 3 days of age
   R/S in V_1 above upper limit for age

Left ventricular hypertrophy

QRS left axis deviation (with no other explanation)
   S wave V_1 beyond upper limit
   R wave V_6 beyond upper limit
   R/S in V_1 below lower limit for age

Chest radiography

A plain chest X-ray gives a great deal of information. Before interpreting an X-ray it is important to note in what position it was taken, whether it was well aligned and what the penetration was. The phase of respiration must also be noted. Variations in these technical aspects can greatly alter apparent heart size (supine, antero-posterior or expiratory films increase the apparent size of the heart shadow) and pulmonary vascular markings; an under-penetrated or expiratory film makes them more prominent. A rotated film alters heart

Table 13.6   Scheme for chest X-ray analysis in cardiac cases.

Heart position in chest
Side of cardiac apex
Heart size (cardiothoracic ratio)
Heart configuration
Side of aortic arch (not always possible)
Pulmonary vascular markings
Bronchial anatomy (not always possible)
Number of ribs
Vertebral abnormalities
Pulmonary collapse, consolidation, focal hyperlucency
Side of liver and stomach shadows

size and shape. Table 13.6 gives a list of features to look for on a chest X-ray in a child with suspected cardiac disease and Figure 13.2 illustrates the landmarks of the normal heart border seen on X-ray. Lateral and occasionally oblique X-rays may add further information. Barium swallow films are useful when aberrant or abnormal vessels are suspected as they often cause oesophageal compression.

Hyperoxia test (nitrogen washout test)

If a normal person breathes nearly pure oxygen for 15 minutes the arterial oxygen tension (Pa_{O_2}) rises massively from the normal 12 kPa in air to 40 kPa or more. If a baby with cyanosis from a cardiac cause breathes 100% oxygen there is only a very small rise in Pa_{O_2}. In respiratory disease, unless extremely severe, the Pa_{O_2} will rise to at least 20 kPa in 100% oxygen. This test is useful when cyanosis is present and there is doubt whether it is cardiac or respiratory in origin, or when cardiac disease is known to be present but it is unclear clinically whether the patient is significantly desaturated. The test is performed either with right radial artery blood gas samples or a transcutaneous oxygen tension monitor on the right upper chest.

Cardiac ultrasonography

This has developed enormously in the last decade. Originally M-mode echocardiography was used to gain anatomical information but this has been replaced by imaging (sometimes called 2D scanning) (Fig. 13.3). Information on cardiac function can be obtained from imaging but M-mode is still used by many for this because measurements are more easily standardized. The Doppler principle allows blood flow direction and velocity to be obtained and this can be used to calculate pressures and

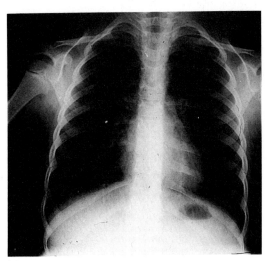

(a)

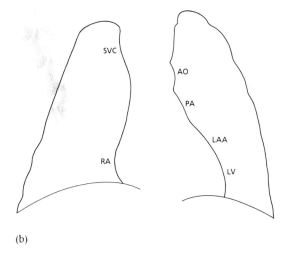

(b)

Fig. 13.2   (a) Chest X-ray (antero-posterior) showing the normal cardiac outline. (b) AO, aorta; LAA, left atrial appendage; LV, left ventricle; PA, pulmonary artery; RA, right atrium; SVC, superior vena cava.

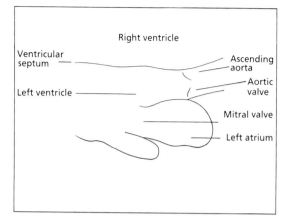

(a)

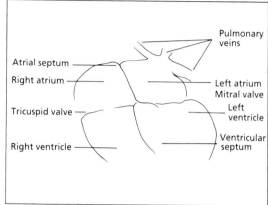

(c)

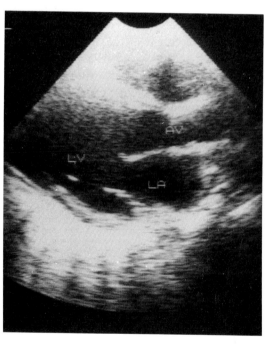

(b)

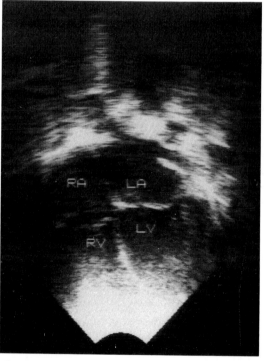

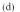

(d)

Fig. 13.3 Cardiac ultrasound imaging of the normal heart. (a,b) Parasternal long axis view; and (c,d) apical four-chamber view.

pressure gradients as well as volume flows in certain circumstances. The increasing availability and non-invasive nature of ultrasound imaging and Doppler ultrasound has made a great contribution to paediatric cardiology but basic history and examination must never be neglected, and in most instances an electrocardiograph and chest X-ray are appropriate before considering an ultrasound examination. Ultrasound scanning of fetal hearts is now being performed in a few places.

Cardiac catheterization

This is the time-honoured gold standard investigation in cardiology, although ultrasound has altered the indication and necessity for its use in many circumstances. Vascular access is gained percutaneously, by cut down or in neonates via the umbilical vein. Catheters are manipulated around the heart and great vessels which allow pressure measurements, sampling of oxygen saturation and the injection of radio-opaque dye to delineate anatomy. Calculations can give pulmonary and systemic resistances, cardiac output and shunt size. The procedure is done either under sedation or general anaesthesia and serious side-effects are rare. Death during cardiac catheterization is very rare, with reported mortality rates of less than 0.1% outside of the newborn period. The risk of death is higher in neonates (up to 2%) but they are of course very sick already if requiring cardiac catheterization. Some of the deaths in the past would have been in children or babies in whom catheterization would no longer be performed at that stage of their illness because sufficient information can be obtained with ultrasound. Cardiac catheterization can be therapeutic in children as well as diagnos-

tic, such uses of interventional cardiac catheterization are given in Table 13.7.

Presentation of cardiovascular disease

Cyanosis

Peripheral cyanosis is a very common normal finding in the first few days of life (p. 56). Central cyanosis can be difficult to recognize in the neonate particularly in babies of pigmented races and may be easily confused with traumatic cyanosis due to multiple petechiae following difficult delivery. It is important to look at the tongue if there is any doubt. Central cyanosis is due to deoxygenated haemoglobin and an otherwise normal baby with polycythaemia who has a normal arterial oxygen saturation will have more deoxygenated haemoglobin than an adult and may occasionally have a blue tongue, especially on crying. This is easily confused with cyanotic congenital heart disease. Furthermore, if a baby or older person is very anaemic, even low arterial oxygen saturations will not produce enough deoxygenated haemoglobin for clear central cyanosis to be recognized easily. If central cyanosis is suspected, but there is doubt, transcutaneous oxygen tension or a saturation monitor may help and arterial blood gas

Table 13.7 Interventional cardiac catheterization.

Well established	
Enlarge foramen ovale	Rashkind ballon atrial septostomy
Endomyocardial biopsy	Post-transplant, unexplained cardiomyopathy
Ballon valvuloplasty	Pulmonary valve
	Aortic valve
Ballon angioplasty	Coarctation and recoarctation, stenosis after intra-arterial repair for transposition
Being explored	
Closure of PDA	
Closure of ASD	
Very rarely in childhood	
Ablation of aberrant conduction pathways	

Table 13.8 Causes of neonatal cyanosis with examples.

Cardiac

Respiratory
  Obstructed airway
  Pneumonia
  Respiratory distress syndrome
  Pneumothorax
  Pleural effusion

Neurological and neuromuscular
  Brain malformation
  Meningitis
  Weak muscles
  Drug depression of CNS

Skeletal
  Small thorax, thoracic dystrophy

Metabolic
  Hypoglycaemia

Methaemoglobinaemia

analysis may be necessary. Cyanosis may be due to cardiac or other causes (Table 13.8). In practice, it is only necessary to distinguish cardiac from respiratory disease and this is not usually difficult. Respiratory disease severe enough to cause cyanosis in the newborn nearly always produces other signs of respiratory distress, abnormalities of lung fields on chest X-ray and elevated carbon dioxide on blood gas analysis. Some improvement in cyanosis or in arterial or transcutaneous oxygen levels is usually seen if high inspired oxygen is provided to babies with respiratory disease, whereas this is less likely and less marked in the majority of babies with cardiac disease. This is the basis of the hyperoxia test. Babies with cardiac cyanosis may or may not have other clear physical signs of cardiac disease. X-ray, electrocardiogram and ultrasound are needed urgently to make a precise diagnosis.

Occasionally, babies with respiratory disease or those who have suffered an asphyxial insult at birth fail to reduce their pulmonary vascular resistance after birth (see Persistent fetal circulation, p. 93). Thus right ventricular pressure remains high and blood goes from right to left across the

foramen ovale and to some extent through the ductus arteriosus. These babies may be profoundly cyanosed with little response to oxygen despite a structurally normal heart and minimal lung disease. They can produce diagnostic difficulties even with readily available paediatric cardiology expertise, although X-ray, electrocardiogram and ultrasound nearly always clarify the issue. The distinction between cyanosis and heart failure is diagnostically important and it should be remembered that cyanosis is only attributable to heart failure if the latter is very gross. Many students and doctors forget this.

There are three basic groups of cardiac abnormality which may cause cyanosis. These are:
1 Transposition haemodynamics.
2 Common mixing situations.
3 Right to left shunting.
A given condition may have more than one of these factors operating.

TRANSPOSITION HAEMODYNAMICS

In transposition, desaturated systemic venous blood returns to the heart but is then pumped back round the body and not into the lungs. Clearly some connection between systemic and pulmonary circulations must exist for life to be sustained. This can be via natural pathways in the form of a patent foramen ovale, an arterial duct, or through a ventricular septal defect.

COMMON MIXING

Common mixing situations are those in which oxygenated and deoxygenated blood are forced to mix thereby resulting in a subnormal systemic arterial saturation. Mixing can occur via abnormalities of venous drainage into the heart (for example, total anomalous pulmonary venous drainage into superior vena cava rather than left atrium) or via an abnormality in the arterial exit from the heart (as in truncus arteriosus) or at any anatomical stage in between at either atrial or ventricular level. Some common mixing situations result in only mild cyanosis and may show a considerable improvement in oxygenation in 100% inspired oxygen.

RIGHT TO LEFT SHUNT

In right to left shunting, deoxygenated blood fails to pass through the lungs before entering the systemic circulation again. This occurs by virtue of partial or complete obstruction to its flow through the right heart and the presence of a way to cross into the left heart, such as patent foramen ovale, atrial septal defect or ventricular septal defect.

More common causes of cardiac cyanosis are given in Table 13.9. In the first instance, precise diagnosis is less important than correct management, stabilization and then obtaining cardiological assessment. On suspecting cardiac disease presenting as cyanosis in a newborn infant, an immediate assessment that respiration and cardiac output are adequate is essential. If they are, physical examination for cardiovascular signs, evidence of congenital abnormalities in other systems and for dysmorphic features pointing to a particular syndrome should be carried out. Chest

Table 13.9 Causes of neonatal cardiac cyanosis with examples.

Transposition haemodynamics
    Simple TGA
    TGA + VSD + PS

Common mixing
    TAPVD
    Tricuspid atresia
    Common atrium
    'Single ventricle' (univentricular atrioventricular
        connection)
    Truncus arteriosus

Right to left shunt
    Tricuspid atresia
    Tetralogy of Fallot
    Pulmonary atresia with intact ventricular septum
    Pulmonary atresia with VSD

TAPVD, total anomalous pulmonary venous drainage; TGA, transposition of great arteries; PS, pulmonary stenosis; VSD, ventricular septal defect.

X-ray, electrocardiogram, four limb blood pressures and usually blood gas analysis with hyperoxia test are then performed. Acidosis and hypoglycaemia should be dealt with, hypocalcaemia and polycythaemia may be relevant to management. Babies with reduced lung blood flow as shown by oligaemic lung fields on chest X-ray and with features of one of the right to left shunting conditions will almost certainly benefit from an infusion or oral administration of prostaglandin E_1 or E_2. These drug re-open or maintain patency of the ductus arteriosus and will in these conditions improve lung blood flow by increasing flow from aorta to pulmonary artery. This will improve oxygenation and help treat or prevent metabolic acidosis secondary to hypoxaemia. Transposition haemodynamics will also respond to prostaglandin by increased systemic arterial oxygen saturation but, on occasions, increasing lung blood flow further in babies with already plethoric lungs may worsen their respiratory function. Babies with common mixing situations and consequent increased lung blood flow do not need prostaglandin. The drug has side-effects including apnoea, pyrexia, jitteriness, diarrhoea and flushing. If a baby is to be transferred to another hospital on prostaglandin infusion the infusion rate should be stable without apnoea for at least an hour before starting the journey.

Cyanosis recognized in infancy outside the newborn period is usually due to those conditions listed in Table 13.9 associated with increased lung blood flow such as total anomalous pulmonary venous drainage, or to conditions in which obstruction to forward flow into the lungs develops progressively as it does classically in tetralogy of Fallot. Presentation with cyanosis after the age of 1 year is rare in developed countries although in tetralogy of Fallot this may occur occasionally.

Cyanosis due to cardiac causes developing after 2 years is likely to be due to shunt reversal. This is called the Eisenmenger complex (p. 228) and may occur in ventricular septal defect, atrial septal defect or patent ductus arteriosus. In developed countries this should be an increasing rarity as such lesions will be detected and treated at an early stage. It may still be seen in very complex lesions with initial large left to right shunts and in children with Down's syndrome and complete atrioventricular septal defect with a common valve ring, in whom the risks of corrective surgery in infancy are considered too great.

Primary pulmonary hypertension without structural heart disease occasionally occurs in paediatric patients and causes cyanosis in its later stages. Clubbing of finger and toe nails is recognizable in late infancy and beyond but does not develop in the first 6 months of life.

Cardiac failure

Symptoms and signs of cardiac failure in the neonate and infant are given in Table 13.10 and it is clear that some of them have a number of causes other than cardiac disease. When cardiac failure is suspected, careful history and examination as described for the cyanosed neonate or infant are indicated. Simple investigations again include four limb blood pressure recordings, electrocardiogram and chest X-ray. Attention to the overall state of the baby is obviously important and hypothermia, hypoglycaemia, electrolyte and fluid imbalance and possible infection should be sought and dealt with. First-line management of a baby in heart failure includes fluid restriction, digoxin and diuretics. Vasodilators such as captopril are also increasingly used. If closure of the ductus arteriosus is thought to have resulted in a critical state being produced, prostaglandin is indicated; this will be discussed again below. Causes of heart failure in the early months of life are listed in Table 13.11. Cardiac failure after infancy is less likely to be due to congenital heart disease except in those with complex lesions who have undergone one or more operations. Acquired heart disease is far more likely to be the cause of heart failure in children and rheumatic fever; viral and other causes of myocarditis and various cardiomyopathies have to be thought of. Acute left ventricular failure is a recognized presentation of acute glomerulonephritis, and children with chronic renal failure may have marked myocardial dysfunction particularly when fluid overloaded prior to intermittent dialysis. Clinical features of heart failure become easier to recognize and, except for infants, are more like those seen in adults beyond infancy (Table 13.12).

Collapse

At any age sudden collapse may be a sign of a cardiac arrhythmia. This is most commonly either extreme bradycardia or tachycardia, particularly

Table 13.10 Features of heart failure in babies.

History	Examination
Poor feeding	Failure to thrive
	Tachycardia
Sweatiness	Tachypnoea with indrawing
	Hepatomegaly
Breathlessness	Gallop rhythm

Table 13.11 Causes of heart failure in neonates and infants.

Hypoplastic left heart syndrome	
Coarctation	*(earlier)*
Critical aortic stenosis	*(later)*
Endocardial fibroelastosis	
Patent ductus arteriosus	
(excluding prematures)	
Ventricular septal defect	
Supraventricular tachycardia	*(any time)*

Table 13.12 Features of heart failure in children.

History	Examination	
Breathlessness	Tachycardia	
	Gallop rhythm	
Lack of energy	Tachypnoea	} Left heart failure
	Indrawing	
Orthopnoea	Crepitations	
	JVP elevated	} Right heart failure
Abdominal pain	Hepatomegaly	
	Peripheral oedema	
Loss of appetite		

ventricular tachycardia. Supraventricular tachycardia if prolonged may cause heart failure in young babies but not usually collapse. Arrhythmias are considered on p. 226.

Duct-dependent lesions

In the neonate some cardiac conditions result in rapid deterioration over some hours in a previously well-looking baby when the ductus arteriosus closes. These are conditions with severe obstruction to, or complete interruption of, the route for blood from the left ventricle to descending aorta and include aortic atresia, and interrupted aortic arch. The most extreme form of these abnormalities is termed the hypoplastic left heart syndrome when mitral valve, left ventricle, aortic valve and ascending aorta may all be atretic or severely hypoplastic (p. 231). In this condition, sepsis is often suspected and metabolic disorders considered because of metabolic acidosis, but careful examination including blood pressures and reference to chest X-ray and electrocardiogram usually alert the clinician to the likelihood of a duct-dependent obstructed left heart or aortic problem. Protaglandin infusion and diuretics with general supportive measures will be likely to resuscitate the baby enough to allow proper cardiac diagnostic assessment. After such collapse renal failure is common and antibiotics, if given, should be carefully monitored as aminoglycosides are frequently used for septic newborn babies. Some of the conditions causing this clinical picture are surgically correctable and full resuscitation is appropriate until diagnosis is clear. It may then be decided that continued aggressive management is contraindicated in some cases.

Murmurs

A heart murmur can be the presentation of cardiac disease at any age. A murmur must always be described carefully (Table 13.13) and placed in the context of the other auscultatory findings, the rest of the cardiovascular examination and the history, all of which are just as important as the murmur itself. It must be remembered that many murmurs do not represent cardiac disease and that some significant cardiac problems produce unimpressive or even no murmurs, particularly in the early weeks of life. Murmurs due to acquired heart disease are accompanied by other clinical features to point to their pathological nature. Murmurs due to particular structural lesions will be dealt with in detail under each lesion but certain helpful principles are listed in Table 13.14. Many murmurs are normal or innocent noises coming from a normal

Table 13.13 Points to note about a heart murmur.

Position in cardiac cycle
Place on praecordium
Radiation
Loudness
Quality
Variation with respiration, posture and valsalva
   manoeuvre

Table 13.14 Simple guide to murmur type.

Timing	Likely source
Midsystolic	Aortic or pulmonary valves, or aorta
Pansystolic	VSD or atrioventricular valve regurgitation
Diastolic	Mitral valve stenosis Ductus arteriosus (also systolic)

Table 13.15 Description of typical Still's innocent murmur.

Midsystolic
Between lower left sternal edge and apex
No radiation
⅙ to ⅗, no louder
Vibratory or twanging
Louder lying down
Quieter during valsalva manoeuvre

heart. They are particularly easily heard when the circulation is hyperdynamic as in fever, excitement, after exercise or some pathological, but non-cardiac, cause of tachycardia such as hyperthyroidism. Many innocent murmurs have definite characteristics as well as there being no features in the murmur or in any other part of clinical assessment of cardiac pathology. Obviously investigations are normal.

Normal murmurs are best considered as they relate to the neonatal period and early infancy and then as they relate to older children. Changes occurring just after birth include closure of the ductus arteriosus and a large increase in volume blood flow through the pulmonary arteries. A murmur from the closing ductus may be heard at the second left intercostal space (pulmonary area) in systole and occasionally in diastole also in the first day or two of life, but not thereafter in healthy term infants. In neonates, a quiet high-pitched midsystolic murmur attributed to blood flowing through the relatively small right and left pulmonary arteries may be heard at both sides of the upper part of the sternum and over the scapulae and upper dorsal spine. If the murmur persists beyond the age of 6 months, then this would be against such a murmur being entirely innocent. In older children a number of innocent murmurs are recognized; four will be mentioned here.

1 *The venous hum.* This is very common. It is heard over the upper chest and upper back, it is continuous throughout the cardiac cycle, very superficial sounding, louder in diastole and on inspiration and it is markedly reduced or abolished by

turning the head, applying gentle pressure to the neck or lying the patient flat or head down.

2 *Still's murmur.* The most common innocent true cardiac murmur is the so-called Still's murmur named after George Still who described it in 1909. It is rarely heard in infancy and usually disappears by the age of 10 years. There are numerous suggested mechanisms for its production. Its positive characteristics are given in Table 13.15.

3 *Innocent pulmonary murmur.* This is heard in the pulmonary area but it is less common and even the experienced may find differentiation from mild pulmonary stenosis difficult. In some children, a bruit is heard when listening above the clavicle, particularly on the right side with the bell of the stethoscope. There may also be a palpable thrill and a bruit may be heard in the neck. It is altered or abolished by backward movement of the elbows and is not heard below the clavicle. This noise is innocent.

4 *Intracranial bruits.* These are common in infants. It is important to check that they are not radiated cardiac murmurs, that there are no other cardiac signs such as those of heart failure and that there are no neurological signs at all. If those criteria are satisfied the systolic intracranial bruit is unlikely to be pathological.

Many innocent murmurs at any age can be positively identified; an electrocardiogram or chest X-ray may add confidence to the diagnosis but are not necessarily indicated. If doubt exists, observation over a period of time in a well patient may be

Table 13.16 Reasons to doubt innocent nature of a childhood murmur.

Accompanied by thrill
Pansystolic
Diastolic (except venous hum)
Radiates widely
Harsh character
Quieter lying down or louder with valsalva manoeuvre
Any symptoms or abnormal cardiovascular findings

all that is needed, although certain features are indications that the murmur is not an entirely normal one (Table 13.16).

Chest pain

Neonates and infants with certain rare cardiac abnormalities develop myocardial ischaemia and infarction. They may get episodes of pallor and sweatiness which presumably mean they are experiencing cardiac pain. Thus cardiac causes must be considered in the differential diagnosis of pallor episodes in babies. Serious ventricular arrhythmias and ischaemia may occur when either the left coronary artery arises from the pulmonary trunk not the aorta, or in coronary artery disease associated with Kawasaki's disease. Examination and an electrocardiogram will give clues for the last two; electrocardiogram recording during a pale episode is necessary to diagnose arrhythmia.

In older children able to describe feelings, chest pain is not rare. If pain is acute, pneumonia and pleurisy, pneumothorax, acute pericarditis and an acute abdominal condition have to be considered. Chest and abdominal pain are common in acute asthma, presumably muscular in origin. Acute cardiac pain in a child not known to have a cardiac condition is exceedingly rare. Kawasaki's disease (p. 478) involves coronary arteries acutely and in some cases chronically when typical angina type pain can occur. Cardiac arrhythmias can cause chest pain or tightness and children with aortic stenosis and hypertrophic obstructive cardiomyopathy may also experience cardiac pain.

Most children with chest pain have chronic recurrent episodes which are not described as typical cardiac pain. Careful history and examination usually allow major disease of cardiovascular, respiratory and gastrointestinal systems to be excluded, but in some, investigations are necessary to reach a diagnosis. Many children appear to have musculoskeletal type pain and, in a few, spinal nerve root pain appears a possibility. This may need expert evaluation, but in most the benign nature of the pain can be readily diagnosed. In some it has become a major emotional or psychological problem, but in the majority reassurance and encouragement suffice.

Palpitations

This is an important symptom which may reflect an underlying significant arrhythmia although sinus tachycardia or harmless ectopic beats can also be a source of anxiety to some children, particularly if they have a cardiac condition even if it is very mild. By the age of 4 or 5 years children can beat out on a table top how their heart thumps. Accompanying symptoms like chest discomfort or giddiness are important to enquire about and whether onset or cessation are sudden can help assess significance, as most arrhythmias have a sudden onset and end. Some children discover for themselves that vagal manoeuvres help terminate episodes. They may take cold drinks or perform the valsalva manoeuvre in some way. Parents may have counted the pulse or praecordial impulse rate although accuracy is by no means guaranteed. Polyuria during or just after an episode points to a true arrhythmia, the mechanism for this is argued over, but relates either to atrial stretching or improved cardiac output when sinus rhythm is restored. If arrhythmia is suspected then electrocardiogram recording during an episode should be obtained, if necessary using repeated 24-hour electrocardiogram monitoring or a telephone electrocardiogram monitor device.

Funny turns

Some episodic symptoms have already been described. Children with funny turns of any kind have a very long differential diagnosis (p. 289) although in a given case the list can usually be reduced very quickly. Cardiac arrhythmias need to be borne in mind in those with convulsions or fainting spells which do not easily fit into other diagnostic categories. Aortic and pulmonary stenosis may present with syncope, classically on exertion, but hopefully in developed countries such children will be detected before these occur. Hypertrophic obstructive cardiomyopathy (HOCM) can present similarly. Aortic stenosis and particularly hypertrophic obstructive cardiomyopathy can present as sudden death in older children. Very occasionally a significant cardiac lesion is found to explain a so-called cot death and sudden death is a recognized occurrence a few weeks into Kawasaki disease when many of the acute features are improving. This is due to myocardial ischaemia and arrhythmia.

Pulse abnormalities

Routine screening of neonates and older children may identify diminished or absent femoral pulses or result in detection of a markedly slower rise in the femoral pulse compared with a radial or brachial one; so-called brachiofemoral delay. These are signs which should never be ignored as they point strongly to coarctation of the aorta. Similarly at screening a bounding pulse or small volume pulses may raise suspicion of a patent ductus arteriosus or aortic stenosis, although in these cases a murmur is more likely to be what arouses suspicion in the first instance.

Arrhythmias

Some arrhythmias are completely harmless and even normal. Thus in a resting child without tachycardia, some acceleration in heart rate in inspiration is to be expected. This is sinus arrhythmia, the absence of which in a school-age child under the above conditions may point to the presence of an atrial septal defect. Occasional supraventricular or ventricular ectopic beats are normal, these are abolished by increasing the heart rate.

Supraventricular tachycardia (SVT)

This may be asymptomatic if short lived. If prolonged it can cause heart failure in early life, even before birth. Older children may be aware of palpitations, chest tightness or pain, light-headedness and polyuria. Underlying structural heart disease is unusual, although accessory atrioventricular pathways are the commonest cause and may declare themselves by resting electrocardiogram abnormalities, including a short PR interval and a delta wave on the upstroke of QRS complexes (Wolff–Parkinson–White syndrome). Such an electrocardiogram may be detected coincidentally in an entirely asymptomatic individual who may or may not be having unrecognized episodes of SVT. Treatment of attacks depends on how ill the patient is, but vagal manoeuvres are always worth trying. These include ice on the face of a baby, cold drinks and valsalva manoeuvre in older children. Direct current cardioversion or intravenous drugs may then be tried in the severely symptomatic. Digoxin, propranolol, verapamil (with great caution in young babies and not after propranolol) and very recently adenosine (not universally available at the time of writing) all have their advocates. Prevention is by avoidance of any recognized precipitant and with drugs, of which digoxin (not in older children with the Wolff–Parkinson–White abnormality) and propranolol are widely used. Many babies with SVT can be successfully weaned from prophylactic drug treatment after 1 year of age. Detailed electrophysiological studies and ablation of accessory pathways are very rarely needed in childhood.

Atrial flutter and fibrillation

These are rare arrhythmias in childhood. Atrial flutter may occur in infants with normal hearts or with myocarditis and the natural history is like SVT in the same age group. These disturbances can also accompany structural heart disease resulting in an enlarged right atrium, such as atrial septal defect in older children and Ebstein's anomaly when an abnormal tricuspid valve produces either regurgitation or more rarely stenosis. Cardioversion may work, digoxin will slow ventricular rate, but restoration to sinus rhythm in older children with structural lesions is unlikely unless surgery results in a smaller right atrium.

Ventricular tachycardia

This is rare in children but is serious. It may present with syncope or fits. The resting electrocardiogram may be normal or may show a long QT interval, in which case a positive family history including deafness, unexplained syncope or sudden death may be present. There may be underlying cardiac disease. Diagnosis in childhood is often delayed and treatment should be undertaken in specialist centres.

Sick sinus syndrome

The so-called tachycardia/bradycardia syndrome can be familial and is only occasionally identified in children with episodes of collapse. Pacemakers for bradycardia and drugs for tachycardia may both be needed.

Heart block

First degree heart block, diagnosed by a long PR interval on ECG, can be a normal and often a familial finding. Some cardiac lesions frequently have a long PR interval of which atrial septal defect is one of the commonest. It is a feature of acute rheumatic and some infective fevers. No treatment is needed for this pattern.

Second degree heart block, with regular or intermittent failure of atrioventricular conduction, more often reflects underlying cardiac disease but of itself is harmless as long as it does not progress.

Third degree or complete heart block is present when atrial electrical activity is totally dissociated from ventricular and may occur following cardiac surgery or be part of a structural cardiac lesion. In these cases a pacemaker is necessary. It is a feature of diphtheria.

Congenital complete heart block may be detected before birth by a slow heart rate or development of fetal oedema, ascites and pleural effusions *in utero* or it may pass undetected until later childhood. Clinically complete heart block can be suspected by a slow heart rate (40–70 beats/min) responding very little to stimuli which should normally raise the rate. Cannon waves will be detected in the jugular venous pulse, the apex may be displaced and the first heart sound varies in intensity. The heart is usually rather large on X-ray even if there is no heart failure. Electrocardiography makes the diagnosis. Underlying cardiac disease must be excluded by echocardiography and those that do not. Some of the commonest congenital defects will now be briefly considered. half of those with structurally normal hearts. This requires a very careful approach to the family as the mother is almost always entirely well. Those without symptoms and with basic heart rate above 55 beats/min with some increase on exercise and with narrow QRS complexes on electrocardiography will probably do well without a pacemaker in early childhood, but their need for one should be kept under review. Cardiac arrest is dealt with in Chapter 14.

Congenital structural heart disease

This is traditionally subdivided into those lesions producing cyanosis, or at least arterial desaturation and those that do not. Some of the commonest congenital defects will now be briefly considered.

Acyanotic lesions with left to right shunt
(Table 13.17)

The lesions to be described have certain features in common. Symptoms are due to increased blood flow through the lungs producing some chestiness or frank heart failure if the shunt is large. Many children with these conditions have no symptoms, especially those with ostium secundum atrial septal defect, small ventricular septal defect and small patent ductus arteriosus.

Table 13.17 Acyanotic lesions with left to right shunt ECG and chest X-ray features.

	ECG	CXR
ASD secundum	± long PR	± Cardiomegaly
	± RAD	PA +
	RSR V_1	PVM +
Primum	LAD	Cardiomegaly
	RSR V_1	PVM +
Complete AV septal defect	RAH	Cardiomegaly
	Superior QRS	PVM +
	RVH	
VSD	Normal	Normal or
	or LAD	cardiomegaly
	or LVH	PVM +
	or L + RVH	
PDA	Normal	Normal or
	or LVH	cardiomegaly
	or R + LVH	PVM +

LVH, left ventricular hypertrophy; PA, pulmonary artery; PR, PR interval; PVM +, increased pulmonary vascular markings; RAD, right axis deviation; RAH, right atrial enlargement; RSR V_1, so-called partial right bundle branch block in right chest leads; RVH, right ventricular hypertrophy.

EISENMENGER COMPLEX

If a large left to right shunt continues for a long period of time, permanent damage occurs to the pulmonary vasculature. The length of time for this to occur is shortest in complete atrioventricular septal defects with common valve ring and longest in small ventricular septal defects or small ostium secundum atrial septal defects. The result of this permanent damage is that pulmonary vascular resistance rises and consequently pulmonary artery and right ventricular pressures rise. When right-sided pressures exceed left-sided ones shunt reversal occurs and cyanosis is noted. Right ventricular failure and death are then the natural progression. This is the Eisenmenger complex. This progression can be prevented if surgical closure of the defect is carried out before significant irreversible damage has taken place. Those children with clinically large shunts, loud pulmonary second sounds or right ventricular hypertrophy on electrocardio-

gram need careful evaluation, usually including cardiac catheterization.

ATRIAL SEPTAL DEFECT

This lesion accounts for approximately 10% of congenital cardiac lesions. Defects may occur at several points in the atrial septum, the two commonest being in the fossa ovalis (ostium secundum atrial septal defect; Fig. 13.4) and low down the septum adjacent to the atrioventricular valves (ostium primum atrial septal defect). The valves themselves are often involved in such primum defects. Ostium primum atrial septal defect may be associated with a large single atrioventricular valve (AV) and a ventricular septal defect; this is termed an AV septal defect with common valve ring (Fig. 13.5) and is one of the cardiac lesions particularly associated with Down's syndrome.

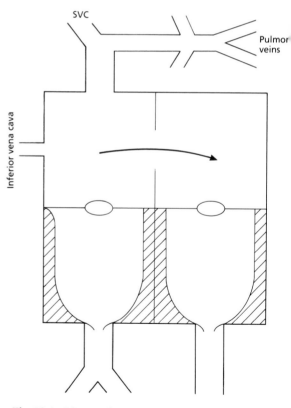

Fig. 13.4 Diagram demonstrating the abnormality in an atrial septal secundum defect.

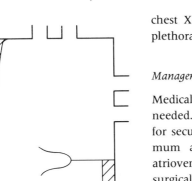

Fig. 13.5 Representation of the abnormality in an AV canal defect.

Clinical features

Blood goes from left atrium to right atrium in atrial septal defect so that timing and severity of symptoms depend on the size of the shunt resulting in increased pulmonary blood flow. Ostium secundum atrial septal defect may be associated with no symptoms in childhood whereas an atrioventricular septal defect often causes severe heart failure in infancy. The ostium primum defect comes somewhere in between in terms of severity of symptoms. Atrial septal defect produces wide splitting of the second sound without respiratory variation in the separation (fixed splitting). There may only be a soft systolic murmur in the pulmonary area. If a shunt is large there is a diastolic murmur at the lower left sternal edge. In primum defects, and more likely in atrioventricular septal defects, a pansystolic murmur of atrioventricular valve regurgitation may be heard at the apex. The

chest X-ray shows cardiomegaly and pulmonary plethora in a large secundum defect (Fig. 13.6).

Management

Medical treatment for heart failure may be needed. Surgical correction carries a very low risk for secundum atrial septal defect and low for primum atrial septal defect but higher risk for atrioventricular septal defect. It can be argued that surgical risk outweighs benefit to the child with atrioventricular septal defect and common valve ring in children with Down's syndrome.

VENTRICULAR SEPTAL DEFECT

This accounts for 15–20% of all congenital heart lesions. There are many forms and single or multiple defects can occur (Fig. 13.7). Some defects form part of a more complex abnormality.

Clinical features

Symptoms vary from none, to heart failure in early infancy. The murmur of a simple ventricular

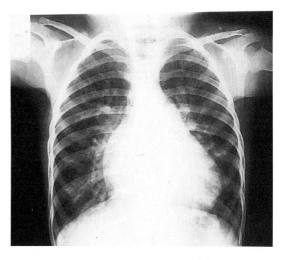

Fig. 13.6 Ostium secundum atrial septal defect in an 18-month-old child. Chest X-ray showing cardiomegaly, pulmonary plethora and a prominent main pulmonary artery.

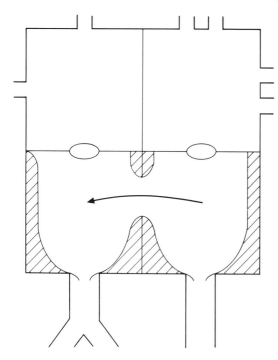

Fig. 13.7 Representation of a ventricular septal defect showing the direction of blood flow.

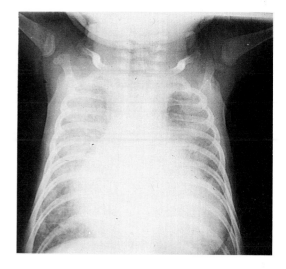

Fig. 13.8 Large ventricular septal defect in a 3-month-old child. Chest X-ray showing marked cardiomegaly and pulmonary oedema.

septal defect is not usually heard in the first week or two of life but becomes apparent as the shunt through it increases with falling pulmonary vascular resistance in the weeks after birth. Heart sounds are normal or the pulmonary component of the second sound (P2) may be loud. There is often a praecordial thrill and a harsh pansystolic murmur is heard loudest at the lower left sternal edge. It may also be heard over the lower thoracic spine. A large shunt causes a diastolic murmur at the apex. Up to 60% of ventricular septal defects close spontaneously, including some which cause symptoms in early life. Most close before 5 years and few after 10 years of age. Some never close, but also never cause symptoms. These may have impressive thrills and murmurs throughout life and are termed *Maladie de Roger*.

Management

Surgical closure is indicated if heart failure is intractable in infancy, if shunt size is shown at cardiac catheterization to be sufficient to cause permanent pulmonary vascular disease if uncorrected, or if another complication such as right ventricular outflow obstruction, aortic regurgitation or infective endocarditis develops.

Radiological features of significant lesions include cardiomegaly, pulmonary plethora and possibly pulmonary oedema (Fig. 13.8).

PATENT DUCTUS ARTERIOSUS

Delayed closure of a normal ductus arteriosus in a pre-term infant with respiratory disease is considered in detail in Chapter 7. Patent ductus arteriosus is a common isolated abnormality (Fig. 13.9); figures for its incidence are difficult because of its frequent finding in pre-term infants. It is very commonly found as part of more complex cardiac lesions.

Clinical features

Symptoms of heart failure may occur but often do not. A classic patent ductus arteriosus murmur is continuous under the left clavicle and also heard over the back. In some cases it is not continuous

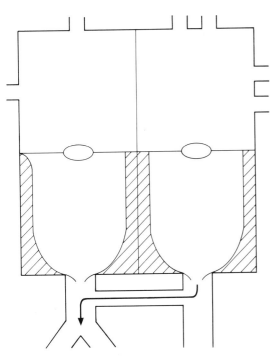

Fig. 13.9 Representation of patent ductus arteriosus showing the level of the left to right shunt.

and a murmur in systole only may be heard. Pulses are full.

Management

Surgical ligation or clipping is a short and safe procedure and should be done to remove the risk of infection in the duct and of pulmonary vascular disease.

Hypoplastic left heart syndrome

This is a condition in which there is obstruction to blood flow through the left heart together with left to right shunting (Fig. 13.10).

Clinical features

If obstruction to blood flow is proximal to the ductus arteriosus, blood will reach the descending aorta from the right ventricle and pulmonary artery via the ductus arteriosus. Thus the baby will remain relatively well until the ductus closes, then rapid shock and heart failure develop. This may occur in the first day or two of life but frequently is delayed until 7–10 days of age. At presentation such babies are pale, cold, poorly perfused, tachypnoeic with hepatomegaly and cyanosed because of their gross heart failure. If cardiac output is very low, all pulses are weak or a difference between upper and lower limbs may be detected, with upper limb pulses being absent or much weaker than lower.

A very large heart is found on X-ray and pulmonary oedema noted. Electrocardiogram shows a virtual absence of left ventricular forces, that is no or very little positive deflection in the left chest leads.

Management

Prostaglandin infusion will resuscitate many such babies but at present surgical intervention is controversial and not widely practised in the UK.

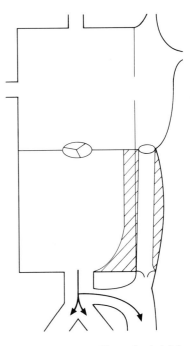

Fig. 13.10 Representation of hypoplastic left heart with mitral atresia.

	ECG	CXR
Coarctation, neonate	RVH	Cardiomegaly
		PVM +
older child	LVH	Normal/cardiomegaly
		Rib notching (rare)
Aortic stenosis	LAH	Cardiomegaly
	LVH + strain	
Pulmonary stenosis	RAH	PA +
	RAD	
	RVH + strain	

Table 13.18 Acyanotic lesions without shunt. ECG and chest X-ray features.

PA, pulmonary artery conus; PVM +, pulmonary vascular markings increased.

Where undertaken, it consists either of neonatal heart transplantation or a major two stage procedure with high mortality and as yet medium-term results which cannot be evaluated properly. Some centres in North America have abandoned this two stage approach.

Acyanotic lesions without shunts
(Table 13.18)

COARCTATION OF THE AORTA

This occurs at various sites in the aorta but usually it is very near the left subclavian artery and the ductus arteriosus may enter the arch before, at or after the coarctation. Abdominal coarctation is rare.

Clinical features

Coarctation may present as heart failure in infancy, particularly if other lesions such as ventricular septal defect accompany it. Ductal closure can precipitate the onset of marked clinical features if blood flow to the lower body is heavily dependent on blood from the pulmonary artery entering the distal aortic arch via the ductus. In infants and children without symptoms, the condition may be detected by the presence of a systolic murmur, often louder over the spine, hypertension or difficulty feeling femoral pulses. Tragically

cases still present with cerebrovascular accidents in young adult life due to undetected severe hypertension. The condition is much commoner in boys and the association with Turner's syndrome should always be remembered if coarctation is diagnosed in a girl. Diagnosis by ultrasound imaging is often possible. Cardiac catheterization is not always needed in symptomatic infants.

Management

Surgery can be performed at any age. There is a small risk of paraplegia both at surgery and also without it. Recurrence of coarctation after successful surgery can occur. Hypertension is not necessarily relieved by surgery and should be treated appropriately.

AORTIC STENOSIS

This can present as heart failure in infancy, as an asymptomatic murmur, as effort syncope or sudden death. A suprasternal and aortic area thrill is present, there may be an ejection click and the aortic component of the second sound (A2) is quiet. Pulses may be small volume. Competitive physical activity is usually advised against. Surgical valvotomy may be only partly successful and valve regurgitaton often occurs as a result of surgery necessitating valve replacement at a later stage.

Supravalvar and subvalvar stenosis also occur

but are rare. One form of subvalvar aortic narrowing is hypertrophic obstructive cardiomyopathy which is considered later. Many stenotic aortic valves are bicuspid instead of the normal tricuspid form. Bicuspid aortic valves are not necessarily stenosed, nor is it clear what proportion of them ever become stenosed in middle age with calcific degeneration. They are clinically apparent by an ejection click in the aortic area and at the apex. Electrocardiogram and chest X-ray are normal; the diagnosis is easily made on ultrasound imaging. No restrictions should be placed on those with bicuspid aortic valves without stenosis, but prevention of endocarditis is important as this is a devastating occurrence on a bicuspid aortic valve.

PULMONARY STENOSIS

Stenosis may occur at, below or above the valve. Only isolated valvar stenosis will be discussed here and is a common lesion. If the stenosis is critical, presentation will be with cyanosis in the newborn period as blood can shunt right to left through the foramen ovale. In this case urgent surgical or balloon valvuloplasty is indicated. Most cases will however be discovered as asymptomatic murmurs in the pulmonary area, often with an accompanying thrill. There is an ejection click. Chest X-ray

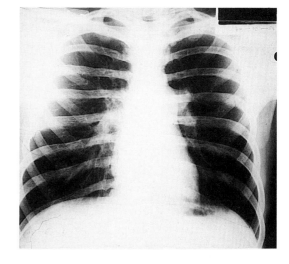

Fig. 13.11 Chest X-ray showing isolated valvular pulmonary stenosis in a 10-year-old child. Note the prominent pulmonary artery due to post-stenotic dilatation.

shows normal or oligaemic lung fields and prominent pulmonary artery (Fig. 13.11). Mild cases with a gradient across the valve of less than 30 mmHg require no treatment. Echocardiography, including a Doppler ultrasound assessment of the

Table 13.19 Cyanotic lesions ECG and CXR.

	ECG	CXR	
TGA	RVH	Cardiomegaly ±	
		Narrow superior	('egg on
		(mediastinum)	side')
		Apex lifted off diaphragm	
TAPVD	RAH	Cardiomegaly	
	RAD	PVM +	
	RSR V_1	After infancy, wide upper mediastinum	
	RVH		
Tricuspid atresia	RAH	Cardiomegaly	
	LAD	PVM −	
	LVH		
Tetralogy of Fallot	RAH	Apex off diaphragm	'boot
	RAD	PA −	shape'
	RVH	PVM −	

PVM, Pulmonary vascular markings; +: increased, and −: induced.

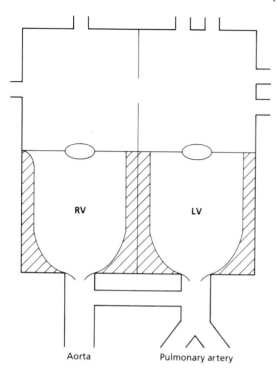

Fig. 13.12 Representation of complete transposition of the great arteries with patent ductus arteriosus.

gradient, taken in conjunction with the electro-cardiogram usually allows mild cases to be identified with confidence. Treatment of first choice in the majority of cases is by balloon valvuloplasty, surgery being reserved for those with very thick dyplastic valves.

Cyanotic lesions (Table 13.19)

TRANSPOSITION OF THE GREAT ARTERIES (TGA) (Fig. 13.12)

Presentation is usually with cyanosis in the newborn period but occasionally it is not detected until a little later if there are large natural mixing pathways via ventricular septal defect and patent ductus arteriosus. Apart from cyanosis, physical examination may be unhelpful unless left ventricular outflow obstruction (pulmonary stenosis) is present to produce a harsh systolic murmur. Chest X-ray shows a large heart (Fig. 13.13). Diag-

nosis is made non-invasively by ultrasound and prostaglandin infusion improves oxygenation.

Management

Classically, the infant's colour is improved by increasing atrial mixing through enlargement of the foramen ovale by balloon septostomy. Intra-atrial redirection of blood by baffles (Mustard or Senning operation) is the established way of producing a pink infant. More recently, certain cases are being subject to an arterial switch operation which reconnects the great arteries to their natural ventricles. This operation is showing encouraging results in appropriately selected patients. Transposition of the great arteries with ventricular septal defect and pulmonary stenosis or with other lesions is a more problematic surgical proposition.

COMMON MIXING CONDITIONS

Total anomalous pulmonary venous drainage (Fig. 13.14). This condition presents with cyanosis at an early stage if pulmonary veins are obstructed, and may mimic respiratory disease. If unobstructed pulmonary venous drainage is present, arterial desaturation is often missed.

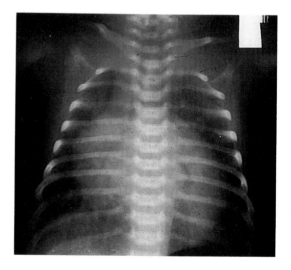

Fig. 13.13 Chest X-ray of a child with transposition of the great arteries.

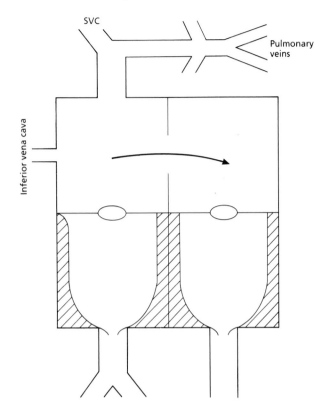

Fig. 13.14 Representation of total anomalous pulmonary venous drainage (TAPVD) of the supra cardiac type with all the pulmonary veins draining into the SVC.

Symptoms include recurrent chestiness and failure to thrive. The signs are of heart failure and a left to right shunt. Auscultation resembles an atrial septal defect. Chest X-ray usually shows massive cardiomegaly (Fig. 13.15). Precise definition of the site of entry of the pulmonary veins into the systemic venous return is important pre-operatively. It can be supracardiac, cardiac or infracardiac. This can sometimes be shown on ultrasound, but catheterization may be required. Surgical correction is appropriate at diagnosis.

Tricuspid atresia. This condition presents with cyanosis in the newborn period unless a large ventricular septal defect and absence of pulmonary stenosis results in high pulmonary blood flow. Specific features on examination are absent, but electrocardiogram is very helpful in the context of cyanosis, usually with reduced lung vascular markings on chest X-ray.

Management

Palliative surgery to increase lung blood flow is usually needed, a systemic to pulmonary anastomosis of the modified Blalock variety being the commonest. In this the subclavian artery is attached, by synthetic graft, side to side with the right or left pulmonary artery. After the age of 4 years or so, some cases are suitable for a Fontan procedure where the right atrium is attached to the main pulmonary artery thereby making the patient pink.

RIGHT TO LEFT SHUNTING

Fallot's tetralogy

The prime example of right to left shunting is tetralogy of Fallot consisting of infundibular pulmonary stenosis, right ventricular hypertrophy,

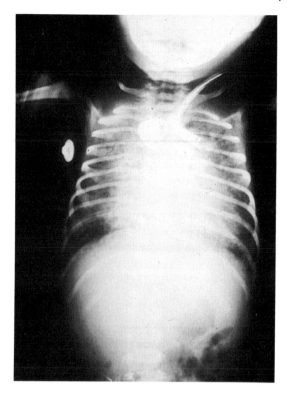

Fig. 13.15 Chest X-ray of a neonate with obstructed TAPVD.

ventricular septal defect under an aorta which overrides the septum so as to arise partly over the right ventricle (Fig. 13.16). A harsh murmur of pulmonary stenosis with absent or quiet and de-layed P2 may be noted in the early days, but cyanosis is not apparent in most cases until after the newborn period. However, in most it is progressively more obvious and avoidance of excessive polycythaemia and iron deficiency, which increases blood viscosity, are important. Dehydration should also be avoided. Chest X-ray may be characteristic (Fig. 13.17).

Some children with tetralogy have so-called hypercyanotic spells in which they are much bluer, hyperventilate and may show altered conscious state. Such episodes can be fatal and are an indication for palliative or corrective surgery. Acutely they are managed by adopting a knee–elbow position and, in hospital, by intravenous morphine. These episodes are thought to be due to increased subpulmonary (infundibular) narrowing through muscle spasm and so producing a greater left to right shunt.

Management

Oral propranolol reduces the incidence and sever-ity of spells until surgery is performed. Total cor-rection of tetralogy of Fallot can be performed in infancy, although some centres prefer to perform a palliative modified Blalock shunt in infancy prior to total correction in the second or third year of life.

PULMONARY ATRESIA

Pulmonary atresia with ventricular septal defect behaves like a severe tetralogy of Fallot with marked cyanosis in the early neonatal period unless collateral arteries from the descending aorta to the lungs exist. Pulmonary atresia with an intact ventricular septum is a much more danger-

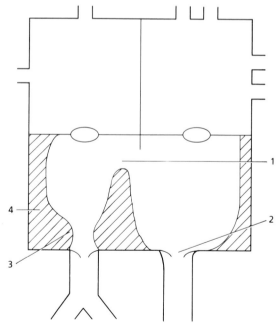

Fig. 13.16 Representation of Fallot's tetralogy.
(1) Ventricular septal defect; (2) overriding aorta;
(3) infundibular pulmonary stenosis; and (4) right ventricular hypertrophy.

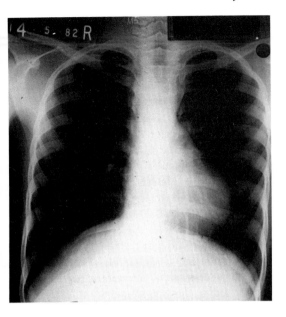

Fig. 13.17   Chest X-ray from a child with tetralogy of Fallot. Note the heart shape is of right ventricular morphology (the apex is off the diaphragm), the pulmonary oligaemia and the right-sided aortic arch.

ous abnormality and no one surgical approach is clearly the best. These infants present very cyanosed in the first day or two and die rapidly unless prostaglandin is given to ensure adequate lung blood flow. Blalock anastomosis and attempts to create a way out of the right ventricle to the pulmonary artery are the common strategies at present.

Miscellaneous congenital abnormalities

Congenital mitral stenosis and regurgitation do occur but are rare. Much commoner is the occurrence of a mild degree of mitral valve prolapse with little or no regurgitation. This condition may be suspected by a middle to late systolic click at the apex, with or without a short murmur late in systole. Diagnosis is made by echocardiography. How many will progress to significant mitral incompetence is not known. Some may develop arrhythmias. Measures to prevent endocarditis are generally recommended. Mitral valve prolapse is

a feature of a number of generalized disorders including Marfan's syndrome and homocystinuria, in both of which other vascular abnormalities can also occur including aortic root dilation and dissection.

Some infants with structural heart disease, particularly coarctation and aortic stenosis, have marked fibrosis of the endocardium, referred to as endocardial fibroelastosis (EFE). This condition is associated with impaired myocardial function. Endocardial fibroelastosis can occur without structural lesions in which case the clinical picture is of cardiomyopathy which may result in gross heart failure in early infancy and death, although prolonged survival can occur.

Acquired heart disease

Pericarditis

Pericarditis is inflammation within the pericardial sac and may be due to a variety of causes (Table

Table 13.20   Causes of pericarditis.

Infective
Bacterial
   Pneumococcus
   β haemolytic *Streptococcus*
   Haemophilus influenzae
   Staphylococcus aureus
   Meningococcus
   Mycobacterium tuberculosis

Viral
   Coxsackie
   Influenza
   Adenovirus

Non-infective inflammation
   Rheumatic fever
   Post-pericardiotomy syndrome
   Systemic lupus erythematosis
   Rheumatoid arthritis

Malignant disease
   Acute lymphoblastic leukaemia

Metabolic

13.20). Typical pericardial pain in uncommon in children; other symptoms and signs are usually more prominent. A pericardial rub may be heard, but if there is an accompanying effusion heart sounds are muffled. Evidence of tamponade should be looked for and includes tachycardia, pulsus paradoxus, elevated jugular venous pressure and hepatomegaly. Chest X-ray may show cardiomegaly if there is effusion, electrocardiography classically shows ST segment elevation initially followed by flattening or inversion of T waves. Ultrasound imaging or M mode will reveal effusion, if present, and warn of imminent tamponade. Tamponade requires urgent pericardiocentesis. Antibiotics given parenterally are essential for bacterial pericarditis; analgesia and anti-inflammatory drugs are needed for non-bacterial causes.

Myocarditis and cardiomyopathy

Myocarditis often accompanies pericarditis and the aetiology is similar. Cardiac failure, gallop rhythm and murmurs from tricuspid or mitral regurgitation may be detected. Poor peripheral perfusion and central cyanosis are grave signs. Arrhythmias can occur. Chest X-ray may be normal or may show cardiomegaly and pulmonary venous congestion or oedema. Electrocardiogram changes, like pericarditis, are non-specific. Echocardiography will reveal further information on cardiac function as well as exclude significant effusion and structural heart disease. Aggressive treatment of the underlying cause, if possible, and of heart failure is appropriate. Digoxin may aggravate arrhythmias and most anti-arrhythmic drugs depress myocardial function further so great care is needed.

Some acute cases of myocarditis recover and some progress to chronic cardiomyopathy requiring antifailure treatment long-term and ultimately heart transplantation may need to be considered. A number of inherited neuromuscular and metabolic diseases are associated with cardiomyopathy and assessment of the cardiac state of children with these diagnoses must not be overlooked. This is particularly important in Duchenne muscular dystrophy (p. 298) where surgery for spinal or other deformity may be made much more hazardous by significant cardiac involvement. One particular cardiomyopathy which has certain characteristic features is hypertrophic obstructive cardiomyopathy. This condition varies in severity but symptoms from left ventricular outflow obstruction, poor ventricular filling and arrhythmias include effort syncope, cardiac pain and sudden death. In some families a clear autosomal dominant inheritance pattern is recognized. Clinical signs include jerky pulses, reverse splitting of the second heart sound, a fourth heart sound and a mid-systolic murmur at the base made softer by lying down and louder by the valsalva manoeuvre. Electrocardiogram is frequently very abnormal showing predominantly left ventricular hypertrophy and strain. Ultrasound shows a thick left ventricle and particularly the septum is sometimes grossly thickened. Arrhythmias should be sought and treated; there is debate about the use of propranolol to limit progressive hypertrophy.

Rheumatic fever

World-wide this remains a major cause of acute and chronic cardiac morbidity and mortality (p. 569). In developed countries it is uncommon but does occur; diagnosis frequently being delayed because of atypical features and a low index of suspicion. Rheumatic fever is considered in detailed in Chapter 26.

Acute episodes may show clinical myocarditis, pericarditis and valve regurgitation, particularly of mitral or aortic valves. Active carditis usually requires steroid therapy. Heart failure and pericardial effusion should be managed as necessary. Follow-up, looking for evidence of chronic mitral and aortic valve disease is necessary. Long-term tricuspid and pulmonary valve damage are much rarer.

Infective endocarditis

Micro-organism infection within heart and blood vessels is a risk for particular groups of people including those with structural congenital heart disease and those with acquired valve lesions.

Corrective surgery does not remove the risk except in those with successful closure of a patent ductus arteriosus. Bacteria are the main causes, but fungi and other micro-organisms can cause infection particularly in the immunocompromised and those with indwelling prosthetic material such as central venous catheters or valve prostheses. Common bacterial causes of endocarditis include *Streptococcus viridans* and *Staphylococcus aureus*. The former tends to cause a chronic illness whereas the latter a devastating acute one. Site of entry of these organisms into the bloodstream is often not determined, but unhealthy teeth, recent dental extraction, infected skin lesions, genito-urinary or gastrointestinal surgery and intravenous drug abuse must always be considered. Diagnosis of infective endocarditis is often the first time that the patient is aware that they have a cardiac lesion as some of the highest risk lesions are haemodynamically trivial, such as bicuspid aortic valve, small ventricular septal defect and possibly mitral valve prolapse. The risk in uncomplicated isolated ostium secundum atrial septal defect is extremely low. Some cases will not have a pre-existing cardiac lesion.

Clinical features are given in Table 13.21. Positive blood cultures and demonstration of intra-

Table 13.21 Clinical features of infective endocarditis.

General
Pyrexia
Confusion
Splenomegaly
Clubbing

Cardiac
Underlying condition
Changing or new murmurs, particularly aortic
 regurgitation
Heart failure

Immunological/embolic
Nail splinter haemorrhages
Skin lesions (emboli, Janeway lesions, Osler's nodes)
Retinal lesions (Roth's spots)
Pneumonia
Microscopic haematuria
Intracerebral haemorrhage or abscess

Table 13.22 Prevention of bacterial endocarditis.

Good dental health

Antibiotic prophylaxis
 Not more than 1 hour before
  dental extraction, gastrointestinal surgery, surgery
  on other infected or heavily colonized regions
 Second dose 6–8 hours afterwards

Prompt treatment of skin sepsis

No tattoos, no ear piercing

cardiac vegetations on ultrasound contribute to a definite diagnosis.

Management

This is a serious illness with at least a 20% mortality, and parenteral antibiotics chosen in the light of culture information with close monitoring of blood levels is essential. Treatment is for 4–6 weeks and, in some cases, oral antibiotics can be used in the second half of the course. If valve destruction occurs, surgery is needed. A haemodynamically insignificant ventricular septal defect which has been the focus for endocarditis should be closed surgically once antibiotic treatment has been successful. Measures to prevent bacterial endocarditis in those known to be at increased risk are shown on Table 13.22 and, although thorough scientific proof of the efficacy of all of them is lacking, they appear sensible.

Further reading

Anderson RH, Macartney FJ, Shinebourne EA, Tynan MN (Eds). *Paediatric Cardiology*, Vols 1 and 2. Churchill Livingstone, Edinburgh 1987.
Miller GAH, Anderson RH, Rigby ML. *The Diagnosis of Congenital Heart Disease*. Castle House Publications, Tunbridge Wells 1985.
Park MK, Guntheroth WG. *How to Read Paediatrics ECGs*. Year Book Medical Publishers, Chicago 1981.
Rosenthal A. *Pediatr Clin North Am* 1984; **31/6**.
Shinebourne EA, Anderson RH. *Current Paediatric Cardiology*. Oxford University Press, Oxford 1980.

14

THE CRITICALLY ILL CHILD

This chapter considers the problem of the critically ill child. The sick newborn infant is considered in Chapter 7. The conditions mentioned in this chapter are discussed in detail elsewhere in this book.

Presentation

Disorders of any body system may produce serious life-threatening illness. In paediatric practice there are only a limited number of ways in which critically ill children present and these are listed in Table 14.1. Although the ill child presents in a limited number of ways, the child must be carefully assessed for evidence of disease in other systems and a comprehensive approach to such patients is essential for proper management. Tables 14.2 and 14.3 give causes for shock and cardiorespiratory arrest in children. At presentation the underlying disease may be obvious, for example trauma and asthma, or it may be less obvious and require detailed history, examination and investigation to elucidate it. The cause of the

Table 14.1 Common clinical presentations of critically ill children.

Coma, altered conscious state
Convulsions
Respiratory failure
Respiratory obstruction
Shock
Trauma
Post-surgical
Post-cardiorespiratory arrest

Table 14.2 Causes of shock.

Haemorrhage from any site
Loss of intravascular fluid
   Vomiting, diarrhoea
   Peritonitis
   Polyuria
   Hypoalbuminaemia
   Burns, scalds
   Leakage from capillaries into tissues
   Excessive peripheral vasodilation
Cardiac arrhythmia
Severe myocardial failure

Table 14.3 Causes of cardiorespiratory arrest.

Primary cardiac disease
   Arrhythmia
   Myocarditis
   Post-cardiac surgery
Primary respiratory disease
Airway obstruction
Neurological disorder
   Raised intracranial pressure
   Head injury
   Drug administration
Severe hypoxic insult
   Drowning
   Asphyxiation
Metabolic disorder
   Hyperkalaemia
   Hypokalaemia
   Hypercalcaemia
Drug or toxin
   Anti-arrhythmic agents
   Solvent abuse
Near-miss cot death

problem does not need to be known in order to initiate life-saving therapy.

Management

This can be considered under a number of sub-headings.

IMMEDIATE

When confronted with a critically ill child certain assessments must be made rapidly and first aid treatment administered. Exact sequences of events will depend on just how ill the child is and in what circumstances the crisis has arisen. Emergency treatment in the home or at the scene of the accident is important but it is not within the scope of this book to consider it in detail here. In some circumstances, when diagnosis is known at the start and when parents are available, history, examination, investigation and treatment can all be taking place simultaneously. Such is usually the case in severe acute asthma. At other times, rela-

tives should be made comfortable in another room while resuscitation takes place, although in these circumstances history taking is just as important and one member of the team should be talking with parents while others are with the child. A first aid approach to immediate assessment and therapy is given in Table 14.4. Most of the actions in Table 14.4 commonly require vascular access to be obtained. If it is not possible to cannulate a peripheral vein quickly there are alternatives and staff dealing with very sick children should become proficient at some of the alternatives (Table 14.5).

The management of cardiorespiratory arrest is given in Table 14.6. Once resuscitation and stabilization have taken place, time should be taken to address the question of diagnosis. At this early stage it may only be possible to consider general categories of disease. This process involves obtaining a full history and performing a careful physical examination so that further investigations such as X-rays, specimens for culture and comprehensive haematological and biochemical tests can be

Table 14.4 Immediate approach to the critically ill child.

Consider	Assess	Action
Cardiac output	Pulse rate, volume, blood pressure Cardiorater for rhythm	External cardiac massage Drugs and plasma Cardioversion
Airway patency	Respiratory noise and effort Cyanosis Indrawing	Suction Laryngoscopy Intubation
Respiratory effort	Cyanosis Respiratory rate Blood gases	Oxygen Artificial ventilation
Neurological state	Fits Coma Evidence of intracranial hypertension	Anticonvulsants Ventilate Mannitol
Trauma	Examination	If suspicion of spinal injury, immobilize
Gross metabolic derangement	Blood glucose stick test Electrolytes Blood gases	If no reaction, measure blood glucose and if possible insulin before giving glucose Correct acidosis, treat hyperkalaemia

Table 14.5 Emergency alternatives to percutaneous peripheral venous access.

Cutdown on peripheral vein
  In antecubital fossa
  Long saphenous vein at ankle
Percutaneous access to
  Internal jugular vein
  Subclavian vein
  Femoral vein
Drug administration via tracheal tube
  (Adrenaline, atropine, not bicarbonate)
Drug administration by deep intramuscular injection
  (Not in cardiac arrest)
Fluid administration into bone marrow
  (Iliac, tibia, sternum)
Fluid administration into peritoneal cavity
Sampling free-flowing capillary samples sometimes
  suitable
Sampling from peripheral arteries

---

arranged. At this point, further treatment might be considered. The need for antibiotic therapy should be carefully assessed and many critically ill children should receive a broad spectrum antibiotic until a specific diagnosis is made. If possible, all samples needed for culture should be obtained before giving antibiotics although notable exceptions to this statement exist. The most clear exception to this is in the case of a critically ill child with probable meningococcal septicaemia to whom penicillin should be given through the same needle as blood cultures are drawn; a lumbar puncture should not be obtained at that stage. This pause for evaluation should also produce a decision about whether there is a need for the child to be transported to an intensive care unit or to another hospital for specialist services if these are not available locally. It is essential to take the time,

---

1 Establish an airway
  Preferably tracheal intubation
  Start ventilation

2 External cardiac massage. Staff should be appropriately trained

3 Put on ECG monitor leads and observe trace

4 Give DC shock if coarse ventricular fibrillation

5 Establish vascular access, check blood glucose

6 Give drugs intravenously for the following rhythm disorders:

Asystole	Calcium
	Adrenaline*
	Isoprenaline*
Bradycardia	Atropine*
	Isoprenaline*
Ventricular tachycardia	Lignocaine

7 Check arterial blood gas if possible
  Give bicarbonate, blind if blood gas not obtainable and no response to first dose of appropriate drugs

8 Glucose – give dextrose if glucose stick test low or no response to first dose of appropriate drugs

---

* These drugs can also be given directly into the trachea through the tube.

Table 14.6 Management of cardiorespiratory arrest.

at an early stage of the child's illness, to let the parents see their child and to update them on the situation.

TRANSPORTATION

If a child needs transporting, even just a short distance, it is important to have stabilized the patient with drips, tracheal tube and monitoring equipment properly attached and working. Adequate staff are needed for transportation, and a speedy but controlled move is the objective and not a disorganized rush. Ensure, too, that equipment and personnel are available to deal with a crisis during transport. These points are even more important if travel some distance in an ambulance is planned.

CONTINUING MANAGEMENT

This is best considered systematically as outlined in Table 14.7 although not every category will always be relevant. Precise details of management of these different aspects will not be discussed here, many of them are dealt with in the other chapters of this book. Each system should be individually

Table 14.7 Systematic approach to continuing management.

Cardiovascular system
Respiratory system
Gastrointestinal tract
Renal function
Fluid and electrolyte balance
Nervous system including patient's awareness, comfort
  and emotional state
Skin
Musculo-skeletal system
Infection
Nutrition
Haematology
Biochemistry
Further diagnostic, progress monitoring or prognostic
  tests
Drug and other therapy review
Patient and family coping, communication, involvement
Communication with other professionals (referring GP
  or hospital, nurses' views, social work involvement)

assessed (cardiovascular, respiratory, renal, neurological, etc.) and close observation for the early detection of changes is a basic part of intensive care. This is monitoring in the broad sense. Appropriate monitoring of each case is part of the skill of intensive care so that important facts are not overlooked, nor the picture confused by unimportant or irrelevant information. Commonly used monitoring techniques are listed in Table 14.8, all of which are used in the context of careful and repeated clinical evaluation which includes conscious state, neurological signs, colour, heart rate, respiratory rate, assessment of abdominal girth, progressive visceral enlargement and detection of tissue oedema.

LONG-TERM MANAGEMENT

Many conditions that cause the child to become critically ill are relatively short-lived and the period during which intensive care is needed should not be protracted. If a child remains very sick for more than a few days it becomes increasingly important to ensure as good a nutritional balance as possible. If feeding can be naso-gastric or naso-jejunal, then this is the preferred method, but in a proportion of children parenteral nutrition is needed either as a complement to gastric feeds or as the total source of nutrients. Other aspects to be dealt with are listed in Table 14.9 and an open mind must be kept in order to detect new developments including complications of treatment. Parental and family needs change if the child remains in intensive care for more than a few days, especially so if the situation is not changing dramatically in either direction. Medical and nursing staff attitudes to situations also evolve if children have a more protracted stay in intensive care and there must be an opportunity to discuss these.

WITHDRAWAL OF INTENSIVE SUPPORT

In the majority of critically ill children, improvement will occur and intensive monitoring and therapy can be gradually withdrawn. It requires as much expertise to know when and how to do this

System	Technique
Cardiovascular	Cardiorater
	Blood pressure (intermittent indirect or arterial line)
	Central venous pressure
	Pulmonary artery wedge pressure
	Cardiac output (toe temperature compared to central temperature, urine output)
Respiratory	Apnoea alarm
	Ventilator alarms
	Transcutaneous blood gas monitoring
	Pulse oximetry
	Sampling from arterial line
Neurological	Apnoea alarm
	Continuous EEG or cerebral function monitor
	Intracranial pressure monitoring
Renal	Urine output
	Regular weighing (practical difficulties)
Laboratory	Acid/base
	Electrolytes, urea, creatinine
	Glucose (use stick tests also)
	Haematology

Table 14.8 Monitoring critically ill children.

as it does to institute intensive care in the first place. The process of getting better must not be held up by continuing too long with what had been a vital part of management, such as endotracheal intubation or regular sedative and analgesia administration. Parents often find this phase of illness very worrying, having presumably become reassured by technological support for their child. On occasions it will be apparent that intensive care is only putting off the time of death or that brain stem death has already occurred. Under these circumstances the most senior doctor should introduce the suggestion of withdrawal of intensive care to the parents. If brain stem death is diagnosed the question of suitability for organ donation must be addressed. In cases where a definitive diagnosis has not been made and death seems inevitable, careful thought must be given to the need for any further diagnostic tests which should be performed before death (such as blood samples for toxins or abnormal metabolites) or just after death (such as liver biopsy for enzyme studies or other special biochemical or histological

Table 14.9 Some common complications of paediatric intensive therapy.

Superimposed infection
Vascular injury related to sampling, infusion and monitoring lines
Pressure sores
Respiratory tract damage from tracheal tubes
Pulmonary collapse
Tissue burns from extravasated injections and infusions
Drug side-effects
Inappropriate treatments from misinterpretation of monitored parameters or investigation results

tests). Many parents cannot face giving consent for autopsy examinations, but do find less invasive procedures such as port-mortem needle liver sampling or skin snips for fibroblast culture acceptable. At times, the coroner may insist on autopsy examination. Reaching a diagnosis is not only valuable to medical staff but may provide information with genetic implications for parents and other family members.

BRAIN STEM DEATH

Most developed countries now recognize both legally and morally the concept of brain death. This refers to irreversible injury to the brain stem rendering the patient dependent on mechanical ventilation for continued support of the cardio-vascular system, and which will inevitably lead to eventual cardiac arrest. This is an important con-cept in order that prolonged ventilatory care is not pursued with no prospect of recovery and so that organs may be removed for transplantation before the heart stops beating.

Brain stem death can be diagnosed in children older than 2 months. Brain stem death cannot be reliably diagnosed in babies below this age. There are preconditions to be met before the diagnosis can be considered. The patient must be comatose for a known reason and apnoeic. It is necessary to ensure that therapeutic agents (barbiturates and neuromuscular blocking drugs) are not the cause of coma and that there is no metabolic disturbance. The test is designed to show loss of brain stem reflexes, no response to pain over the trigeminal nerve area and apnoea persisting, despite a rise in $PaCO_2$ to >50 mmHg (6.6 kPa) and not in the presence of simultaneous hypoxia. The tests should be carried out by two experienced clinicians at least twice with an interval of 12–24 hours between tests. In the UK it is not necessary to use EEG to support the diagnosis of brain stem death.

Follow-up

Whether the outcome is complete recovery or death of the child, follow-up is important for many reasons. Many serious acute illnesses may have long-term sequelae and most parents appreciate the opportunity to return to discuss aspects of their child's fatal illness some weeks afterwards.

Further reading

Rogers MC. (Ed.) *Textbook of Paediatric Intensive Care*, Vols I and II. Williams and Wikins, Baltimore 1987.
Orlowski JP. (Ed.) *Paediatr Clin North Am* **34/1**. W B Saunders, Philadelphia 1987.

15
DISORDERS OF THE URINARY TRACT

Abnormalities of the urinary tract are relatively common and are being increasingly recognized antenatally with the more widespread use of obstetrical ultrasound. Previously undiagnosed problems in the urinary tract may be suspected on routine examination in the newborn infant or more rarely in the older child. Obvious physical abnormalities such as spina bifida or a chromosomal abnormality or syndrome should alert one to the possibility of an associated urinary tract problem.

Infection in the urinary system may cause an acute septicaemic illness in the young child but more commonly the symptoms are vague such as vomiting, poor feeding and unexplained temperatures. In the older child there may be more recognizable symptoms such as dysuria, frequency, incontinence, abdominal pain or haematuria. In all situations it is important to consider and *positively diagnose* a urinary tract infection as further investigations will be required. This is particularly true in the younger child where there is the greatest potential for preventing renal damage.

Kidney development and function

The formation of nephrons is usually complete by 34 weeks of gestation with the overall cellular content being less than 20% of the adult kidney. Although the term infant has the same number of nephrons as an adult (approximately 1 million per kidney) the renal vascular resistance is high and a combination of factors is responsible for the low glomerular filtration rate of 20 ml/minute/1.73 m^2 at term. This compares to adult values of 110−120

ml/minute/1.73 m^2 which are only achieved in the second year of life.

There is also immaturity of tubular function. Neonates are very prone to dehydration and metabolic abnormalities because of a combination of high metabolic rate in relation to body weight, greater insensible losses and inability to control their oral intake. Very strict attention to fluid and electrolyte balance is also required with the sick infant.

Renal function tests and investigations

URINALYSIS

The first investigation of any suspected renal problem should be urinalysis combined with microscopy. The tendency to delegate these tasks to the laboratory should be reversed as much can be learnt from these simple tests.

Urinalysis should always be done on a *fresh* urine sample. Many urine-testing sticks are available and the majority incorporate pH, protein, blood and glucose. Newer sticks also test for leucocytes and nitrite, which if positive, may indicate urinary tract infection.

pH and osmolality

Normal urine pH is between 5 and 7 but is affected by dietary intake. A high urinary pH in the right clinical context might suggest the rare problem of renal tubular acidosis (p. 268). A first morning urine sample after fasting overnight provides a

246

useful screening test for concentrating ability with normal values being above 800 mosmol/kg (specific gravity above 1.020).

Glycosuria and aminoaciduria

Tubular defects can give rise to glycosuria and aminoaciduria which may also be secondary to elevated serum levels.

Proteinuria

The urine normally contains a small amount of protein and transient proteinuria (+ or ++) is common and may occur in association with fever, stress or after heavy exercise. There is a poor correlation between proteinuria and urine infection.

Persistent proteinuria in a well child should be investigated further. It may be the clue to underlying renal disease, especially if associated with haematuria.

Postural or orthostatic proteinuria is suggested by the absence of significant proteinuria on a first morning specimen compared to one tested after the patient has been ambulant. Orthostatic proteinuria is relatively common in older children and can be confirmed by taking formal daytime and night-time urine protein collections. Urine protein excretion should be less than 4 mg/hour/m^2 (<0.1 g/l) during the night but may be ten times higher during the day. Orthostatic proteinuria is generally accepted as a functional variant of no clinical importance. There should be no limitation of the child's activity and repeated assessments are not necessary.

Very heavy proteinuria and oedema suggest nephrotic syndrome (see p. 262).

Haematuria

Macroscopic haematuria is a dramatic symptom and is quickly brought to the doctor's attention. Often the description is of 'tea' or 'coke' coloured urine. A careful history should be taken to elicit whether there has been any preceding upper respiratory tract infection (to suggest nephritis),

Table 15.1 Causes of haematuria.

Infection
Bacterial
Viruses
Tuberculosis
Schistosomiasis
Trauma
Glomerulonephritis
Post-streptococcal
Mesangial IgA nephropathy (Berger's disease)
Calculus
Congenital abnormality
Hydronephrosis due to PUJ obstruction
Tumour
Wilms'
Vascular
Arteritis
Infarction
Bleeding disorder
Drug induced
Cyclophosphamide
Exercise induced
Fictitious (Munchausen by proxy)

urinary symptoms (to suggest infection), or abdominal pain (to suggest stones or obstruction). A careful family history should be elicited particularly with respect to stones or obstruction. All children with haematuria need to be fully investigated and the potential causes are shown in the Table 15.1.

Microscopic haematuria may also be a transient finding like proteinuria and it is being increasingly detected on routine urinalysis. It may occur in association with heavy exercise and only if it is confirmed in one or two samples should further investigations be carried out. Urine microscopy should reveal the presence of red blood cells and exclude a false positive test due to free haemoglobin, myoglobin, beeturia or confectionary dyes. It is important to test the urine of other family members to recognize a familial nephritis or benign familial haematuria.

Urine microscopy

This may give useful information especially in the presence of persistent proteinuria or haematuria. Fresh urine should always be used when examining

for casts. Red blood cell casts suggest glomerulonephritis. The presence of increased white blood
cells above five/high-powered field or motile
bacteria suggests urinary tract infection but this
requires confirmation by urine culture.

There have been several recent reports of looking at red cell morphology in patients with haematuria using phase contrast microscopy. The
presence of crenated and distorted cells suggests
upper tract bleeding while normal red cell morphology suggests a lower urinary tract source.
There is a great deal of overlap, however, and the
test is unlikely to be of much help in paediatric
practice. Fictitious haematuria has been recognized as part of the Munchausen syndrome by
proxy (p. 528). One needs to remember this as a
possibility if other clinical pointers are present.

FURTHER INVESTIGATIONS

Biochemical tests

Plasma urea, electrolytes and creatinine are usually checked when a renal problem is suspected. The
blood urea is easily affected by a number of factors
such as meals and the creatinine level varies with
age. It should be remembered that the plasma
creatinine can remain within the normal range
until the glomerular filtration rate is less than
50% of normal. Hence the need for an accurate
measurement of glomerular filtration rate if a
significant renal problem is suspected.

Glomerular filtration rate (GFR)

Traditionally this has been done by collecting a
24-hour urine sample and measuring plasma and
urine creatinine levels. In children, however, the
technique is liable to errors because of the
difficulties in collecting reliable samples.

The approximate GFR can be derived from the
plasma creatinine using the equation:

$$\text{GFR (ml/minute)}/1.73\ m^2 = \frac{38 \times \text{height (cm)}}{\text{plasma creatinine (}\mu\text{mol/l)}}$$

This approximation is most valid in children
between 2 and 10 years of age.

When an accurate GFR is required the child
should be admitted to a unit accustomed to using
multiple blood sampling techniques of radio-
nuclides such as chromium 51 EDTA or 99 technetium DTPA.

Radiological techniques

Ultrasound. This has been a great boon to the investigation of urinary tract problems and being
non-invasive it is now the first choice investigation
in most instances. An experienced radiologist with
a good machine can provide details about kidney
size and structure, dilatation of pelvis or ureters as
well as bladder size and structure. The patency of
blood vessels and, with Doppler techniques, renal
blood flow, can also be assessed. Renal calculi may
be recognized but the technique is not sensitive
enough at present for scars or vesicoureteric
reflux.

The intravenous urogram (IVU). This has been the
traditional technique for outlining the structure of
the urinary tract and may be better than ultrasound at detecting duplex systems and ectopic
ureters. It incorporates an initial plain abdominal
X-ray which has to be requested separately with
the use of ultrasound if stones or spinal abnormalities are not to be missed. However, an IVU does
involve an injection which can cause morbidity
and very rarely mortality in children. The renal
outlines may not be adequately defined because of
faecal loading and this is especially true in small
children. An IVU should not be requested within
48 hours of birth in any neonate.

The micturating cystourethrogram (MCU). This remains the main technique by which the bladder
and urethra are outlined and potential ureteric
problems such as vesicoureteric reflux are detected. It does involve bladder catheterization and
the technique needs to be carried out with some
sensitivity by radiologists familiar with working
with children. Too many children have been
traumatized in the past by this technique. The
procedure needs to be covered with 48 hours of

antibiotics if the child is not already receiving them.

Although an initial MCU is required in the investigation of a proven urinary tract infection in the young child the need for repeat procedures requires careful consideration.

Dimercaptosuccinic acid (DMSA) scan. This involves one injection of a radionuclide and it outlines the functioning renal tissue in each kidney. It is a good investigation to study scarring of kidneys as well as detecting parenchymal defects following pyelonephritis. The differential function between the two kidneys can also be assessed and this is useful when contemplating or following-up surgical procedures (Fig. 15.1).

A 99 technetium diethylenetriaminepentacetic (DTPA) scan. This also involves the injection of a radionuclide and this technique is a better functional assessment of the urinary tract than the DMSA in that the renogram curves allow comparison between the uptake and excretion of the radionuclide by both kidneys and the detection of any obstruction (Fig. 15.2). The differential uptake between the two kidneys can also be measured. Some units have successfully used a DTPA technique to follow problems such as vesicoureteric

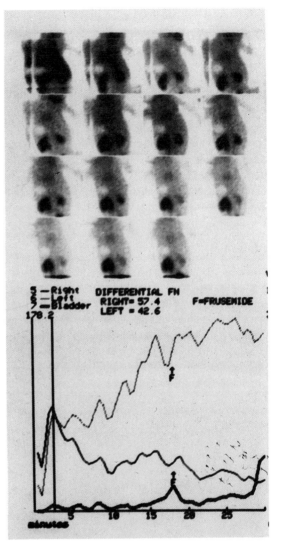

Fig. 15.2 ^{99}Tc DTPA scan of an infant with suspected PUJ obstruction on ultrasound examination. The radionuclide curve continues to rise on the left side with no response to frusemide (F), suggesting a significant PUJ obstruction which was confirmed at operation.

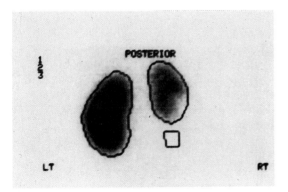

Fig. 15.1 DMSA scan of an infant with bilateral vesicoureteric reflux. The left kidney is normal but the right kidney shows decreased size and loss of parenchyma in its lower pole. The differential function of the two kidneys can be calculated and the right contributes 20.8% and the left 79.2% of the total.

reflux. If a child has received an injection of DTPA which has been cleared by the kidneys and is then able to pass urine in front of the gamma camera, reflux should be detected as an increase in counts over the kidneys during micturition. This technique is known as an indirect micturating renogram.

Computerized tomography (CT) and magnetic resonance imaging (MRI). CT scanning will certainly give very good details of the kidneys but most children will require a general anaesthetic for this procedure. The development of MRI may enable kidney detail to be defined even better in the future.

Renal biopsy. This is only undertaken in specialist centres and for indications such as atypical nephritis, suspected chronic nephritis, steroid-resistant nephrotic syndrome and unexplained persistent haematuria. Most biopsies can be performed under sedation and ultrasound control.

Abnormalities of the urinary tract

These may be recognized *in utero* either because of oligohydramnios in the mother or with increasing frequency as a result of the use of antenatal ultrasound. Fortunately most of these abnormalities are unilateral and can be dealt with after the baby is born.

If both kidneys are abnormal then the resulting oligohydramnios (urine production from the fetus is 28 ml/hour at term) may cause a Potter type syndrome (Fig. 15.3). Such fetuses may be aborted spontaneously or electively. If the fetus survives then death usually ensues in the neonatal period from associated lung hypoplasia (p. 91). The presence of a reduced liquor volume or bilateral hydronephrosis *in utero* has led some centres to contemplate an aggressive approach with intra-uterine intervention including shunts between the bladder and amniotic fluid, but there is little evidence that these procedures do any good and are probably not justified.

Congenital abnormalities of the urinary tract may be single or multiple. They may be asymptomatic and go undetected, e.g. renal duplication, or they can be associated with severe infections and renal damage, e.g. posterior urethral valves. Urinary tract abnormalities are often associated with abnormalities of the genitalia due to their common embryological origins.

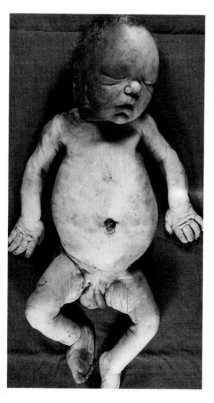

Altered facies
  low set ears
  receding chin
  broad flattened nose

Small chest and lung
  hypoplasia

Urogenital abnormalities

Limb deformities

Fig. 15.3   Potter syndrome. (Reproduced with permission from Dr J. Rapola.)

It has long been recognized that some abnormalities such as ureteral duplications, vesicoureteric reflux and hypospadias are familial disorders. Exact genetic patterns are imprecise but the detection of a major abnormality such as bilateral vesicoureteric reflux in one child should lead to the consideration of non-invasive screening of other siblings by urine cultures and ultrasound examinations.

UNILATERAL RENAL AGENESIS

The incidence is about 1:1500 births and is often found in association with other congenital abnormalities, e.g. oesophageal atresia, anorectal atresia, congenital heart disease. The remaining kidney undergoes hypertrophy but it may be subject to other abnormalities such as vesicoureteric reflux or pelviureteric junction obstruction. If no other abnormality exists the patient and family should be given a good prognosis.

HYPOPLASIA/DYSPLASIA

Hypoplasia (a decreased number of nephrons) will result from abnormal development in the first trimester. Obstruction of the collecting system anywhere from the pelvis to urethra can result in cystic dilatation of the nephrons and de--differentiation with cartilage deposition and

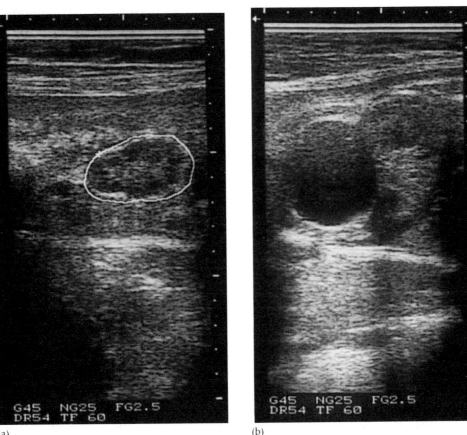

(a) (b)

Fig. 15.4 Antenatal ultrasound (34 weeks gestational age) showing: (a) normal right kidney, and (b) multicystic dysplastic left kidney.

primitive mesenchyme (dysplasia). If the abnormality is unilateral there may be little consequence for the fetus. Severe bilateral involvement would result in a Potter type syndrome or, if the child survives, chronic renal failure requiring dialysis and transplantation later in life.

A non-functioning *multicystic dysplastic kidney* is one of the commonest urinary tract abnormalities detected on antenatal ultrasound (Fig. 15.4). Multicystic kidney is an extreme form of dysplasia with no functioning renal tissue and atretic ureter. The appearances of multiple cysts should not lead to confusion with polycystic kidney disease which is bilateral and has a different prognosis and inheritance pattern. Although there have been rare reports of tumour development in multicystic dysplastic kidneys many centres have a non-operative policy unless there is an obvious mass or obstruction. The child can be followed serially by ultrasound. Again with one abnormal kidney care should be taken to exclude an abnormality such as reflux on the apparently good side.

Children with bilateral hypoplastic/dysplastic kidneys will need constant assessment as the majority of patients will proceed inexorably into chronic renal failure in late childhood.

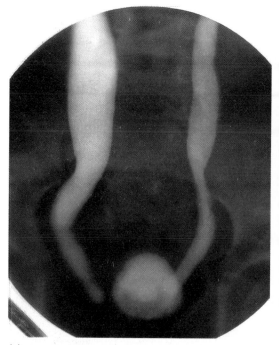

(a)

PELVIURETERIC JUNCTION (PUJ) OBSTRUCTION

This is again one of the commonest abnormalities and may be detected *in utero* or on postnatal examination as an abdominal mass. Presentation later in childhood may be in association with a urinary tract infection, haematuria, abdominal pain or hypertension. The problem may remain undetected into adult life where loin pain is the commonest symptom. Dilatation of the pelvis does not necessarily equate with obstruction and careful radiological investigation is required. If there is unequivocal evidence of obstruction or symptoms then referral for pyeloplasty is required.

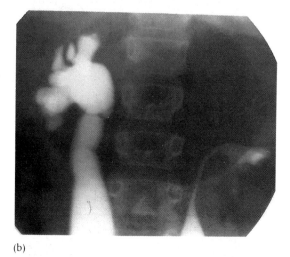

(b)

Vesicoureteric junction obstruction

This is much less common than PUJ obstruction and hydronephrosis and hydroureter may only be

Fig. 15.5 Micturating cystogram in a 5-year-old girl investigated for repeat urinary tract infection. There is bilateral vesicoureteric reflux (a), but note also the 'drooping flower' appearance (b) on the left side suggestive of a duplex system with reflux into the lower pole moiety only.

discovered when the child is investigated for urinary tract infection. Reimplantation of the ureter is usually required.

URETERIC DUPLICATION

This condition has a strong familial incidence. Bifid ureters are commoner than complete duplication. Many patients are asymptomatic but the incidence of complications is high.

When the ureters enter the bladder separately the ureter draining the upper pole moiety is situated in a lower position or may be ectopic. It is liable to become obstructed with hydronephrosis of the upper pole while the ureter draining the lower pole moiety is prone to reflux because of its short intravesical course (Fig. 15.5).

A truly ectopic insertion of a ureter into the urethra or vagina will result in dribbling of urine night and day. This is a rare abnormality but one that needs to be considered if the child is constantly wet night and day. Sometimes the parents even report that urine can be seen dribbling down the legs of their child. Since the ectopic ureter may be associated with a poorly functioning upper pole several radiological investigations may be required and this is one situation where an intravenous urogram may be better at revealing the abnormality than ultrasound. Heminephrectomy can provide dramatic relief of the symptoms.

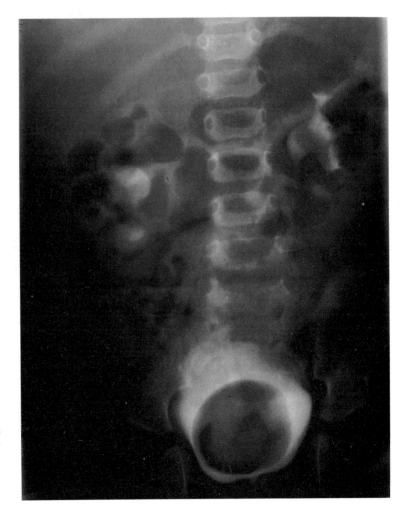

Fig. 15.6 Intravenous urogram (45 minutes after injection) in a 10-month-old female infant. The left kidney shows a normal pelvicalyceal pattern, but the right kidney shows hydronephrosis due to an obstructed ureter. There is also a large filling defect in the bladder due to a right-sided ureterocoele.

Ureterocoele

Sometimes an ectopic ureter is associated with a *ureterocoele* (Fig. 15.6) which affects girls more than boys and is bilateral in 10% of cases. The abnormality may appear as a filling defect in the bladder but occasionally it can prolapse through the bladder neck and in girls even appear as a mass in the vagina. There are a number of surgical approaches and the reader should refer to a paediatric urology text.

HORSESHOE KIDNEY

This results from fusion of the lower poles of both kidneys which are usually situated lower in the abdomen than normal (Fig. 15.7). Horseshoe kidneys are commoner in males but there is a well-known association with Turner's syndrome. The abnormality may be entirely asymptomatic or may be associated with infection, vesicoureteric reflux or obstruction.

MEGACYSTIS–MEGAURETER SYNDROME

Occasionally the investigation of a child with a urinary tract infection (UTI) reveals gross dilatation of the ureters and bladder without any identifiable obstruction. Treatment is by conservative methods using prophylactic antibiotics and a regime of double or triple micturition (emptying the bladder and then waiting before attempting re-emptying).

Megacystis and megaureters may also occur in the rare Triad or Prune Belly syndrome which consists of absence of abdominal muscles, cryptorchidism and urinary tract abnormalities (Fig. 15.8). There may be a number of associated chest and orthopaedic abnormalities and the prognosis will depend largely upon the degree of associated renal dysplasia.

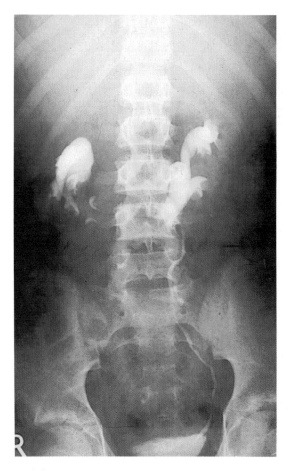

Fig. 15.7 Horseshoe kidney showing calyceal rotation and lower pole fusion.

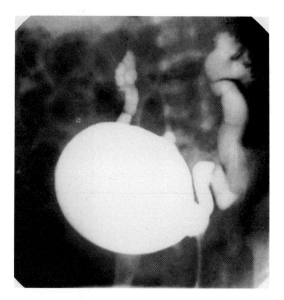

Fig. 15.8 Micturating cystourethrogram showing a huge bladder and gross bilateral vesicoureteric reflux into dysplastic kidneys in a male infant with Prune Belly syndrome.

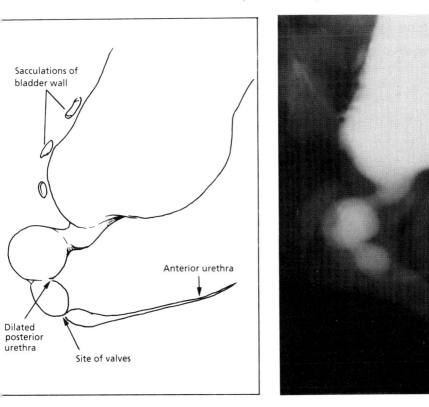

Fig. 15.9 Posterior urethral valves seen on a micturating cystourethrogram.

POSTERIOR URETHRAL VALVES

Posterior urethral valves are the commonest cause of lower urinary tract obstruction in the male child (Fig. 15.9). The diagnosis may be suspected on antenatal ultrasound because of bilateral hydronephrosis with an enlarged bladder and urethra. Postnatally the infant may have a poor urinary stream with palpable kidneys or bladder but the condition is easily overlooked and the infant may present with urinary tract infection, septicaemia and renal failure. The prognosis for patients with this condition has improved considerably with expert neonatal care. There is a spectrum of involvement, from the child who dies in the neonatal period with severe pulmonary and renal dysplasia to the child who presents with a urinary tract infection and intermittent stream later in child-hood when the valves are detected on a micturating cystourethrogram. This investigation should be carried out by an experienced paediatric radiologist so that the child is spared repeated X-ray examination.

Treatment of the valves is by ablation either transurethrally or occasionally suprapubically. The prognosis for renal function will depend upon the degree of hydronephrosis and renal dysplasia. Unfortunately a significant number of these children will require dialysis and transplantation later in childhood.

BLADDER EXTROPHY

This results from failure of midline fusion of the infra-umbilical midline structures. It is twice as common in males where complete epispadias is almost always present. At birth the bladder mucosa is often bulged outwards by intra-abdominal pressure, the umbilicus is normally low and the pubic bones are widely separated. In girls the clitoris is duplicated and the labia are widely separated anteriorly. In both sexes the anus lies in an unusually anterior position. Surgical management consists of abdominal wall closure with an attempt at reconstruction of the bladder and bladder neck. However, full continence is achieved in only a minority of patients and urinary diversion is often required.

POLYCYSTIC KIDNEY DISEASE

This term should be restricted to the two main types: infantile polycystic disease (IPCD) and adult polycystic disease (APCD) which can present in childhood. The term should not be applied to other cystic kidney problems such as multicystic dysplastic kidneys referred to previously.

Infantile polycystic disease (IPCD)

This rare disease is inherited in an autosomal recessive fashion. It may be associated with a Potter

syndrome or severe respiratory distress in th newborn period. IPCD, however, is not uniform fatal and there is a spectrum of involvement an hence a variable prognosis. One constant feature involvement of the liver and this may be a distir guishing feature from APCD which can rarel present in the newborn. IPCD tends to hav characteristic radiographic appearances of a brigt echogenic pattern on ultrasound or a mottle nephrogram on delayed IVU films (Fig. 15.10 Progressive renal insufficiency occurs in childre surviving the newborn period and renal replace ment therapy will be required.

Adult polycystic disease (APCD)

This is inherited as an autosomal dominant cond tion and can present in childhood either wit symptoms (haematuria, hypertension, rena masses) or may be recognized as a result of famil screening by ultrasound or the new gene probe APCD accounts for 8% of adult patients requirin dialysis and transplantation in Europe but rena function impairment is rare in childhood. Fev cysts are visible before the age of 10 years an affected children should be monitored for hyper tension (Fig. 15.11).

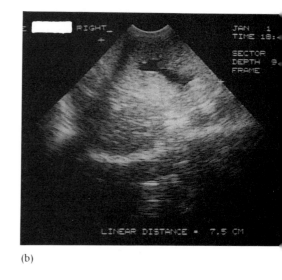

(a)

(b)

Fig. 15.10 Ultrasound of a neonate with bilaterally enlarged kidneys. There is nephromegaly with increased medullary echogenicity.

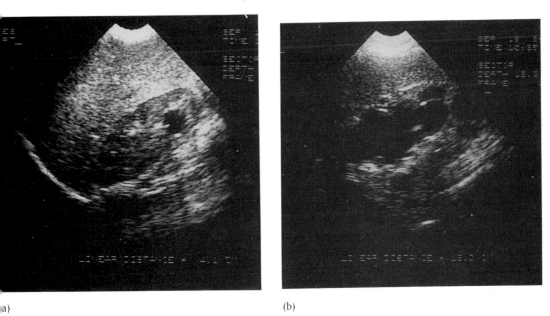

(a)   (b)

Fig. 15.11 Adult-type polycystic kidney disease. (a) Ultrasound scan of an 8-year-old boy showing a single cyst in the upper pole. (b) Scan from the boy's father showing numerous cysts.

Urinary tract infection

This is a common and important paediatric problem because not only may it be associated with considerable morbidity in children but infections may be the pointer to underlying urinary tract abnormalities. One of the most important of these is vesicoureteric reflux which can lead to renal scarring and later hypertension and if severe bilateral, chronic renal failure. Chronic pyelonephritis, or the more appropriate term *reflux nephropathy*, accounts for 25% of children and adults who develop end-stage renal failure under 40 years of age.

However, approximately 0.7% of boys and 2.8% of girls are at risk of a symptomatic urine infection in childhood. About one-third will have an underlying urinary tract abnormality which may be minor or major. It is important that any child with a *proven* UTI (bacterial count $>10^8$ organisms/l) has appropriate investigations which should be more comprehensive in the younger child (<5 years) where renal damage is most likely to occur.

A newborn infant with a urinary infection may present with prolonged jaundice, weight loss or a frank septicaemic episode. Again in the young child the symptoms may be non-specific such as poor weight gain, irritability, fever, vomiting and diarrhoea. Only occasionally in childhood does one recognize the classical picture of pyelonephritis with high temperature, rigors and loin pain. Any child in whom there is an unexplained fever or illness should have a urine culture taken and antibiotics should not be given blindly.

Obtaining urine samples

It is again important to stress that a UTI can only be *proven* on properly taken urine samples which may need to be repeated if unsatisfactory. The midstream urine is the ideal, but is only practicable in the older, continent child. In the younger child, a clean-catch urine into a sterile container such as a cardboard dish may suffice and the child may be encouraged to pass urine by stroking or tapping in the suprapubic region. Collecting bags placed over the genital area are popular in infants but are prone to contamination. The newer bags allow the urine to pass into a lower chamber where it can be drained from the end of the bag instead of pouring the urine through the upper seal which is likely to be contaminated by the groin flora. If an infant is ill or septicaemic and warrants urgent investigations including blood and/or lumbar puncture cultures then a suprapubic aspiration of the urine should be attempted. Occasionally a catheter specimen of urine using a fine feeding tube is justified.

Organisms derived from patient's own bowel flora are the commonest infecting agents and *E. coli* is by far the most likely. Some children develop recurrent urine infections without an underlying problem and this may be associated with abnormal Gram-negative colonization of the introitus and peri-urethral areas. It is important to stress general prevention measures to the parents of any child who develops a urine infection. It is helpful if these instructions are written down (Table 15.2) as well as being discussed in the clinic situation. Studies showing increased adherence to uroepithelial cells by pyelonephritogenic bacteria may allow improved preventative measures in the future.

Management

When the child is acutely ill and a urine infection strongly suspected (urgent urine microscopy is helpful), antibiotic treatment should be started without delay. The initial treatment should be with intravenous antibiotics (Table 15.3). Depending upon culture reports and sensitivities as well as clinical response, oral therapy can then be introduced and continued for 7 days before reducing to a prophylactic dose until investigations are complete.

Oral antibiotics are generally sufficient for the less ill child and follow-up urine cultures

Table 15.2 Information leaflet for parents: prevention of urinary tract infections.

When your child has a urinary tract infection, the doctor will prescribe antibiotics. As well as the antibiotics, there are also some things you can do to help the infection to get better and also to prevent another infection.

1 *Avoid constipation.* You can do this by giving your child a high fibre diet to include plenty of fresh fruit and vegetables and eat wholemeal bread instead of white bread. Ensure that your child drinks a lot and has regular exercise. The doctor may also give your child a medicine to soften the stools.

If your child has any problems with *worms* let the doctor know.

2 In young girls the tube to the bladder is very close to the back passage. *Wiping* should be done in a front to back direction.

3 It is better to take a shower rather than a bath. Always avoid irritating soaps and bubble baths. *Cleanliness* is very important to help prevent infection.

4 *Emptying the bladder properly is very important.* Encourage your child to sit on the toilet regularly and empty the bladder. Sometimes we ask that your child will double-empty the bladder. The child will pass water then wait a few minutes before trying to pass water again.

5 Always encourage your child to *drink* as much as possible during the day, and to *empty the bladder properly* last thing at night.

6 *Correct underwear.* Avoid tight underpants or pantyhose. They prevent air from circulating freely and encourage the warm, moist environment which favours infection. Soft cotton briefs, changed daily, are a far better choice. Consider changing the washing powder you use for the pants if irritation persists.

7 When taking antibiotics the full course must be taken at the time required. Any *problems* such as burning when passing water, going to the toilet often or blood in the water *should be reported* to the doctor.

We hope that these ideas will help you to help your child. Please do not hesitate to ask questions or contact us if you are worried.

Table 15.3 Antibiotics used in urinary tract infection.

	Dose (mg/kg/day)	Dose interval (hour)	Prophylaxis (mg/kg/day)
Gentamicin	2 mg/kg/dose IV	Depends upon renal function and levels	—
Ampicillin	50	6	—
Amoxycillin	20	8	—
Trimethoprim	4	12	2
Nalidixic acid	50	6	20
Nitrofurantoin	3–5	6	2
Cephradine	50	6	—

should be obtained to ensure eradication of the organism.

Investigations

The choice and extent of investigations are still debated but I usually request a plain abdominal X-ray and ultrasound as the initial investigations in children with a *proven* UTI. Hopefully with the increased availability of, and expertise in the use of ultrasound there will be less need to carry out IVUs on children. If these investigations are normal then one can wait and see, but in children under 5 years of age (and especially in males) a micturating cystourethrogram is also carried out to rule out vesicoureteric reflux or bladder and urethral problems. An MCU may be required in an older child if there is a history of repeated UTIs or a suspicious ultrasound or IVU. Further investigations such as DMSA and DTPA scans will depend upon the initial tests and whether one wants to rule out obstruction or scarring. Reflux can be a familial problem and it may be justified to at least screen other family members by ultrasound or less invasive radionuclide methods if available.

VESICOURETERIC REFLUX

The management of reflux is a controversial area. A great number of reports have emanated from surgical centres where there has been an obvious bias to reimplantation operations. The only proper controlled trial reported to date was by the Birm-ingham Reflux Study Group which showed no difference between operative or conservatively managed groups in terms of breakthrough infections, new scarring or progression of scarring or other complications. However, it should be said that the question is still very much open in the very young child, especially those with Grade III reflux (Fig. 15.12) and further studies are underway. In the meantime, in the absence of some complicating urological pathology such as a duplex system or bladder diverticulum, most children with reflux are managed conservatively by continuous prophylaxis with antimicrobial agents such as trimethoprim or nitrofurantoin. Surgery is contemplated if there are symptomatic breakthrough infections on prophylaxis or recurrent abdominal symptoms.

URETHRAL SYNDROMES

These do occur in childhood and are analogous to recurrent cystitis in adults. Only 25% of children with dysuria and frequency have a confirmed bacterial infection of the urine. While viral infections may play a role, acute vulvitis or balanitis may be associated with poor hygiene, perineal candidiasis or contact sensitivity to nylon pants. Attention should therefore be directed to sensible advice. Some children present with a frequency syndrome with no proven urinary infection. Usually the problem is self-limiting but occasionally an anticholinergic drug may be required.

Recurrent urine infections associated with

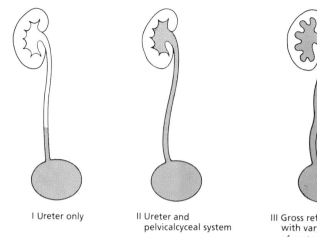

I Ureter only   II Ureter and   III Gross reflux
                        pelvicalcyceal system   with varying degrees
                                                       of ureteric and
                                                       calcyceal distension

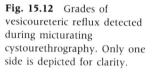

Fig. 15.12 Grades of vesicoureteric reflux detected during micturating cystourethrography. Only one side is depicted for clarity.

persistent vulval or perineal signs must also raise the suspicion of sexual abuse (p. 524).

Acute nephritic syndrome

This is characterized by:
1 Haematuria.
2 Oliguria.
3 Oedema.
4 Hypertension.

Urinalysis will show a large amount of blood with a lesser amount of protein. Microscopy reveals red blood cells with haem granular and red cell casts.

Classical post-streptococcal glomerulonephritis is now regarded as an uncommon problem in the UK and Western countries due to improved nutrition and hygiene standards and/or changes in the prevalence of the nephritogenic strains of Group A beta haemolytic *Streptococcus*. We have recently noticed an increase in the number of cases in our area, however, and the condition still needs to be considered in any child with haematuria. Post-streptococcal nephritis is very common in developing countries where the nephritis may follow skin infection such as impetigo on top of scabies.

Many affected children are asymptomatic apart from the haematuria which may be reported as 'tea' or 'coke' coloured. Typical complaints include malaise, headache and vague loin discomfort. Oedema tends to collect around the orbits and the back of the hands and feet. In the majority of cases the oliguria is only mild but severe fluid retention can occasionally produce acute hypertension with encephalopathy and seizures or very occasionally pulmonary oedema. Characteristically the infection has followed on 7–14 days after a Group A beta haemolytic streptococcal infection (Fig. 15.13). A number of acute glomerulonephritides are assumed to be post-infectious as a variety of bacteria and viruses can cause a similar picture (Table 15.4).

It is important to carry out the appropriate investigations (throat swab, complement levels, anti-streptolysin O and viral titres) to try to prove the aetiology of the glomerulonephritis as post-streptococcal disease usually has a very good prognosis. A 10-day course of penicillin should be commenced while awaiting the result of the throat swab and other family members should have swabs taken. Hospital admission is advised if there is any suggestion of oliguria, fluid overload, hypertension or significant renal impairment. Management of these complications is as for acute renal failure (see later).

A biopsy in a child with nephritis is only justified if the clinical presentation is very atypical, the serum complement is normal in the presence

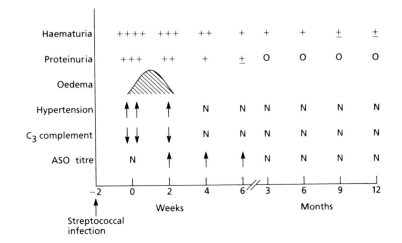

Haematuria	+ + + +	+ + +	+ +	+	+	+	±	±
Proteinuria	+ + +	+ +	+	±	O	O	O	O
Oedema								
Hypertension	↑ ↑		↑	N	N	N	N	N	N
C₃ complement	↓ ↓		↓	N	N	N	N	N	N
ASO titre	N	↑	↑	↑	N	N	N	N

Fig. 15.13 Clinical course of
acute nephritis.

Streptococcal
infection

of renal insufficiency (which makes post-streptococcal nephritis unlikely) or there is persistent hypocomplementaemia. The long-term prognosis of post-streptococcal glomerulonephritis is assumed to be excellent with over 90% of cases resolving without significant renal impairment. There is still some caution about the eventual status of the non-streptococcal group.

Mesangial IgA nephropathy

Some children, particularly in adolescence, have recurrent episodes of macroscopic haematuria usually precipitated by incidental infection with no evidence of renal impairment or complement activation. The likely diagnosis is mesangial IgA nephropathy (Berger's disease). Mesangial deposits of immunoglobulin A are found on renal biopsy which is generally performed if there are any signs of renal impairment or if the haematuria is persistent for over 1 year. The presence of persistent haematuria may have implications for future job prospects such as the armed forces. The prognosis is again very good but the children need to be followed long-term as some can have a progressive lesion.

HENOCH–SCHÖNLEIN PURPURA (HSP)

In this condition there is involvement of the skin, intestine, joints and kidney, either singly or together. Henoch described the intestinal, and Schönlein the joint features. Seventy per cent of children with this condition have haematuria and/or proteinuria and this is the complication which has the most important long-term significance.

HSP is due to a vasculitis and often occurs after an upper respiratory tract infection. No specific organism has been implicated in its causation. The term 'anaphylactoid purpura', used occasionally, is unfortunate since there is no connection with anaphylaxis.

Clinical features. The disease may occur at any age, but is rare under 2 years. The rash is typical, start-

Table 15.4 Causes of post-infectious
glomerulonephritis associated with infection.

Bacteria	Viruses
Staphylococcus spp.	Echo
Pneumococcus spp.	Coxsackie
Klebsiella spp.	Hepatitis B
Meningococcus spp.	Epstein–Barr
Salmonella typhi	Influenza
Mycoplasma pneumoniae	Mumps
	Rubeola
	Varicella

ing as an itching urticarial eruption which changes to form pink maculopapules which are usually a deeper red at the centre than at the periphery. These lesions become progressively less raised and more dusky, so that by the following day the rash is composed of dusky red macules which do not fade on pressure and may coalesce to form large patches. The rash occurs predominately on the buttocks, the lower back, and the extensor aspects of the arms and legs.

The knees and ankles are the joints most commonly affected, though these are usually only slightly swollen, as joint effusion occurs very rarely. Intestinal involvement causes abdominal pain from submucosal haemorrhages which may cause intestinal bleeding, sometimes leading to intussusception.

The condition is very liable to relapse, so that for several weeks crops of the typical maculopapules appear and gradually fade. With each new crop there may be a recurrence of the abdominal and joint symptoms. Recurrences seldom occur after 3 months of freedom.

Renal involvement

Although almost three-quarters of children with HSP have evidence of glomerulonephritis on investigation of their urine, the renal involvement is usually asymptomatic and non-progressive. Haematuria is usually microscopic. Despite this, however, chronic HSP nephritis accounts for 5% of children requiring dialysis and transplantation. Children presenting with an acute nephrotic syndrome or rapidly progressing to a nephrotic state require assessment in a paediatric renal unit. Renal histology is some guide to prognosis with glomerular lesions varying from minimal change to crescentic nephritis. It is this latter group that give rise to concern and in whom immunosuppressive treatment might be considered. Children with urinary abnormalities after HSP should continue to undergo urine examination and blood pressure measurements at periodic intervals in order to detect the late development of hypertension and renal impairment.

SYSTEMIC LUPUS ERYTHEMATOSUS (see also p. 478).

The incidence of renal disease in this uncommon condition of childhood is 75%. Again the involvement may be mild to severe and a renal biopsy and close monitoring of the clinical and biochemical parameters will be required. The prognosis will depend upon the degree of involvement and response to immunosuppressive treatment.

Nephrotic syndrome

This is characterized by:
1 Heavy proteinuria (>40 mg/hour/m^2 and usually >400 mg/hour/m^2).
2 Hypoalbuminaemia (albumin <25 g/l).
3 Oedema.
4 Hypercholesterolaemia.

It is an uncommon condition with an incidence of 2:100 000 Caucasian children. This incidence appears to be increased in Asian populations where 9–16:100 000 may be affected. Males are more commonly affected (2:1) with a peak age incidence between 1 and 5 years.

Despite extensive research the cause is unknown and approximately 85% of Caucasian children with nephrotic syndrome have the so-called minimal change type (MLNS). This is not the case in African children where nephrotic syndrome in association with quartan malaria or schistosomiasis are commoner.

The usual presenting feature is periorbital or dependent oedema (Fig. 15.14). Since it is such an uncommon condition many children are treated as having an allergy until someone performs a urinalysis. Abdominal ascites may also be present and occasionally there is abdominal pain, vomiting duced circulating plasma volume any additional dehydration can result in hypovolaemia, circulatory collapse and pre-renal failure. It is only in this situation that intravenous plasma infusions may be required.

Children with ascites or gross oedema are prone to sepsis particularly pneumococcal peritonitis and urinary tract infection. Some children have

Clinical features

Gross generalized oedema
 (anasarca)

Periorbital oedema

Pleural effusion

Ascites

Sacral oedema

Peripheral oedema

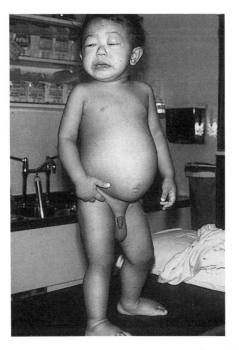

**Potential complications
of steroid therapy**

Depression or agitation
Posterior capsular
 cataracts
Moon face
Growth impairment
Obesity
Thin extermities and
 buffalo hump
Striae
Myopathy
Osteoporosis
Glucose intolerance
Decreased resistance
 to infection

Fig. 15.14 Nephrotic syndrome showing the clinical features and the potential complications of treatment.

actually had laparotomies for peritonitis before the underlying nephrotic syndrome has been recognized.

Pathology

The term minimal change lesion is derived from the light microscopy appearances. It is the electron microscope which shows fusion of the epithelial cell foot processes which is now recognized as a non-specific consequence of proteinuria. Recent research has suggested that there may be reduction in the fixed negative charge on the glomerular capillary wall with a resultant protein leak but the exact cause for this condition is still unknown.

Management

In the child who is oedematous, moderate fluid restriction can be prescribed. Initial bed rest may be beneficial but this should never be enforced and can be guided by the patient's wishes. Diure-

tics should be used with care as powerful loop diuretics such as frusemide can cause hypovolaemia. There is probably little to be gained by trying to push an unpalatable high protein, salt-restricted diet which the child will not tolerate. Instead we prefer a reasonably well balanced diet with no added salt. Prophylactic penicillin is usually prescribed while the child is grossly oedematous but it must be remembered that a primary peritonitis may be due to Gram-negative organisms.

The most potent diuretic for the nephrotic syndrome is prednisolone as the majority respond to this therapy by losing their oedema within 7–10 days. There is little need for albumin infusions unless clinical and biochemical parameters indicate pre-renal failure in which case salt-poor albumin followed by frusemide will generally maintain an adequate urine output.

There is still a 1–2% documented mortality from this condition due to infection and thrombosis. A number of coagulation problems can occur with nephrotic syndrome and careful clinical assessment of the circulatory status is required during the initial oedematous phase and at times of potential dehydration such as with diarrhoea and vomiting.

Unfortunately at least 75% of children who respond initially to prednisolone will have a subsequent relapse (recurrence of proteinuria). It is important that the parents carry out regular monitoring of the urine and record it in a diary. Children who are frequently relapsing and becoming steroid-dependent or manifesting toxic effects from the steroids may be considered for cytotoxic therapy such as cyclophosphamide. As long as the child responds to steroids the prognosis for renal function is still excellent and relapses become less frequent as the child grows older. A few children continue to have relapses into late adolescence and adulthood.

A biopsy is not usually undertaken in a child with nephrotic syndrome unless there is no response to prednisolone or if the child has unusual features such as being very young or old (only 10% of adult nephrotic patients have minimal change), or has atypical features such as persistent heavy haematuria, hypocomplementaemia or hypertension. Steroid unresponsiveness may point to a more sinister underlying pathology such as focal glomerulosclerosis which is a cause of chronic renal failure in children (see later).

CONGENITAL NEPHROTIC SYNDROME

This is very rare and either presents at birth or develops in the first few months of life. It may be familial with an autosomal recessive inheritance pattern such as the Finnish type where there are microcystic changes in the renal cortex. Previously the condition was fatal before 2 years of age but dialysis and transplantation is now available. Antenatal diagnosis may be possible based on alphafetoprotein estimations in maternal serum and amniotic fluid.

SECONDARY CAUSES OF NEPHROTIC SYNDROME

It should again be pointed out that any chronic nephritis may give rise to a nephrotic state if the proteinuria is sufficiently heavy to result in hypoalbuminaemia. Examples already quoted are Henoch–Schönlein purpura, SLE, quartan malaria and schistosomiasis. Heavy metal poisoning, congenital syphilis and drugs are other potential causes.

Renal failure

ACUTE RENAL FAILURE (ARF)

This is an uncommon but important problem in which the kidneys are no longer able to maintain biochemical homeostasis. It is usually associated with oliguria (urine output <1 ml/kg/hour) but

Table 15.5 Causes of acute renal failure.

Pre-renal
Acute hypovolaemia
    Haemorrhage
    Gastro-enteritis
    Third space losses (burns, gut)
Peripheral vasodilatation
    Sepsis
Low cardiac output
    Cardiac failure
Bilateral renal vessel occlusion
    Renal artery/vein thrombosis

Intra-renal (renal parenchymal)
Haemolytic uraemic syndrome
Acute glomerulonephritis
Acute interstitial nephritis from drug hypersensitivity
Nephrotoxins
    Antibiotics
    Anti-cancer drugs
Vasculitis
    Polyarteritis
Bilateral acute pyelonephritis
Myoglobinuria haemoglobinuria
Acute crystalline nephropathy
    Uric acid
    Oxalosis

Post-renal
Posterior urethral valves
Bilateral obstruction
    Pelviureteric junction, or vesicoureteric junction
        obstruction
Neurogenic bladder
Stones

polyuric acute renal failure may also occur when urea and other waste products continue to accumulate despite an apparently good urine output. The causes of ARF can be considered in three main groups as shown in Table 15.5.

Investigation and management

The main priority is to distinguish pre-renal from established renal failure, as fluid and diuretic therapy in the former situation can reverse the impairment. The clues may well be in the history and examination. Urinalysis and urine microscopy should always be attempted. Comparison of the plasma and urinary electrolytes and osmolality may also give important clues because in pre-renal failure the urinary sodium will be low, creatinine high and the urine concentrated. Interpretation of the urinary electrolyte results, however, is difficult when there has already been administration of fluids and diuretics. An ultrasound examination of the abdomen is invaluable in helping to exclude obstructive lesions of the urinary tract that may require surgical intervention or other problems such as renal vein thrombosis and calculi.

Pre-renal failure. Volume expansion is required using plasma, mannitol or blood and this can be combined with powerful loop diuretics such as intravenous frusemide to improve urine output.

Established renal failure. Management requires strict fluid input and output monitoring with frequent weighing. The fluid input should be restricted to the previous day's urinary output plus insensible losses (400 ml/m^2) which should be increased if the child is pyrexial or decreased if the child is on a ventilator. Fluid-overloading the patient should be avoided as this will lead to hypertension requiring drug treatment or dialysis if pulmonary oedema threatens.

Attention to nutrition is important as children become hypercatabolic very quickly and the assistance of a dietitian is essential. Nasogastric feeding may be required to ensure a high carbohydrate, restricted protein, low potassium, low phosphate and no-added salt diet. Correction of metabolic abnormalities such as acidosis, hypocalcaemia and hyperphosphataemia are very important. Hyperkalaemia is particularly dangerous because of potential cardiac arrythmias and the risk of sudden death. Urgent steps should be taken to reduce an elevated plasma potassium level including dialysis.

Post-renal (obstructive) renal failure. This should always be suspected in high risk patients such as a male infant with sepsis and a poor urinary stream when posterior urethral valves would be high on the list (see Fig. 15.9). If an ultrasound examination suggests obstruction then urethral, suprapubic or nephrostomy drainage may be required. There may be a marked diuresis with relief of the obstruction and the fluid balance must be *strictly monitored*.

Dialysis

Indications for this procedure will include uncontrolled hyperkalaemia, acidosis, uraemia, hypertension and fluid overload. Peritoneal dialysis is the initial method of choice. When there are contraindications such as recent intra-abdominal surgery then the more difficult technique of haemodialysis may have to be undertaken. This requires good access to the circulation and can only be carried out in specialist centres. Haemofiltration using a highly water permeable membrane connected between the patient's artery and vein may be considered for fluid overload states.

Prognosis

The prognosis for acute renal failure in childhood is generally good but it will depend upon the underlying condition. Whereas a child with acute glomerulonephritis may recover completely, the prognosis for a child developing ARF following complex cardiac surgery will depend upon whether the heart recovers to perfuse the kidneys adequately.

HAEMOLYTIC URAEMIC SYNDROME (HUS)

In the UK this is probably the commonest cause of acute renal failure in childhood. It consists of a triad of haemolytic anaemia with fragmented red cells and burr cells on the blood film, thrombocytopenia and acute renal failure. Typically there is a diarrhoeal prodrome and although small outbreaks may occur in the UK the condition is endemic in other parts of the world such as South America. The enteropathic form of HUS has been associated with a variety of bacterial and viral agents and current interest has been focused on verotoxin-producing *E. coli*. The toxin may cause damage to vascular endothelial cells in a number of organs and severe neurological impairment and death can result from widespread vessel involvement.

Clinically the child has vomiting and diarrhoea which is frequently blood stained. Usually, as the diarrhoea settles the child becomes pallid, lethargic, oliguric and oedema develops as acute renal failure supervenes. It is important to think of this condition in any child with a history of bloody diarrhoea who is slow to recover as undetected hypertension and electrolyte disturbances can result in seizures. These may also reflect underlying central nervous involvement.

The enteropathic form of HUS generally has a good prognosis with supportive treatment alone (dialysis is usually undertaken at an early stage) and recurrences are extremely rare (Fig. 15.15). There has been no proven benefit from therapeutic interventions such as plasma infusions. Sporadic cases of HUS are sometimes associated with recurrences and there may be a familial tendency.

CHRONIC RENAL FAILURE (CRF)

Chronic renal failure may proceed inexorably into end-stage failure requiring dialysis and trans-

plantation in childhood. The causes are shown in Table 15.6.

Chronic renal failure may be recognized shortly after birth in a neonate whose mother had oligohydramnios or in whom there are obvious clinical problems such as Prune Belly syndrome. However, a number of children with hypoplastic/dysplastic kidneys or chronic reflux nephropathy only present later with growth failure, anorexia, or an acute or chronic crisis. This may be precipitated by either infection in the urinary tract or with extrarenal infection which results in increased metabolic demands and an acute decline in the glomerular filtration rate. The commonest group cause of CRF is chronic nephritis of which focal sclerosis is the most prevalent. Inherited and metabolic problems are important because genetic counselling and ante-natal detection can be offered.

Chronic renal failure can have a profound effect on growth and development in children and their long-term supervision should be undertaken in a paediatric nephrology unit which can provide the optimal care (see Table 15.7). This will involve specialist dietary and nursing support, surgical liaison and psychosocial preparation if dialysis and transplantation become imminent. In order to prevent growth failure in these children, aggressive feeding regimes and/or early dialysis may need to be undertaken thereby hopefully preventing the short stature which has been a feature of such children in the past. Chronic bone disease and anaemia can be prevented using vitamin D analogues and the recently developed human recombinant erythropoietin, respectively.

The number of children who develop end-stage renal disease requiring dialysis and transplantation is approximately 4–6:1 000 000 child population.

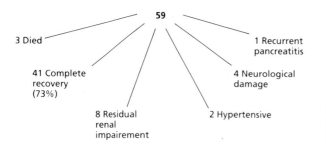

Fig. 15.15 Outcome following haemolytic uraemic syndrome in 59 children (Birmingham data).

Table 15.6 Causes of end-stage renal failure in children under 15 years. (European Dialysis and Transplant Association.)

Cause	%
Chronic glomerulonephritis, e.g. focal glomerulosclerosis	32
Reflux nephropathy and urinary tract malformation	22
Hereditary – familial, e.g. Alports syndrome	16
Renal hypoplasia/dysplasia	12
Other diagnoses, e.g. Henoch–Schönlein purpura	12
Uncertain	6

Table 15.7 Problems and management of chronic renal failure.

Problem	Cause	Treatment
Anaemia	Nutritional Reduced erythropoeitin Blood loss (on haemodialysis)	Iron and folate if deficient Transfusion Human recombinant erythropoeitin
Hypertension	Renin secretion from kidney Salt retention Artery stenosis (post-transplant)	No added salt diet Diuretics Anti-hypertensives Surgery
Growth failure	Poor intakes, especially calories Metabolic factors, e.g. acidosis Salt and water loss Anaemia	Dietary supplements orally or via naso-gastric/gastrostomy feeding Vitamins, Na, HCO_3 Early dialysis
Renal osteodystrophy	Phosphate retention Lack of $1,25\,(OH)_2D_3$ Secondary hyperparathyroidism	Reduce phosphate in diet Calcium carbonate phosphate binders $1,25\,(OH)_2$ vitamin D_3 supplements

Dialysis should only be seen as a temporary measure while the possibility of transplantation is actively pursued. However, because of the shortage of cadaveric kidneys a child may have to spend some time on chronic dialysis. This is preferably continuous ambulatory peritoneal dialysis (CAPD) which the child and parents can carry out at home with three or four bag changes a day. Recently continuous cycling peritoneal dialysis (CCPD) has been introduced where the child has most of his dialysis overnight using an automatic cycling machine. This enables him to avoid bag changes during the day either at home or school and we feel this makes CCPD the home dialysis therapy of choice. Haemodialysis is technically more difficult and generally has to be done in hospital although home dialysis is feasible in

some instances. One of the major problems with haemodialysis is obtaining access to the circulation. Traditionally this was by means of an arteriovenous fistula but we prefer the use of indwelling jugular venous (WBW or Hickman type) catheters which with local anaesthetic (EMLA) creams have considerably reduced the trauma of repeated venepunctures.

Dialysis and transplantation is now feasible at any age (preferably greater than 10 kg body weight) but it does impose considerable demands upon the patient, family, staff and resources. It requires a fully integrated team approach to decide the best treatment options for each individual. Transplantation undoubtedly offers the best chance of full rehabilitation and present cadaveric graft survival rates are in the region of 85% at 2

Type	Radio-opaque	Causes
Magnesium ammonium phosphate	Variable	Urinary infection particularly proteus species
Calcium phosphate	Yes	Renal tubular acidosis Idiopathic hypercalciuria Vitamin D toxicity Immobilization Hyperparathyroidism
Calcium oxalate	Yes	Idiopathic Oxalosis (1° or 2°) 'Dietary' bladder stone
Cystine	Variable	Cystinuria
Uric acid	No	Haematological malignancies Dietary Inborn errors (Lesch–Nyhan syndrome)

Table 15.8 Common types of urinary tract stones.

years with 93% graft survival at 5 years using living related donor transplants.

Renal stones

The incidence of renal stones in children in the UK is approximately 1.5:1 000 000 population but in other parts of the world stones are much commoner and probably attributable to higher infection rates and dietary factors. Nephrocalcinosis is the deposition of calcium salts within the renal parenchyma and it is associated in most instances with urinary tract stones (urolithiasis). The characteristics of the common types of urinary stone are shown in Table 15.8.

Stones may be asymptomatic or result in haematuria, abdominal pain, urinary infection or even renal failure (Fig. 15.16).

Investigations should be thorough to elucidate the aetiology and will include urinary pH measurements (to exclude renal tubular acidosis), urine culture and 24-hour excretion of calcium, oxalate, cystine or uric acid. The finding of cystine, ornithine, lysine and arginine ('COLA') on an amino acid screen of the urine suggests cystinuria. Obviously any stone passed should be analysed.

Stones causing obstruction or associated with infection require removal by pyelolithotomy or ureterolithotomy. Small cystoscopes are available for use in children and low ureteric stones can be captured in a Dormia basket. Shock wave lithotripsy has been carried out in children and its increasing usage will avoid the need for operative intervention.

A high fluid intake is always advised in any child at risk of stone formation and occasionally thiazide diuretics may be contemplated in patients with hypercalciuria.

Renal tubular disorders (Fig. 15.17).

These need to be considered whenever there is a persistent urinary abnormality such as aminoaciduria or an impaired ability to concentrate or acidify urine. The rare inborn error of cystinosis (not cystinuria) is now one of the most common causes of a Fanconi type syndrome and can present with rickets and failure to thrive. Children with the nephropathic form of cystinosis almost invariably progress to chronic renal failure.

Renal tubular acidosis (RTA) is a very rare condition and distinction of the various types will depend upon carefully conducted urinary acidification tests. Distal RTA (type I) is an inability to acidify the urine and is commonly recognized because of failure to thrive associated with

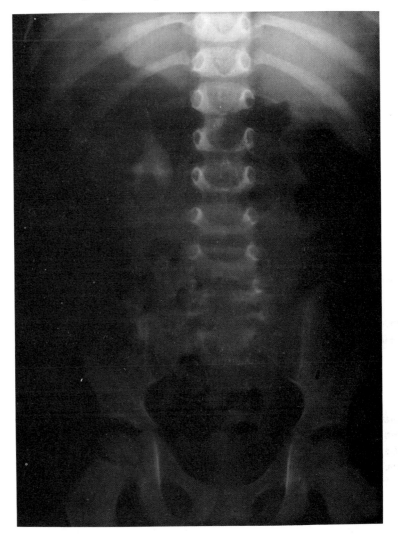

Fig. 15.16 Staghorn calcu in the pelvis of the left kidn plain abdominal X-ray in a old boy with a recent Prote infection.

nephrocalcinosis. The urine is always alkaline but in proximal RTA (type II) there is a low renal threshold for bicarbonate and the urine pH may be normal when the plasma bicarbonate is below the renal threshold.

Nephrogenic diabetes insipidus is an important condition to remember in male infants who present with unexplained fevers and bouts of dehydration who are persistently hungry, i.e. thirsty. It is a preventable cause of mental retardation as recurrent hypernatraemia can result in brain damage.

Hypertension

There is a lack of awareness that hypertension can and does occur in children, and measurement of the blood pressure should be routinely included in the examination of all children. Blood pressure varies with age and sex and reference should be made to appropriate centile charts just as for growth (Fig. 15.18).

The prevalence of hypertension in childhood is probably between 1 and 3%, but the majority of children will have mild increases and can be

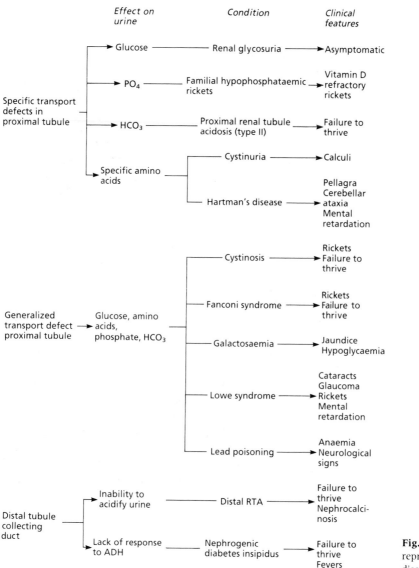

| Effect on urine | Condition | Clinical features |

Fig. 15.17 Schematic representation of renal tubular disorders.

garded as having primary (essential) hypertension. Primary hypertension in childhood is being increasingly recognized and is found to cluster in families and be associated with obesity. An elevated blood pressure in childhood may persist into adult life where it is a risk factor for cardiovascular disease and early recognition may enable appropriate advice and monitoring to be offered.

A much smaller number of children will have severe hypertension which carries a high risk of morbidity and mortality. The causes are shown in Table 15.9 and renal diseases account for 80–90% of cases with the commonest problem being the coarse renal scarring of reflux nephropathy. There may be little clue to this problem in the history, but there could be a story of previous urinary tract infections or unexplained fevers. Investigations will be tailored to the severity of the hypertension

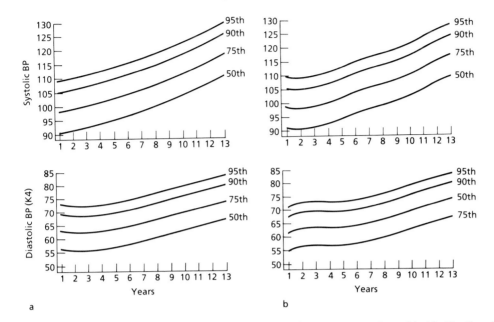

Fig. 15.18 Age-specific percentiles of blood pressure in children aged 1–13 years. (a) Boys. (b) girls. The Korotkoff phase IV was used for determination of the diastolic value. (Reproduced with permission from the report of the Second Task Force on Blood Pressure Control in Children. *Pediatrics* **79**, 1:1987. American Academy of Pediatrics.)

and the suspected lesion, e.g. a radiofemoral arterial pulse difference will suggest coarctation while renal bruits may suggest renovascular disease.

Management

If hypertension is diagnosed, evidence should be sought for chronicity and severity by fundoscopy and electrocardiographic evaluation of left ventricular hypertrophy and strain. In mild hypertension, with absence of underlying cause and no signs of cardiac strain, repeated measurements over some months should be made before drug therapy is considered. Weight loss should be encouraged where appropriate and smoking stopped.

Table 15.9 Causes of severe or sustained hypertension in childhood.

Renin-dependent
Renal parenchymal disease
   Renal scarring due to reflux or obstructive uropathy
   Chronic glomerulonephritis
   Polycystic kidneys
   Renal dysplasia
   Haemolytic uraemic syndrome

Renovascular disease
   Renal artery stenosis
   Renal artery thrombosis
   Polyarteritis nodosa
   Arterio-venous fistula

Renal tumours
   Nephroblastoma

Catecholamine excess
Phaeochromocytoma
Neuroblastoma

Coarctation of aorta

Chronic renal failure
Post-renal transplant

Corticosteroid excess
Congenital adrenal hyperplasia
Conn's and Cushing's syndrome

If severe hypertension is present, then blood pressure needs to be adequately controlled while investigations proceed. Drugs such as vasodilators (nifedipine, hydralazine), beta blockers (propranolol, atenolol) and diuretics (frusemide, thiazides) can be used individually or in combination. Hypertensive emergencies may require temporary treatment with controlled doses of diazoxide or nitroprusside infusions, but in most instances sublingual nifedipine is sufficient. An angiotensin converting agent inhibitor such as captopril is logical treatment for a high-renin state and some cases of hypertension such as renal artery stenosis are amenable to percutaneous balloon angioplasty or a direct surgical approach.

FLUID AND ELECTROLYTE PROBLEMS

The younger the child the more vulnerable he is to fluid and electrolyte disturbances because of the difference in body water composition, higher metabolic rates and larger surface area to volume ratio compared to adults.

Water is the most abundant component of the human body and the distribution between the two main compartments at various ages is shown in Table 16.1. The fall in the total body water with age is due to the accumulation of fat.

The extracellular compartment can be further divided into intravascular and interstitial compartments separated by the capillary membrane. The principal cation of the extracellular fluid is sodium while bicarbonate is the main anion. Intracellular fluid has potassium and magnesium as principal cations and phosphate, protein, sulphate and bicarbonate as anions. Despite the differences in body water the electrolyte concentrations of intracellular and extracellular fluids are similar in both infants and adults.

Normal water and electrolyte requirements

Water turnover and hence requirements are directly related to energy expenditure. Mainten-

Table 16.2 Maintenance fluid and electrolyte requirements.

	Weight (kg)	Daily requirements
Water	3–10	100 ml/kg
	11–20	1000 ml plus 50 ml/kg for each additional kg above 10 kg
	> 20	1500 ml plus 20 ml/kg for each additional kg above 20 kg
Sodium and potassium	3–10	2.5 mmol/kg
	11–30	2 mmol/kg
	> 30	1.5 mmol/kg

ance fluid requirements have been computed to include insensible water losses (skin and respiratory tract), obligatory urine volume and small amounts of water lost in the stool (Table 16.2).

The maintenance requirements need to be 20–25% higher for oral fluids because of the increased solute load in the diet. Maintenance requirements for premature and term infants vary according to the postnatal age but are generally

Table 16.1 Body water composition at different ages.

Age	Total body water (% body weight)	Extracellular fluid (% body weight)	Intracellular fluid (% body weight)
Pre-term	85	55	30
Term	80	45	35
1–3 years	65	25	40
Adult	65	25	40

150 ml/kg up to 6 months of age. It is important to remember that the fluid requirements need to be *increased* in the following situations.

1 Pyrexia – increase by 12% for each degree above 38°C.

2 Abnormal fluid and electrolyte losses, e.g. gut, fistulae, burns.

3 Tachypnoea from acute respiratory infections may increase requirements by 25–50%.

4 In newborns who are under radiant heaters there is an increased requirement of 25%.

Fluid requirements should be *reduced* in:

1 Ventilated patients and those who receive humidified air.

2 Oedematous patients and those in whom there is likely to be release of ADH, e.g. post-operative patients and those with central nervous system trauma or infection.

3 Heavily sedated or paralysed patients.

4 Patients with established renal insufficiency.

Electrolyte and fluid disturbances

CLINICAL FEATURES

The limitations of electrolyte studies in the assessment of these patients is apparent and urgent cases must be treated without waiting for the results. Clinical assessment is therefore of prime importance, close attention also being paid to the weight, temperature and intake and output of fluids; the mother should always be asked the time since the child last passed urine.

Dehydration is the feature of a serious case (Table 16.3). It causes sunken eyes, depressed anterior fontanelle, dryness of the mouth and loss of skin elasticity. When testing this elasticity, the skin over the ribs should be used rather than the abdominal skin which can give fallacious results. A marasmic baby may have loose abdominal skin from loss of weight rather than loss of fluid; lack of potassium can cause abdominal distension with consequent stretching of the skin.

The relative loss of sodium and water is seldom the same as their proportions in the extracellular fluid. Consequently, isotonic dehydration is rare. It is necessary, therefore, to differentiate hyponatraemic and hypernatraemic dehydration since their clinical management is totally different.

Hyponatraemic dehydration

This is defined as serum sodium <130 mmol/l and occurs when the relative loss of sodium exceeds the loss of water; it is the commoner of the two types of dehydration. Thirst is not a feature, the baby being limp and apathetic. Anorexia and vomiting are common. The skin is dry and inelastic. Convulsions may occur. In the most severe cases the infant is ashen grey and cold, lying with half open eyes in a state of shock; death frequently follows.

Hypernatraemic dehydration

This is defined as a serum sodium >150 mmol/l and occurs when the relative loss of fluid exceeds the loss of sodium. It results from three situations particularly.

1 Simple fluid depletion associated with inadequate replacement of excessive insensible loss in a feverish or comatose baby.

2 Excessive administration of sodium, particularly

Sign	5% dehydration	10% dehydration
Mental state	Lethargic	Prostration, coma
Skin	Loss of elasticity	Mottled, poor capillary return
Fontanelle	Depressed	Deeply depressed
Eyes	Sunken	Deeply sunken
Peripheral pulses	Normal	Tachycardia, poor volume

Table 16.3 Clinical assessment of dehydration.

caused by incorrect preparation of powdered milk feeds.

3 Mixed fluid and electrolyte loss when the loss of fluid predominates.

Thirst is very marked, the baby being restless, irritable and sometimes developing convulsions. The peripheral signs of dehydration are less marked than in hyponatraemic dehydration since the increased osmolality of the extracellular fluid causes a shift of water out of the cells into the extracellular compartment. The skin may therefore have a rubbery or doughy feel. The fluid lack commonly causes fever. Hypernatraemic states cause shrinkage of the brain with meningeal congestion and vascular stasis which may lead to thrombosis. Cerebral thrombosis may leave the child mentally retarded and spastic. In general, the changes in hypernatraemic dehydration are more profound than those in hyponatraemic dehydration and peripheral circulatory failure occurs often despite a brief history. Acidosis is common. The blood sugar is commonly raised, sometimes to very high levels, making a mistaken diagnosis of diabetes mellitus possible.

Acidosis. This causes deep sighing respirations termed 'air hunger'. Acidotic patients are usually dehydrated and may be comatose.

Alkalosis. This causes few symptoms, dehydration being minimal. The respirations are shallow, the cry feeble and less frequent. The alkalotic baby, since he cries less often, may mistakenly be believed by his mother to have improved.

Lack of potassium. This causes flaccid muscular weakness; peristalsis is inhibited, leading to gaseous distension of the small intestine. In almost all cases of dehydration there has been loss of potassium as well as sodium and fluid. Since potassium is mainly intracellular the plasma potassium may not be reduced. In severe cases the full clinical picture of paralytic ileus is present. Changes in the electrocardiogram, resulting from low potassium, may be present. These comprise a lowered T-wave and depression of the S–T segment.

MANAGEMENT

This requires careful repeated clinical assessment (including accurate weighing) as well as monitoring of plasma electrolytes. Random measurements of urinary sodium are not useful except in the *initial* assessment of an oliguric clinically dehydrated patient *not* on fluid therapy, in which a low urine sodium concentration is diagnostic of reduced effective intravascular volume whereas a high urine sodium concentration implies impaired renal or adrenal function.

Replacement of losses

Mild dehydration (under 5%). This can usually be managed by oral rehydration therapy using a range of formulations which include glucose or sucrose in addition to electrolytes.

Moderate to severe dehydration (over 5%). Intravenous therapy is usually administered in this situation especially when there are signs of peripheral circulatory failure. A shocked patient requires an urgent infusion of plasma or normal saline 20 ml/kg body weight followed by 0.45% saline in 5% dextrose at 10 ml/kg/hour for the first 4 hours until plasma electrolytes are available. In hyponatraemic dehydration it is appropriate to give the remainder of the total fluid requirements (maintenance + deficit + ongoing losses) to restore a normal extracellular fluid (ECF) volume over the first 24 hours using 0.18% saline in 4.3% dextrose. Potassium chloride (20–40 mmol/litre of fluid) can be added once urine output is established and acidosis can be corrected using sodium bicarbonate.

Hypernatraemic dehydration. This should be corrected with caution as a rapid return of water to the brain cells causes cerebral oedema. After the initial resuscitation the fluids should be restricted to 100 ml/kg in the first 24 hours using 0.18% saline in 4% dextrose and total correction should take at least 48 hours.

Hyponatraemia. A low plasma sodium should not automatically be equated with sodium deficiency. If there is a true sodium loss, e.g. diarrhoea, then there is usually a reduction in extracellular fluid volume recognized as thirst, dehydration and hypovolaemia.

Fictitious hyponatraemia can occur with the presence of a relatively impermeable solute in the extracellular space, e.g. glucose and mannitol. Pseudohyponatraemia can also occur as a result of replacement of plasma water by lipids or protein.

There may also be a gain of water in excess of sodium to account for the hyponatraemia. This occurs in oedematous states, renal failure with salt and water retention, excessive water intake and the syndrome of inappropriate ADH secretion following surgery and CNS lesions.

Acid–base balance

The plasma pH is normally maintained between 7.32 and 7.45, the normal arterial $Pa\mathrm{co}_2$ is 4.6–6.5 kPa (35–50 mmHg) and the normal plasma bicarbonate is 24–34 mmol/l. Acids are produced as a result of metabolism, and the kidneys and lungs are ultimately responsible for the excretion of these acids. Maintenance of acid–base status is finely balanced by a variety of buffering mechanisms, of which carbonic acid-bicarbonate is the most important buffer in the plasma. Protein is the most important intracellular buffer.

Carbon dioxide is produced from the Krebs' cycle as the result of aerobic metabolism. The principal acid produced from this process is carbonic acid derived from carbon dioxide. Carbonic acid can be excreted by the kidneys as bicarbonate ions or by the lungs as carbon dioxide. Quantitatively the latter route is responsible for the greatest excretion:

$$CO_2 + H_2O \rightleftharpoons H_2CO_3 \rightleftharpoons HCO_3^- + H^+$$

The enzyme carbonic anhydrase is responsible for this reaction. With reference to the Henderson–Hasselbach equation:

$$pH = pK + \log \frac{(HCO_3^-)}{(K_1 \; Pa\mathrm{co}_2)}$$

acidosis may result from an increase in $Pa\mathrm{co}_2$ or reduction in plasma HCO_3^-. Aklalosis may result from a reduction in $Pa\mathrm{co}_2$ or an increase in HCO_3^-. On this basis acidosis and alkalosis can be referred to as either respiratory or metabolic (Table 16.4).

Compensatory mechanisms exist within the kidneys and respiratory system to minimize these forms of alkalosis and acidosis. In the presence of normal lungs, metabolic acidosis is rapidly compensated by hyperventilation and a reduction in the $P\mathrm{co}_2$, with a fall in plasma carbonic acid. In metabolic alkalosis, hypoventilation occurs which causes retention of CO_2 and an increase in carbonic acid. If the respiratory system is damaged, compensation fails and there may be a mixed respiratory and metabolic acidosis.

In the presence of respiratory acidosis due, usually, to respiratory failure the kidney will retain bicarbonate and excrete chloride ions. This is done by exchanging a hydrogen ion for a sodium ion. The H^+ is generated by the carbonic anhydrase enzyme which simultaneously generates HCO_3^- and this is reabsorbed into the plasma at the expense of Cl^-. This mechanism is not as rapid as occurs with respiratory compensation. The reverse renal mechanism will compensate for respiratory alkalosis due to hyperventilation from fever raised intracranial pressure, etc.

Table 16.4 Typical plasma findings in clinical disturbances of acid–base balance (compensated).

	pH	$P\mathrm{co}_2$	HCO_3
Metabolic acidosis	↓	↓	↓
Metabolic alkalosis	↑	↑	↑
Respiratory acidosis	↓	↑	↑
Respiratory alkalosis	↑	↓	↓

METABOLIC ACIDOSIS

This is a primary reduction in plasma bicarbonate which can be due to:

1 Bicarbonate loss
  Gastrointestinal, e.g.
    Diarrhoea, small bowel drainage, ureterosigmoidostomy
  Renal, e.g.
    Proximal renal tubular acidosis, chronic renal failure, renal insufficiency
2 Reduced hydrogen ion excretion
  Distal renal tubular acidosis
  Acute or chronic renal failure
  Carbonic anhydrase inhibitors
3 Excess hydrogen ion load
  Endogenous, e.g.
    Inborn errors of metabolism such as disorders of amino acid or organic acid metabolism
    Lactic acidaemia
    Ketoacidosis
    Renal failure
  Exogeneous, e.g.
    Salicylate
    Methyl/ethyl alcohol
    Organic acids

A recent concept which has helped to classify metabolic acidosis is that of the anion gap. This can be calculated as follows:

$$\text{Anion gap} = Na^+ - (Cl^- + HCO_3^-) \text{ mmol/l}$$

There is normally a balance between plasma anions and cations but a number of anions such as phosphate, sulphate, creatinine and protein are not usually measured and these are represented in the normal anion gap of 10–14 mmol. When bicarbonate is lost either via the gastrointestinal tract or the kidney there is usually compensatory hyperchloraemia and consequently there is a hyperchloraemic acidosis with normal anion gap. When there is accumulation of acid it is usually directly buffered by bicarbonate and hence there is a normochloraemic metabolic acidosis with increased anion gap. The anion gap is usually greater than 20 mmol in this situation.

Management

Correction of severe acidosis is important to prevent clinical deterioration. An approximate formula for total correction would be:

$$\text{Amount of base in mmol} = 0.3 \times \text{base deficit} \times \text{body wt (kg)}$$

Usually this is given as 8.4% sodium bicarbonate (1 mmol/ml) by slow intravenous injection correcting half the deficit initially and rechecking blood levels and pH.

Metabolic acidosis is associated with a number of rare inherited disorders of metabolism which can render the child acutely ill in the newborn period (p. 378). There may be vomiting, lethargy, hypotonia, seizures and coma with the onset towards the end of the first week after the introduction of milk feeds. The clinician needs to maintain a high index of suspicion and the presence of a previous neonatal death, strange odours, e.g. maple syrup in maple syrup urine disease, and ketonuria should result in an urgent request for plasma and urine amino and organic acid analysis.

METABOLIC ALKALOSIS

This is characterized by a primary elevation of plasma bicarbonate and a rise in blood pH. As a compensatory mechanism alveolar hypoventilation leads to a rise in $P\text{CO}_2$ in an attempt to lower the pH to normal.

The main causes are:
1 Excessive intake of base preparations.
2 Selective chloride depletion (chloride responsive).
3 Direct stimulation of H^+ secretion by the kidney (chloride unresponsive).

An excessive intake of bases is rarely seen in childhood compared to adults who are more prone to consume antacid preparations. Chloride depletion is the commonest cause of alkalosis in children. When a child is vomiting due to pyloric stenosis there is loss of hydrogen and chloride ions. The loss of sodium and potassium leads to extracellular volume contraction. The kidney responds by enhanced tubular sodium reabsorption but the disproportionate loss of chloride as HCl, NaCl and KCl means that Na^+ can only be retained at an accelerated rate of exchange with K^+ and H^+ in the distal tubule, hence the hypokalaemic alkalosis. The alkalosis is 'chloride responsive' because as soon as chloride is made available to the kidney it is retained at the expense of bicarbonate. Other causes of a 'chloride-responsive' alkalosis include congenital chloride diarrhoea, diuretic therapy and rarely cystic fibrosis.

Chloride unresponsive metabolic alkalosis is so-called because chloride replacement does not alleviate the alkalosis. Causes include Cushing's syndrome, some types of congenital adrenal hyperplasia, hyperaldosteronism, Bartter's syndrome and severe potassium deficiency.

Management

Severe metabolic alkalosis is rare but central nervous changes similar to hypocalcaemia may occur. Gastrointestinal losses can be replaced by sodium and potassium chloride if renal function is satisfactory. Ammonium chloride may also be given orally or intravenously.

17
DISORDERS OF THE NERVOUS SYSTEM

Disorders affecting the brain, spinal cord, peripheral nerve and muscle are amongst the most important in childhood when considering their implications for subsequent function. Disorders affecting the brain are common, but the ways in which they present are relatively few. This chapter reviews the commoner manifestations and causes of neurological illness occurring in children.

Investigating the nervous system

Lumbar puncture

Examination of the cerebrospinal fluid (CSF) is of fundamental importance to the diagnosis of many disorders of the nervous system. CSF is most conveniently obtained by lumbar puncture. This must be performed aseptically by an experienced doctor. The child lies on his side and the back is tightly curved. The L4–L5 interspace is palpated in the line of the iliac crests. A 22-g styletted spinal needle is inserted in the midline aiming towards the umbilicus. A give is felt as the needle penetrates the dura and the stylette is then removed. The CSF pressure should be measured and fluid taken for microbiological, chemical and cytological examination. In infants, a higher interspace (L3–L4) may be used as the spinal cord has not descended as far in babies.

The suspicion of raised intracranial pressure is a definite contraindication to lumbar puncture as this may cause the brain stem to herniate through the foramen magnum with fatal consequences.

Imaging

Modern imaging techniques allow the investigator to obtain remarkable structural detail of the brain and spinal cord. X-ray computerized tomography (CT) will give serial slices through the brain and the investigator can build up a three-dimensional picture of the organ. More recently, magnetic resonance imaging (MRI) has been developed and is now in routine use to provide scans of the central nervous system. This principle is based on the proton density of the organ and it will provide structural information on the progress of myelination. In infants with an open fontanelle, ultrasound is a very valuable imaging technique.

Function

Although imaging has changed the whole approach to neurology, techniques to assess function of the nervous system are also valuable. These include electroencephalography and electrical evoked potentials. This latter technique measures the neuronal response to a stimulus by averaging the minute electrical potentials produced by the stimulus. Visual, auditory and somatosensory evoked potentials all give useful information non-invasively and can be used in infants and children.

Infections of the central nervous system

Meningitis

Meningitis is most commonly caused by bacterial or viral infectious agents and is a common condition in childhood. The term refers to infection of the meninges which surround the brain and spinal cord. Bacterial infection is usually confined to the meninges, but viruses not infrequently involve the underlying brain and the condition is then referred to as meningoencephalitis.

BACTERIAL MENINGITIS

The prevalence of this condition in childhood is approximately 0.5%. Distinction must be made between neonatal meningitis (including infants up to 3 months of age) and infection occurring in children older than this.

In older children there are only three organisms likely to cause meningitis:
1 *Haemophilus influenzae.*
2 *Neisseria meningitidis* (commonest in the UK).
3 *Streptococcus pneumoniae.*

The commonest route of spread to the meninges is via the blood stream. In cases of recurrent infection or infection by organisms other than the three mentioned above, careful investigation to ascertain an anatomical defect or sinus to account for the repeated infections must be undertaken. Tuberculous meninigitis still occurs in Britain and is common elsewhere in the world and is discussed on p. 562.

Clinical features. The classical features of neck stiffness and head retraction as seen in the adult are late features in children and seldom seen in infants. In children and especially infants, the most frequent symptoms are irritability, vomiting and anorexia. Older children usually complain of headache. Drowsiness is an early feature; the infant has a vacant expression with staring eyes and, in severe cases, may present in coma. A reduction in the normal level of consciousness is always a serious sign. If the fontanelle is still open the tension may be sufficiently increased to cause bulging, but this is often a late sign.

The cry is high pitched ('meningeal'). Convulsions are common in infants, and may be the presenting feature, although a history of the child being off colour and refusing feeds for a few hours before is usually obtained. An acute onset squint is common. Petechial haemorrhages may be present in the early stages of meningococcal infection (see p. 366). Papilloedema is not usual in children and Kernig's sign, although present in older children, is often absent or a late sign in infancy.

Differential diagnosis. In infants the clinical picture is that of an acute infection and the condition must be differentiated from other forms of sepsis. Signs of raised intracranial pressure are ominous and although meningitis may be the cause of this, a lumbar puncture should not be performed until a CT scan has been done to exclude a space-occupying lesion. Subarachnoid haemorrhage, although rare in childhood, may cause very similar symptoms to meningitis. CT scanning will distinguish the two.

Meningismus causes considerable diagnostic difficulties in children. This name is given to the neck stiffness which may accompany the onset of any acute infection in childhood, especially tonsillitis, otitis media, pneumonia and pyelonephritis. Its cause is unknown. Children with meningismus are alert and show signs of the primary infection, but examination of the CSF, which is normal, may be essential to establish the correct diagnosis.

Investigations. The diagnosis is made at lumbar puncture and in most cases an organism can be identified. Table 17.1 summarizes the different findings at lumbar puncture. The appearance of the CSF should be noted. Bacterial meningitis often causes the fluid to be cloudy. Microscopy is essential to count and identify the cells. In some cases of fulminating bacterial meningitis there may be few cells or none at all, but the fluid is teeming with bacteria. Polymorphs suggest bacterial and lymphocytes suggest viral infection. In the early stages of viral meningitis, polymorphs may be seen

Table 17.1 The characteristic findings at lumbar puncture in children with different forms of meningitis.

		Type of meningitis	
	Bacterial	Viral	Tuberculous
Cells	Polymorphs (in early stages, cells may be absent)	Lymphocytes (in early stages polymorphs may be present)	Lymphocytes (in early stages polymorphs may be present)
Protein	Elevated	Mild elevation	Elevated
Glucose	Reduced	Normal	Often normal but may be reduced

and lymphocytes are characteristic of tuberculous meningitis (see Table 17.1). The fluid must be cultured to obtain confirmation of the infecting organism.

The glucose level should be measured and compared to that of the blood. The usual ratio between blood glucose and CSF glucose is 5:3. Bacterial and tuberculous meningitis are associated with low CSF glucose and it is usually normal in viral infection.

Protein estimation is usually raised in bacterial meningitis and may be slightly elevated in viral meningitis. It is characteristically extremely high in tuberculous meningitis.

Aseptic meningitis refers to those cases where an organism is not isolated on routine microbiological investigation. This is most commonly the case in viral meningitis, although a virus may subsequently be identified. Partially treated meningitis may also produce an aseptic picture. In such cases immunological investigations may be helpful in identifying the organism. Counter immunoelectrophoresis (CIE) may determine the infecting organism in cases of partially treated meningitis.

Treatment. Treatment of bacterial meningitis is directed towards anti-microbial sterilization of the CSF and avoiding or managing the complications of meningitis. The organism should be fully sensitive to the antibiotic and it should achieve adequate levels in the CSF of the subarachnoid space.

If the organism is recognized on Gram staining then the antibiotic management is straightforward

Table 17.2 Antimicrobial treatment of meningitis. The management of tuberculous meningitis is discussed on p. 565.

Haemophilus influenzae	Ampicillin Chloramphenicol
Neisseria meningitidis	Benzyl penicillin
Pneumococcus	Benzyl penicillin
Partially treated (no organism seen on Gram stain)	Ampicillin Chloramphenicol
Neonatal meningitis Organism unknown	Gentamicin Ampicillin
Staphylococcus	Cefotaxime

(Table 17.2). Antibiotics must be given intravenously for the first 5−7 days and thereafter if the child has recovered, they may be given orally for a further 5−7 days. A complete course should last 2 weeks. There is no advantage in giving intrathecal antibiotics.

Some children with meningitis may have been partially treated with antibiotics before reaching hospital and identification of the causative organism may not be possible. In these cases a combination of intravenous ampicillin and chloramphenicol should be used for 14 days.

Meningococcal meningitis is associated with a high carrier rate in the nasopharynx of contacts and prophylactic rifampicin should be given for 2 days to all household contacts to reduce the risk of cross-infection (see p. 366).

Neonatal meningitis

The incidence of neonatal meningitis in the UK is 1:4000. Neonatal meningitis differs from meningitis in older children in a number of ways. The neonate is relatively immuno-incompetent and is more at risk of all types of infection. He is exposed to a variety of potentially pathogenic organisms on passage through the birth canal. Consequently the organisms causing neonatal meningitis vary considerably from those causing meningitis in older children.

In neonates a wide variety of organisms cause infection but the Group B beta haemolytic *Streptococcus* and *E. coli* are the most common. The organism usually reaches the neonatal meninges by blood borne route, but direct penetration through a dermal sinus or spina bifida lesion is possible.

Symptoms associated with neonatal meningitis include unstable temperature, lethargy, vomiting, convulsions, apnoea and irritability. In the neonate there may be no localizing features at all and it is always important to consider meninigitis in all ill neonates and to perform a lumbar puncture to exclude the condition (see p. 95).

The treatment of neonatal meningitis depends on the organism. As stated above there is a much wider group of potential infecting agents and the choice of antibiotics needs to cover the possibility of other bacteria. A combination of ampicillin and gentamicin is the best first line treatment even if the organism is unknown. If staphylococci are suspected a cephalosporin such as cefotaxime is indicated.

The prognosis depends on how early the diagnosis is made and effective treatment instituted. The mortality rate is of the order of 25% and one-third of survivors are likely to be handicapped.

VIRAL MENINGITIS

The diagnosis of viral meningitis is initially presumptive based on the clinical features, the CSF cytology and the absence of recognizable bacterial organisms (aseptic). Unfortunately it may be difficult to be sure that this pattern is not due to partially treated bacterial meningitis, tubercul-ous meningitis or infection due to some other organism. A high level of clinical suspicion must be maintained in the early stages of aseptic meningitis.

The pathology and symptomatology in this group is similar to bacterial meningitis. Some viruses show an affinity to grey matter and are called neurotropic. Viruses most likely to cause meningitis or meningoencephalitis are mumps, poliomyelitis, Coxsackie, ECHO, herpes simplex, lymphocytic choriomeningitis and rabies. A variety of rare arthropod-borne viruses are also neurotropic and cause epidemic encephalitis.

Clinical features. Viral meningitis is often preceded by a mild pharyngitis or gastrointestinal upset. The child then develops fever, headache and neck stiffness. The sensorium is clear unless encephalitis develops when coma may occur. Involvement of the brain may cause ataxia and cranial nerve palsies.

Treatment. Viral meningitis is usually self-limiting and requires no specific treatment. Viral encephalitis due to herpes simplex may be treated with antiviral agents such as acyclovir.

COMPLICATIONS OF MENINGITIS

Hydrocephalus

This is a relatively common complication of bacterial meningitis and is due to obstruction and fibrosis of the intracerebral drainage system, particularly blockage at the exit of the fourth ventricle (see also p. 295).

Subdural effusion

This is a common complication, especially in infants with severe meningitis. It occurs most often with *Haemophilus influenzae* meningitis and to a lesser extent with pneumococcal infection. Effusion is most often situated over the frontal or parietal region and has a high protein content. This may cause the effusion to expand by an osmotic effect.

The possibility of its existence must be considered if the signs, particularly fever, fail to settle within 72 hours of the beginning of adequate therapy. An effusion must also be suspected if culture of the CSF remains positive or if focal neurological signs develop.

Diagnosis is made by CT scan. If treatment is required repeated subdural taps will be necessary. If daily taps continue to produce 20–30 ml of fluid then neurosurgical treatment will be necessary.

Acute adrenal failure

This is a serious complication of systemic meningococcal disease and is discussed in Chapter 21.

Deafness

This is an important complication of both bacterial and viral meningitis. It is particularly associated with mumps meningitis (see also Chapter 18).

Major cerebral deficit

Meningitis is still an important cause of cerebral palsy, mental retardation and major seizure disorders. Up to one-third of children with bacterial meningitis may be left with some impairment after recovery from the acute illness.

The factors which determine outcome are the infecting organism, the age at infection and the rapidity of effective treatment. The prognosis of neonatal meningitis has certainly improved with more awareness of the condition and earlier diagnosis.

Encephalitis

This form of infection is invariably due to a virus and as mentioned above may present initially with features of meningitis when the term meningo-encephalitis may be more appropriate.

Encephalitis may be due to direct invasion of the brain by a virus (primary) or be due to an allergic vascular reaction within the brain. In these cases the virus has not penetrated the blood–brain

Table 17.3 Viruses causing encephalitis.

Primary	Secondary
Herpes simplex	Measles
Mumps	Varicella zoster
Enteroviruses	Rubella
Arboviruses	Infectious mononucleosis (Epstein–
Rabies	Barr virus)

barrier and the condition is referred to as post-infectious encephalitis. Table 17.3 lists the commoner viruses which cause primary encephalitis as well as post-infectious encephalitis.

Primary encephalitis presents dramatically with severe illness, reduction in the level of consciousness and other signs of encephalopathy including seizures and cranial nerve palsies.

MEASLES

Post-infectious encephalitis

This common infectious disease is dealt with in Chapter 21. Measles virus does not invade the brain directly but post-infectious measles encephalitis occurs in approximately 1:1000 cases of measles. Convulsions and coma develop in the second week after the rash develops and the CSF may be normal. Steroids (dexamethasone) have been used to treat this condition but up to 20% of survivors are left severely disabled. Measles vaccination prevents this complication and post-infectious measles encephalitis does not seem to develop as a result of the vaccination.

Subacute sclerosing panencephalitis

This is a very rare condition and on average occurs 5–15 years after primary measles infection. It is due to direct invasion of the measles virus into the brain and is associated with progressive neurological and intellectual deterioration.

Initially the children show deterioration in their school work and then curious backward stumbling movements and myoclonic jerks. Later, characteristic sudden movements of the arms occur, these being raised to shoulder height where they remain 'hung up' for a few seconds. The disease progresses to spasticity, dementia and eventually death. There is a characteristic EEG pattern and focal retinitis may help to confirm the diagnosis.

POLIOMYELITIS

This important cause of encephalitis is discussed in Chapter 29.

Cerebral abscess

The commonest cause of cerebral abscess is in association with cyanotic congenital heart disease. Cases are also seen following otitis media, mastoiditis and sinusitis. Cerebral abscess following meningitis is a very rare complication.

The commonest presentation is with symptoms of raised intracranial pressure (vomiting and headache) and papilloedema is often present. Focal neurological signs may be seen. Diagnosis is made by CT scan examination and the abscess is well visualized following enhancement with radio-opaque dye.

Treatment involves neurosurgical drainage or excision and prolonged use of appropriate antibiotics.

Convulsions

Epilepsy is a disease of great antiquity, recognized by Hippocrates and other ancient physicians. Convulsions, however, are not the same as epilepsy and the terms seizure, fit and convulsion are often used synonomously. Neonatal convulsions are discussed on p. 100.

Convulsions are due to synchronous discharge of electrical activity from a group of neurones. The observed seizure is the clinically apparent result of this discharge through the central and peripheral nervous system. It may be generalized or partial; simple or complicated.

Neurones have an excitatory and/or inhibitory function. Cerebral activity is the result of a fine balance between these two types of control. Factors that stimulate the excitatory neurone or depress the inhibitory neurone may throw the system out of balance and may precipitate rhythmical firing which may in turn cause a clinically observed convulsion. The immature brain is particularly liable to be subject to imbalance as a variety of insults may disturb the equilibrium and precipitate convulsions. Neonatal seizures are particularly common and fits occurring in the first 5 years may be precipitated by relatively minor insults such as fever or sleep deprivation.

Convulsions may be due to a large number of cerebral insults such as birth injury, meningitis, encephalitis, metabolic disorders, hypoglycaemia, vascular accidents, trauma, congenital malformations and neoplasms. Much more commonly the cause is idiopathic.

Epilepsy

Epilepsy is the term used to describe a chronic state where convulsions may occur at intervals and is due to a disorder of the control of neuronal electrical discharge. A child should never be labelled as having epilepsy following a single convulsion, nor should neonates with frequent seizures be regarded as having epilepsy. The convulsion is a symptom and epilepsy may subsequently be found to be the disease label. The fear of epilepsy in the community is high and the condition is often misunderstood and equated with being 'mental', retarded or otherwise brain damaged. Many epileptic children and adults lead completely normal lives and many great figures in history were epileptic.

Epilepsy takes many forms and the various seizure types are discussed below. The electroencephalogram is an extremely useful diagnostic tool and contributes to the diagnosis. EEG alone, however, cannot be used to make the diagnosis of epilepsy; it can only support it. A normal EEG between seizures does not exclude epilepsy. In addition, approximately 4% of normal children have an abnormal EEG and never show evidence of epilepsy.

Children with epilepsy are usually entirely neurologically normal, but perhaps one-quarter have other features of cerebral compromise including cerebral palsy or mental retardation. The epileptic child should be encouraged to lead as normal a life as possible but some activities are unacceptably dangerous. Bicycle riding on the main road may be fatal if the child has a convulsion and similarly unsupervised swimming is clearly proscribed. The persuance of potentially dangerous activities where falling from some height is a possibility should be discussed with the child and his parents and the relative risk considered. If undertaken it should be in the presence of a responsible adult.

There is commonly a genetic predisposition towards epilepsy. The risk of a child developing epilepsy if one parent is epileptic is about 3%, rising to 25% if both parents are affected. It is likely that such a child is born with the predisposition towards epilepsy but a precipitating event is necessary to trigger it. Epileptic seizures in children are very rarely due to a cerebral tumour and are more commonly associated with tuberous sclerosis.

There is no entirely satisfactory classification of convulsions but they can be simply divided into generalized and partial seizures.

GENERALIZED CONVULSIONS

Grand mal seizures

This is the form of seizure generally considered by the public to be epilepsy. It is the commonest form of convulsion seen in childhood and follows a typical pattern.

It is usually preceded by an aura. In young children this may not be described but the mother can often recognize a typical pattern of behaviour. The child then loses consciousness, falls over and becomes stiff. This is the tonic phase and rapidly gives way to clonic spasms with rhythmical contraction and relaxation of the limb and facial muscles. There is the attendant risk of biting the tongue at this time. The usual timing of the jerks are 1–2 per second. During the clonic phase the child may be incontinent. The duration of the clonic phase is variable but if prolonged the child is said to have status epilepticus (see p. 286). The fit is usually followed by a period of deep sleep. The child may be confused or irritable after this.

Grand mal spasms, particularly the first one, are very frightening to the parents. They often think the child is going to die and this feeling continues for many attacks until they can accept the benign nature of the convulsions. They should be warned not to leave the child during a seizure and to avoid airway compromise by putting him on the floor in a semi-recumbent position. They should be warned not to force anything into his mouth as this well-meaning manoeuvre may cause more trauma than the risk of him biting his own tongue.

Grand mal convulsions usually occur in children with idiopathic epilepsy and otherwise functionally normal brains. Children with underlying cerebral disorders such as cerebral palsy or hydrocephalus are much more likely to develop grand mal seizures. A careful developmental history and neurological examination must be performed on all children who present *de novo* with any form of convulsion.

Grand mal seizures as a feature of idiopathic epilepsy have a relatively good prognosis when presenting in childhood. Presentation between the age of 5 and 15 years is unlikely to be associated with epilepsy in later life. Presentation before the age of 3 years carries a worse prognosis.

Reflex epilepsy. Grand mal seizures can be triggered by sensory stimulation and this is referred to as reflex epilepsy. This is most commonly due to the flickering of a television screen and typically occurs in the early teenage years. Children with this form of epilepsy should be warned to sit well back from the screen and to watch the television in a well-illuminated room.

FEBRILE CONVULSIONS

These are seizures which occur in children between the age of 6 months and 5 years and are due to fever. As mentioned above the immature brain is more unstable to environmental factors and fever may precipitate a massive electrical discharge with the clinical features of a grand mal convulsion. They occur in approximately 5% of all children of this age and there is often a strong family history. It is important to remember that convulsions themselves, particularly if prolonged, produce a temperature due to the increased muscle activity. It is always important to consider whether the temperature is the cause or effect of the convulsion. Similarly, children with severe infection such as meningitis may have both fever and convulsions and this must always be carefully considered.

The seizure is usually grand mal in nature. They are often short-lived, lasting only a few minutes. In some children the seizure may be prolonged and the child may develop status epilepticus. Febrile convulsions lasting longer than 20 minutes are potentially damaging and must be stopped pharmacologically.

Management. The management of an established febrile convulsion depends on its duration. If the child has had previous fits the mother can be given diazepam for rectal administration. This is a safe procedure but the child should be seen and examined by a doctor following the fit. The management of status epilepticus is discussed below.

Prophylaxis is extremely important in all children who have had one febrile convulsion or those with a first degree relative who had this form of seizure. The parents must undress the child and give paracetamol elixir as soon as the temperature is recognized. Sponging with tepid water, particularly in the flexures, groin and axillae will also help to keep the temperature down. These methods are often very successful, but the parents must not be made to feel guilty if the child goes on to have a convulsion. In some children the convulsion occurs almost as soon as the fever develops.

Children with frequent febrile convulsions may need continuous anticonvulsant treatment and this is discussed below. The indications for continuous medication in these children are:

1 More than four febrile convulsions per year.
2 Prolonged seizures.
3 When they occur in the presence of underlying neurological abnormality.
4 A strong first degree family history of epilepsy.

Following the first febrile convulsion the parent will want to know what the risk of further febrile convulsions is and the risk of non-febrile epilepsy later in life. The prognosis following the first febrile convulsion depends on a number of factors. Bad features (high risk of recurrence) include onset below the age of 1 year, prolonged single convulsion (more than 15 minutes), multiple convulsions in one febrile illness, unilateral seizure, previous evidence of neurological impairment and family history of epilepsy. Low-risk children will have a 10–15% chance of further febrile convulsions and the risk of non-febrile epileptic seizures is about 2–5%. Girls have a higher risk of repeated febrile convulsions than boys.

A particularly well-recognized complication of prolonged febrile convulsion is damage to the hippocampus. This has been described as *mesial temporal sclerosis* and is an important cause of subsequent temporal lobe epilepsy (see p. 288).

STATUS EPILEPTICUS

This is defined as a prolonged single convulsion lasting 20 minutes or more, or a series of shorter convulsions with failure to regain consciousness between them. It is a potentially very serious problem and may be life-threatening if breathing is impaired. Prolonged seizure activity may cause irreversible cerebral injury. Status epilepticus may also refer to status petit mal or partial seizures.

Rapid treatment of prolonged seizures is necessary. In hospital, medication such as diazepam can be given intravenously. Parents with a child at risk of prolonged seizures can be given rectal diazepam (Stesolid) to give before the doctor arrives. Continuous anticonvulsant medication is necessary in all children with regular epileptic fits (see below).

INFANTILE SPASMS

This condition, also known as West's disease, affects infants most commonly between 3 and 6 months of age. The diagnosis is strongly suggested by the pattern of the seizure. Characteristically the child suddenly flexes the neck and trunk as if bowing. For this reason they have been called

Table 17.4 Causes of infantile spasms.

Congenital cerebral anomaly
Prenatal infection
Cerebral birth injury
Tuberous sclerosis
Post-pertussis vaccination
Post-meningitis
Untreated phenylketonuria
Hypoglycaemic cerebral injury
Idiopathic

salaam attacks. The arms fly out and the legs are drawn up or extend and may resemble a spontaneous Moro reflex. The attack only lasts a second and is often followed by a cry as though the child is in pain. The spasms may be very frequent and occur in runs.

Infants with infantile spasms fall into one of three groups. The most common is the symptomatic group where a clear diagnosis can be made to account for the spasms. Table 17.4 lists the more commonly recognized causes. A small group of children who develop infantile spasms show clear evidence of a preceding neuro-developmental disorder with severe retardation or cerebral palsy. No definite cause for the developmental problems or the spasms can be found. In approximately one-third of cases the children may appear to be developing normally until the onset of the spasms and this is referred to as the idiopathic group. The prognosis in this group may be relatively good.

The diagnosis is confirmed by EEG examination which shows a very disorganized trace which is referred to as hypsarrhythmia. All children with infantile spasms should be carefully examined and investigated for the conditions listed in Table 17.4.

A course of ACTH by intramuscular injection is often effective in reducing or stopping the fits. Sometimes the EEG may normalize with little in the way of clinical improvement and vice versa.

The prognosis is usually very poor. This is particularly the case where the child showed abnormalities prior to the onset of the infantile spasms. Idiopathic cases and those occurring after immunization have the best prognosis and up to one-half of these will recover completely.

PETIT MAL

This condition is a relatively rare cause of generalized seizures, most commonly seen in girls between the ages of 5 and 10 years. It accounts for about 5% of all childhood epilepsy and there is a family history of epilepsy in one-third of cases. The diagnosis is usually suspected on taking a clinical history and confirmed on EEG.

Petit mal presents with absences lasting 5–15 seconds but never longer than 30 seconds. The eyes stare vacantly and there are no associated movements of the limbs but there may be flickering of the eyes. The child may have frequent attacks and this is usually noticed at school as performance in class deteriorates. Attacks can often be produced in the clinic by inducing the child to hyperventilate. This is most easily performed by asking him to keep the wheel of a toy windmill turning by blowing on it.

Diagnosis is confirmed by EEG examination. This characteristically shows a symmetrical three cycle per second spike and wave pattern throughout both hemispheres.

Treatment is considered later.

Prognosis is usually good. Petit mal disappears spontaneously by 15 years in about 75% of cases. Some children go on to develop grand mal epilepsy, and this is more likely in those who present with petit mal after the age of 10 years.

MYOCLONIC SEIZURES

This is a relatively vague group of disorders which occurs in a variety of forms. It is often associated with pre-existing neuro-developmental disorders, commonly mental retardation. In some cases no underlying cause can be found.

Myoclonic fits may occur at any age but are most commonly seen in young children and infants. Characteristically the children present with sudden symmetrical mass jerking often involving all limbs. The head may jerk forward and they may be confused with infantile spasms. They may be very frequent and appear to distress the child.

Another type of myoclonic epilepsy is akinetic attacks. In these the children lose consciousness transiently and may fall to the ground, immediately get up and resume what they had been doing. Sometimes these falls may produce severe lacerations particularly to the unprotected face and head. Very brief episodes may be confused with petit mal.

There are no typical EEG abnormalities in this condition but the trace is usually abnormal and may show slow spike and wave discharges or diffuse slowing.

Drug treatment is discussed later but intractable cases may respond to a ketogenic diet. This is a diet low in carbohydrate and high in fat which induces the production of endogenous ketone bodies and these inhibit neuronal discharge. Ketogenic diets may be of value in many forms of epilepsy where drug treatment is unsuccessful.

Prognosis is poor particularly in children who present early in life; within 2 years of birth. Those presenting at an older age may have a relatively good prognosis particularly if there is a family history of epilepsy.

Partial seizures

This refers to focal epileptic seizures and in children without neurological handicap they are relatively uncommon. They are also called partial seizures. Partial seizures are due to some underlying cerebral injury or malformation that produces an epileptic discharge in a particular region of the brain. If this focus is in the motor cortex then the seizures will affect a limb or the facial muscles controlled by this area. If the focus is in the temporal lobe then bizarre sensations, smells or emotions may be the effect of the epileptic discharge. For this reason many children with focal seizures have pre-existing cerebral injury, most commonly cerebral palsy or hydrocephalus.

Rarely epileptic discharges occur in a localized area of cortex with no spread to adjacent areas. This causes clonic movements of a limb which may last for hours or sometimes days. This is called *epilepsia partialis continua*. Todd's paralysis is the result of a grand mal focal fit and can leave the child with temporary paralysis of the affected side that may last for minutes or hours.

BENIGN FOCAL EPILEPSY OF CHILDHOOD

This is a relatively common form of partial epilepsy occurring in childhood and there is often a strong family history of epilepsy. It usually develops in children between 7 and 10 years of age and the seizures occur almost exclusively at night. The timing of the convulsions often makes an exact description of their focal nature difficult. EEG confirms the focal nature of the spike and wave discharges. The seizures respond well to standard anticonvulsant therapy and almost all the children are free of convulsions in their adult years.

TEMPORAL LOBE EPILEPSY (TLE)

This is the commonest form of partial seizure and accounts for about 10% of all types of childhood epilepsy. It is usually due to a focus within the temporal lobe although some children also have a more diffuse form of cerebral injury with developmental delay and/or cerebral palsy. A particularly important cause of TLE occurs following prolonged febrile convulsions. Prolonged seizure activity is most likely to selectively damage the areas of brain with the highest metabolic demands such as the hippocampus which lies within the temporal lobe. This lesion is referred to as mesial temporal sclerosis. Gliosis and 'scarring' results which later serves as the focus for seizures.

The onset of TLE may be difficult to determine particularly in young children because the symptoms are so vague and beyond their description. TLE may take many forms. The child may have frightening visual or auditory hallucinations causing them to become inexplicably terrified. There may be an intense sense of smell or forboding. In milder cases there may be a sensation similar to *déjà vu*. As the viscera are controlled by the temporal lobe, strange abdominal symptoms may be described, such as pain or an unpleasant churning sensation.

Major behavioural problems may be related to TLE. Some children and adolescents develop 'fits' of uncontrolled rage often with no precipitating cause. These children may be referred to the psychiatric department before making the diagnosis.

Some children have more complicated TLE with extension of epileptic activity beyond the temporal lobe into the motor cortex, and grand mal convulsions may occur following the sensory disturbance. Automatic actions, sometimes quite complicated, may also occur with TLE. Sometimes these may be very brief and can be confused with petit mal.

An EEG may be particularly helpful in confirming the diagnosis, but if the focus is deep within the temporal lobe special techniques may be necessary to obtain EEG support for the diagnosis. An X-ray CT scan may show some evidence of focal pathology or atrophy within the temporal lobe.

Drug treatment is discussed on p. 290. Surgical removal of part of the affected temporal lobe which is precipitating the epilepsy can be performed in some cases of intractable TLE where there is clear evidence of a discrete lesion causing the fits.

The prognosis varies depending on the extent of the underlying cerebral damage. One-third of children are subsequently seizure-free, one-third are independent but need to remain on anticonvulsant therapy for life, and one-third die or are severely disabled and require constant supervision for life.

Differential diagnosis of convulsions

The diagnosis of convulsions in children is usually fairly clear from the history but sometimes major difficulties may occur. A careful history is the most important method by which to determine the

Tabl 17.5   Differential diagnosis of convulsions.

Faints
Breath-holding spells
Reflex anoxic seizures
Cardiac arrhythmias
Vertigo
Migraine
Masturbation
Hypoglycaemia
Hysteria
Drugs (oculogyric crises)
Munchausen syndrome by proxy (p. 528)

nature of the episode. Table 17.5 lists the common conditions that can be mistaken for convulsions.

FAINTS

These are the commonest events confused with seizures. They are often preceded by some precipitating event or circumstance such as prolonged standing, unpleasant sights or a vivid imagination. The feature of faints is that the child suddenly becomes very pale immediately before falling and slowly sinks to the ground. In a faint he may make an attempt to save himself from injury which does not happen in convulsions. Faints are due to sudden cerebral ischaemia and recovery occurs very rapidly when blood supply to the brain is restored as the victim lies prone. Occasionally a faint may be followed by a few clonic movements and there may rarely be urinary incontinence.

BREATH-HOLDING ATTACKS

These are common in infants below the age of 3 years and take two different forms. In one type, the child once angered takes a deep breath and holds it on inspiration, goes intensely blue in the face and may lose consciousness at the end with rapid recovery (see also p. 31).

A second form is described as *pallid syncope* or *reflex anoxic seizures*. They are not convulsive but due to vagal stimulation precipitating a short period of asystole. This is always self-limiting. The child starts to cry vigorously, then goes deathly pale, is cold and clammy and completely floppy. A few beats of clonus are not uncommon and there is rapid recovery.

CARDIAC ARRHYTHMIA

Sudden asystole occurs rarely and may be associated with an abnormality of cardiac conduction such as prolonged Q–T interval (p. 226). They may be precipitated by vigorous exercise. Asystole may also occur as the result of vagal stimulation and this has been reported to be associated with breath holding.

Table 17.6 The first line anticonvulsant drugs in the management of various forms of convulsions in childhood.

Type of convulsion	First line drugs
Neonatal seizures	Phenobarbitone Clonazepam
Grand mal epilepsy	Sodium valproate Phenytoin Carbamazepine
Febrile convulsions (prophylaxis)	Phenobarbitone Sodium valproate
Infantile spasms	ACTH Clonazepam Nitrazepam
Petit mal	Ethosuximide Sodium valproate
Myoclonic seizures	Clonazepam Sodium valproate
Partial seizures	Carbamazepine
Temporal lobe epilepsy	Carbamazepine Phenytoin

Treatment

The keystone in the management of seizures is anticonvulsant medication of which a variety of very effective agents exist. The drug selected for first use depends on the type of epileptic convulsions that the child manifests. Table 17.6 lists the most appropriate anticonvulsants for different forms of epileptic seizures. One drug should be used to maximum tolerance before a second anticonvulsant is introduced.

Monitoring of the serum level of most anticonvulsants is now possible on a routine basis with the exception of the benzodiazepines. The metabolism of the major anticonvulsants is often unpredictable and the only way to ensure optimal use of these drugs is to monitor serum levels on a regular basis. Too low a level of anticonvulsant and adequate control may not be achieved. Too high a level may cause major toxic effects. The dosage of all the antibiotics is age-related and increments on a regular basis should be made in light of the serum levels which must be kept in the therapeutic range.

The duration of anticonvulsant therapy depends on the indications for treatment. Febrile convulsions are not likely to occur after the age of 5 years and prolonged prophylactic treatment beyond this time is of little value. Petit mal and grand mal convulsions in children who are otherwise normal carry a good prognosis in terms of spontaneous termination of seizures. For these children cessation of therapy 3–4 years after the last convulsion is recommended. Children who have cerebral palsy or other developmental problems as well as convulsions are likely to require anticonvulsant medication for a considerably longer period of time and this may need to be life-long.

Phenobarbitone. This is the oldest of the effective anticonvulsants and is still used as the first line anticonvulsant in the neonatal period. It may cause hyperactivity in some children even in therapeutic dosage and it is best to change the infant to an alternative medication at 6 months of age if continuous medication is still required.

Phenobarbitone is also a very effective prophylactic drug for use in febrile convulsions, but this role may be superceded by sodium valproate.

Sodium valproate. This is a very effective anticonvulsant for use in children. The dosage is gradually built up over several weeks and it is usually well tolerated. It is known to be associated with severe and sometimes fatal hepatic necrosis but this is very rare. It should not be used in children with known impairment of liver function.

Carbamazepine. This is an effective and well-tolerated anticonvulsant, particularly useful in the management of partial seizures and temporal lobe epilepsy. It is also very effective in the treatment of grand mal epilepsy. It appears to be a remarkably well-tolerated and safe drug in childhood.

Headaches

This is a very common symptom and rarely indicates severe disease. Pain referred to as headache may arise from the intracranial blood vessels (migraine), the meninges, stretch of the dural membranes (raised intracranial pressure), the muscles of the scalp, the facial sinuses, temporomandibular joints or referred from other sites.

In the evaluation of the child with headaches the following points should be clarified:
1 Whether the headaches are acute or chronic.
2 Is the headache of sudden onset suggestive of a vascular cause?
3 Are there associated features such as vomiting, photophobia, or alteration in conscious level?
4 Is the headache worse in the mornings?
5 Whether there is a family history of headaches.
6 Visual disturbances such as occur in migraine.

Headache can be divided into three main groups; primary due to disorders of function, secondary due to intracerebral disease, and headaches due to referred pain (see Table 17.7).

The child should be examined carefully and the fundi visualized. Papilloedema requires immediate CT scan. Fever and neck stiffness suggests meningitis and the child should have a lumbar puncture. Sinuses, ears and teeth should all be carefully examined to exclude referred pain.

MIGRAINE

This is a common condition and may occur in children as young as 5 years. Migraine is due to disorder in control of the size of the larger cranial arteries. Initially there is vasoconstriction which causes the aura, followed by vasodilatation and headache. Migraine may occur several times a week or considerably less frequently. There are often precipitating factors such as following a period of stress, or a sensitivity to certain foods such as dark chocolate. The aura most commonly produces visual symptoms. These include flashing lights, fortification spectra around bright objects and scotomata. The latter is a blind area in the centre of the visual field. Rarely, migraine may be associated with aphasia or hemiplegia, but this is almost never permanent.

There is no confirmatory test and the diagnosis is made on the following features:
1 Episodic nature.
2 Aura.
3 Nausea in 90% of cases.
4 The headache is usually unilateral.
5 Strong family history.
6 Impairment of normal function during the attack.

Management. The acute headache is treated by simple analgesics such as paracetamol and an antiemetic may also be helpful.

Prophylactic treatment should be considered for regular attacks. Useful continuous medication includes propranolol, clonidine and pizotifen (Sanomigran).

CLUSTER HEADACHES

This is a separate entity to migraine but the two are often confused. In this condition the child complains of frequent headaches lasting over a period of weeks or months which then fade away

Table 17.7 Causes of headache.

Primary	Secondary	Referred
Migraine	Hypertension	Sinusitis
Cluster headaches	Hydrocephalus	Otitis
Tension headaches	Post-lumbar puncture	Caries
Periodic syndrome	Intracranial haemorrhage	Temporomandibular
Reflex (ice cream	Post-traumatic	joint
headache)	Benign intracranial	Glaucoma
	hypertension	
	Tumour	

perhaps to recur the same time the following year. The characteristic features of these headaches are that they occur behind the eye and are unilateral. Sometimes there is redness and watering of the affected eye.

TENSION HEADACHES

These are well recognized in adults but may occur in older children. They are due to stress and sustained contraction of the temporalis muscle and muscles of the neck. The headache is diffuse and the child cannot localize it as he can for migraine or cluster headaches.

'PERIODIC SYNDROME'

Headaches occur as part of the so-called periodic syndrome which includes recurrent abdominal pain, vomiting and often limb pains. An individual child often focuses on one particular type of pain and complains frequently of it. The pains rarely seem to disable the child and they frequently occur during school, rarely at weekends and holidays.

There is a strong emotional overlay to this condition and it is discussed elsewhere. In all children with headaches other causes must be considered.

RAISED INTRACRANIAL PRESSURE (see also p. 296)

A variety of important conditions cause intracranial hypertension and headache. The headache is usually constant but may be worse in the mornings. It is associated with vomiting and the conscious level may be depressed. Careful neurological examination usually reveals some deficit, often ataxia. Papilloedema is usually present except in infants.

Ataxia

Ataxia is a disorder of movement involving incoordination and disturbance of balance. It is age-dependent in that the child must have achieved the neurological maturity to be able to sit, stand, reach or walk before degrees of ataxia can be

Table 17.8 Causes of ataxia in childhood.

Acute ataxia
Drugs
   Phenytoin
   Piperazine
Toxins
   Alcohol
Cerebellar infection (abscess)
Varicella (chicken pox) encephalitis
Acute cerebellar ataxia of childhood
Tumour
Head trauma
Acute hydrocephalus
Vascular accident

Chronic ataxia
Friedreich's ataxia
Ataxia–telangiectasia

---

identified. The co-ordination of movement is a complicated neurological process involving the integration of a number of systems including proprioception, and cerebellar function.

Clinical features suggestive of ataxia include titubation (persistent head wobbling) and wide-based gait. Observation of the handwriting is useful to identify relatively mild ataxia. The ataxic child cannot walk a straight line heel-to-toe and limb tone is usually reduced.

The causes of ataxia can be divided into acute and chronic and these are listed in Table 17.8. Many of these conditions are discussed elsewhere.

ACUTE CEREBELLAR ATAXIA

This is a condition that affects relatively young children. It usually occurs after a viral infection, particularly varicella. The child becomes acutely ataxic involving the trunk and limbs, often with titubation and nausea. Ataxia worsens over several days before stabilizing and gradually improving. The child is uncommonly left with residual deficits.

The CT scan is normal (this must be done to exclude a posterior fossa tumour) and lumbar puncture contains a relatively small number of white cells. There is no specific treatment.

FRIEDREICH'S ATAXIA

This is the commonest cause of progressive ataxia in childhood and is an autosomal recessive disorder. The first symptoms occur between 5 and 15 years with ataxia and absent tendon reflexes. Progression is relatively slow and affected patients develop clumsiness, scoliosis, pes cavus, dysarthria and muscle weakness. Electrocardiography shows abnormalities due to cardiomyopathy in the majority of cases.

Independent walking gradually deteriorates and the patient becomes wheelchair bound at an average age of 25 years. There is no treatment.

ATAXIA–TELANGIECTASIA

This is an autosomal recessive disorder characterized by features involving both brain and skin. Ataxia is first noticed when the child starts to walk and becomes progressively more severe to involve trunk, hands and articulation leading to dysarthria. The children become wheelchair bound in their second decade. Death occurs in the third decade due to innanition.

This disease is associated with features in other systems. Telangiectasia affecting the conjunctiva appear at about the time the ataxia is noticed and later develop on the skin. There is often a disorder of eye movement. Other associated conditions are an immune deficiency and predisposition to neoplastic disorders.

Involuntary movements

This is a complicated group of disorders in which the children show abnormal and involuntary movement at rest. This must be distinguished from ataxia where the abnormal movement is only apparent during voluntary muscle activity.

The abnormal movements are described by a number of terms:

Tic or habit spasm. These are common and usually benign. They are described in detail on p. 28.

Tremor. This refers to fast repetitive movements usually of the hands when held out straight and away from the body. They may be of a fine or coarse nature. Tremor may be entirely benign and familial.

Athetosis. These are writhing movements of the limbs, particularly the hands. The affected person is constantly moving and the fingers hyperextend as if playing the piano and bridging the keyboard. Facial grimacing also occurs.

Chorea. This refers to irregular, involuntary movements more spasmodic and violent than athetosis. There is a gradation between athetosis and chorea and the term choreo-athetoid is usually used to describe these movements.

Abnormal movements are usually due to disorders involving the basal ganglia. In the past the two commonest causes of choreo-athetosis were cerebral palsy due to kernicterus (p. 108) and Sydenham's chorea. These are now rarely seen. Wilson's disease (p. 212) is associated with choreo-athetosis but abnormal movements in Huntington's chorea are rarely seen in childhood.

SYDENHAM'S CHOREA

This is now a rare condition and in 75% of cases there is a previous history of rheumatic fever (p. 476). It may be an allergic reaction to the haemolytic *Streptococcus*.

The patients present at an average age of between 10 and 15 years and there is a striking predilection for girls. The onset is insidious, the child develops uncontrollable fidgets and drops things, often incurring punishment from unsuspecting parents. On examination there are involuntary, purposeless movements which are non-repetitive and are increased when the child is aware of being watched or asked to do a manual task. Rarely the movements only affect one side and this is referred to as hemichorea. Facial grimacing is common and dysarthria may occur. If the child squeezes the examiner's hand there is inconstancy of grasp. The fingers assume the piano playing posture described above. The limb tone is reduced and the muscle power weak.

The choreiform movements may respond to sedation with phenobarbitone or chlorpromazine. A course of penicillin should be given to eradicate the haemolytic *Streptococcus*.

The condition may last for months, with relapses being common. Progress can be followed by weekly records of the child's handwriting. Eventually the movements subside completely but some patients are left with residual cardiac damage due to coincidental rheumatic carditis. Recurrences are relatively common but rare if the child has been normal for 2 years after the initial episode.

Hyperactivity

Hyperactivity is a much misused term and many normally active, but disobedient children are mistakenly labelled as hyperactive. The main features of hyperactivity are lack of concentration, impulsivity and distractability. If a child can sit and concentrate on television, or other passive activity for more than 5 minutes then he is most unlikely to be clinically hyperactive. Mentally retarded or psychotic children show features of hyperactivity but this should be obvious on historical enquiry and examination.

The nature of true hyperactivity is unknown. There may be abnormality in the processing of sensory input into the brain and the child cannot habituate to many minor or irrelevent stimuli. This may be a form of discrete cerebral injury or biochemical dysfunction. An alternative hypothesis is that the child becomes hyperactive as the result of toxic substances presented to him in the environment. In particular, food additives have been implicated including naturally occurring salicylates and tartrazine.

Emotional disturbance and drug ingestion (particularly phenobarbitone) can also result in hyperactive behaviour and these should be considered. Bizarre behaviour has been reported in children with iron-deficiency anaemia.

Amphetamines have been used to treat hyperactivity. Withdrawing additives from the diet has also benefited some children. The natural history of hyperactivity is to improve as the child matures.

Coma

Coma is a poorly understood condition in which the brain drops its metabolic rate and cerebral function falls to minimal levels with little or no conscious activity. This may be a protective state and occurs following a large number of insults.

Altered states of consciousness exist between coma and normal awake cerebral activity and these abnormal states can be described as encephalopathy. Onset of coma may be rapid or delayed and the child passes through stages of lethargy, obtundation and stupor into coma. Table 17.9 lists the commoner causes of coma in children.

The diagnosis of coma is not difficult, but discovering the cause of it may require many investigations. The depth of coma can be measured objectively using the Glasgow coma scale which

Table 17.9   Causes of coma and encephalopathy in children.

Rapid onset
Head trauma
Vascular accident
Hypoxic-ischaemic encephalopathy
Status epilepticus

Slower onset
Drug induced
Raised intracranial pressure
   Tumour
   Hydrocephalus
Infection
   Meningitis
   Encephalitis
Hypertensive encephalopathy
Metabolic disorders
   Hypoglycaemia
   Diabetic ketoacidosis
   Organic acidurias
   Amino-acidurias
   Lactic acidaemias
   Dehydration
   Uraemia
Reye's syndrome
Hepatic encephalopathy
Water intoxication
Hysteria
Burns

records motor responses to command or painful stimuli, the best verbal response of the patient and the degree of eye opening to command or pain.

The management of coma must be in an intensive care unit with facilities for investigating neurological function (see Chapter 14). Accurate prognosis may be extremely difficult but the concept of irreversible brain stem death is now accepted in most countries and life support can be withdrawn in such patients despite continued cardiac activity.

The child with a large head

A large head is referred to as macrocephaly, and a large brain as megalencephaly. Hydrocephaly means an excess of CSF and this is usually associated with macrocephaly. Head size is clearly age-dependent. It is necessary to refer to centile charts in order to establish whether a child's head is abnormally large for his age. Measurements within two standard deviations of the mean are generally taken to be normal.

The clinical assessment of large head includes a careful developmental assessment and neurological examination. The head circumference of both parents should also be measured as familial macrocephaly is common.

The simplest classification of the child with a large head is to divide the condition into:
1 Hydrocephalus.
2 Hydranencephaly.
3 Macrocephaly without hydrocephalus.
4 Megalencephaly.

Hydrocephalus

Hydrocephalus is the end result of a number of different pathological processes as listed in Table 17.10. Hydrocephalus as a cause of enlarged head size only occurs in infants with unfused sutures. Accumulation of CSF under pressure will cause the sutures to separate and the head size will increase disproportionately. The infant may be born with overt hydrocephalus (p. 146) and this condition is most commonly due to spina bifida. Hydrocephalus occurring in older children will cause

Table 17.10 Causes of hydrocephalus.

Communicating
Post-haemorrhagic
Post-meningitic
Choroid plexus tumour

Non-communicating
Arnold–Chiari malformation and spina bifida (p. 146)
Post-meningitic
Post-haemorrhagic
Intracranial tumour
Aqueduct stenosis
Dandy–Walker malformation
Achondroplasia

an increase in intracranial pressure (ICP) because the head size does not increase and this is dealt with in the next section.

The management of hydrocephalus is to insert a ventriculo-peritoneal shunt to by-pass the obstruction to CSF drainage.

DANDY–WALKER MALFORMATION

This is due to a cystic malformation in the posterior fossa which is almost always associated with hydrocephalus due to blockage of the intracerebral CSF drainage system. Hydrocephalus may not develop for several months after birth.

STENOSIS OF THE AQUEDUCT OF SYLVIUS

After neural tube defects this is the commonest cause of isolated congenital hydrocephalus. Although it is usually sporadic it may be inherited as an X-linked condition.

Hydranencephaly

In this condition there is complete loss of cerebral tissue above the basal ganglia due to infarction of the internal carotid arteries in the first trimester of pregnancy. Cerebral structures supplied by the vertebral arteries are spared. The head size may be normal at birth, or enlarged, but the prognosis is hopeless and there is no treatment. It may be difficult to distinguish severe hydrocephalus from hydranencephaly on imaging techniques.

Macrocephaly without hydrocephalus

This is a common condition and refers to a child with head size above the limit of 'normal' for his age. The head growth is usually parallel but above the 97th centile. There are no signs of progressive increase in size.

It is most commonly due to a condition referred to as *external hydrocephalus*. This is due to an excess of CSF over the surface of the brain but the intracerebral ventricles are not particularly dilated. It is probably due to mild impairment of CSF absorption at the arachnoid granulations. There is almost always one parent with an abnormally large head. Provided the child is developmentally normal, no treatment is required.

Infants who have a rapid growth spurt after premature birth and those with severe intra-uterine growth retardation may have disproportionately large head size compared to body weight. This is because brain growth is the last to slow down under conditions of starvation. In these children it is not that the head is too big, but rather that the body is too small.

Megalencephaly

This is a rare condition and is usually due to abnormal deposition of material in the brain associated with a genetically inherited disorder. These children usually have severely abnormal development. CT scans will show a large brain with no evidence of excess CSF within the ventricles or subarachnoid space.

Raised intracranial pressure

This is an important paediatric problem which must be recognized rapidly and treated effectively. The brain is contained within a rigid box (the skull) and if brain swelling occurs following an insult then at a point the space within the skull will be completely taken up and further swelling

Table 17.11 Causes of raised intracranial pressure.

Hydrocephalus
Cerebral oedema
 Post-traumatic
 Post-hypoxic
Tumour
Intracranial haemorrhage
Cerebral abscess
Meningoencephalitis
Reye's syndrome
Status epilepticus
Benign intracranial hypertension
Hypertensive encephalopathy
Lead encephalopathy

will cause the intracranial pressure to rise. Initially the systemic blood pressure will rise to maintain blood perfusion through the brain and the heart rate falls. This is known as *Cushing's response*. The time will however come when cerebral perfusion falls and the brain is further damaged by ischaemia.

The causes of raised intracranial pressure (ICP) are listed in Table 17.11. Raised ICP is usually associated with abnormal neurological signs and the conscious level is depressed. In younger children, the sutures are not fused and the head size may increase to compensate to some extent for brain swelling. If there is slow onset of intracranial hypertension as occurs in hydrocephalus then the anterior fontanelle bulges and the head size will increase and the child shows the classical sunsetting sign (Plate 5). In young children raised ICP will be accompanied by systemic disturbance including vomiting, irritability and possibly changes in conscious level.

Older children with slow onset of intracranial hypertension will complain of headache, which is often worse in the morning. Rapid onset of raised ICP usually causes the child to become lethargic, obtunded and finally comatose. Papilloedema is seen in older children but may be a late sign in infants.

Urgent investigation is necessary in these children. Lumbar puncture is contraindicated in any child with suspected intracranial hypertension and a CT scan is essential to diagnose or exclude hydrocephalus or tumour as the cause of the brain swelling. Severe meningitis may also cause cerebral oedema and raised ICP may cause coning if a lumbar puncture is attempted.

Treatment of intracranial hypertension involves stabilizing the patient and if respiration is compromised he should be mechanically ventilated. The $Paco_2$ should be kept low (about 3.5 kPa) to reduce brain swelling. Mannitol is useful as an osmotic agent to reduce the extracellular fluid within the brain. Treatment is directed towards the cause of the intracranial hypertension wherever this is possible.

BENIGN INTRACRANIAL HYPERTENSION

In this condition the child presents with signs of raised intracranial pressure but neither evidence of hydrocephalus nor cerebral tumour is present on CT examination. It is most commonly seen in the presence of chronic otitis media, but may also develop during the course of steroid treatment. The administration of tetracycline has also been implicated.

The children present with headache most commonly, but visual disturbances and vomiting are also seen. Overt papilloedema is rare, but blurred disc margins is relatively common. The diagnosis is made by exclusion of other conditions and CT scan examination is essential. The condition is generally self-limiting and requires no specific treatment.

The child who is weak

Persistent weakness is not a common symptom in childhood and when present may be due to a large number of disorders. Weakness may be due to pathology involving almost every level of the nervous system from upper motor neurone to muscle fibre. Table 17.12 summarizes the causes and anatomical site of weakness in children.

CLINICAL FEATURES

The features of the floppy neonate and infant are described below. In older children weakness may

Table 17.12   Causes of weakness in children with the anatomical level of the disease process.

Brain
Cerebral palsy
Vascular accident

Spinal cord
Transverse myelitis
Cord compression
  Tumour
  Abscess
Trauma

Anterior horn cell
Spinal muscular atrophy
Poliomyelitis

Peripheral nerve
Guillain–Barre syndrome
Polyneuropathies
  Charcot-Marie-Tooth disease

Neuromuscular junction
Myasthenia gravis
Botulism
Drugs

Muscle
Muscular dystrophy
Myotonic dystrophy
Mitochondrial myopathies
Metabolic myopathies
Periodic paralysis
Dermatomyositis
Polymyositis

not occur until somewhat later in life. The child may achieve independent locomotion before weakness is apparent and then gradually loses the ability to walk. There is often a family history of weakness.

Each muscle group should be assessed separately. Some disorders involve proximal muscle weakness and others affect distal musculature preferentially. Observing the child rising from the floor to stand upright is a good test of proximal weakness as those who are weak show Gowers' sign. Special note must also be made of sensation, tendon reflexes, the presence of fasciculation and myotonia.

INVESTIGATION

Investigation of the weak patient includes assessment of both muscle and nerve function. The electromyogram (EMG) is elicited by a fine needle electrode inserted into a weak muscle, often the quadriceps. Motor or sensory nerve conduction velocity measurements determine whether a peripheral neuropathy exists. Definitive diagnosis of muscle disease can only be made after examination of a needle biopsy from an affected muscle using appropriate staining techniques. This is performed in specialized centres.

Muscular dystrophy

This is a group of genetically inherited disorders in which there is progressive weakness due to atrophy of skeletal muscle. Different types are classified according to the muscle groups involved. The muscle fibres swell, then undergo hyaline degeneration, being replaced by connective tissue and fat. This connective tissue and fat take up more space than the muscle it replaces, giving the limb the impression of being enlarged, hence the term 'pseudohypertrophy'.

PSEUDOHYPERTROPHIC MUSCULAR DYSTROPHY (DUCHENNE TYPE)

This form occurs only in boys, usually presenting during the first 5 years of life and is transmitted as a sex-linked recessive character with a high mutation rate. Approximately 30% of cases arise as the result of a new mutation. The disease starts with symmetrical involvement of the pelvic girdle muscles and spreads up to the shoulder girdle. Pseudohypertrophy occurs mainly in the calf muscles, giving a false appearance of muscle strength. The gait first becomes waddling, and then the child has difficulty climbing stairs. Weakness of the pelvic and spinal muscles leads to marked lordosis and difficulty in getting up from the ground and he demonstrates Gowers' sign.

The disease progresses steadily and relatively rapidly, the child usually being unable to walk within 10 years of the onset. The intelligence is usually below average. Involvement of cardiac muscle by the dystrophic process is common and this may cause death.

Patients have an increased serum level of creatine phosphokinase (CPK), this being elevated before the onset of symptoms and can be used as an early diagnostic test in male infants of affected families. It is only positive if the CPK level is increased 1 month after birth. Some female carriers may also be recognized by this test, but 30% have normal levels. Reliable DNA techniques are now available to recognize the female carriers.

There is no treatment and death, usually from pneumonia, occurs during the late teens.

FACIOSCAPULOHUMERAL MUSCULAR DYSTROPHY

This type may start at any time from early childhood to late adult life, occurring both in boys and girls. It is usually transmitted by an autosomal dominant gene, but occasionally by an autosomal recessive gene. The muscles of the face and shoulder girdle are involved and the facial expression becomes mask-like. The eyes cannot be closed completely, the mouth droops so the child looks as if he is pouting, and weakness prevents him from whistling when requested. Involvement of the shoulder girdle causes 'winging' of the scapula, and the hand can be raised to the head only by swinging the arm round. Pseudohypertrophy is rare in this form of dystrophy.

Progression of the disease is very slow so that the disability is slight; most patients remain active to a normal age.

BECKER-TYPE DYSTROPHY

This is similar to Duchenne-type dystrophy in that it is inherited as an X-linked condition but usually presents in the second decade and has a much slower progression. Pseudohypertrophy is less obvious than in Duchenne dystrophy, but pes cavus is often a prominent feature.

LIMB GIRDLE MUSCULAR DYSTROPHY

This type of muscular dystrophy starts in late childhood or shortly after puberty. It is usually transmitted as an autosomal recessive gene but is occasionally dominant. Both the shoulder and pelvic girdle muscles are affected. The disease is slowly progressive so that the patient is usually unable to walk within 20–30 years of onset.

MYASTHENIA GRAVIS

This is a rare disease in children and is due to an abnormality of the neuromuscular junction causing abnormal fatigability of the voluntary muscles. There are a number of forms of this condition.

Transient neonatal myasthenia

This is due to antibodies acquired from the mother who has the disease but who may be asymptomatic at the time of delivery. The infant presents with weakness which is relieved by neostigmine. It is a transient self-limiting condition with an excellent prognosis.

Congenital myasthenia

In this condition the mother is normal and the child shows weakness from birth. Ptosis and paralysis of certain eye movements (ophthalmoplegia) are a particular feature.

Juvenile onset myasthenia gravis

This condition is due to the production of antibodies against the post-synaptic acetyl choline receptors. The child usually presents with ptosis or ophthalmoplegia. Trunk and limb muscles are affected later. Muscle strength is at its best in the morning and the child becomes weaker as the day progresses. A simple test for fatigue is to ask the child to grip the doctor's hand repeatedly. The thymus may be enlarged on radiological examination and abnormalities are present in the gland in the majority of patients.

There is a dramatic improvement in muscle strength after the intramuscular injection of 1–2 mg edrophonium (Tensilon). The long-term treatment is with neostigmine which acts for longer than edrophonium. It works by depressing the activity of cholinesterase which normally destroys acetylcholine.

TRANSVERSE MYELITIS

This is due to an auto-immune post-infectious aetiology. The child presents with loss of function usually of the lower limbs together with some bladder dysfunction. It is often preceded by paraesthesia. Both a motor and sensory level can be found on clinical examination which is usually symmetrical. Rarely the myelitis may ascend with upper limb involvement.

The prognosis is good in the majority of cases with complete spontaneous improvement to normal function.

Other conditions to be considered in the differential diagnosis of transverse myelitis are cord compression due to a tumour, abscess or trauma. Myelography will detect cord compression.

GUILLAIN–BARRÉ SYNDROME

This is the commonest form of peripheral neuropathy affecting children. It is an auto-immune post-infectious condition and there is commonly a 10–14 day history of preceding upper respiratory tract infection.

The child presents with acute onset of symmetrical limb weakness, the legs often being weaker than the arms. In severe cases the respiratory muscles may be affected and cranial nerve involvement (particularly VII) may also occur. Sensory involvement may also occur with tingling or pins and needles.

Examination reveals weakness with absent or diminished tendon reflexes. Sensory loss is often present in a 'glove and stocking' distribution.

The CSF findings are usually characteristic with very high protein levels and few or absent cells.

The tendency is for this condition to improve spontaneously and specific treatment is probably unnecessary. Steroids have been used in some cases that are slow to resolve. In severe cases, ventilatory failure may develop due to respiratory muscle weakness and mechanical ventilation will be required.

The differential diagnosis of this condition includes poliomyelitis (not associated with sensory nerve changes) and dermatomyositis/polymyositis (see p. 477).

PERONEAL MUSCULAR ATROPHY (CHARCOT-MARIE-TOOTH DISEASE)

This is the commonest cause of chronic, progressive polyneuropathy seen in children. There is usually a positive family history and it is inherited either as an autosomal dominant or recessive condition.

The children present in the first decade with clumsiness, particularly on running, pes cavus and sometimes scoliosis. On examination they have distal weakness, loss of sensation and absent reflexes. Characteristically there is wasting of the distal lower limb muscles and this has been likened to an upside-down champagne bottle.

The prognosis is often very good with normal life expectancy and near normal function.

Other causes of polyneuropathy in childhood are *Déjérine–Sottas disease* (sensory neuropathy), *Refsum's disease*, and *Riley–Day syndrome*.

FACIAL NERVE PALSY

This is a cause of weakness isolated in one region of the face. It is seen most commonly in the newborn period following birth trauma (p. 112) or very rarely may be bilateral and involve other cranial nerves (the *Möbius syndrome*).

In older children facial nerve palsy may arise as a complication of meningitis or otitis media. Rarely facial nerve palsy may be spontaneous and is referred to as *Bell's palsy*. The onset is always sudden, sometimes a few minutes only, and complete lower motor neurone paralysis of the facial nerve occurs. Pain may precede the onset of paralysis but is otherwise not a feature of the condition.

The prognosis for spontaneous recovery is very good and no form of treatment has been shown to be of benefit. Systemic steroids are used in some cases.

The floppy infant

The earliest presentation of neuromuscular disease is in the newborn period. The infant may develop respiratory problems due to diaphragmatic or intercostal muscle weakness. He may be born with contractures due to lack of movement *in utero*. At, or shortly after birth, the child is seen to be floppy and may have restricted limb movement. A distinction must be made between the child who is floppy (hypotonic) but not weak, as is seen in Down's syndrome, and those who are floppy and weak. These children may have no anti-gravity movements at all. Table 17.13 lists the causes of the floppy infant.

SPINAL MUSCULAR ATROPHY (WERDNIG-HOFFMANN DISEASE)

This is due to progressive degeneration of the anterior horn cells within the spinal cord. This is one of the commonest causes of weakness at birth but symptoms may not develop until later on in

Paralytic	Non-paralytic
Spinal muscular atrophy (Werdnig–Hoffmann disease)	Hypotonic cerebral palsy
Congenital muscular dystrophy	Down's syndrome
Dystrophia myotonia congenita	Birth asphyxia
Congenital myopathy	Prader–Willi syndrome
Myasthenia gravis	Nutritional and metabolic disorders
	Skeletal and connective tissue disorders
	Drugs
	Benign congenital hypotonia

Table 17.13 Causes of congenital hypotonia.

the first year of life and rarely later still. The condition is inherited as an autosomal recessive disorder.

When the disease presents in the first few months of life it is known as Werdnig–Hoffmann disease. The infant is profoundly weak and can make few spontaneous movements and has no antigravity power. Despite this the child remains intellectually normal and he has a bright facial expression. The arms lie out abducted on the mattress and the legs take up the characteristic abducted 'frog posture' with external rotation of the hip.

The prognosis in Werdnig–Hoffmann disease is hopeless, the child dying of pneumonia in his first or second year. There is no effective treatment.

Spinal muscular atrophy may rarely present later in life and is less rapidly progressive.

CONGENITAL MUSCULAR DYSTROPHY

This autosomal recessive condition presents at birth with severe hypotonia and little spontaneous movement, but unlike spinal muscular atrophy is usually non-progressive. These infants often show severe contractures and represent one cause of arthrogryposis multiplex.

Treatment involves physiotherapy and the prognosis is good for independent walking in the majority of cases.

DYSTROPHIA MYOTONIA CONGENITA

Infants with this condition are often profoundly weak at birth but the diagnosis should be made on the basis of the clinical examination of the mother.

She demonstrates facial weakness and myotonia and is often unaware that she has a muscle disease. The infants show no myotonia.

Dystrophia myotonia is an autosomal dominant condition, but infants with congenital dystrophia myotonia are invariably born to mothers rather than fathers with this condition. This, together with gradual improvement in the infant with advancing age, suggests the effect of an, as yet, unknown transplacental agent which affects the baby's muscles.

Rarely this condition presents in older childhood. Weakness may be present in the face or limbs. Muscle stiffness resulting from myotonia is the presenting symptom and this can be demonstrated by tapping with a patellar hammer and observing a sustained muscle contraction. In adults the intelligence is usually impaired.

CONGENITAL MYOPATHY

This is a heterogeneous disorder due to a variety of biochemical abnormalities, all of which are rare. The diagnosis can only be confirmed by muscle biopsy and sophisticated histochemical staining techniques may be necessary. The prognosis is usually poor.

The neurocutaneous disorders

These are a group of genetically inherited disorders where there is involvement of both the nervous system and the skin. They commonly present in childhood and may produce symptoms in the neonatal period. Table 17.14 lists these conditions together with their mode of inheritance.

Table 17.14 The neurocutaneous conditions with their mode of inheritance.

Condition	Inheritance
Neurofibromatosis	Autosomal dominant
Tuberous sclerosis	Autosomal dominant but with high degree of mutation
Sturge–Weber syndrome	Usually sporadic
Ataxia–telangiectasia (p. 000)	Autosomal recessive
Incontinentia pigmenti	X-linked dominant; lethal in males

NEUROFIBROMATOSIS (VON RECKLINGHAUSEN'S DISEASE)

The neurological features of this condition include multiple benign neurofibromas of the peripheral nerves as well as neuromas and meningiomas. The peripheral neurofibromata may involve the skin; they are violet coloured at first, sometimes producing large, fleshy, pedunculated masses which are very unsightly. Other cutaneous manifestations include multiple *café-au-lait* spots and axillary freckling.

The first sign is often pigmented skin lesions and more than five such lesions, each over 0.5 cm in diameter, is strongly suggestive of neurofibromatosis. The child may present with convulsions. Neurological involvement is due to neuromas of the optic or auditory nerve or neurofibromas of the spinal cord causing compression. Mental retardation is more common in patients with neurofibromatosis.

TUBEROUS SCLEROSIS

The neurological features of this condition are due to small benign tumours or 'tubers'. They may be the focus of convulsions which often start in the first year of life. Infantile spasms are the classical neurological feature of tuberous sclerosis. Mental retardation is common and occurs even in children without convulsions. Rarely the tubers may cause obstructive hydrocephalus. Small white tumours may be seen in the retina.

The skin manifestations include de-pigmented (ash-leaf) patches, shagreen patches, and in older children an acne-like condition on the butterfly area of the face referred to as adenoma sebaceum. De-pigmented patches are most easily detected, particularly in small children, with a Wood's ultraviolet light.

Rhabdomyomata may be found in the heart and adenomata in the kidneys.

STURGE–WEBER SYNDROME

In this condition there is characteristically a congenital port wine naevus involving the mid-part

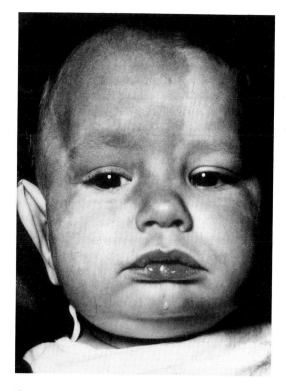

Fig 17.1   Right-sided port wine naevus in a child with Sturge–Weber syndrome.

of the face (Fig. 17.1), convulsions and spastic hemiplegia. The neurological effects result from angiomatous malformation of the leptomeninges on the same side as the capillary naevus. The angiomatous malformation tends to calcify and can be seen on X-ray CT examination. The major clinical effect is convulsions which may be difficult to control. Mental retardation is relatively common and glaucoma may occur.

Disorders of speech and language

Speech is the oral expression of language. The acquisition of language which is so important to our development as human beings requires the ability to hear and comprehend spoken words, to process such information and then to formulate and verbally express thought. Speech therefore ensues from a complicated process involving both comprehension and expression of the spoken word and results from the integration of complicated auditory, neurological and structural factors.

It is vital that parents are aware of the importance of their child's vocal play from a very early stage. If encouraged this leads the baby to be able to identify strings of sounds (i.e. words) with actions, objects and feelings. Gradually, as parents and others reinforce and reward the baby's babble by their responses, the foundations of speech and language development are laid down. Providing the child with a stimulating verbal environment will ensure that this gives the child the best chance of normal speech and language development.

Children with speech and language problems usually present to the doctor in one of three ways as shown in Table 17.15.

1 The child with little or no speech.
2 The child with unclear speech.
3 The child who is non-fluent.

Table 17.15 Modes of presentation of speech disorders in children together with the main causes.

Little or no speech
Familial speech delay
Hearing impairment
   Sensorineural
   Intermittent conductive
Lack of stimulation
Mental retardation (p. 327)
Autism (p. 345)
Congenital auditory imperception
Idiopathic

Unclear speech
Hearing impairment
Mental retardation
Structural abnormalities
   Cleft palate
Dysarthria
   Cerebral palsy
     Spasticity
     Athetosis
Dyspraxia

Non-fluency
Normal non-fluency
Stress
Stuttering

A speech and language problem may also be an important factor in a child who presents with behavioural problems.

Little or no speech

There is considerable variation in the age at which normal children speak, but if a child has no words at all by 18 months then this should be taken seriously. Speech delay may be due to the child being able to communicate adequately by means of gesture. Speech will also be slow to develop if the child has little incentive for speech. This may occur if his needs are constantly anticipated by others such as siblings or parents. Twins often attain speech at a later age than singletons because they develop their own language and spend the day in each other's company with less need to communicate in words.

NEGATIVISTIC BEHAVIOUR

Some children refuse to speak as a negativistic reaction to parental concern that they should speak well; they have become 'word-holders' comparable to other negativistic forms of behaviour such as stool-holding (p. 28). They should be encouraged to mix with other children to whom their noises are unintelligible. Such situations can be well managed by the speech therapist supporting and advising parents and acting more directly with the child if he thinks this necessary.

DEAFNESS

The most important cause of severe delay in speaking is deafness (p. 308). Normal speech depends on normal hearing. High-tone sensorineural hearing impairment is particularly liable to be overlooked as the cause of delayed speech. Consonants are carried on the high frequencies and are more distinctive in character than vowels; they must be heard if words are to be intelligible. Recurrent otitis media and glue ear (p. 155) may cause intermittent conductive hearing loss which if severe or unrecognized may cause speech delay.

MENTAL RETARDATION

Children with mental retardation are slow to acquire speech. History and developmental assessment will reveal a global delay (p. 41).

LACK OF STIMULATION

The child's ability to develop speech is dependent on a close relationship with an adult care-giver, usually the mother. Positive reinforcement of normal babbling encourages a child to learn to speak. A child deprived of this close one-to-one relationship at this stage receives fewer opportunities to learn than one with a normal mother–child relationship. In the most severe case, the maternally deprived child remains apathetic and silent.

Maternal deprivation can occur without physical separation from the mother. Many mothers fail to understand normal child development and the importance of play in order to learn, perhaps because they were not played with as children. A child who is left on his own shows little impairment of motor function but is retarded in language and in the personal and social areas of behaviour. It is the attainment of language which is particularly affected so that although the child has the potential ability to understand, he falls behind in comprehension of speech and can only express himself poorly.

FAMILIAL SPEECH DELAY

A family history may reveal that some close relatives were late in speaking. This may make the family particularly anxious about the child's speech development and negativism may be an additional factor in the slow acquisition of language.

CONGENITAL AUDITORY IMPERCEPTION
(DEVELOPMENTAL DYSPHASIA)

This is a complex group of disorders which is not yet fully understood, nor is terminology uniform. The children are brought to medical attention because they are late in talking but their intellect and hearing are normal. Lack of speech results from an inability to comprehend the spoken word (dysphasia or word deafness), and later there may be associations with failure to understand the written word (dyslexia or word blindness). It is sometimes ascribed to a lag in the maturation of the appropriate brain centres, but some of these patients never acquire these skills. It is more probable that there is a defect in cerebral organization analogous to the clumsy child (p. 331). The condition is commoner in males and may be familial.

The patients often develop emotional disorders as a result of their difficulties. Such emotional problems, being more easily diagnosed, are often regarded as the cause instead of the result of the speech difficulty.

Unclear speech

Causes of unclear speech vary from the clearly pathological such as occurs with cerebral palsy, cleft palate and hearing loss, through to poor auditory perception and on to relatively straightforward immature speech patterns. A list of causes is shown in Table 17.15.

DYSARTHRIA

This is a neurological deficit with impairment in the control of both voluntary and involuntary oral musculature. It is most commonly associated with cerebral palsy, either spastic or athetoid. Depending on the severity of the motor involvement the speech may be very indistinct and effective oral communication may be difficult. Feeding problems are commonly associated with dysarthria. Speech therapists are trained to deal with problems in both these areas.

VERBAL DYSPRAXIA

This condition refers to impaired control of the voluntary oral musculature. There is no demonstrable upper or lower motor neurone lesion since individual movements are intact but articulation is imperfect.

Non-fluency

Non-fluency is an extremely common phase in speech development and is normally seen in children of between 3 and 4 years. The young child may have difficulty in formulating or expressing his words and the concept of 'normal non-fluency' must be understood by all those involved in child health care. Stress is an important factor contributing to non-fluency as all those who have been called upon to speak publically will know! Parents anxious for their child to speak may produce a stressful environment and make him self-conscious. This has the reverse of the desired effect and non-fluency may result. It is essential in such a situation that the parents are given advice and support.

STAMMERING

Stammering or stuttering usually begins between the ages of 3 and 4 years and is initially indistinguishable from normal non-fluency. It is more common in boys than girls. A family history of stammering is frequent, but it has not been possible to establish whether this is due to heriditary factors or imitative influences. Despite much research the causes of stammering are not clear.

The disorder occurs in two stages. In the primary stage there is usually excessive repetition of syllables and words. At this stage, the child is often unconscious of what he is doing. Stress is again an important factor and should be discussed with the parents and teachers. Steps can then be taken to alleviate tension where this is possible. If attention is not drawn to the non-fluency itself then the condition should resolve spontaneously. An over-anxious parent making the mistake of trying to correct the child's speech will make him conscious of the problem and is likely to move him into the more serious second stage.

In the secondary or more established phase the child has become aware of what he is doing and, fearful of his mistakes, tries to correct them by voluntary effort. This results in tonic spasms of the muscles involved in speech, especiany those of the lips, throat, larynx and diaphragm. Speech be-

comes entirely blocked and the child may perform accessory actions such as clenching the fist, closing the eyes, whistling and facial contortions. He may also become involved in complex circumlocutions to avoid certain feared words.

Treatment

In the primary stage no attention should be paid to speech but emotional tensions should be relieved. The advice and support of a speech therapist is recommended at this early stage. Once the secondary stage has started speech therapy is certainly necessary.

Degenerative disorders

Degeneration of the nervous system is amongst the most distressing of disease processes for families and their medical attendants. Children may present with failure of development, arrest of established development or regression of learned skills. The age at presentation depends on many factors including the severity of the illness and the powers of observation of the parents.

The approach to the diagnosis of degenerative conditions is difficult partly because of our limited

Table 17.16 Causes of degenerative disorders of the nervous system.

Neuronal storage disorders (p. 373)
Tay–Sachs
Gaucher's disease
Batten's disease
Niemann–Pick disease

Leukodystrophies (p. 374)
Metachromatic
Krabbe's
Pelixaeus–Merzbacher

Mucopolysaccharidoses (p. 375)
Hurler's syndrome
Hunter's syndrome
Sanfillippo syndrome

Mucolipidoses
'I' cell disease

---

understanding of the processes involved in many of these conditions. A large number of different conditions, all of which are very rare, may cause degeneration of the nervous system. The majority are inherited in an autosomal recessive manner. Table 17.16 lists the major groups of these conditions.

NEURONAL STORAGE DISEASES

These involve deposition of complicated compounds within neurones. In Tay–Sachs disease (p. 373) lipid gangliosides are deposited, and in Gaucher's disease (p. 373) glucocerebrosides are laid down in the neurones. All these conditions are progressive, incurable and fatal. Severe mental retardation is inevitable.

LEUKODYSTROPHIES

Unlike the storage diseases which largely affect neurones, the leukodystrophies such as meta-chromatic leukodystrophy, Krabbe's disease and Pelizaeus–Merzbacher disease affect predominantly white matter. These are discussed on p. 374.

MUCOPOLYSACCHARIDOSES

In this condition mucopolysaccharides are deposited in a variety of organs and in some cases the brain may be spared. Table 17.16 lists only those types directly involving the brain. In these, severe neurological abnormalities usually occur, but the age at which mental retardation develops varies with the different types. These disorders are discussed on p. 374.

Further reading

Brett EM. *Paediatric Neurology*. Churchill Livingstone, Edinburgh 1983.
Levene MI, Bennett MJ, Punt J. *Fetal and Neonatal Neurology and Neurosurgery*. Churchill Livingstone, Edinburgh 1988.

18
DISORDERS OF
THE SPECIAL SENSES

The special senses refer to vision and hearing. It is possible to demonstrate clinically that the newborn infant can both see and hear and an assessment of these functions should be included in all routine newborn examinations. Visual impairment or a deficit of hearing, if untreated, may cause very serious disability and it is essential that children with abnormalities involving the special senses should be detected early and appropriate treatment offered.

Disorders of balance and hearing

The ear is a complicated organ involved not just with the conduction of sound waves and their conversion to nervous stimuli, but also with balance. Figure 18.1 illustrates the structures of the ear together with nerve pathways to the auditory cerebral cortex. The structures can be divided into the external, middle and inner ear. Disorders of the outer and middle ear have been discussed in Chapter 10.

VERTIGO

The vestibular apparatus or sense organs of balance are part of the inner ear structure. The semicircular canals are closely related to the cochlea and comprise three loops, containing endolymph, orientated at right angles to each other. Disorders of the semicircular canals may cause dizziness or vertigo.

Balance is maintained by three different sense organs; vision, proprioception and the vestibular apparatus. Disorders of any one of these may cause disequilibrium. Vertigo is the inappropriate sensation of movement. If mild, the disorientation may be described as dizziness or giddiness and if severe the term vertigo is used which implies the sensation of gross swinging movements of the world in relation to the subject. Vertigo is not often seen in children. Table 18.1 lists the commoner causes.

Benign paroxysmal vertigo

This is a rare condition and usually starts at between 2 and 3 years of age. The episodes of vertigo start suddenly and the child may appear to be acutely disorientated and unsteady. He may not be able to communicate the sensation and becomes upset and frightened. The episode lasts up to 5 minutes, but sometimes only a few seconds. Nausea and vomiting may occur with it. There is no loss of consciousness or abnormal movements

Table 18.1 Commoner causes of vertigo in children.

Otitis media
Intoxication with drugs and alcohol
Concussion
Trauma
Vestibulitis
Migraine
Benign paroxysmal vertigo
Tumour
Epilepsy
Hypoglycaemia

307

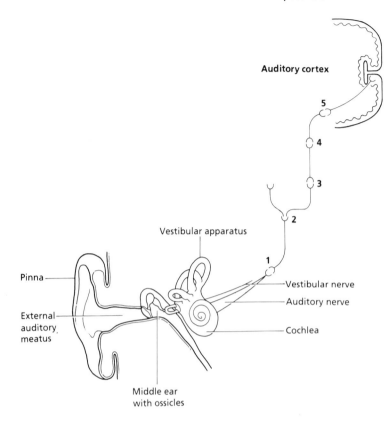

Fig. 18.1 The anatomy of
hearing. 1–5 refer to the nuclei of
the brain stem and thalamus.

which distinguishes it from epilepsy. The prognosis is good with complete recovery, usually before 5 years of age.

Deafness

SCREENING FOR HEARING IMPAIRMENT

Newborn

It is possible to assess clinically the hearing of a newborn infant. With the infant in an appropriately alert state, a loud rattle (80 dB) is sounded 12 inches from his ear but out of sight. The infant will still or startle and make some effort to turn his head towards the source of the sound. It is necessary to be patient and wait for the infant to be appropriately alert for the test to be performed successfully.

A number of methods have been devised to test hearing routinely in all newborn infants. At present these are not widely used, but the principle of routine screening of infant's hearing is very important as early diagnosis and treatment of deafness will significantly improve the quality of subsequent speech.

Infant

Distraction testing of hearing is routinely performed by the health visitor at between 6 and 10 months of age and is designed for the child up to 30 months of age where co-operation is unlikely.

The child sits on the mother's lap facing forward with his back against the mother's chest. Two people are necessary to perform a distraction test; the first attracts the child's attention with a visually interesting toy, but makes no noise. The second person stands behind the child and when the

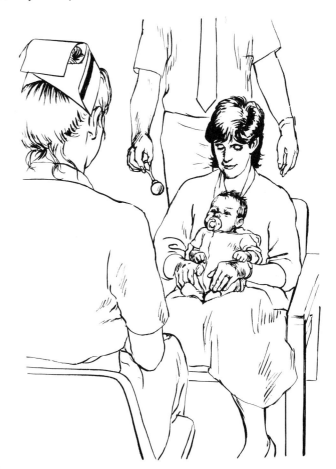

Fig. 18.2 Distraction test of hearing in an 8-month-old infant. Two people are necessary to perform this test.

child's visual attention is obtained the visual object is removed and simultaneously a test sound is delivered 3 feet from the child's ear and out of sight (Fig. 18.2). The test is positive if the child turns to the sound. It is best to use a high-frequency rattle, shaken gently to give a very soft sound. Impairment in the appreciation of high-frequency sounds is the commonest form of frequency rattle effectively excludes this.

Children

In children old enough to co-operate, hearing can be tested by conditioning the child to respond to a command. This must be performed in a quiet, preferably sound-proof room. The child is given a toy (or a small brick) and asked to operate the toy (or drop the brick into a pot) on a verbal command. In the older child this is best done with the child wearing headphones when sounds of different frequencies can be tested down to low sound thresholds.

AUDIOMETRY

This is the standard method to test hearing in children from 5 years and up and should be performed as a formal procedure where careful assessment of hearing is necessary. A chart is produced of both the frequency of the sound (measured in Hertz or cycles per second) and loudness (measured in decibels or dB). Assessment of both

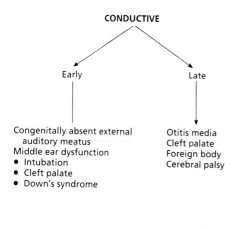
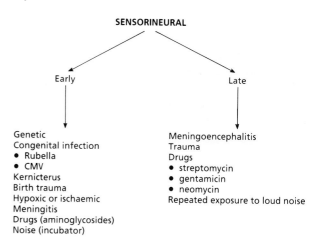

Fig. 18.3 Causes of hearing impairment.

air and bone conduction can be made separately. Failure to respond to sound levels of 30–35 dB does not constitute a clinically important deficit.

AETIOLOGY OF DEAFNESS

Deafness can be conveniently divided into two types: conductive (middle ear disease) and sensorineural (nerve) and these can be further subdivided into those which occur early in life (congenital) and the later acquired causes (Fig. 18.3). Many of these are discussed elsewhere in this book.

The commonest cause of hearing impairment occurring after the neonatal period is otitis media, particularly following frequent, or partially treated infections (see p. 154). This may cause intermittent deafness and the child may at times have relatively normal hearing. Deafness may be a sequel of meningitis or encephalitis. It is a particularly important complication of mumps, usually developing during the first 2 weeks of the illness when it may be associated with mumps meningitis or is due to isolated involvement of the eighth cranial nerve.

MANAGEMENT OF THE DEAF CHILD

Early diagnosis is essential for successful treatment and the normal development of speech. All babies

should be given a screening test at the age of 8 months (see p. 308). Particular attention should be paid to children who are considered to be 'at risk' for hearing impairment as described in Table 18.2.

Mothers are extremely competent at appreciating the inability of their young children to hear normally, seldom being wrong unless the child is mentally handicapped; their complaint must therefore be treated very seriously. They are less competent at appreciating acquired partial loss of hearing so that a careful follow-up of children who have had otitis media is needed. Bright deaf children are particularly easy to miss because, being clever, they can compensate almost as though they have eyes in the back of their heads.

In understanding the management of the deaf

Table 18.2 Conditions which should alert the clinician to the need for careful assessment of hearing.

Family history of deafness
Premature birth
Hyperbilirubinaemia
Cleft palate
Down's syndrome
After meningitis infection
History of recurrent otitis media
Delayed or unclear speech
Cerebral palsy
Parental anxiety

child it is vital to appreciate that the normal child has to learn to hear, the first year of life being the most crucial for this. Their ability to learn auditory discrimination diminishes as the child grows older. The deaf child must be taught to hear as early as possible. Delays cause diminished capacity for hearing, the consequent impairment of speech being seen in its most severe form in the deaf-mute. Total deafness is exceptional and only 1–2% of deaf children have no hearing at all. All children should therefore have a 2-year period of auditory training before being regarded as totally deaf.

The prevalence of profound deafness is approximately 2 : 1000 school-age children. An estimate of 1 : 1000 infants are born profoundly deaf. Babies born very prematurely are most at risk of having severe hearing impairment due to a number of risk factors. Hearing loss of up to 35 dB is classified as mild, between 40–60 dB it is moderate and loss over 70 dB is described as severe.

Parental guidance starts from the day deafness is diagnosed, being undertaken by the audiologist and by the specialist teacher of the deaf. This teacher will visit the home in addition to her work at the auditory training centre. By visiting, she not only learns about the home circumstances, but is able to relate her advice to the actual needs of a particular home and a particular mother. She will also train the other children so that they can help the deaf child.

For the first 1–2 years of life, all auditory training will be given by the mother under the supervision of the peripatetic teacher of the deaf (also called an advisor to the hearing impaired). She will be taught how to handle her child so as to bring sound to him. She must speak very close to her child's ear, repeating sounds again and again so that he can learn auditory discrimination.

A hearing aid should be fitted at the earliest age at which the child will accept it, this often being as young as 3–4 months. The aid should be a double one, since two ears are better than one, and must be worn continuously. It is particularly important that he should be wearing an aid when he starts to crawl since he will no longer be close enough to his mother for full instruction. Children of this young age enjoy their aids and do not pull them off. It is the child who has not been given an aid until later in life who refuses to wear it since sound means nothing to him, not having been taught how to hear. The function of a hearing aid is to make sounds louder. The child must still go through the lengthy process of learning to appreciate the sounds which now reach him.

The child should be kept in a normal environment so that he is able to listen to speech all day long; with auditory training it will be found that his capacity to hear, as measured by audiometry, improves. Lip reading should also be taught in order to fill in any gaps in his hearing. Children with a hearing deficit over 70 dB are unlikely to acquire reasonable speech even with optimal sound amplification and teaching. Controversy exists as to whether these severely disabled children should be taught to communicate by sign language. This is very successful but limits the ability to communicate with those who are unable to sign.

If possible, the child should be taught in an ordinary school. This can often be achieved by means of a hearing aid and sitting him in the optimal position in the classroom. If specialized training is required he may need to be sent to a school for deaf children, but outside school hours he should be in contact with normal children as much as possible. It is very important to assess accurately the intelligence of hearing-impaired children, and this should be done by special tests which have been standardized for deaf children.

Disorders of the eye

Vision is the most important sense in perceiving the world and impairment of vision is a major handicap in any child. The eye is the sense organ of vision, but blindness may be due to an abnormality anywhere in the visual pathway.

The eye is a globe that focuses the visual image on to the retina. Light penetrates the clear cornea, is focused by the lens and the image is converted into a series of electrical stimuli by the rods and

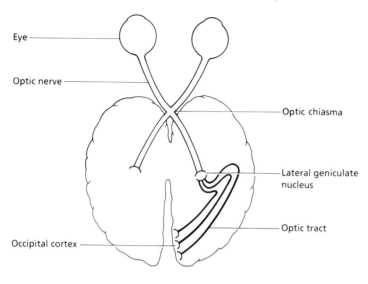

Eye

Optic nerve

Optic chiasma

Lateral geniculate nucleus

Optic tract

Occipital cortex

Fig. 18.4 Anatomy of vision.

cones of the retina. The image is conducted from the retina via the optic nerve to the lateral geniculate body. The optic nerves decussate at the optic chiasm; the fibres from the two nasal sides of the retina cross to the opposite hemisphere and the fibres from the temporal fields radiate to the same hemisphere (Fig. 18.4). There is point-to-point projection of nerve fibres from the retina to the lateral geniculate body and also from there to the occipital cortex. The sensation of vision is appreciated in the occipital cortex. Disorders of vision may occur at any point from the cornea to the occipital cortex. Visual disturbances must be detected early and therefore routine assessment of vision is performed regularly in infancy and childhood.

ASSESSMENT OF THE EYE AND VISION

The methods used to assess vision depend on the age of the child and the degree to which he will co-operate with the tester. In general, all children should have screening tests in the newborn period by a paediatrician, and by health visitors, GPs or community paediatricians at 6 weeks, 8 and 18 months and again at 3 years. In school, children should be assessed regularly for disorders of refraction.

Newborn examination

All neurologically normal newborn infants will be able to fix and follow a visually interesting object. The human face is such an interesting object and with the infant in an appropriately alert state the examiner should be able to get the infant to fix on his face. The examiner should directly face the infant and hold him about 12 inches from his face with his hands supporting the infant's back and head. The infant will be observed to follow the examiner's face when his head is moved from side to side. The most important condition to exclude in the examination of the newborn eyes is congenital cataract. The red reflex must be elicited from both eyes of every newborn baby.

The red reflex. This is performed in a dimly lit room with a direct ophthalmoscope held 18 inches from the infant and directly in front of him. The examiner holds the ophthalmoscope in front of him looking down the beam of light and particularly notes the reflection of the light from the baby's retina. Normally a red reflection is seen (the red reflex). If the reflex is darkened or white then the test is abnormal and the child should be referred to an ophthalmologist urgently for further assessment. The most important cause for loss of the red reflex is cataract, but severe retinopathy of pre-maturity or the rare retinoblastoma may also cause this abnormal appearance.

Pre-school screening

The detection of squint (strabismus) is extremely important in young children and these techniques should be learnt by all those involved with child health screening programmes. The simplest method for assessing squint is to get the child to look directly at the examiner. Note whether the visual axes appear to be parallel. Whilst looking at the eyes, note whether the visual axes remain parallel when the child's vision is directed at the eight positions of gaze (Fig. 18.5). The eyes should then be tested for the corneal light reflex. A bright torch is reflected into the child's eyes from 18 inches distant. The point of light reflection in the cornea should be noted and should be symmetrical in the two eyes. The torch is then moved through the eight positions of gaze with the infant's head remaining still. Note that the light remains symmetrically reflected in the eyes.

Some children show 'pseudosquint'. This refers to an apparent squint which is due to a wide nasal bridge or epicanthic fold giving the appearance of squint, but if the corneal light reflex test is normal in these children then parents should be strongly reassured that the child does not have a squint.

The cover test. This is a sensitive test for children suspected of having a squint. The child's attention

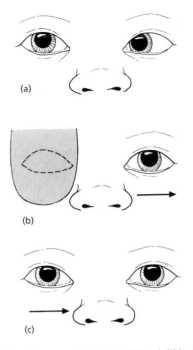

Fig. 18.6 The cover test. (a) With the child looking at the examiner there is an apparent squint of the left eye. (b) The right eye is covered and the left moves to the point of focus. (c) With the patch removed the right eye moves to be the dominant eye of vision again. This confirms that the left eye is abnormal.

is attracted to a visually interesting object held 18 inches from his face. The position of the eyes is noted and then one eye is covered without touching the child's face. The examiner watches the other (uncovered) eye to see if the visual axis changes. If the eye moves then the test is positive and the child has a squint involving that eye (Fig. 18.6). The other eye is then tested in a similar way by covering the eye that was just tested. If a child fails this test he should be referred to an ophthalmologist for further assessment including fundoscopy.

ASSESSMENT OF VISUAL ACUITY

In addition, assessment must include both near and distant vision. In children of between 5 and 6 years, distance vision can be assessed by Snellen's

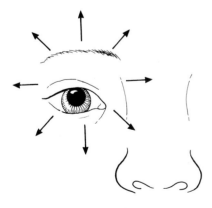

Fig. 18.5 The eight positions of gaze.

chart or an equivalent test for younger children based on matching shapes rather than letters. Each eye should be assessed separately with the child 6 metres from the chart. In very young children the Stycar test is used. This involves white balls of different sizes rolled against a black background. The infant should sit 10 feet from the tester who remains out of sight of the child. The balls are either rolled or moved on black sticks against a black background.

Fine vision in small infants can be tested with minute sweets such as 'hundreds and thousands' or small pellets. In older children picture matching can be used for the assessment of fine vision or by asking them to read from a book with letters of different sizes.

COLOUR VISION

Colour blindness affects about 8% of males and less than 1% of females. It is not usually a disabling condition but may limit the choice of occupations the individual may enter in later years. The commonest colour defects are for red and green. Colour vision can be screened by the use of special colour charts such as those produced by Ishihara. These are now well adapted to the requirements of young children.

SQUINT (STRABISMUS)

Binocular vision is achieved by means of both eyes focusing on the same object. Squint refers to failure of both eyes to work together in this manner and one eye deviates away from the point of focus. Binocular vision is not attained until about 3 months and up to that time squint is not abnormal. The clinical detection of squint is described above. There is a strong genetic influence on squint; up to 25% of squinting children have a family history of this condition.

Amblyopia

Persistent squint will cause diplopia and the occipital cortex will suppress the image from the squinting eye. This eventually leads to amblyopia or blindness in the affected eye. The eye is anatomically normal yet becomes irreversibly blind unless the amblyopia is detected at an early stage. For this reason squints in children older than 3 months must be carefully assessed and managed by an ophthalmologist and orthoptist to prevent amblyopia from developing. Parents should be told that children do not 'grow out' of squints. The term 'lazy eye' is misleading and dangerous. Amblyopia which has not responded to treatment by 8 years of age is irreversible, but squint developing *de novo* after 8 years does not cause amblyopia. Although squint is the commonest cause of amblyopia, any cause of unilateral visual impairment may produce it including ptosis, cataract or vitreous opacity.

Clinical features

Squint is demonstrated by the cover test (p. 313). Squints can be divided into paralytic and non-paralytic.

Paralytic squint. This is much less common in children than non-paralytic squint. It is due to ocular nerve or muscle paralysis. It is often congenital or may develop as the result of cerebral tumour. The affected eye does not have a normal range of movement through the eight positions of gaze.

Non-paralytic squint. This is usually due to an imbalance in the muscle control of the eye and each eye individually can move through the normal positions of gaze.

Squint can be further divided into concomitant or incomitant forms.

Concomitant squint. The angle of squint remains the same irrespective of the position of gaze.

Incomitant squint. The angle of squint varies with the position of gaze. This occurs in paralytic forms of squint.

The direction of the squint can be further described as either horizontal or vertical. In the horizontal plane, the squint is said to be convergent if the squinting eye turns inwards towards the nose, or divergent if the squinting eye turns outwards.

Some children adapt to a squint by holding their heads in a peculiar position to bring the direction of gaze in the two eyes into a parallel plane. Head tilt in children should always suggest squint and the eyes must be carefully examined. When a squint is diagnosed, the child's eyes should be carefully examined following pupillary dilatation to exclude lens opacity (cataract) or fundal abnormalities. As the commonest cause of squint is a refractive error careful testing of visual acuity is also necessary.

Management

If the child has a disorder of refraction, appropriate glasses should be prescribed. The normal non-squinting eye is patched to encourage vision in the squinting eye to develop normally or to recover if there is some degree of amblyopia. Once optimal vision has been obtained then surgery is carried out to repair the muscular imbalance of the eye. After this, a further period of careful supervision, sometimes with additional patching, may be necessary to ensure that normal vision is maintained.

Blindness

Blindness is imprecise and it is better to use the term severe visual handicap (SVH) to describe children with a deficit in vision severe enough to require special education. The prevalence of blindness or SVH in Britain is 1 : 3000 children. There are many causes and these are listed in Table 18.3. Many of these are discussed elsewhere in this book.

Diagnosis

Parents usually suspect severe visual handicap from an early age. The child shows no visual interest and does not fix or follow his parent's face. In infants with cortical blindness, they may fix and follow for the first few months and then appear to become blind. This is because cortical vision probably does not develop until 3 months of age. Almost 75% of infants with SVH have additional

Table 18.3   Causes of apparent blindness in children.

Congenital glaucoma
Cataract
Severe myopia
Retinal pathology
　Retinopathy of prematurity
　Leber's amaurosis
　Retinoblastoma
　Prenatal toxoplasma infection
　Retinitis pigmentosa
Optic nerve pathology
　Optic nerve hypoplasia
　Trauma
　Cerebral infarction
　Congenital cerebral anomaly
Albinism
Cortical blindness
Delayed visual maturation

disabilities and it is important to assess neurological function in such children carefully. One-third of blind children are also mentally retarded. Formal assessment of hearing is particularly important.

Blind babies are usually alert and bright, but a proportion may be withdrawn and 'strange' presumably due to lack of visual stimuli. Developmental skills including motor skills are usually somewhat delayed, also due to impairment of sensory input. Many congenitally blind babies show a form of 'roving eye' nystagmus. Others may have marked squint.

CATARACT

An opacity in the lens is referred to as a cataract. One-third of babies born with visual impairment have bilateral cataracts as the cause of their disability. Cataracts may be congenital or occur secondary to some other disease process. Table 18.4 lists the commoner causes of cataracts.

All infants should be tested at birth for cataracts and the red reflex detected in each eye separately. Elicitation of the red reflex is described on p. 312. If there is any doubt as to whether this test is normal or not, the child should be referred to an ophthalmologist. Unilateral cataract may lead to

Table 18.4 Causes of cataracts.

Congenital
Prenatal infection
  Rubella
  Cytomegalovirus
Trauma
Prematurity
Down's syndrome
Other syndromes (rare)

Acquired
Trauma
Inborn errors of metabolism
  Galactosaemia
  Hypophosphataemia
  Mucopolysaccharidoses (p. 374)
Juvenile chronic arthritis
Diabetes mellitus
Drugs (steroids, chloroquine)

amblyopia and this is a preventable condition.

Management is by means of surgical removal of either the opacity or the lens together with optical correction by means of contact lenses or glasses. Vision can be restored in the majority of children born with cataracts if they are detected early.

REFRACTIVE ERRORS

Refractive errors (particularly myopia) in children are very common and may affect up to 20% of school-age children. Errors of refraction are usually due to a deviation in shape of the eye ball. If the eye is too flat from front to back the image

focus will be behind the fovea (hypermetropia or long sightedness) or if it is too long the focus will occur in front of the fovea (myopia or short sightedness) (see Fig. 18.7). Severe, unilateral refractive error may cause amblyopia. Astigmatism refers to an irregularity in the shape of the globe producing difficulties in both vertical and horizontal planes simultaneously.

Errors of refraction can be corrected with appropriate prescription lenses. These may be provided as either glasses or contact lenses.

GLAUCOMA (BUPHTHALMOS)

This condition accounts for 5–10% of children admitted to schools for the blind. It is familial in 10% due to a recessive gene. The disorder is due to a developmental anomaly of the filtration angle which impedes the flow of aqueous humour from the anterior chamber. Clinical features may be present at birth and 80% develop during the first 3 months, the rest during the remainder of the first year.

Clinical features include enlargement of the globe (buphthalmos) and clouding of the cornea due to oedema. There may be excessive lachrymation and photophobia. The condition is bilateral in 80% of cases, but in unilateral cases a difference in ocular tension is appreciated by comparing the two eyes. Obvious pain is not a feature of the disease in infants.

Management. As treatment may be curative, early detection is essential to avoid permanent visual

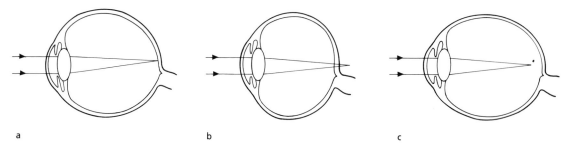

a   b   c

Fig. 18.7 Disorders of refraction. (a) Normal focusing on the retina. (b) The hypermetropic eye focuses the object beyond the retina; the eye is too short. (c) The myopic eye focuses the object too short; the eye is too long.

impairment. Goniotomy is the operation of choice, an incision being made into the blocking tissue so as to open up a channel through which the aqueous fluid can drain.

LEBER'S AMAUROSIS

This is an autosomal recessive disorder and is associated with blindness from shortly after birth. It is associated with a form of retinitis pigmentosa, but this does not become clinically apparent until the child is about 2 years old. The infants show roving nystagmus with no visual attention. The fundus usually appears normal initially but diagnosis can be made on the basis of electrical testing of the retina and visual cortical responses. There is no treatment.

ALBINISM

This is a genetically determined condition that exists in a number of forms. The most usual form is tyrosinase negative and these children have no melanin production. Their hair is white and irises blue or grey and they show nystagmus. They initially appear to be quite blind with no visual contact, but this gradually improves and by school age they have some useful vision, although their vision for distant objects is usually severely impaired and they are often registered as blind. It is inherited as an autosomal recessive condition.

The tyrosinase positive form of the condition may be difficult to distinguish from tyrosinase negative disease but in the positive form vision is usually not as severely affected. The defect may be confined to the fundus which shows a deficit of pigment (ocular albinism). These children present with nystagmus and impaired vision. Ocular albinism is inherited as an X-linked condition. The prognosis in tyrosinase positive albinism is better than for the tyrosinase negative form.

CORTICAL BLINDNESS

This is due to congenital absence of the occipital cortex which is usually associated with a very poor prognosis, or an acquired defect of the cortex. The latter occurs in infants who have developed extensive periventricular leukomalacia (p. 102). These conditions are evident on brain imaging. The children may initially fix and follow but later have no visual interest. The fundi show optic atrophy or hypoplasia.

DELAYED VISUAL MATURATION

This is a curious condition in which otherwise developmentally normal infants appear to be blind. No abnormality can be detected either clinically or on investigation of the eyes. Between the ages of 3 and 6 months vision suddenly develops and parents sometimes describe this as occurring overnight. The diagnosis of permanent blindness should not be made in young infants without demonstrable ocular abnormality because the visual impairment may be due to delayed maturation. Some children with generalized developmental delay may also show this condition but the prognosis in these may not be as good.

NYSTAGMUS

This is a disorder in eye movement characterized by abnormal oscillatory movements, often in the horizontal plane or more rarely involving vertical or rotating movements. The neurology of nystagmus is very complicated and may represent severe disease in the cerebellum, brain stem or vestibular apparatus. Nystagmus is seen in blind babies, as well as in albinism and other disorders.

Congenital nystagmus is an inherited, benign form of nystagmus which is rarely present at birth and usually develops between 1 and 2 months of age. Vision is not significantly impaired.

COLOBOMA

This is a notched defect which may involve the iris, choroid or eye lid (Fig. 5.5). The abnormality may occur as an isolated lesion or in association with other malformations, especially cleft lip or palate, mandibulo-facial dystosis or arachnodactyly. If the cleft involves the choroid, vision may be severely impaired.

Management of SVH

The child must be looked after by a multi-disciplinary team involving paediatrician, oph-thalmologist, occupational therapist and the peripatetic teacher of the blind. The child's development should be assessed regularly and the parents encouraged in ways of assisting their child's development which is impaired by his visual disability. A child is registered as blind by the Director of Social Services on the recom-mendation of a consultant ophthalmologist.

Further reading

Hall DMB. *The Child With a Handicap*. Blackwell Scientific Publications, Oxford 1984.

19

THE CHILD WITH A HANDICAP

The World Health Organization has defined the ways in which a condition can interfere with normal function:

Impairment

Any loss or abnormality of psychological, physiological or anatomical structure or function.

Disability

Where an impairment causes restriction of the ability to perform any activity in a normal manner or a manner considered to be within the limits of normality.

Handicap

A disadvantage bestowed on the individual by virtue of an impairment or disability that limits or prevents the achievement of a role that is normal for that individual.

It is clear that many children have an impairment and some may be disabled by it. The responsibility of paediatricians and therapists is to prevent these from causing the child to be handicapped so that the child can fulfil his potential to his own satisfaction.

Handicap is a term used to describe a large variety of conditions that interfere with a child's growth, development or learning. Handicap in childhood may be due to either physical, psycho-logical or developmental causes and the incidence of physical handicap in young children is 1–2%. This chapter concentrates on some of the causes of disability affecting the brain.

The nature of handicap resulting from cerebral causes is extremely heterogeneous and the clinical manifestation of these lesions also varies. Major handicap can be considered in the context of cerebral palsy, mental retardation, visual impairment (p. 315), hearing deficit (p. 308) and severe epilepsy (p. 284). These latter three conditions are considered elsewhere. Blindness may be due to a peripheral problem such as retinal detachment following retinopathy of prematurity and if the brain is unaffected the child is likely to show no other disability. The cause of cerebral palsy, however, is likely to involve structures other than just the motor pathways and consequently the child may also show mental retardation, epilepsy or possibly cortical blindness. All children with any disability of neurological function must be carefully assessed in all aspects of cerebral function as they may have multiple disabilities (Fig. 19.1), each of which can be modified to reduce the degree of eventual handicap.

Management of the handicapped child

The age at presentation of the child with a disability depends on the nature of the problem. Down's syndrome and spina bifida will be obvious at birth but conditions such as mental retardation or cerebral palsy may not be diagnosed for years. The diagnosis is usually made by a hospital or

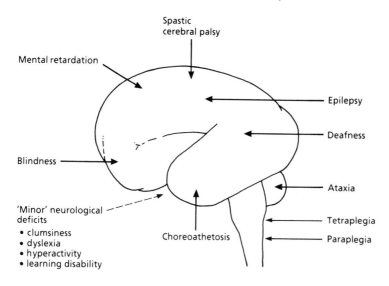

Mental retardation

Spastic
cerebral palsy

Epilepsy

Deafness

Blindness

Ataxia

'Minor' neurological
deficits
• clumsiness
• dyslexia
• hyperactivity
• learning disability

Choreoathetosis

Tetraplegia

Paraplegia

Fig. 19.1 The manifestation of different forms of disability affecting the brain.

community paediatrician, but services for the child must involve the hospital, community, and school as well as a wide range of other professional groups. There must be multi-disciplinary integration of all these services. Once a disability is diagnosed or strongly suspected the child should be referred to the district handicap team (DHT) which usually works in the context of a child development or assessment unit. The DHT should comprise a paediatrician, social worker, educational psychologist, senior nurse and a teacher.

EDUCATION

In Britain, every effort is made to educate disabled children with their able-bodied peers in normal schools. Such children are recognized to have 'special educational needs' irrespective of the nature of their disability. This term is defined as a child who finds learning significantly more difficult than the majority of children of his age or one with a disability that makes it hard for him to make use of ordinary local schools.

The local education authority (LEA) must provide free full-time education for all children with special needs from the age of 2 until the age of 16. In addition, all babies whose special needs are identified must also be provided for.

Each child is formally assessed to discover his special educational needs. A statement is prepared by all those involved with the child including paediatricians, therapists, teachers, and psychologists. The parents have the right to appeal if they disagree with the statement or the decision made by the LEA in deciding at which school the child is to be enrolled. The concept is that there is a partnership between the medical services, educational authorities and the parents to provide the most appropriate educational facilities and to try and minimize the child's disability becoming a handicap to him or his parents. The child's statement must be reviewed every year and there is a statutory requirement for reassessment between the ages of 12 and 14 years.

Cerebral palsy

Cerebral palsy is the term used to describe the clinical effects of a *non-progressive* lesion within the brain which causes impairment of motor function. The cause of the cerebral lesion develops in fetal or early neonatal life and its effects are obvious by 5 years of age. Lesions occurring in older children, those of the spinal cord and progressive disorders of the brain are excluded from this definition. Although the disease is not progressive, the

Table 19.1 A classification of cerebral palsy with the prevalence of each type.

Spastic – total	85%
Hemiplegia	30%
Diplegia	20%
Quadriplegia	35%
Choreoathetosis	5%
Ataxic	5%
Hypotonic	2%
Unclassifiable	3%

manifestations appear to change in the first few years due to maturation of the nervous system.

A variety of classifications of cerebral palsy based on the patterns of movement disorder have been described. Table 19.1 summarizes a relatively simple classification and indicates the relative frequency of the various types.

AETIOLOGY

The prevalence of cerebral palsy in developed countries is approximately 2.5:1000 school-age children. It is not possible to diagnose cerebral palsy at birth as the nervous system is not mature enough for the clinical signs to be manifested.

Cerebral palsy is much commoner in infants who were born prematurely. Approximately 80:1000 infants of birth weight 1500 g and below develop this condition compared with only 1:1000

infants of birth weight above 2500 g. Within the group of children born prematurely and who develop cerebral palsy, spastic diplegia is the most common form of this condition. It is tempting to assume that the complications of being born prematurely cause cerebral palsy and this may be true in some cases, but it is also possible that the underlying cause for the premature delivery may also be the cause of the motor disorder.

The cause of cerebral palsy can be considered to have occurred either prenataly, during the course of delivery or in the early months after birth. Table 19.2 lists the possible causes of cerebral palsy. In a significant proportion of children with cerebral palsy, no obvious cause can be determined.

ASSOCIATED FORMS OF HANDICAP

If cerebral palsy is due to a discrete lesion within the pyramidal tract, then the child may show no abnormality other than the disorder of movement. Brain injury, however, is rarely this specific and function in other parts of the brain may also be abnormal. Approximately one-half of children with cerebral palsy also have mental retardation and one-quarter have epilepsy. Hearing impairment is common with athetoid cerebral palsy and this is usually due to kernicterus (p. 108). Conductive hearing loss is particularly common in children with incoordination of the bulbar musculature and this should be anticipated. Severe

Table 19.2 Specific causes of cerebral palsy related to the timing of the insult. Associated factors such as intrauterine growth retardation and prematurity have not been listed as they are risk rather than causative factors.

Prenatal	Perinatal	Postnatal
Genetic	Intracranial haemorrhage	Kernicterus
Dominant	Peri-ventricular leukomalacia	Cerebral traumatic injury
Recessive	Birth asphyxia	Meningitis
Congenital cerebral anomaly	Cerebral artery infarction	Hypoxic-ischaemic injury
Iodine deficiency		
Teratogens		
Mercury		
? Alcohol		
Prenatal infection		
Cytomegalovirus		
Toxoplasmosis		

visual impairment is rare in all but the most severe forms of cerebral palsy but when it does occur, cortical blindness is the commonest cause (see p. 317).

Clinical features

As indicated in Table 19.1, a variety of clinically recognizable patterns of cerebral palsy exist.

SPASTICITY

Spasticity refers to increased tone or spasm within a muscle or muscle group. The increased tone is described as 'clasp-knife' as it is only detectable in one direction of joint movement. It occurs as the result of a lesion in the motor cortex or pyramidal tract.

Spasticity is associated with increased tendon reflexes, clonus and extensor plantar responses. Clonus can occasionally occur in normal individuals from nervous tension and may be seen in an ill-sustained form in normal infants. In most cases it is evidence of a pyramidal lesion.

Spasticity is further defined in terms of limb involvement.

Spastic hemiplegia

In this condition the cerebral lesion affects only one hemisphere with involvement of the contralateral side of the body. The limb involvement may be relatively different depending on the precise position of the cerebral lesion. One lower limb may be considerably more affected than the ipsilateral upper limb and if the involvement of the arm is minimal the child may show signs sometimes referred to as spastic monoplegia.

In spastic hemiplegia the arm is held close to the chest in a position of adduction, flexion and internal rotation. The leg is adducted at the hip, partially flexed at the knee and the foot is plantar flexed (see Fig. 19.2). The affected limbs grow more slowly than the unaffected side. The face is seldom severely affected. Speech may be affected in right-

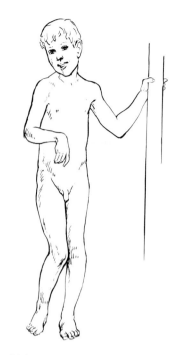

Fig. 19.2   Right spastic hemiplegia.

sided hemiplegia of postnatal origin, but in congenital right-sided hemiplegia no speech defect occurs, presumably because the speech centre on the other side can take over at that stage of development. Intelligence in this group is variable; it may be normal and the patients are seldom severely mentally handicapped. Convulsions are common.

Spastic diplegia

This is due to a symmetrical bilateral cerebral lesion, but the corticospinal tracts to the lower limbs are particularly affected. This is the condition that characteristically occurs in infants born prematurely. In practice, all four limbs are affected, but the upper limbs are usually only mildly or minimally involved. The lower limb involvement is symmetrical.

The children show adduction of the thighs with internal rotation so that the knees are touching. The calf muscles are tight and the child stands

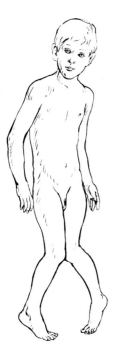

Fig. 19.3 Spastic diplegia.

on his toes with bent knees and toes pointing together (see Fig. 19.3). Intelligence is usually normal but convulsions may occur.

Spastic quadriplegia

This is also referred to as double hemiplegia implying that the condition is asymmetrical. The upper limbs may be more severely affected than the lower. Some children with spastic quadriplegia show a mixed picture with athetoid movements.

This condition is due to severe and extensive injury to the motor pathways in both hemispheres. It is likely that injury has involved other parts of the brain and the child may also be severely mentally retarded. Severe speech and swallowing problems may also exist. Convulsions occur commonly.

Assessment of intelligence in young children is very dependent on motor and speech function. Children with severe spastic quadriplegia may find it very difficult to express their intelligence to their parents and medical attendants. It must always be assumed that these children are intelligent until they are old enough to have accurate psychometric testing.

ATHETOSIS

This condition is due to an abnormality of the basal ganglia and is characterized by bizarre involuntary movements which may be slow and writhing, or jerky as in chorea, and are described in detail on p. 293. The movements are always grossly exaggerated as soon as voluntary movement is attempted.

The commonest cause of athetoid cerebral palsy has in the past been due to neonatal kernicterus (p. 108), but is now rarely seen in Western countries. Athetosis does not usually develop in the first year of life and may be delayed as late as 3 years. Prior to the development of abnormal movements the child is usually hypotonic. The longer this stage of hypotonicity lasts, the more severe the athetosis is likely to be.

Athetoid patients are often of normal intelligence although the associated dysarthria may give the appearance of impaired intellect and careful developmental assessment is necessary.

Children with athetoid cerebral palsy are usually very thin as a result of excessive muscular activity. If due to kernicterus, deafness commonly occurs in conjunction with the athetosis. Convulsions are rare.

ATAXIA

This is a rare type of cerebral palsy and is often due to an acquired defect of cerebellar function (see also p. 292). Although genetic causes of cerebral palsy are rare, an ataxic form is the most likely to occur.

Ataxia may affect the arms, interfering with the precision of their movement, or the legs causing an unsteady tremulous gait. In some cases all limbs are involved, in which case the legs are usually more severely affected than the arms. Occasionally, the ataxia is central so that the child is ataxic when sitting. There is nystagmus and an intention tremor. Incoordination from abnormalities of muscle tone or athetosis must be excluded. Ataxic children have a natural tendency to improve as they get older.

HYPOTONIA

Hypotonia is a common precursor of both spastic and athetoid cerebral palsy. A small proportion of patients remain hypotonic and other causes of hypotonia must be excluded (see p. 300) as the diagnosis of hypotonic cerebral palsy is usually made by exclusion.

MIXED PATTERNS

The majority of patients fall into one predominant category but mixed types exist. These result from extensive brain lesions and are less common since these children are less likely to survive.

Early diagnosis

The diagnosis of cerebral palsy is often preceded by identification of the infant who is at high risk; those who have sustained severe birth asphyxia, those born very prematurely with evidence of intracranial pathology such as cystic periventricular leukomalacia (p. 102) or kernicterus. Such children should be seen and examined frequently. Feeding difficulties are common from a very early age.

Most children develop spasticity from a background of hypotonia. The floppy infant is one in whom increased tone may develop in the first 4–8 months. Limb tone is assessed by stretching the limbs through the normal range of movements. Lower limb hypertonia is often first elicited by showing some spasm in the hamstring muscles. This is detected with the infant lying supine and the thighs flexed on to the abdomen. The lower limb is then extended and the angle of the knee joint is measured. The lower limb adductor muscles are the group next most commonly showing increased tone. This is assessed by rapidly abducting the legs when held straight in extension. There

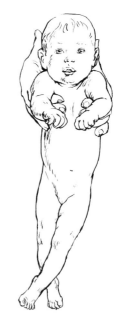

Fig. 19.4 Scissoring in a child with spastic quadriplegia.

is a feeling of increased resistance when this is done. When held in an upright position with the legs off the couch increased adductor tone is demonstrated by the child 'scissoring' (Fig. 19.4). The legs are held in extension and cross each other.

Evidence of hypertonia in the upper limbs in children with spastic quadriplegia usually becomes apparent after increased tone is detected in the lower limbs. Persistent adduction of the thumb into the palm of the hand (fisting) is an early feature of upper limb hypertonia. The combination of limb hypertonia with trunk and neck hypotonia is an ominous feature in the early prediction of severe spastic cerebral palsy.

Tendon reflexes are exaggerated and this is often a very early sign of cerebral palsy. A crossed adductor reflex is an ominous sign. This is elicited by testing for a knee jerk and if present there is adduction of the opposite thigh. As long as this is not obligatory it may be normal in the first 6 months of life.

The persistence of primitive reflexes is also an early feature of cerebral palsy. These include the presence of an obligatory asymmetrical tonic neck reflex (Fig. 4.4), persistence of the Moro reflex after 6 months, and the grasp reflex after 4 months.

The important parachute reflex develops in a normal baby at about the age of 9 months and is described on p. 8. The normal baby puts out both his arms to protect himself and absence or asymmetry of this reflex is very suggestive of upper motor neurone lesion involving the upper limbs.

Once the child is old enough to reach for objects the hand movements should be observed. A child with cerebral palsy moves his hand in one piece like a mechanical grabber, instead of using more sophisticated and independent finger movements. In testing the hands it is useful to flap them rapidly, since this exaggerates the diminished movement of spasticity, or to ask the child to make rapid tapping movements with both hands alternately.

The child with mild cerebral palsy may achieve independent walking at a relatively early age. His walking posture should be carefully observed. Failure to swing one or both arms, or the asymmetrical wearing out of shoes at a faster rate than normal may be early evidence of relatively mild cerebral palsy.

Testing for sensory defects is not practicable in babies but is essential in older children. Many of the difficulties of the child with cerebral palsy result from a loss of discriminative sense and an absence of the normal body image, so that the child does not realize the position of his limbs in space. This is particularly important in spastic hemiplegia.

THE LATE-WALKING CHILD

Three per cent of children fail to walk independently by 18 months of age and this is often an isolated delay in gross motor development. Cerebral palsy must always be considered as a cause for this. Other important organic causes of failure to walk are mental retardation and, in boys, muscular dystrophy (see p. 298). There is, however, a group of children with benign causes of failure to achieve independent locomotion and 'bottom shuffling' is the best recognized condition.

Bottom shuffling

This condition occurs in up to 10% of normal children and is particularly common in boys. They rapidly move around the floor by propelling themselves in a kicking fashion whilst sitting upright. They show the characteristic 'sitting on air' sign when held in an upright position off the couch. Bottom shuffling is a benign condition in the majority of children.

Cerebral palsy must be carefully considered in all late-walking children, including those who bottom shuffle, as some are subsequently found to have this condition, but it may be very difficult to exclude cerebral palsy in mild cases before the age of 3 years. Serum creatine kinase should also be measured in late-walking boys (after 18 months) to exclude Duchenne muscular dystrophy.

Treatment

Cerebral palsy is a condition that directly affects the pyramidal tracts, but often indirectly produces profound effects throughout the body. The abnormal posture may result in secondary orthopaedic deformations. Dislocated hips are particularly common. If the spine is affected with severe scoliosis, restrictive airway disease may occur with eventual respiratory failure. Feeding and speech may be severely abnormal due to the involvement of bulbar musculature. Many children with cerebral palsy become extremely frustrated and behaviour difficulties are common.

Early assessment and treatment is essential for the prevention of deformities and the provision of experiences required for normal development but denied to the child with cerebral palsy. The secret of success lies as much in the successful handling of the parents as of the child.

The management of cerebral palsy is really the management of the whole child. This should be undertaken in the context of a multi-disciplinary child development centre. The child and his parents are evaluated over a number of days by a

physiotherapist, occupational therapist, specialist
health visitor, psychologist, speech therapist, social
worker, a dentist, and a paediatrician experienced
in the problems of handicapped children and their
families. At the end of the assessment a conference
is held to which the parents and the child, if this is
appropriate, are invited. The child's problems are
identified and a therapy plan drawn up. Many
therapists or just one may be involved depending
on the child's problems. A date for reassessment
should be fixed at the first conference.

Although the management of the child with
cerebral palsy is a multi-disciplinary one, particular therapeutic interventions can be identified.

PHYSIOTHERAPY

There are a number of different methods of
physical therapy aimed at the child achieving his
maximal potential. Physiotherapy should be introduced as soon as the child shows signs of abnormal tone or movement. There is no evidence that
physiotherapy started before this stage is of further
benefit. Abnormal postures are discouraged and
normal patterns of posture and movement are encouraged. Many children with cerebral palsy are
severely disabled by the persistence of primitive
reflex postures. One aim of physiotherapy is to
inhibit these postures and to facilitate more

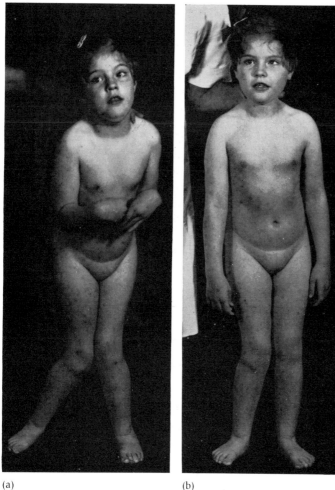

(a) (b)

Fig. 19.5 Spastic quadriplegia.
(a) Before physiotherapy. (b) Same
child after 30 minutes of postural
physiotherapy to inhibit the
increased tone.

normal movements. Figure 19.5 demonstrates the difference in posture before and after 30 minutes of physiotherapy in a young child with bilateral hemiplegia.

Mothers can easily be taught these methods and this is important in encouraging the family that they are all making an important contribution to the child's progress.

OCCUPATIONAL THERAPY

This is a most important aspect of the child's management and should be undertaken in conjunction with physiotherapy. Initially the child must be encouraged to sit in a position of maximum advantage to eye and hand control and to minimize spinal curvature. The design of the chair is also particularly important for feeding. A head rest to prevent excessive neck flexion and a table bar to fix the hand is important for athetoid children. A specially designed chair built to the specifications of the child is necessary and a walking or lying frame may also be built so that the child can make maximal use of his hands.

Splints may be necessary for some children to aid walking. Well-fitting boots with good ankle support are particularly important. The child should be helped to become independent as early as possible. To make this easier, crockery, eating implements and clothes should be suitably modified.

SPEECH THERAPY

Children with feeding problems related to cerebral palsy can be helped by both the speech therapist and the physiotherapist. In the field of communication, the speech therapist encourages verbal skills as well as introducing alternative methods of communication such as signing or microcomputers if the child is severely disabled.

ORTHOPAEDIC INTERVENTION

Some children with severe spasticity may benefit from the use of drugs which reduce muscle spasm. Baclofen (Lioresal) has been most widely used but unfortunately it may exacerbate a tendency towards convulsions.

Spastic cerebral palsy may cause permanent postural changes due to the long-standing effects of increased tone. In children who achieve independent walking, splinting may be necessary to control the leg in a normal posture. Tendon lengthening, especially the tendo Achilles, may help provided that maximum improvement from physiotherapy has been achieved first. Surgery to stabilize joints such as ankles and hips may also be particularly helpful. Whenever possible surgery should be delayed until after adolescence, so that growth has ceased.

Surgery may also be undertaken in severely handicapped children in whom independent walking is not likely to be achieved. Adductor tenotomy will allow thigh abduction and lessen the risk of hip dislocation. Scoliosis is an important condition in this group of children and the spine must be regularly assessed. Scoliosis should be managed by an experienced orthopaedic team.

Mental handicap

A distinction must be made between developmental delay and mental retardation. Mental retardation implies an impairment of reasoning ability and can only be diagnosed when the child is old enough for his reasoning ability to be tested. The earliest age at which intelligence testing is possible is between 2 and 3 years. Intelligence is expressed as an IQ (intelligence quotient). This was standardized on an average score of 100 for the population at large, but now the norm is closer to 110. Intelligence testing is a complicated and controversial subject and there are a large number of tests, many of which are only appropriate at a specific age. The best known British psychometric tests include the Wechsler Intelligence Scale for Children (WISC), the Merrill Palmer, the British Ability Scales and the Griffiths Developmental Scale. Some children with a possible combination of developmental problems require specific tests to assess intelligence adequately. The Reynell Developmental Language Scale is used for children with speech and language problems and children who are deaf or blind must be tested with scales appropriate to their disabilities.

By contrast, development is tested by observing the developmental skills of a child and does not necessarily reflect reasoning ability. Developmental age is expressed as a DQ (developmental quotient) based on the observed developmental skills compared to the chronological age corrected for prematurity if this is appropriate.

Intelligence in a community is represented as a Gaussian curve (Fig. 19.6) and a proportion of 'normal' children will fall into the mildly subnormal range. Children with mild mental subnormality therefore represent a very heterogeneous group. They may have no reason for being subnormal other than genetic or environmental influences. Unfortunately, those who are most socially disadvantaged are also those least likely to be stimulated as babies and to have the least good educational opportunities.

Children may be classified on the basis of intelligence testing into two classes of educational subnormality depending on their IQ:

Educationally subnormal, IQ 50–70
  mild – ESN(M)

Educationally subnormal, IQ < 50
  severe – ESN(S)

The severely subnormal child is defined as one who is 'incapable of living an independent life or of guarding himself against serious exploitation'. In Britain the terms ESN(M) and ESN(S) are no longer used in an educational context, but they serve to describe the severity of the mental impairment.

Aetiology

This is a much more heterogeneous condition than cerebral palsy and may have diverse causes. Mental handicap may be due to cerebral abnormality either congenital or acquired, genetic conditions, environmental, metabolic or traumatic lesions. In a significant number of cases no specific cause can be identified. Table 19.3 lists the commoner causes of severe mental retardation.

For a child to achieve his full intellectual potential a variety of factors must operate optimally on his genetic background. There is a very rapid brain growth spurt in the mid-trimester of pregnancy which is maintained for the first 2 years of life. Malnutrition during this time may cause permanent restriction of brain growth which cannot be corrected by subsequent adequate nutrition. Severe intrauterine growth retardation may cause a child's eventual IQ to be significantly lower than a child with similar socioeconomic background who has not been starved *in utero*. It is unlikely that this form of nutritional inadequacy alone will be enough to cause severe subnormality.

Learning opportunities are essential for normal intellectual development. The child who is totally deprived of stimulation will be severely subnormal in later years. Complete lack of any form of stimulation will cause severe delay in speech and intellectual development but little impairment of motor development.

PREVALENCE

The prevalence of severe mental subnormality is approximately 3:1000 school-age children. The commonest single cause is Down's syndrome which accounts for up to 30% of children with mental handicap. Amongst males the fragile X syndrome is the next most common cause of severe mental retardation and this is discussed fully on p. 126. Approximately 10:1000 children fall into the ESN(M) group.

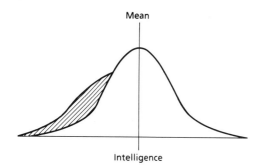

Fig. 19.6 The normal (Gaussian) distribution for intelligence. The shaded area to the left of the curve represents 'abnormal' cases of mental retardation in which a cause can be found.

Table 19.3 Causes of mental retardation.

Chromosomal*
  Down's syndrome
  Fragile X syndrome
  Cri du chat syndrome
Genetic
  Autosomal recessive*
  X-linked recessive*
  Tuberous sclerosis
  Neurofibromatosis
Cerebral malformations*
Metabolic
  Hypoglycaemia
  Hypothyroidism*
  Phenylketonuria, including undiagnosed maternal
    disease
  Galactosaemia
  Mucopolysaccharidoses
  Amino-acidurias
  Organic acidurias
  Mucolipidoses
  Peroxisomal disorders
Prenatal infection
  Cytomegalovirus
  Toxoplasmosis
  Rubella
Infective
  Meningitis
  Encephalitis
  Cerebral abscess
Environmental
  Starvation*
  Alcohol*
  Lead*
  Severe emotional deprivation
Perinatal
  Birth asphyxia
  Intracranial haemorrhage
  Cerebral infarction
Psychosis
  Autism

* Represents those conditions in which mental retardation may occur in isolation from other neurological deficits.

Diagnosis

Diagnosis is made by psychometric testing. There is always a history of developmental delay unless there has been a postnatal cause for the cerebral damage which has led to mental handicap. Diagnosis is particularly difficult if there are associ-ated defects such as cerebral palsy. In severe cerebral palsy it may be extremely difficult to detect the child's intellect which is locked up inside an impotent body. A number of other conditions can lead to a false impression of mental retardation; these must be considered in every case. They include visual and auditory defects, emotional disorders, speech defects, autism (p. 345), developmental aphasia and the syndrome of the clumsy child.

It is essential to take a careful family history in every case. Many causes of mental handicap, particularly severe, are genetically inherited. Thorough physical examination of the child is also essential. Dysmorphic features such as occur in Down's syndrome should be considered and the occipito-frontal head circumference should be measured to exclude microcephaly. Chromosome analysis is mandatory in all cases of mental retardation with special attention to the fragile X syndrome. Prenatal infection screening is also important but of limited value in older children.

Every mentally handicapped child must be investigated to determine whether there is an underlying metabolic defect. These disorders include enzyme defects affecting amino acid, carbohydrate, lipid or mineral metabolism. In addition, an increasing number of other rare metabolic disorders are being recognized which cause mental retardation or regression of learnt skills. These disorders may be associated with subtle dysmorphic features, organomegaly (particularly hepatosplenomegaly) or retinal abnormalities. Biopsy of liver, bone marrow or rectal mucosa may confirm the diagnosis in some of these conditions.

Undiagnosed maternal phenylketonuria should be considered in all mentally handicapped children. The mothers have impaired intellectual ability but this may not be severe. They usually suffer from epileptic convulsions. The mother's serum or urine should be tested for an excess of phenylalanine.

Associated problems

Table 19.4 lists the major associated problems which are relatively commonly seen in children who are

Table 19.4 Problems associated with mental retardation.

Visual defects
Hearing impairment
  Sensorineural
  Conductive
Epilepsy
Behaviour disorders
Sleep problems
Hyperactivity
Speech and language disorders
Dental caries

mentally handicapped. Many of these are· discussed elsewhere in this book.

Patterns of behaviour that are common in mentally handicapped children include head banging, repetitive rocking movements, masturbation and self-stimulation including eye kneading and mutilating picking. Many mentally handicapped children show behaviour patterns considered to be antisocial when considered in the context of children of normal intelligence. This may be acceptable in small children but can cause problems when the child is adolescent. Excessive masturbation or inappropriate affection may be particularly embarassing to the family and may put the child at risk of sexual abuse by adults. Unwanted pregnancy is always a risk in sexually mature mentally handicapped girls.

Management

Early detection of mental handicap is important, not only for the rare treatable cases but also for the opportunity of offering the child and his parents the most appropriate forms of intervention. In the case of Down's syndrome the diagnosis is obvious from birth and the parents should be told immediately of the doctor's suspicions. Confirmation will come later once the chromosomes have been examined. In most other cases of mental retardation the diagnosis is not made suddenly, but the child's delay becomes progressively more apparent as his chronological age outstrips his developmental and intellectual achievements. The

doctor should discuss with the parents the possibility of mental retardation relatively early when the diagnosis is first seriously considered. The parents may fear this diagnosis and a frank and open discussion often clears the air. An honest relationship with the parents serves as a very important foundation to the relationship that the doctor and therapists will build with the child and his family and which will lasts for many years.

It is misleading to tell the parents that the child's development is half his chronological age. If this statement is left unqualified, many parents will believe that at 10 years of age their child will be like a 5-year-old and so on. Other parents told that their child is mentally handicapped will believe this means a standstill in further development. Parents should be helped to understand that all children progress to some extent each year, though the rate varies with the intelligence quotient. Over a period of years they will appreciate some development, even though this may only be slight.

Parents' reaction to the diagnosis will vary from aggressive rejection to pathological attachment associated with feelings of guilt. The first stage is to help the parents mourn the loss of the perfect child they had expected. Once they have accepted the fact that their child is retarded, they are in a position to work out with the doctor and therapists the best way to help the child.

EDUCATION

It is an attractive proposition that early detection of mental retardation will allow a programme of early stimulation to improve the developmental milestones. Down's syndrome is the condition that lends itself best to this approach as the diagnosis is obvious at birth. The best-known method is the Portage scheme which was developed in the USA and has been adopted in many parts of Britain. The children (from an age of between 9 and 12 months) are set goals to achieve in directed play activities. These are reviewed weekly and further goals given once the earlier ones are achieved. The philosophy involves the setting of realistic objectives that the child can achieve in a relatively short period of time. This method depends on a large parental input and a supervisor keeping very close contact, together with a supply of appropriate toys. The method is very popular amongst a group of parents but there is little convincing evidence that it does actually improve the IQ of these children in later childhood or adolescence.

There can be no doubt that children with intellectual impairment do better in a loving and stimulating environment and this usually means the child's own family home. Residential accommodation is recommended only for the needs of parents or siblings, not for the patient. A period of 2–4 weeks to give the parents a holiday is often the greatest help.

Educational needs of the mentally handicapped child will be determined by the local authority and the child will undergo the process of 'statementing' as described on p. 320. Many children who are ESN(M) may be educated in a normal school but receive additional remedial teaching sometimes in the context of a class for children with special needs. Children who are ESN(S) will need special education in a school for severely mentally handicapped children which is staffed by teachers specially trained to meet their needs.

MEDICAL SUPPORT

A high proportion of mentally handicapped children show emotional disturbance. Doctors must be aware of this and offer advice to parents on behaviour modification. Many parents have unknowingly reached the point where they respond only to their child's 'bad' behaviour. For example, unless he cries or shouts they take no notice of his requests for help and it is little wonder that he shouts and cries so much. Once the parents are helped to understand what is happening and to respond to good behaviour rather than to negative behaviour, the child's performance improves. Sometimes more formal family psychotherapy is necessary to help a complicated crisis in the home.

Epilepsy is common in mentally handicapped children and careful pharmacological management is necessary to control seizures as well as possible. Careful assessment of vision and hearing is also necessary to avoid the child being more disabled by a treatable reduction in sensory input.

PROGNOSIS

It is very difficult to give accurate information as to prognosis in children who are severely mentally retarded. Much depends on the family background and educational opportunities. In general terms, one-third will be totally dependent and two-thirds will achieve a degree of independence as adults and some may be able to live alone with community support.

'Minor' neurological deficits

This term has been used to describe a group of children with a constellation of features which together suggest that there is failure of normal cerebral integration. These children have also been described as having 'soft neurological signs', minimal brain dysfunction and the clumsy child also fits into this group. The term minimal brain dysfunction has been criticized by the late Dr Tom Ingram who claimed that it is not used to make a diagnosis, but to escape from making one. Whether these children have organic pathology or whether this condition just represents one end of a normal range has never been satisfactorily resolved, but it is considered to be an entity by some and is therefore discussed here. It would, however, be wrong to believe that the term minor neurological deficit describes a single disorder or even a consistent pattern of abnormal behaviour.

THE CLUMSY CHILD

Normal motor co-ordination and adroitness develops rapidly between the ages of 3 and 8 years and it is the child who fails to show this maturation who is referred to as clumsy. This affects about 5% of school-age children and is much commoner in boys. It has been suggested that this is simply a problem of maturation and in time dexterity will improve, but the follow-up evidence for this is lacking at present. If not a failure of maturation, clumsiness may be due to a minor motor disorder (dyspraxia), in other words a sub-clinical form of cerebral palsy, or alternatively a disorder of sensation and perception (agnosia). Clumsiness occurs more frequently in children who have been born prematurely and in those who have suffered intra-uterine growth retardation suggesting that there are organic factors in terms of the child's cerebral organization.

The child is awkward in all motor activities and has great difficulty in dressing, especially with buttons and laces, ball catching and writing. He may show features of hyperactivity with a short attention span and get blamed in school for fidgeting. Many of the children have perceptual difficulties and left–right confusion. Spatial relationships and the concept of their body image may be disturbed.

Objective neurological testing of dexterity may be helpful in showing particular deficits. There is often impairment in the ability to tap the index finger on the thumb, rapidly and repeatedly, and also to pronate and supinate the forearm rapidly. These items are of course age-related and comparison must be between children of similar ages. Gross motor function is also diminished. They find it more difficult to stand on one leg, jump and hop. Clumsy children usually have above average reading skills and their verbal ability is good.

Management is difficult and may not be particularly effective. Clumsy children require infinite patience from everyone around them. At first it may help if new skills are broken down into simple parts so that they can be taught separately and then recombined into a whole.

LEARNING DISABILITY

This concept describes the child who has normal intelligence as assessed by psychometric testing, yet has difficulty in understanding or processing the spoken or written word. The child with a learning disability is therefore one who has a discrepancy between IQ and achievement. It has been suggested that children with learning disabilities show more 'soft neurological signs' such as clumsiness but this has been disputed. There is a subgroup of children with mild cerebral palsy or epilepsy who show significant learning difficulties and this should be anticipated.

If this condition exists as a pathological disorder it is certainly heterogeneous and children may fail to achieve for many reasons. Such children should be very carefully assessed by an educational psychologist and remedial teaching by an experienced teacher may be of great help.

Children with learning disability may present with anxiety, depression or behaviour problems due to frustration. Learning disorders may include the highly intelligent or 'gifted' child who can cope in a normal class no better than a subnormal child and who may present with major behavioural disturbances.

HYPERACTIVITY

This is also discussed in Chapter 17. There is considerable difficulty as to the definition of hyperactivity but it is generally considered to be associated with a short attention span, increased distractability and impulsiveness. There is evidence that children who are clinically hyperactive also show an increased number of 'soft neurological signs'.

DYSLEXIA

Dyslexia refers to children who have specific difficulties with reading but are of normal intelligence. A reading age 2 years behind the chronological age may occur in up to 10% of 10-year-olds and is three times commoner in boys than girls. There is often a family history of reading problems. Dyslexia is due to a variety of poorly understood conditions including inability to recognize the written word, inability to relate the written word to visual or auditory memory or integration of the senses involved with reading and writing. In addition to dyslexia, these children often have left–right confusion, poor handwriting, mirror writing and they may be extremely clumsy.

Dyslexia does not have a single cause and in view of the heterogeneous nature of the problem there can be no uniform management strategy. The specific problems of the individual child must be assessed and tasks designed to reinforce more normal processing. Positive reinforcement is essential but progress is often slow and the children, who may be highly intelligent, may continue to have severe problems throughout life.

Further reading

Hall DMB. *The Child With a Handicap*. Blackwell Scientific Publications, Oxford 1984.

20
EMOTIONAL AND
BEHAVIOURAL DISORDERS

A separate chapter on emotional disorders in a book on child health is something of an artefact since, as implied in Chapter 1, any episode of ill health in children will have an impact on the emotional life of both the child and his family. In many cases the impact is mercifully brief but in others, particularly where chronic disorder and disability are involved, the emotional reaction of the child and family can critically influence the extent of the resulting handicap.

Emotional and behavioural disorders are extremely common. Community studies have identified prevalence rates of between 6 and 21% in different communities, with a strong tendency for high rates in groups subject to social deprivation. The child psychiatrist will only see a small fraction of these problems, others will come to the attention of the family doctor or paediatrician. For this reason, a comprehensive, if highly condensed overview of children's emotional and behavioural problems will be presented here, then some particularly relevant disorders will be picked out for more detailed discussion.

Developmental psychopathology

Some elements of developmental psychology were introduced in Chapter 4. Childhood disorder can best be understood by reference to the way that development has deviated from the normal in particular children. There are two situations that should be carefully distinguished in the clinical situation. First, some 'symptoms' are indeed passing phases; fears and tantrums in 3-year-olds are a

good example. The paediatrician should know when to expect a function to be within the child's capabilities, for example, efforts to treat enuresis under 5 years are likely to fail because nocturnal dryness as a stage is often not reached until after this age. The second situation is where deviations in development may indicate more serious problems. By considering development under a few simple headings, we can point out ways in which deviant development can lead to problems.

ATTACHMENT AND EARLY SOCIAL RELATIONSHIPS

Here deviations from normal development can take two forms: *exaggaration of attachment* and *detachment*.

Exaggaration of attachment

In this case, emotional tension in the child's early attachment to parent figures can give rise to either clinging behaviour or to angry turning away from the parent. This is beautifully shown in the classic films of children in brief separation by James and Joyce Robertson. These difficulties, if not corrected at an early stage can lead to a vicious circle of difficulties with the parent, resulting in chronic emotional tension, increasing naughtiness and antisocial behaviour by the child and rejection and despair by the parent. These reactions have major implications for the young child admitted to hospital, undergoing fostering or entering children's homes. Reluctance and tears on arrival at school is another manifestation of attachment. It is common and not particularly significant at 5 years old when the child first goes to school, moving out of the ambit of the parent into a new, demanding environment for the first time. At 15, when the need for such attachment represents a major deviation from normal development, school refusal it is often a portent of severe psychiatric difficulties extending into adult life.

Detachment

In detachment, repeated disruption of the parent–child bond, e.g. by admissions into local authority care, seems to be an important ingredient. It is the parental rejection and discord that is associated with the difficulty rather than the separation in itself, since separation under happier circumstances, such as the mother working, doesn't have the same adverse consequences. The types of disturbance that can arise include conduct disorder (described below) or nocturnal enuresis. Intellectual retardation can result from understimulation of the child in the early years.

OTHER SOCIAL DEVELOPMENT

The birth of a younger sibling results in dramatic changes in the relationship of the older child to the mother. This can result in more confrontations and naughtiness which, if the mother is having other difficulties and doesn't have enough emotional support, can result in continuing behaviour problems. Play relationships with other children develop in the first few years in a sequence from no interaction to parallel play and finally co-operative play. Disturbed children often demonstrate the greatest difficulty in sharing and co-operation with other children of their own age.

PSYCHOSEXUAL DEVELOPMENT

This is a particularly important issue since recent discoveries about the extensiveness of child sexual abuse (p. 524). For example, flirtatious and provocative behaviour towards her peers is normal in an extrovert 15-year-old girl whereas it would be abnormal, indeed very worrying, in a 7-year-old, or if directed exclusively towards older men.

LANGUAGE DEVELOPMENT

Language is the ability to receive, process and transmit symbolic information to others. It has many components: hearing behaviour, reception of language, the ability to use 'inner language' which is necessary for any but the most primitive thought, speech and other forms of language production, which would also include sign language. Delays can arise as a specific developmental problem or as a component of general intellectual retardation. More complex disorders include early childhood autism and specific language delays which are sometimes associated with educational difficulties in later childhood and conduct disorders.

TEMPERAMENT

Another set of issues in development is the individuality of a particular child through the developmental process. It will be no surprise to the reader to be told that human behaviour alters out of all recognition between the ages of 0 and 21 years. The next question is whether there is any continuity in the individual though this period and, if so, has this any significance? Infant temperament has been intensively studied from this point of view, and it is clear that some children are more difficult to bring up than others because they are active, irregular in their biological rhythms such as sleep and feeding and tend to be negative in mood. The parent–child relationship is more liable to go wrong in these children who also react more adversely to parent–child separation. Information about the temperament of the child is an important part of the developmental history.

Assessment

Chapter 1 was devoted to history taking and examination, however, it is necessary to devote a little space to examine the art and discipline of good history taking when the prime object is to assess an emotional problem. This should include an interview with the child and with the parents. Interviewing children is not easy. One may see the parents as providing more 'objective' information and thus give great weight to their account. The fact is, however, that parents often come to the doctor when they are angry with, or worried about, their child and this concern may lead to the adult giving a coloured account of events. This is not a reason to dismiss the parental history but rather to see it as one part of an assessment that should also include an interview with the child. It is also essential to get an account from the school since behaviour of children at school is usually sharply different from behaviour at home. Where relevant, other professionals such as the health visitor should also be consulted. Some aspects of psychological function can be assessed more rigorously; intellectual level and educational attainment are common examples, but other aspects of relationships can also be assessed formally, and, in particular, direct observation of behaviour and social interaction. A popular approach to assessment with a rather different purpose is the whole family interview but this will not be described in detail here.

TALKING TO CHILDREN

Distraught parents, bewildered doctors and puzzled teachers utter the same cry: 'how do you get through to this child?'. The masters of child psychiatry, such as Winnicott, have written detailed transcripts of encounters with children in which they really do seem to have 'got through' to them in just this way. For most of us, however, it is as well to have a framework for our interview with the child at our fingertips just as one does for any other case history or examination. Talking to children repays practice. Here are some of the special problems together with ways of coping with them. A summary of the areas that should be covered in a routine child interview can be found in Table 20.1.

Table 20.1 Format for interviewing children.

Child welcomed and set at ease. Go to waiting room and observe interaction with parent. Play or interview? Reassure that confidences will not be betrayed.

Establish relationship
Ask about hobbies and activities. What TV programmes do you like? What do your enjoy at school? Pop music, football, etc.

Presenting problem
'What did you hear about why you have come here?' When you have their account, share your knowledge of why they have come. Be prepared with face-saving explanations for embarrassing problems.
   Ask for concrete detail about the problem.

Exploration of life areas
To be approached from least emotive moving to more emotive areas.

School
   General attitude to teacher, to work and to peers. Attitude to any problems that have arisen at school. What do you like best/least? Anybody at school helpful to you?

Peers
   General report about friends. What do you do together? Any special friends? Fall out with friends? Visit each other's homes? Etc.

Family
   Relationship with siblings, things they do together, quarrels, etc. Parents: their health? Who are they closest to? What do you do together? Who is the strictest? Any arguments with either parent?

Table 20.1 (cont)

Psychopathology and health

Physical symptoms
    How is your health? Do you have any aches or pains: tummy aches, headaches, growing pains? Does it get worse
        when you are upset? Do you worry about your health? Ascertain whether they have hypochondriacal fears and
        ideas.

Sleep and appetite
    Going to sleep? Wake at night? Wake early? Any dreams or nightmares? Any tiredness and lassitude? Eat OK? Enjoy
        food? Likes and dislikes?

Concentration
    Can you concentrate on things you like doing? What about schoolwork?

Activity
    Do you get restless and fidgity? Do you get into trouble for running about or being restless?

Depression
    Do you get fed up and miserable? How long does it last? Find you don't enjoy things as you used to?

Anxiety
    Are you a worrier? Get nasty thoughts you can't get rid of? Afraid of particular things like spiders, dogs, etc?

Direct observations

Speech
    Articulation, maturity, amount.

Activity level
    Attention, distractability.

Relating to examiner
    Eye contact, spontaneity, responsiveness.

Mood
    Anxiety, depression, anger.

Activities
    Jigsaws, imaginative play, paints and crayons.

Children may be shy of revealing their more personal thoughts and, indeed, they may be unaware of more painful feelings and conflicts. It may be possible to understand children by the way they cope with feelings rather than to rely on their reporting them. To take a simple example, a friendless child may give a vivid account of how many friends he has and how he is a leader of his group. Phenomena such as these, ways of coping with conflict and failure, were recognized many years ago by Anna Freud and were called 'defence mechanisms'.

Children are brought to the doctor because an adult is annoyed with them or worried about them. They may not know why they have come but will likely have some half-formed suspicions that it is because they have been a nuisance. The visit may have been presented as some kind of punishment. For this reason, it is best not to ask the child about the problem immediately, but to concentrate on establishing a warm and friendly relationship. The use of toys, painting and other play materials is a great help. Later in the interview, when the child has had a chance to get to know you, you can ask about the reason for the referral. A good approach is to ask: 'what did you hear about why you have come here today?'.

Young and disabled children may have limited understanding of language. They will be made anxious if you use words they don't understand, and will 'best guess' the answers. If set in context, very simple language can tell the whole story, e.g. 'what was it like when the time came to go to school — good or bad?'. Direct observation of behaviour is very important in children for the same reason.

Under the age of about 7 years, and even in some much older children, play is an essential component of any interview. Apart from being enjoyable and relationship building, the play sessions can develop into an interaction where the children can communicate their concerns in their own way.

Painful feelings in a child are very near the surface. Just talking about an adverse experience can re-evoke the accompanying affect with great intensity with the result that the child becomes uncontrollably distressed or will not want to 'talk to that doctor again'. The art is to keep the interview on a generally light note but to probe emotive areas at the right moment. It is useful to warn and ask the child if you can talk about a particular topic, e.g. for a bereaved child it might be appropriate to ask 'could we talk a bit about your grandma?'. If the child says no, you can ask if you could come back to the topic later. If the child is prepared to discuss the topic, be ready to move off it quickly if they seem to be getting upset. There is nothing to be gained by sending a distressed and decompensated child back to his parents; it is likely to be the last time you see him.

PARENT INTERVIEW

When emotional problems are suspected, the case history format outlined in Chapter 1 can be extended in three main directions. First, it is clearly appropriate to spend more time on the family and social history and to follow leads in these areas more fully. Secondly, more time should be given to asking the parents to describe the child's mood and behaviour as well as any physical symptoms they may have. Thirdly, there is the importance of listening to the parents' account with the 'third ear'. The way the parent tells the story of their difficulties has been found to be more meaningful in predictive studies than the content of what they say. Ask yourself:

'does this parent get any pleasure from their child?',

'are they critical of the child?',

'do they seem to be over-involved, so that you feel that they are suffering more than the child itself from the painful symptoms?',

'do they present an emotional and dramatic display?'.

These factors are helpful both in psychodiagnosis and management. As in any other good history, it is best to have a format of areas that you always cover. This is covered in Table 20.2.

CONJOINT FAMILY INTERVIEW

Seeing the whole family together for assessment of emotional problems and for therapy has become popular with some child psychiatrists and social workers. In the hands of the well trained and experienced, this approach can be very effective. It is based on the idea that the family is the main socializing organization in society and that this socialization occurs in the context of the largely unconscious every-day interaction in the family. An interview with the whole family seen together can help in understanding the structure and relationships of the family. For the clinician with little experience in this area, whole family interviews are best confined to occasions where the meeting has a very specific purpose.

Diagnosis and classification

The bald statement of a diagnosis has a less important function in emotional disorders than in physical disorders. This is because the problems

Table 20.2 Format for parent interview.

Try to see both parents. Explain the form the consultation will take. Introduce yourself.

Reason for referral and presenting problem
Spend time here. Ask open questions. Establish motivation behind referral. Explore time relationships. Precipitants.
How was the problem handled? What impact did it have on others, including parents?

Feeling and attitude of parents
How do the parents tell the story? Do they express concern? Over-involvement? A rejecting attitude? Do they display
warmth and sympathy towards the child?

Systematic exploration

Health
  Somatic pains, sphincter control, fits and 'blackouts'. Episodes in hospital.

Motor
  Clumsiness or over-activity.

Relationships
  Siblings, peers, teachers and other adults, parents. Any special attachments to adults?

Psychosexual
  Relationships with opposite sex, sexual precocity or other concerns of parents.

Moral development
  Aggression or other antisocial behaviour.

Education
  Attitudes (of parents and child). Attainments. Do parents visit the school?

Family structure
  Parents' ages, occupations and health. Grandparents, aunts, uncles and cousins and their relationship to nuclear
    family.

Family relationships
  Communication about family problems, sharing of roles. Satisfaction within the family.

Child's development
  Any other aspects of development, separations, etc.

encountered tend to have many interacting causes and it is thus more helpful to develop a diagnostic formulation which gives a fuller account of the many roots of the disorder and develops a hypothesis of how the problem came about and how it can be solved (see below for an example of how this works). Some clinicians and social scientists decry the whole idea of classification in emotional disorders on the grounds that it dehumanizes the individual. The classification of child psychiatric disorders is, however, essential because not all emotional problems have the same causes, implications and outcome. What is important is to remember that problems can be considered in several ways simultaneously; as unique predicaments and in a systematic framework. This presentation is based on the World Health Organization ICD-9 system, which is in widespread use at the time of writing. This system allows the clinician to classify the disorder under five separate

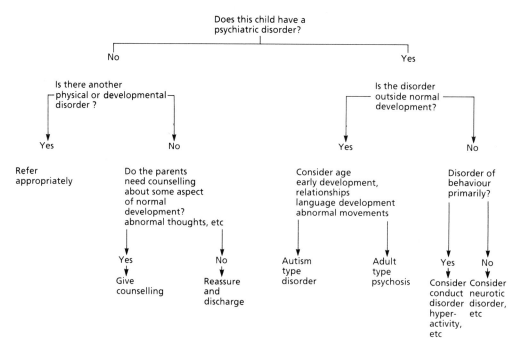

Fig. 20.1 Flow diagram of diagnosis. In all cases consider whether there are developmental problems: either as a global feature or isolated delays. Are there other medical problems? What is the social context? The ultimate aim is to arrive at a formulated treatment hypothesis and treatment plan.

headings simultaneously; it is therefore a multi-axial classification system (Fig. 20.1). The headings are:

1 Psychiatric disorder.
2 Specific developmental problems.
3 Intellectual level.
4 Medical conditions.
5 Abnormal psychosocial factors.

This presentation will help to highlight some of the underlying principles.

A sequence of questions can be asked while carrying out an assessment.

Does the child have a psychiatric disorder?

This first question should differentiate disorder from mild difficulties that are part and parcel of development. A psychiatric disorder can be defined as a persistent disorder of behaviour, emotions or relationships which is abnormal in the context of the child's sociocultural background

and developmental stage. It should be accompanied by an impairment of personal and social functioning, cause significant ongoing distress and/or interfere with the development of the child to a handicapping degree.

Is the disorder an exaggeration of behaviour seen in ordinary development or something outside normal development?

The most prominent example of this latter much less common situation is *childhood autism*. This is present from birth or becomes manifest in the first 30 months. There are a triad of features of the condition, in the fields of language, social behaviour and repetitive stereotyped behaviour (see below).

Other disorders which have features outside normal development are older children with adult-type psychiatric disorders such as *schizophrenia* and *manic depressive psychosis*. These are rare in children but more common in adolescents. They show the usual features of these conditions, but it is more difficult to distinguish between the different forms of psychosis, thus mania may present as a delusional psychosis rather similar to schizophrenia.

If the disorder can best be described as an exaggeration of normal development, does it take the form of disturbance of emotions within the child or of disturbance of conduct?

These are the most common problems in child psychiatry. The young child with an *emotional disorder* will be anxious, unhappy, shy, sensitive, fearful or withdrawn to a degree where their symptoms give rise to concern or impair their progress. The problems may arise around particular situations, school being a common one, or there may be a more general withdrawal. Hysterical conversion states are much more common in children than they are in adults. They may present as fits, paralyses, painful symptoms such as arthritis, excessive fluid intake, vomiting and a host of other conditions.

Emotional disorders may give rise to a lot of individual and family distress but the prognosis is generally good, school progress is unaffected and the disorders are not generally associated with severe family problems. In teenagers, emotional disorders assume characteristics more akin to adult neuroses; anxiety states, obsessional illness and reactive depression. In recent years, a lot of research attention has been directed at whether depression occurs in childhood in the way it does in adult life. There is no resolution of this problem but it is clear that children's unhappiness often goes unrecognized and that it often coexists with or underlies other behaviour problems.

Conduct disorders. This refers to persistent aggressive or destructive behaviour, stealing, setting fires and other bad behaviour. They may be associated with official delinquency, and are often associated with other signs of maladjustment such as difficulty in getting on with other children. Such problems are commonly associated with a family history of disturbed relationships, along with criminality and instability in other ways. Children with severe conduct disorders may have life-long problems of adjustment, unstable relationships, tendency to substance abuse and other health problems. Another rather different disturbance of conduct is *hyperactivity* (see also p. 332). Here the child has a short attention span, is disinhibited and impulsive. There has been a considerable difference between the USA, where this disorder is reported as being very common, and the UK, where it is far less common. Is this a difference in national character, or the way we bring up children? Probably neither, but rather a difference in the way disorder is reported and interpreted. American child psychiatrists pay great attention to *attention deficit disorder* which is sometimes associated with hyperactivity and sometimes not. Hyperactivity has been seen as a sign of brain damage in the past, but this is now seen as true in only a minority of cases. It seems likely that some children are merely temperamentally overactive and this may be exacerbated by family difficulties.

Other disorders. A number of other disorders are likely to present to the clinician. *Anorexia nervosa* is a persistent and active refusal to eat based on the mistaken idea of being overweight (see p. 348). *Tics* are quick, involuntary and apparently purposeless movements which are not part of any neurological disorder. The face is most frequently affected and there may be just one or multiple tics. On rare occasions the tic extends to vocalizations which may be in the form of grunts or may be recognizable words, often with an obscene content. This is *Gilles de la Tourette syndrome.*

Consideration of the other four axes of the classification prompts further questions and extends the systematic framework, thus assisting systematic assessment.

What is the child's general intellectual level?

Children with mild intellectual retardation are more likely to have emotional and behaviour problems than their brighter peers. Severely retarded children have a high rate of additional problems such as autism and hyperactivity.

Are there any specific delays in development?

Child development can be seen as an ordered sequence of events, but language, reading, arithmetic or motor functions can sometimes be delayed past their correct point in this timetable. This is a specific delay in development. Some of these, such as language and reading problems are rather commonly associated with conduct disorders and hyperactivity.

Chronic medical disorders and disabilities

Chronic medical disorders and disabilities have many links with emotional problems and a variety of routes of causation can be postulated in the individual case. The disorder may have affected the child's self-esteem and self-confidence, the burden of care on the parents may encourage over-protectiveness or may have triggered family break-up. The behaviour problem may have precipitated the medical problem, such as when accidents are caused by a child's oppositional or impulsive behaviour. Children with *disorders that effect brain function* such as underlying epilepsy or cerebral palsy are particularly vulnerable to psychiatric disorders.

The social sphere

The social sphere is the one that is most closely associated with child disturbance in the public and professional mind. Comments such as 'what can you expect with parents like that' or 'when the child has a problem, treat the parents' are still prevalent. These represent less-than-helpful generalizations from undoubted truths. Thus there is strong evidence that conduct disorder and delinquency are transmitted through family culture and discord, although even here there is some evidence from twin and adoption studies for a genetic influence, perhaps operating through some indirect mechanism. In childhood emotional dis-

orders, there is a weaker link with social factors.

As with the rest of the classificatory framework, this social description does not imply that the social situation causes the child's disorder, merely that a description of social problems is a necessary part of any formulation of a child's problem. The social problems concerned may be within the family or difficulties in the wider community, such as migration or a natural disaster.

DIAGNOSTIC FORMULATION

This consists of a summary of the essential features of the problem in all its facets: psychiatric, developmental, medical and social. This is followed by a differential diagnosis, a hypothesis regarding the way the disorder developed and is maintained, together with recommendations for treatment. The procedure is best illustrated by an example.

Kevin is a 6-year-old boy who has been a focus of concern since infancy. He now presents with ceaseless over-activity which is present in all situations. His parents are most concerned about outbursts of aggression directed at his younger brother. This leads to major tension and discord within the home. Kevin has global developmental delay with a social age of around 18 months. There is no speech. The cause of his mental retardation is tuberous sclerosis, which is also the origin of his focal fits. The parents are at present getting little family support with this boy, although the school offers some relief. There are signs that the family relationships are being adversely affected by the management problem he presents and this is a cause of major concern. Treatment will need to involve the whole family and be angled towards social and material support rather than major family change, although methods of control of children could be usefully explored further. Behavioural methods should be tried and also a cerebral stimulant and major tranquillizers. The disorder appears to be the result of a new mutation.

Two points about the formulation should be noted:
1 That the axes in the classification offer an excellent framework in developing the formulation.

2 That the treatment plan has several components to it; in this case a mixture of supportive counselling, direct help in modifying the environment and drug treatment. In child psychiatry there is no place for giving drug treatment unless the social, developmental and medical situation has been properly assessed and a full treatment plan considered.

Principles of treatment

The most usual form of treatment is psychotherapy of various types. Psychotherapy is the use of psychological principles to relieve a problem of living. Medical or non-medical members of the child psychiatric team are skilled in the application of this technique. The history of psychology can be seen as the development of a variety of theories about the basis of human behaviour, motivation and feelings. By and large, the different forms of psychotherapy are based on these rather different ways of looking at the human psyche and it is important to understand the theoretical framework when applying the therapy.

Mental health consultation

In a book for the non-psychiatrist, it is appropriate to start the presentation of treatment principles with the theme of mental health consultation. This is because, as outlined above, there are many more children with psychiatric problems than will ever, or should ever, be seen by child psychiatrists. On the other hand, a very wide group of professionals offer therapeutic help to children in related areas. This argues for collaboration. Mental health consultation can be defined as a discussion between professional equals where the consultant has some skills or knowledge that may be useful to the consultee. The consultee describes the problem and the consultant then asks for elaboration, offers insights, makes suggestions, etc., that may help the consultee with the child or family problem. There are many examples in medical practice where consultation can occur: the psychosocial ward round or a service to a particular clinic such as a child development centre or a diabetic clinic are good examples. Some medical settings are very stressful working environments. In these cases, mental health consultation can be helpful in that a skilled consultant can offer a degree of objectivity in situations where feelings run high. This approach has been used in special care baby units.

The other treatment types to be presented require a degree of special training. They are presented here so that the general doctor can understand some of the principles involved and thus engage in a more informed dialogue with the therapist who is carrying out the treatment, or may become a partner in a consultation process.

Drug treatment

Drug treatment has a limited but important role in child psychiatry. The most carefully researched situation is the use of amphetamines in attention deficit disorder. This has been shown to improve concentration in the short-term although the long-term advantages of treatment are not clear. Antidepressants are used, but there is a need for rigorous clinical trials to assess effectiveness. Tics and Tourettes syndrome respond to haloperidol and pimozide, and phenothiazines have been used for aggressive behaviour. Overall, there is a need for more research to establish the place of drugs in child psychiatry.

Psychodynamic therapies

Psychodynamic therapies take as their starting point that the behaviour we see is merely the tip of the iceberg of human feeling, motivation and potential behaviour. The main aim of therapy is to understand the child and get in touch with their deeper, often unconscious longings, frustrations and feelings which are expressed indirectly as symptoms. The acknowledgement of feelings that are unacceptable and which give rise to guilt and shame is particularly valuable. There are a variety of different psychodynamic therapies, the most well known being based in some way on psychoanalysis, the system of psychology developed by

Sigmund Freud and his disciples, including his daughter referred to earlier. Other psychodynamic approaches include the technique developed by Virginia Axline which is a particularly useful and practical approach. The core of this therapy is the relationship between the therapist and the child. This is seen as a learning situation where the child has an opportunity to learn how to establish healthy relationships. Psychodynamic therapy is usually scheduled in meetings of standard length (20 or 50 minutes) which may be once a week or more frequently. Less often than once a week is less helpful. In the meetings the therapist allows space for the child to express himself. In younger children, play is a particularly valuable medium for therapy. Regular supervision from an experienced therapist is particularly important. Dynamic therapies are useful, particularly for emotional difficulties in childhood.

Behaviour therapy

In the case of behavioural therapy it is the behaviour itself that is considered important, rather than unobservable underlying feelings. Behaviours are seen as learned responses which can be strengthened if the consequences of the behaviour are rewarding to the child. Abnormal behaviour is seen as being maintained by rewards that are naturally occurring, e.g. if a neglected child can get attention by misbehaviour, he is rewarded for misbehaving. The therapy *must* start out with an analysis of these natural reinforcers and this can be done best by direct observation of the child in the natural situation, e.g. the home or the classroom. The therapist then has to find a way to replace the natural reinforcers with an alternative regime which will reinforce desirable behaviour. This analysis of the natural reinforcers of behaviour is called a functional analysis. It leads to a treatment hypothesis and the divising of ways in which alternative reinforcers can be established. Recently, behaviour therapists have developed a number of new techniques. These include cognitive therapies, where the thoughts as well as the behaviour of the patient are considered. Also, social skills training, which is particularly helpful for

adolescents who have problems with social relationships. Behaviour therapies can be useful for a variety of disorders. They have a place in the treatment of disruptiveness in school, in early mother–child behaviour difficulties, in childhood autism and a host of other disorders.

Family therapy

In the case of family therapy the family is seen all together and is considered as a small social system that influences the behaviour of the family members and so contributes to the problems that they have with the child who has been identified as the patient. By altering these habitual relationships between family members, the family environment and thus the behaviour of the individual will be modified. The social system that constitutes the totality of family relationships is not easy to change because it is made up of habitual patterns of behaviour that are part of daily life, are deeply ingrained, and operate at an unconscious level. The techniques that are used to change families are based on getting the family to enact modes of behaviour that lie outside their habitual style, or that demonstrate in some vivid way where their difficulty lies. This may be in terms of giving the family homework assignments or of role play in the family meeting. A clinic where thorough training and ongoing supervision is available is necessary for the proper conduct of family therapy. The technique is useful for a variety of disorders which involve family dysfunction. Contraindications include situations of gross family disorganization and where child abuse is suspected.

Educational therapies

All psychotherapies can be seen as learning experiences so it seems logical that some could be linked to special education. There is a long tradition of special schools for maladjusted children, but recently note has been taken of how much ordinary schools can help children in difficulties. Highly structured education has been found to be particularly helpful for children with autism.

In-patient management

In-patient management is only likely to be required for a small number of children with particularly complex or serious problems. An in-patient unit in child psychiatry is very different from an ordinary paediatric ward. The nurses are active therapists, observing the way the children behave and relate to others in the relatively controlled in-patient environment and developing treatment programmes to counter the difficulties. They may use psychodynamic or behavioural techniques.

Specific problems

There are some problems that are particularly likely to present to the doctor or that may present special difficulties. These are the subject of this final section.

Child abuse

All doctors who have dealings with children and families must be conversant with the presentation and the management of the various forms of child abuse and should be prepared to be actively involved when a case comes to their attention. This subject is discussed in detail in Chapter 28.

MANAGEMENT

The psychological needs of the abused child must be carefully considered. The decisions of the case conference (see p. 524) may be various, including whether the matter is taken to Court for the child's protection and whether the child is separated from the family. In some cases, psychotherapeutic approaches, particularly behavioural therapies, can play a useful role in the family while psychodynamic play therapy can be useful to help children overcome the trauma of the abuse. The overall thinking in the management of child abuse should be guided by what are basically quite simple principles of child care. These are:
1 The child's psychological parent may not be the same as the biological parent.
2 Long-term plans need to be developed as soon as possible for the child.

3 The child victims in these situations are, unfortunately unlikely to have a perfectly happy childhood: rather, we must look for the least detrimental alternative for them.

It is essential that the doctor maintains an ongoing interest in the child's welfare and ensures, through regular follow-up, that normal development is taking place.

Autism

Language development is severely delayed as shown by inability to use gesture, and speech delay and abnormality, including echolalia, reversal of pronouns, immature grammer and inability to use abstract terms. Social impairments include abnormal eye-to-eye gaze and lack of social attachments and of co-operative play. They are greatest below 5 years of age. Behaviour problems include rocking, attachment to inanimate objects and repeated behaviour such as pirouetting. General intelligence may be in the normal range, but is usually depressed. Some of the features of autism are common in mentally handicapped children and also in children who have degenerative disorders of the brain, such as subacute sclerosing panencephalitis (p. 283). In this case the features are called *disintegrative psychosis*. Another related but controversial disorder is so-called *Asperger's syndrome* where the child's language is normal but they have social difficulties including a lack of empathy and unusual and obsessive interests.

Aetiology

This disorder may coexist with known brain damage, with deterioration sometimes occurring in the teenage years, or there may be a hereditary link, including the chromosomal abnormality, fragile X (p. 126). In other cases the cause is unknown.

Management

There is no known treatment for the basic defect. Treatment should be a total approach to the family. Home treatment by the parents using behavioural-based approaches is of proven value as is a structured educational regime. With these approaches over time significant relief can be gained from the behaviour problems and social withdrawal and useful advances can be made in language acquisition.

Depression, suicide and attempted suicide

Depressive feelings are common in childhood as in any other age period. In recent years, much attention has been paid to depressive disorders.

Clinical features

The diagnosis is often not considered because it masquerades as other disorders and is not recognized by parents. Psychosomatic symptoms, social withdrawal and school difficulties are common presentations. Children will complain that they do not derive pleasure from usual activities and may withdraw from peer contact. They may show irritability and fits of crying, agitation and lack of energy. The child may regress and show the behaviour of a younger child, e.g. anxious attachment. They may show antisocial behaviour and in older children, there may be feelings of worthlessness, hopelessness and suicidal ideas. The disorder is less clear cut in younger children while in adolescents it approximates to the adult condition. Profound depressions in younger children are rare but can occur.

Aetiology

It has recently been recognized that *bereavement reactions* can be profound in children and this should always be considered. A positive family history may draw attention to a possible *genetic* link in aetiology. Poor family *communication* of feelings in the family may mean that the child's distress has gone unrecognized and has developed into a major disorder. *Post-viral* states can be associated with severe depressions.

Management

Drawing the parents' attention to the nature of the problem can often be of help. Dynamic or non-directive therapy can give the child space to express his feelings. Often the mere fact that the child knows that someone impartial is listening to them and understands is more help than anything. Family therapy can help improve faulty family communication, while cognitive therapy may be tried with adolescents. Antidepressants can make a contribution in severe cases.

SUICIDE AND ATTEMPTED SUICIDE

Successful suicide in children is rare, becoming commoner through the teenage years. The very young case may have above average intelligence. It is often associated with depression but can also be associated with other types of distress, such as family discord. Family difficulties are extremely common and here the attempt represents a faulty method of communication where more adaptive approaches, such as an intimate chat with a parent, are not available because of family problems. Attempted suicide most often consists of overdoses, but the problem merges imperceptibly into other types of self-harm such as wrist cutting.

Management

This is often extremely difficult since the families are often uncooperative and don't keep appointments. For this reason it is advisable that all suicidal attempts should be seen by a child psychiatrist in the acute stage, since if there is any possibility of detecting the underlying problem and establishing treatment, it will be in this crisis period. The initial approach should be that the gesture must mean that the child is seriously distressed; emphasizing the feelings and not the behaviour. Depending on the underlying problem, family or individual therapy may be of help.

School refusal and truancy

With compulsory education to the age of 16 the problem of children who do not attend school arises. In some cases they are kept at home to help an inadequate or disabled parent with younger children and these cases should be recognized.

There are two psychological reasons for school non-attendance.

TRUANCY

With truancy the picture is of an underachieving child, possibly from a large, underprivileged family, who may also show other types of antisocial behaviour. These youngsters may leave home in the morning in the normal way but spend the day with their friends rather than at school. Their absence may escape detection for many months, witness to the fact that parental interest and supervision is limited and that the absence may be secretly welcomed by school staff because the children are so disruptive when at school.

SCHOOL REFUSAL

School refusal presents a different picture. The disorder often follows a move to a larger school or an intercurrent illness and the child may have shown reluctance and anxiety about school for some time. In the acute state, the child will do anything to avoid going to school, including suicide threats and locking themselves away. Unlike truancy, the parents are only too aware of the problem but seem powerless to re-establish attendance. The child is likely to be a high achiever at school and the family may show signs of over-involvement and anxiety.

Aetiology

This is quite different for the two conditions. The truant develops the problem, often as part of a general picture of antisocial behaviour, and the multi-problem picture in the family goes along with this. School refusal on the other hand, occurs in small over-involved and anxious families. The child may show the signs of depressive disorder.

Management

The aim of management is the same in each case; reintegration into school.

Truancy. In this condition, counselling approaches have been found not to be effective. Coercion, in the form of repeated periods of remand by the court is one way of ensuring attendance at school. In some cases, special units have been tried where the curriculum is less demanding and the child can be given remedial help. The problem comes when the child has to be reintegrated into the ordinary classroom.

School refusal. Here a therapy approach is needed, and, depending on the severity and chronicity of the disorder, a period of therapy before the planned return to school may help. In some very severe cases, rehabilitation in a child psychiatric unit with therapeutic education in the programme may be necessary. In milder cases, or where he can be caught early, a quick return to school is the best approach, possibly using a graded approach so that the child returns part-time at first, progressing later. Coexistent depression should be treated, as outlined earlier.

Somatic pains in childhood

Recurrent abdominal pain and headaches are extremely common in childhood, afflicting some 10–20% of children at some time. A minority will be found to have organic disease. In a further proportion of cases, psychological causes are suggested by an association with adverse life events, by the finding of depressive or anxiety disorders at assessment or by characteristic temperamental traits; over-activity and anxiousness. Follow-up studies suggest that the condition can become chronic and persist into adult life. Investigation should exclude physical disorder and a careful psychiatric history and interview should then be undertaken.

Treatment for uncomplicated cases consists in giving the firm message that the symptoms are real, but not an indication of serious illness. If the child is under stress, non-medical but face-saving ways of coping should be developed, gently moving the problem into the psychological sphere. In some children, the symptoms are a warning sign of more severe problems, such as child abuse. This may only be detected after a proper diagnostic assessment and psychosocial investigation.

Anorexia nervosa

The key characteristic here is that the patient has a mistaken idea that they are too fat and, with it, an overwhelming desire to lose weight. This often leads to secretive dieting and to other ways of loosing weight such as excessive exercise and self-induced vomiting. The disorder is primarily one of girls, with a sex ratio of 1:8. In post-pubertal girls, there is secondary amenorrhoea while in younger girls the menarche is delayed.

Aetiology

This remains a mystery although there are no shortage of theories. The condition seems to be more common in upper social classes and in situations where slimness is admired, as among fashion models and ballet dancers. Theories have pointed to over-involvement in the families of anorexics and to the way in which the condition can be used as an attempt at avoiding the difficult task of growing up. On some occasions a major depression or obsessional disorder is evident in the early stages which seems to merge into the compulsion to slim. In some younger children there is a life-long history of faddiness.

Management

At the first interview the family may seen co-operative and well motivated but it is common for a wall of denial of the problem to appear as soon as the therapist attempts to change the status quo. In investigation, a thorough physical examination should be carried out as well as the history and if there is any doubt, a full differential diagnosis should be considered. Rarely bowel disorders such as Crohn's disease or a cerebral space-occupying lesion can mimic anorexia. Once the diagnosis is established, this needs firmly stating and the main aim of treatment in the early stages must be weight gain. In severe cases this may mean admission to a psychiatric unit and bed rest until a target weight has been achieved. Increased activity and freedom can be made contingent on the achievement of target weights. In agitated or depressed patients, a phenothiazine or antidepressant can be helpful, although caution must be exercised as hypotension can be a major problem and drug clearance is altered in the condition.

The other mainstay in management is psychotherapy. A family approach has been found to be particularly helpful in younger, acute cases. In the early stages, the family is forcefully encouraged to insist on the child taking a proper diet, while later other family difficulties, including over-involvement are addressed. Individual therapy can also be extremely useful and it can be helpful to the young person to help them uncover their fears about growing up.

Encopresis

This is the passage of faeces in inappropriate places, either the pants, hidden in the house or smeared on the walls. The condition may be continuous from birth or constitute a relapse from previously attained continence. The disorder may be superimposed on chronic constipation.

Aetiology

Disturbance in the child and the family is extremely common in encopresis. Two common patterns can be identified. One is the over-hygienic, over-achieving family where the parents have, often from an early stage, got into a conflict with the child that revolves around bowel training. The other pattern is of faulty bowel training where no routine has been established.

This is commonly only one component of generally chaotic family relationships.

Management

Many children with encopresis prefer to deny to themselves that they have such an unpleasant and socially handicapping habit, particularly as they are likely to have been subject to repeated attempts to train them. The management is a direct physical approach to the symptom as well as both general and specific psychological approaches. There is a need to keep the bowel clear, since chronic constipation and impacted faeces are common. There is little hope of establishing training if the rectum is loaded. Useful agents are Senokot, or a bulking agent such as Normacol granules. In very severe cases an enema may be needed, this should be carried out in a different setting to that of the subsequent psychological management.

Psychological management should take account of the fact that the child may have had the unpleasantness of his disorder drummed into him. A psychodynamic approach in the first instance can convince the untrusting patient that someone is listening to his point of view rather than just trying to train him. It is important that the therapist and child acknowledge what the problem is, but in the relaxed, non-confrontational atmosphere of the therapy session the child may begin to reveal extraordinary fears and fantasies. For example, they may seem to feel that their faeces are alive or that they will• disappear down the toilet. In cases of any severity, this non-directive phase should precede a behavioural approach. This is carried out in the form of a training programme. Shaping methods can be used with appropriate rewards first to develop a habit of sitting on the toilet and then of depositing faeces in the correct place.

Enuresis

This is involuntary emptying of the bladder, either day or night over the age of 5 years, and is discussed fully in Chapter 3. However, it has also been mentioned here as it is sometimes an indication that the child is under psychological stress.

Management

This is a frequently under-treated condition, either because it is applied by over-stretched staff or because the family are insufficiently organized or motivated to co-operate properly. Time and care are needed and an intensive programme over a relatively short time is likely to achieve the best results. An account of previous treatment should be sought since valid approaches may have been discredited in the parents' eyes by unsystematic application. The approaches that are likely to be helpful are to start with a star chart which will record how many nights the child is wetting. It is a good idea to put the child in charge of the chart. The detailed management of enuresis is discussed on p. 26.

Drug taking

The drug taking career generally starts with alcohol and tobacco, progresses to marijuana and then to other drugs, including hard drugs. Choice of drug is influenced by fashion and opportunity. Peer support is said to influence marijuana use, but not the progression to other drugs. Sufficient funds to support the habit can be important. Family factors are important, both through learning drug taking behaviour from parents and through the sort of lack of family support which exposes the youngster to antisocial peer group influences. Delinquent conduct commonly coexists with drug taking, together with a generally alienated and antisocial attitude.

GLUE SNIFFING

Glue sniffing became popular in the mid-1970s, particularly in deprived inner city areas. For many youngsters it constitutes a phase of group experimentation, while a few apparently become psychologically dependent. Such young people may come to medical attention during acute intoxication, which compared to alcohol may cause a more severe ataxia or a hallucinosis, incidently in other emotional or behavioural disturbance, or occasionally in connection with liver or kidney damage. These latter adverse effects are associated with inhalation of chloro- or fluoro-carbon gases in aerosols. Treatment is difficult unless the young person can be provided with a sense of direction or meaning to their life. Prevention, by making solvents less easy to obtain, may be better than attempted cures.

ALCOHOL

Alcohol constitutes the drug that is most woven into the fabric of western societies. There has been recent concern at the rise in teenage drunkenness, associated with the relative availability and cheapness of alcohol. It is likely that early use of alcohol has some relationship with problem drinking later, but it is unclear how strong this relationship is.

TOBACCO

Tobacco is seen by many as a major drug of dependence with well-known and serious effects on health. Twenty-five to 30 per cent of 15-year-olds smoke up to 1 cigarette a week, often prompted by peer group pressure.

OTHER DRUGS

These include amphetamines which can induce a psychotic state, barbiturates and benzodiazepines which induce major dependence. Incidence probably fluctuates from year to year. Use of heroin and cocaine emerge later in adolescence.

Further reading

Barker P. *Basic Child Psychiatry*, 5th Edn. Blackwell Scientific Publications, Oxford 1988.

Graham P. *Child Psychiatry: A Developmental Approach*. Oxford University Press, Oxford 1986.

Herbert M. *Behavioural Treatment of Children with Problems: A Practice Manual*. Academic Press, London 1987.

Rutter M, Hersov L. *Child and Adolescent Psychiatry: Modern Approaches*, 2nd Edn. Blackwell Scientific Publications, Oxford 1985.

Winnicott D.W. *Therapeutic Consultations in Child Psychiatry*. Hogarth Press, London 1971.

21
IMMUNIZATION AND
INFECTIOUS DISEASES

Diagnosis of infection

Many infections in childhood can be diagnosed on clinical grounds alone, but for others the laboratory plays an essential role and treatment with antibiotics should only begin after appropriate tests have been initiated. Table 21.1 summarizes the laboratory features of the major types of bacterial infection.

Blood. Blood cultures are an essential investigation in the diagnosis of septicaemia in childhood. They should be taken before antibiotics are given in the newborn and early infancy and in children with fever in whom bacterial infection is suspected but not localized to a particular site (such as the urinary tract), as well as in children where the site of infection is known but identification of the organism may play a crucial role in treatment (as in osteomyelitis). Adequate skin sterilization with antiseptics prior to drawing blood is essential because of the ease with which skin commensals contaminate blood cultures. Under some circumstances, interpretation may be difficult but a pure bacterial growth in two or more bottles is diagnostic of infection.

Urine. Care must be taken in the collection of urine specimens for culture (see p. 257) as they may become contaminated easily. Infection is confirmed on culture of a pure bacterial growth of greater than 10^5 organisms/ml and is unusual in the absence of pyruria (>50 WBC per high-power field).

Cerebrospinal fluid. The diagnosis of meningitis is confirmed by examination of cerebrospinal fluid taken at lumbar puncture. It should be examined immediately and bacterial culture performed (see Table 21.1). Contamination of CSF during collection is so unusual that any bacterial growth should be considered significant.

Identification techniques

Identification of bacteria is by culture on agar; rapid diagnostic methods such as antigen agglutination tests are also available and are sometimes used when specimens are collected after antibiotic treatment has been started, such as in the diagnosis of bacterial meningitis. Rapid diagnostic tests can be used to detect chlamydial infection with a fluorescent-labelled monoclonal antibody. Similar techniques allow detection of viruses such as respiratory syncytial virus (RSV) and herpes. Electron microscopy is of particular value in the identification of viruses causing diarrhoea, such as rotavirus and the Norwalk agent. Techniques such as DNA and RNA hybridization are being used increasingly for viral detection and are of particular use where viruses may be difficult to culture.

The immune response

The immunological response to infective agents is of two main types:

Natural immunity. This is relatively non-specific and includes:

Table 21.1 Features suggestive of bacterial infection in children with meningitis, bacteraemia or urinary tract infection.

Meningitis		Bacteraemia	Urinary tract infection	
Test	Abnormality	Test	Test	Abnormality
CSF microscopy	Presence of bacteria diagnostic	Blood culture		
Gram stain	" "			
CSF culture	" "	Pure bacterial growth in two or more bottles diagnostic		
CSF WBC	>20 mm³ polymorphs Mononuclear cells predominate in TB meningitis and partially treated meningitis		Urine WBC Culture	>50 WBC per high power field associated with: >10⁵ bacteria mm³ in pure growth diagnostic
CSF glucose	Less than 50% of blood value			
CSF protein	>0.4 g/l			

1 Polymorphonuclear leucocytes and macrophages which are scavengers of bacteria.
2 Complement which when activated results in bacterial lysis assisted by opsonins.
3 Lysozyme which attacks bacterial cell walls.
4 Interferon which inhibits viral replication.

Adaptive immunity. This is based on the specific response to individual antigens mediated by antibodies which are secreted by B lymphocytes. The antibody response is crucial in defence against bacterial infection. Thymus-derived lymphocytes (T cells) produce cell-mediated immunity (CMI) which is of special importance in immunity to viral infection.

Antibody

There are five classes of antibody which are proteins of the gamma globulin type:
1 IgM which is the first antibody produced following exposure to antigen.
2 IgG is produced as part of the amnestic response. Transplacentally acquired IgG provides immunity during the first few months of life at a time when the immunological system is undergoing maturation.
3 IgA is secreted into the lungs, gut and breast milk. Levels are particularly high in colostrum which is swallowed by the newborn and remain in the gut providing protection against gastrointestinal infection. This antibody is produced following immunization with oral polio vaccine (OPV).
4 IgE or reaginic antibody combines with antigen on mucosal surfaces resulting in the release of histamine, and other vasoactive amines which are chemotactic for granulocytes, leading to an influx of plasma IgG, complement, polymorphs and eosinophils. This antibody is of importance in immunity to helminthic infections.
5 IgD is present on the surface of lymphocytes where it acts as a lymphocyte receptor.

Immunization

The introduction of vaccines to combat serious infectious diseases has had a profound effect on mankind. Smallpox has been eradicated; polio virus and diphtheria and infection are now very rare in Britain and are in decline in the many developing countries where comprehensive vaccination programmes are available. Such diseases would become rife in the event of nuclear war or other catastrophe, resulting in the breakdown of sanitary systems and interruption of vaccine supply and administration. Fatal and preventable infections, however, still occur commonly in the developing world (see Chapter 29), but even in Britain, six deaths from measles in the first half of 1988 were reported. Although there may be contraindications to immunization these are few; failure to immunize without good reason is a serious omission.

The World Health Organization have recommended immunization targets, that is the propor-

tion of the population to be immunized to achieve eradication of infection as a result of herd immunity. This proportion varies according to the infection involved, but other factors, such as state of nutrition are also important. These targets for Europe are a 90% uptake rate for polio, diphtheria, and pertussis by the age of 2 years. These targets can easily be exceeded even when contraindications to vaccination are considered.

Immunity to infection can be achieved artificially in two ways; by active immunization in which an agent stimulates natural immunity, and by passive immunity which results from the administration of antibody and which is short-lived.

Active immunity follows injection, or ingestion of an attentuated living organism (measles and polio vaccine), injection of killed organism (pertussis vaccine) or injection of a modified product (tetanus and diphtheria toxoid).

The nationally recommended immunization schedules for immunization of children in Britain are given in Table 21.2. As can be seen, the first

Table 21.2 Recommended immunization schedules in childhood in the UK.

Age	Antigen	Dose	Route
2 months	Polio	3 drops	Oral
	Diphtheria/tetanus/pertussis (DTP)	0.5 ml	Intramuscular (IM) or
	DT (where pertussis contraindicated)		deep subcutaneous (SC)
3 months	Polio	3 drops	Oral
	DTP	0.5 ml	IM or deep SC
4 months	Polio	3 drops	Oral
	DTP	0.5 ml	IM or deep SC
15 months	Measles/mumps/rubella (MMR) or measles	0.5 ml	IM or deep SC
4–5 years	Polio	3 drops	Oral
	DT booster	0.5 ml	IM or deep SC
	MMR (if not given before)		
10–14 years (neonatal period in special groups)	BCG	0.1 ml	Intradermal
10–14 years	Rubella (girls only, where no previous MMR)	0.5 ml	SC
15 years	Polio	3 drops	Oral
	Tetanus	0.5 ml	IM or deep SC

dose should be given at 3 months. This applies to the pre-term infant irrespective of gestation. All vaccines should be given into the lateral aspect of the thigh or deltoid muscle of the arm and not the buttock because of the risk of sciatic nerve damage at this site.

Those vaccines given routinely are now described in detail.

DIPHTHERIA TOXOID

This infection still occurs in Britain and five cases in children were reported in 1985. The vaccine is a toxoid prepared from the diphtheria toxin. When cases occur attempts should be made to ensure protection of the local population by giving diphtheria vaccine to:
1 Non-immunized children and adults who have not received vaccine over the past 10 years.
2 Where the immunization history in children and adults is unclear. In this case a low-dose vaccine is available.

In the past a Schick test was performed to evaluate whether the individual was immune and prevent a hypersensitivity reaction to the vaccine but this is now unnecessary. With an increasing proportion of the population immunized against diphtheria, the number of natural infections which in the past have served to boost immunity have declined, which has resulted in increased susceptibility of the adult population to infection. It is possible that booster immunizations will be recommended for adults over the next few years.

PERTUSSIS VACCINE

This is a suspension of killed *Bordetella pertussis* organisms and is available either as a constituent of triple vaccine, with diphtheria, and tetanus absorbed to aluminium hydroxide (DPT) or on its own as a plain vaccine. Pertussis immunization uptake in Britain in 1985 was only 65%, largely as a result of publicity over possible damage produced by the vaccine. A childhood encephalopathy study suggested that at the most 1:110 000 injections was associated with transient neurolo-

gical abnormality and 1:330 000 associated with residual neurological sequelae such as developmental delay and seizures. Many so-called vaccine reactions in the past have been falsely attributed to the vaccine. Signs of cerebral palsy may only reveal themselves at the age when pertussis immunization is performed and this vaccine has been unfairly blamed.

Contraindications

Contraindications to immunization include:
1 An acute febrile illness. Immunization should be deferred until recovery.
2 Previous history of a severe local reaction (induration of most of the antero-lateral aspects of the thigh or arm).
3 Severe general reaction with a high temperature within 48 hours of injection.
4 Anaphylaxis or convulsions following a previous immunization.

If any of these reactions occur with the triple vaccine it is assumed that they are a result of the pertussis component and only tetanus and diphtheria vaccine (DT) should be given subsequently.

Special consideration should be given to the immunization of certain children. These include children with a history of cerebral damage during the neonatal period, or where the child has had convulsions, or family members have a history of idiopathic epilepsy. This may require discussion with a paediatrician who will weigh the risks of immunization against risks of infection. Infants with a history of birth asphyxia can be immunized, as can those with stable neurological conditions, such as cerebral palsy.

A homoeopathic oral pertussis vaccine is available but is of no proven benefit.

TETANUS TOXOID

Tetanus immunization is with a toxoid and is highly effective. Disease follows release of exotoxin from *Clostridia tetani* and occurs in the non-immunized and newborn. The neonate is particularly vulnerable in some parts of the world where it is caused by dressing the umbilical cord with cow dung (p. 534).

Tetanus toxoid is available combined with DP or alone. If a non-immune child is injured and thought to be at low risk of tetanus (clean wound) then a catch-up schedule should be given. A dirty wound in a non-immune child should be treated with debridement and anti-tetanus serum (ATS). If the previous dose of tetanus vaccine was given more than 5 years previously, then a booster dose should be given.

POLIO VACCINE

This is available as either oral polio vaccine (OPV) combining the three live attenuated strains of polio virus or as inactivated polio vaccine (IPV). Very rarely (less than one in a million doses) the live vaccine reverts to the wild form causing poliomyelitis in the vaccine recipient and close contacts infected from virus excreted in the stools.

OPV has not been demonstrated to cause disease in children with human immunodeficiency virus infection (HIV) but it should not be given where the infant or other family members have symptomatic infection. IPV is also indicated when immunosuppressed children need to be immunized.

MEASLES VACCINE

Until the autumn of 1988 this was given to children in their second year as a single agent but it is now combined with mumps and rubella vaccine as 'MMR'. The measles component of MMR is an attenuated live virus which is grown on chick fibroblasts. The vaccine is contraindicated where there is a history of anaphylaxis (rather than allergy) to eggs. Some children develop a mild illness with fever and rash 8–12 days after immunization and although a history of febrile convulsions is not a contraindication to immunization, parents of such children should be warned and have an antipyretic agent available. The risk of febrile convulsion is higher following wild measles infection than occurs following vaccination. The risk of subacute sclerosing encephalitis

(SSPE) is much reduced following immunization. Measles vaccination in developing countries is discussed in Chapter 29.

MUMPS VACCINE

Although there is no evidence that mumps causes fatal infection in children, the complications of illness (principally meningoencephalitis) have led to more than 1000 hospital admissions each year in Britain. This is a live attenuated virus which is normally combined with measles and rubella as MMR.

RUBELLA VACCINE

This is an attenuated live vaccine which until recently was administered to schoolgirls in their early teens. Unfortunately the uptake of rubella vaccine was too low and cases of congenital rubella infection remained all too common; 20 live-born infants per year in England and Wales and many terminations of pregnancy were performed following intra-uterine infection. In the USA a different immunization policy was introduced in the early 1970s with immunization of all infants with MMR during the second year of life. There, a very much lower rate of intra-uterine rubella infection has allayed fears that immunity would not persist into adult life. Although infants are now immunized with MMR the rubella component of the vaccine is still available for older children and adults. Rubella vaccine, like all viral preparations, should not be given before conception or during pregnancy, but there is no evidence from over 1000 doses given inadvertently at this time that intra-uterine infection has occurred. There is no justification for termination of pregnancy in these circumstances.

BACILLUS CALMETTE-GUÉRIN (BCG) VACCINE

This vaccine is an attenuated mycobacterium in a freeze-dried form. Tuberculosis (TB) is now very uncommon in children in Britain and routine Heaf testing and BCG immunization has been abandoned in many areas. Children born in Asia, or those born in Britain with parents from the Indian subcontinent, however, have a higher risk of infection and this should be taken into account when immunization policies are considered. These children should be given BCG after birth. Immunized infants have a significantly lower risk of infection but at the same time 20% remain susceptible to disease. In some areas of Britain BCG is given to children in their teenage years after a tuberculin skin test (Heaf test) has been performed and shown to be negative. Children may have a positive Heaf test because of active TB infection, previous infection or following BCG.

BCG should be given intradermally to avoid ulceration and lymphadenitis which occurs with subcutaneous injection. A fatal 'BCG' infection has been reported in adults with AIDS and therefore HIV-positive children should not be immunized.

OTHER VACCINES

Hepatitis B

This is an inactivated vaccine made from the surface antigen of the hepatitis B virus. It should be given in three doses to infants whose mothers are surface and e antigen positive (see p. 210 for a more detailed description). Those infants at greatest risk are those whose mothers come from South–east Asia where hepatitis B infection is endemic or where there is a history of maternal abuse of intravenous drugs.

Meningococcal vaccines

These are available for the A and C serotypes and are used following outbreaks of *Neisseria meningitidis* infection.

Pneumococcal vaccine

This is a polysaccharide vaccine and is used in children at increased risk of *Streptococcus pneumoniae* infection, children following splenectomy and those with sickle cell disease.

NEW VACCINES

Haemophilus influenzae

This is administered routinely in the USA between 18 and 24 months.

Varicella

This is an attenuated live viral preparation and is likely to be of value in the protection of children with malignant disease who may be at risk of fatal varicella infection.

Specific infectious diseases

Viral infections

RUBELLA

This infectious disease is endemic in Britain but epidemics occur every few years. The virus is transmitted in nasopharyngeal secretions and can be isolated from the urine of infants with congenital infection. The incubation period is 16–18 days. In children the rash appears first but in adolescents and adults there is a prodrome of 1–5 days with fever, headache, coryza, mild conjunctivitis and lymphadenopathy. These symptoms disappear following eruption of the rash. Red spots may be seen on the soft palate during this prodrome but they cannot be distinguished from those seen in scarlet fever and measles. The lymph nodes most commonly involved are those in the sub-occipital, posterior auricular and cervical groups. A pinky-red maculo-papular rash appears first on the face and then spreads rapidly downwards to the neck, arms and lower parts of the body. The lesions on the trunk may coalesce but those on the limbs remain discrete unlike the lesions of measles. Although the lesions may be difficult to distinguish from those of scarlet fever, in rubella infection the area around the mouth is not spared. There may be a low-grade fever at the time the rash appears, but this is not a consistent finding. An important complication is an arthritis which is normally polyarticular and associated with pain and sometimes joint effusion. This develops as the rash is fading and may last 5–10 days. Thrombocytopenic purpura may also occur.

The diagnosis should be made on clinical grounds but serology is indicated where a pregnant woman has been exposed to rubella infection. When a woman has been exposed in the first 18 weeks of pregnancy and it is not known whether she is already immune, blood should be taken for measurement of IgG antibodies and then repeated 2 weeks later. A four-fold rise in titre is indicative of infection, as is the presence of IgM antibodies which are sometimes measured. If a woman is known to be immune prior to exposure, then reassurance can be given because reactivation or recurrent infection does not occur. Rarely infections may occur in the absence of rash which means that all susceptible women should be tested when exposure to infection occurs.

Diagnosis in children can normally be made on clinical grounds. As with many viral infections, the total white count is usually low.

MEASLES (see also p. 553)

This is caused by a paramyxovirus. It is a highly contagious virus which causes a high mortality among children in developing countries and immunosuppressed children in Britain. Infections are unusual among infants less than 6 months old because of the acquisition of maternal antibodies. The incubation period is approximately 10 days. Coryza, conjunctivitis and cough are the first symptoms with a rash developing on the fourth day. About 2 days before the rash develops 'Koplik's spots' can be seen on the buccal mucosa close to the molars. They look like grains of sand and are pathognomic of measles. Koplik's spots disappear by the end of the second day of the rash which is itself present for about 5 days. The rash is erythematous and maculopapular (Plate 6) and is first seen on the forehead, behind the ears and on the upper part of the neck. It then spreads downwards but is less confluent on lower parts of the body. As the rash fades a brown staining of the skin appears and desquamation may occur, although in contrast to scarlet fever the hands and feet are spared.

Complications of measles include:
1 Otitis media.
2 Pneumonia, either viral (characterized pathologically by giant cells) or a secondary bacterial pneumonia due to *Staphylococcus aureus* or *Haemophilus influenzae*.
3 Laryngitis and tracheitis which may necessitate endotracheal intubation.
4 Haemorrhagic measles resulting from disseminated intravascular coagulation and which is normally fatal.
5 Measles encephalitis (p. 283).
6 Subacute sclerosing encephalitis (p. 283).

Management. Treatment of measles is symptomatic. Antipyretic agents and plenty of fluids should be given. Antibiotics should only be given where there is suspected secondary bacterial infection. Immunosuppressed children with no history of measles or previous immunization should be given gamma globulin to reduce the risk of pneumonia and encephalitis, either on exposure to an infected case or following onset of infection. Children with uncomplicated measles should not be admitted to hospital because of the risk to any immunosuppressed child already on the ward.

A modified relatively mild measles illness may follow the administration of the vaccine 8–12 days later. Parents should be warned and be ready to administer antipyretics particularly when there is a history of febrile convulsions.

ERYTHEMA INFECTIOSUM (FIFTH DISEASE)

This was the fifth exanthem to be described and is caused by the human parvovirus B19. Infection is commonest in late winter and early spring and is spread in secretions from the respiratory tract. It tends to occur in school-age children and is a mild, usually afebrile, illness with an incubation period of 1–4 days. Initial features include a maculopapular rash most vivid on the face with circumoral pallor; the so-called slapped cheek syndrome (Plate 7). Similar lesions may also occur on the forehead and chin. A maculopapular rash with a lace like appearance appears on the arms and spreads to the trunk and lower limbs.

Children with inherited disorders of red cells have developed aplastic anaemia following infection with B19 parvovirus. There is evidence that intra-uterine infection may lead to non-immune hydrops.

ROSEOLA INFANTUM, EXANTHEM SUBITUM OR SIXTH DISEASE

This is an illness which is thought to be viral in origin. Attempts to isolate infective agents from children with this disease have failed but the leucopenia which develops is suggestive of a viral aetiology. In a questionable experiment in the USA, serum from an infant with roseola infantum was injected into handicapped children who developed this condition with onset of symptoms 9 days later. In a recent Japanese study, human herpes virus-6 (HHV) was isolated from the lymphocytes of a group of children with roseola infantum.

This condition is seen in infants and young children between 6 months and 2 years of age. The illness begins with an abrupt rise in temperature to at least 40°C, sometimes associated with a febrile convulsion. Fever persists for 3–4 days and then subsides as the rash develops. This appears as discrete rose-pink macules which fade without trace in about 2 days. There may be generalized lymphadenopathy and mild inflammation of the middle ear and tonsils. The main complication is febrile convulsions which, as might be expected, occur early in the illness when fever is present.

MUMPS

This is caused by a paramyxovirus and infection is endemic in Britain. It is hoped that with the introduction of MMR immunization, infection rates will fall to the low numbers seen in the USA. Aerosol spread of the virus occurs from respiratory tract secretions and the incubation period is 16–18 days. The infection is uncommon in children under the age of 1 year and in older children it may be subclinical.

At the onset of illness there is fever and headache and this is followed by pain in the affected salivary gland (normally the parotid). A day later parotid enlargement occurs with resulting upward and outward deviation of the ear lobe and the gland reaches its maximum size over the next 2 days. The fever subsides by the sixth day of illness. Usually both parotids enlarge but at different stages of the illness. In a minority of infections, the parotid glands do not appear to enlarge but submandibular glands are affected. The orifices of the ducts draining the salivary glands may appear inflamed. Abdominal pain associated with mumps may result from pancreatitis; plasma amylase is elevated following both parotitis and pancreatitis so measurement of this enzyme does not help in the diagnosis. Meningoencephalitis occurs in about 10% of children and occurs in the period when parotid gland enlargement has reached its peak. Deafness is a rare complication. Symptoms include headache and vomiting and signs include neck stiffness sometimes with a reduced level of consciousness. Cerebrospinal fluid has the characteristic features of a viral meningitis with pleocytosis (predominantly lymphocytes), an elevated protein level and normal CSF glucose. In adolescents epididymo-orchitis may be the only clinical feature of mumps or may complicate parotitis. Partial atrophy of the testis is said to occur but this is rarely bilateral and has not been shown to be associated with infertility.

There is no convincing evidence that mumps infection during pregnancy is associated with congenital abnormality. Mumps does not cause death in childhood but is responsible for approximately 14 000 admissions to hospital in Britain (children and adults) each year. Diagnosis should be on clinical grounds, but in children with complications, viral isolation and serology can be performed.

VARICELLA (CHICKEN-POX) AND HERPES ZOSTER (SHINGLES)

These infections are caused by the herpes zoster virus. Varicella infection may have a grave prognosis in the newborn, and the immunosuppressed, but in most children it is benign.

Infection is spread by direct contact with the vesicles and from respiratory secretions in children before the onset of rash. The incubation period is 14–16 days but may be as long as 20 days.

At the onset of illness there is a low-grade fever and mild coryza. Within 1–2 days a rash develops. The lesions progress rapidly from macule to papule and then vesicle before crusting over. A characteristic feature of infection is the cropping of lesions; usually three crops over as many days with vesicles congregating on the trunk and upper parts of the arms and legs. Once the vesicles crust the child is no longer contagious. Small de-pigmented scars on the skin of many children bear evidence of previous infection. Diagnosis of varicella should be on clinical grounds, although the virus can be identified by electron microscopy or cultured on cell monolayers. Treatment is symptomatic; children with varicella treated with aspirin have developed Reye's syndrome (p. 211) so this agent should not be used in the symptomatic management of this infection. Children with chickenpox should not be admitted to hospital unless they have one of the rare, but serious, complications of infection such as encephalitis or secondary bacterial infection of the skin lesions. This is because of the risk of transmission of infection to immunosuppressed children, particularly those with malignant disease undergoing treatment with cytotoxic drugs. These children may develop haemorrhagic lesions and a fatal disseminated varicella associated with pneumonia. Such children exposed to varicella should be given Zoster immune globulin (ZIG) in an emergency and the anti-viral agent acyclovir should varicella infection occur.

Most adults of child-bearing age are immune to varicella so that infection during pregnancy is uncommon and neonatal infection rare because of the passive transfer of antibodies. However, intra-uterine varicella infection does occur following infection during the first half of pregnancy but in only a small proportion of cases. The characteristic abnormality is a cutaneous scarring with a segmental distribution. Infection during late pregnancy puts the fetus at greater risk, particularly when this occurs in the period of 5 days before

delivery or 7 days after. Both the mother and the newborn infant should be given ZIG in these circumstances and if the infant shows evidence of cutaneous lesions, acyclovir should also be given intravenously.

Reactivation of varicella may occur with resulting zoster (shingles) in immunosuppressed children and this requires treatment with acyclovir. Zoster may also occur in normal children but does not appear to be associated with malignancy.

ECZEMA HERPETICUM OR KAPOSI'S VARICELLIFORM ERUPTION

This is caused by herpes simplex virus, with vesicles developing in children with eczema (see also p. 491). The appearance of vesicles is preceded by a high fever. These lesions often appear in crops (Plate 8) over a period of about a week. In severe infections, large numbers of vesicles break down with resulting fluid loss and risk of bacterial infection. This condition should be regarded as a medical emergency requiring hospitalization and treatment with anti-viral drugs and antibiotics where necessary, as well as management of possible dehydration. Superinfection is normally caused by *Staphylococcus aureus* or *Streptococcus pyogenes*. Skin swabs should be sent to the laboratory for bacterial culture so that appropriate antibiotics can be selected.

SMALLPOX

This disease has now been eradicated as a result of immunization. Stocks of virus remain in four laboratories around the world. Smallpox is a highly contagious disease with a mortality rate of approximately 50%. The incubation period is about 12 days. In the prodromal period there is fever, headache, vomiting and seizures. Two to four days later ulcers occur in the mouth and pharynx followed by macules on the face and then lesions on the back and legs. These progress to papules, vesicles and pustules on the seventh to ninth day of illness. The fever is biphasic and rises during the pustular phase. Death, when it occurs, is from haemorrhage into the lesions and from mucous membranes. The lesions differ from those of varicella in that they do not crop and have a peripheral distribution with few lesions on the trunk.

INFECTIOUS MONONUCLEOSIS (GLANDULAR FEVER)

This is caused by the Epstein–Barr virus. Infection may be subclinical in infancy and childhood but commonly produces illness in the adolescent. The infection is thought to be spread in saliva; the infection has been named the 'kissing disease' for obvious reasons. The incubation period is 30–50 days. Glandular fever presents with fever, headache and malaise and is followed by a sore throat and lymphadenopathy. The period of fever is variable but may last for up to 14 days. The lymphadenopathy is generalized but more pronounced in the cervical glands. A thick white exudate may be present on the enlarged tonsils and petechiae on the soft palate. An erythematous maculopapular rash is seen in children given ampicillin, or its derivatives, for what was mistakenly considered to be a bacterial infection. Splenomegaly may occur and is a more consistent finding that hepatomegaly associated with hepatitis. Rare complications include pneumonia, aseptic meningitis and transverse myelitis. Pneumonia is a feature of EBV infection in children with acquired immunodeficiency deficiency syndrome (AIDS).

The diagnosis may be difficult in the absence of splenomegaly and tonsillitis cannot be distinguished clinically from that caused by other viruses or streptococcal infection. The haematological changes are non-specific; there may be a leucopenia but atypical lymphocytes are normally increased. Children with this infection develop high titres of agglutinins to sheep red blood cells detected in the 'monospot' or 'Paul Bunnell' tests, often only 3–4 weeks after the onset of symptoms. Glandular fever may need to be distinguished from diphtheria and streptococcal tonsillitis. Treatment is symptomatic. If resolution of tonsillitis and regression of fever does not occur within 10 days then acute lymphoblastic leukaemia should be considered as a possible diagnosis.

CYTOMEGALOVIRUS

This is a DNA virus and is a member of the herpes group. Up to 40% of individuals have acquired the virus by adulthood. Virus may be spread in saliva and urine; it may be present in vaginal secretions and semen and can be transmitted during sexual intercourse. Congenital infection develops *in utero* as a result of blood-borne spread from the placenta. Acquired infection of the newborn may follow contamination of the infant with genital secretions during delivery, ingestion of breast milk or blood transfusion. In most children and adults CMV infection is asymptomatic although pneumonia may develop in the immunosuppressed. The main importance of CMV is in immunosuppressed patients and as a cause of congenital infection. The latter is discussed in detail on p. 367.

INFLUENZA

The influenza viruses are orthomyxoviruses. They are classified into three major groups (A, B, C) according to the ribonucleoprotein antigen. Subclassification is then made according to the types of haemagglutinin (H) and neuraminidase (N) antigen. Epidemic infections are caused by types A and B. These viruses undergo minor changes in their antigenic composition (H, N) almost annually and this is known as antigenic drift. Approximately every 10 years major changes occur in the H or N antigen with even more widespread epidemics of infection.

The virus is spread by droplets from the respiratory tract of infected children and adults. The incubation period is from 1 to 3 days. Illness is characterized by the sudden onset of fever often associated with chills and rigors, headache, cough and myalgia. Children may subsequently develop conjuctivitis and tonsillitis. In some cases there may be associated vomiting and diarrhoea. Influenza during early infancy may result in pneumonia and apnoea. Children with congenital heart disease are at risk of severe infection associated with cardiac failure. Secondary bacterial infection of the lungs is uncommon, but may occur in cystic fibrosis. Cases of Reye's syndrome have been reported following influenza infection in children given aspirin as an antipyretic.

The diagnosis is normally made on a clinical basis. The virus can be identified in tissue culture and a rapid diagnosis made with an immuno-fluorescent technique on nasopharyngeal secre-tions. Treatment is symptomatic with antipyretics and antibiotics are only indicated in children with cystic fibrosis or where there is evidence of secondary bacterial infection. Children at increased risk of severe infection should receive influenza vaccine effective against the particular type of influenza virus prevalent in the community.

HUMAN IMMUNODEFICIENCY VIRUS INFECTION (HIV)

This virus was discovered in isolates from a patient with persistent generalized lymphadenopathy by Montagnier at the Pasteur Institute in Paris in 1983. It is a retrovirus and binds to lymphocytes, monocytes and macrophages. Most cases of infec-tion in children result from maternal transmission of virus; either *in utero*, intrapartum or post-partum. Preliminary data suggest that approxi-mately 25% of infants delivered from HIV-positive women become infected with the virus. Although HIV has been isolated from breast milk and in at least one case, HIV infection developed in a breast-fed infant following transfusion of HIV-contaminated blood to the mother post-partum, there is no evidence of increased risk to breast-fed infants when the mother is already infected during pregnancy. There may, however, be a risk to the baby if a breast-feeding mother were to become infected post-partum. Other routes of infection in childhood are from contaminated blood. Although factor VIII and IX concentrates for transfusion to haemophiliacs are now heat-treated and con-sidered safe, a large number of haemophiliacs be-came infected from blood products before the risks of infection became known. In the period to December 1987 there were 253 reported cases of children up to the age of 14 known to have been HIV positive in Britain; most of the 170 children infected from blood products had haemophilia. It is likely that some HIV infection will occur in children following transmission by the sexual route. Those adults at highest risk of HIV infection are intravenous drug abusers, sexual partners of drug abusers, bisexual men and haemophiliacs. Women who have had sexual relations with men from countries in Africa where AIDS is endemic or were transfused with blood in these areas are also at risk.

There are a number of different manifestations of HIV infection in children. Congenital HIV infec-tion is discussed in detail on p. 367. AIDS is char-acterized by opportunistic lung infection with agents such as Epstein–Barr virus, *Pneumocystis carinii* and cytomegalovirus. In childhood, most cases of AIDS-related complex (ARC) progress to AIDS which has a high mortality. A neurological presentation has been described with acquired microcephaly, encephalopathy and transverse myelitis.

Diagnosis of infection may be difficult during infancy and at the time of writing there is no reliable antigen detection test. At other times de-tection of HIV antibodies is diagnostic of infection; seroconversion occurs any time from 8 weeks after transmission of virus. Supportive evidence of symptomatic infection comes from a reduced T_4 lymphocyte (helper cells) to T_8 lymphocyte (killer) cell ratio.

There is no treatment for HIV infection. Mea-sures taken to reduce the risk of infection in-clude heat treatment of blood products, the screening of donor blood for HIV antibodies and the use of condoms during sexual intercourse. HIV infection is of low infectivity compared to hepatitis B virus for instance and although special precau-tions should be taken in the handling of body fluids from infected patients, children should not be excluded from school or nursery and normal social physical contact should be allowed. When a mother is HIV positive, her infant should be bottle fed with formula milk, but only in areas where this is a safe alternative to breast feeding. These children should not be given BCG.

Bacterial infections

SCARLET FEVER

The Group A beta haemolytic *Streptococcus* is a cause of acute tonsillitis, impetigo and scarlet fever. Untreated streptococcal infection may result in glomerulonephritis and rarely rheumatic fever.

The incubation period of scarlet fever is 2–4 days but may be as long as 7 days. Initial features of illness are tonsillitis, fever, vomiting and abdominal pain. The fever reaches its peak by the second day of illness and the temperature falls to normal over the next 5 days. The tonsils become reddened and may be covered with exudate. During the first 2 days of illness, the dorsum of the tongue is coated in a white fur, but the edges are red. The papillae become reddened and oedematous to produce the 'white strawberry tongue'. The white coat peels off over the next few days leaving a red tongue covered with prominent papillae and this is known as the 'red strawberry tongue'. An erythematous and punctiform rash appears normally on the first day of illness. This is punctate and gives the skin a rough feel. Certain features of the rash are distinctive. The punctiform rash does not develop on the face but instead the forehead and cheeks are flushed and the area around the mouth is spared to give circumoral pallor (Plate 9). The rash becomes generalized within 24 hours of its first appearance. It is more intense in the skin folds and desquamation is a consistent feature, starting at the end of the first week of illness and persisting for several weeks after the fever and sore throat have disappeared.

Diagnosis is based on clinical features. Rubella and measles are the most easily confused conditions, but circumoral pallor is not seen with these infections and in rubella desquamation is unusual and measles rash does not occur on the hands and feet.

Infection can be confirmed by isolation of Group A *Streptococcus* from throat swab culture. There will be a significant rise in the antistreptolysin titre following infection and this test may be helpful if culture is not possible because of previous antibiotics. Scarlet fever should be treated with oral phenoxymethyl-penicillin for 10 days. A course of this length has been shown to lessen the risk of rheumatic fever but shorter courses have not been properly evaluated. When it is thought likely that the parent will not give the complete course of antibiotic the first dose of penicillin can be given as intravenous or intramuscular benzyl-penicillin.

DIPHTHERIA

Diphtheria is caused by a Gram-negative rod *Corynebacterium diphtheriae*. There are three strains: 'mitis' produces mild disease and gravis and intermedius, severe infection. Illness can be devastating and is produced by an exotoxin to which the vaccine is directed. Only strains of the bacteria associated with bacteriophage mutancy produce toxin. The disease is very rare in the developed world; in Britain, there were only five cases in children during 1985, but it is a significant cause of morbidity and mortality in developing countries.

Infection is spread in droplets from nasal and throat secretions or by direct contact with the skin of someone with cutaneous diphtheria. Fomites, such as handkerchiefs, may also be a source of infection and food-borne infection may also occur. Infection can be transmitted from both colonized asymptomatic individuals and those with infections. Infection occurs when diphtheria bacilli adhere to the nasopharynx, replicate and produce toxin with resultant tissue damage which allows further invasion and bacterial growth. The necrotic epithelial cells and inflammatory exudate make up the membrane which is the hallmark of the disease. The incubation period of diphtheria is 2–4 days. Infection is classified according to the site of the membrane; on occasions more than one site is affected.

Nasal diphtheria presents with a nasal discharge and low-grade fever. The discharge is initially serous but then becomes purulent and may be associated with epistaxis. A membrane forms on the nasal septum and is difficult to see. There is little absorption of toxin from this site and so the disease is mild. Untreated, the discharge may persist for many weeks.

Tonsillar and pharnygeal diphtheria has a gradual onset of symptoms with malaise, anorexia, sore throat and low-grade fever. During the first day of illness a membrane develops on the tonsils or fauces. It enlarges to cover the uvula and pharyngeal wall. The membrane is normally a dirty grey colour and bleeding follows its removal from the pharynx. Associated lymphadenopathy results in a 'bull neck'. A striking feature of the illness is the high pulse rate associated with a normal or only slightly elevated temperature. In severe cases death occurs in 6–10 days following cardiac failure, arrhythmias and haemorrhage. Recovery in the survivors may be complicated by myocarditis usually in the second week of disease and is more likely to occur when anti-toxin therapy has been delayed. Toxin-induced paralysis of the soft palate may occur producing a nasal voice and nasal regurgitation of imbibed fluids. Blurred vision may develop following paralysis of eye muscles and diaphragmatic paralysis may occur from phrenic nerve involvement up to 6 or more weeks after the onset of infection.

Laryngeal diphtheria is often an extension of pharnygeal infection. Fever and cough are the initial features but as the membrane develops stridor occurs. In mild cases, the membrane is sloughed around the end of the first week as with pharyngeal diphtheria, but in severe cases fatal obstruction of the airway may occur. There is limited absorption of toxin through the mucous membrane of the pharynx.

An early diagnosis of diphtheria is essential to prevent the more severe complications. A Gram smear may not be helpful and culture takes a minimum of 15 hours on Loefflers medium. Treatment should start once a clinical diagnosis has been made. Diphtheria anti-toxin should be given intravenously where possible and the dose is calculated according to the site of involvement. Penicillin should also be given. Supportive treatment may be required for children with myocarditis or paralysis.

PERTUSSIS

Infection with the Gram-negative bacteria *Bordetella pertussis* results in an illness called 'pertussis' or whooping cough. This is a common infection of childhood in Britain with epidemics occurring in 4-year cycles with a peak incidence in the winter months. In the period from 1976 to 1985 there were 64 deaths from such infection. Transmission is by droplet spread or direct contact with discharge from the nose or mouth and the incubation period is 7–10 days. Children remain infectious for 3 weeks from the onset of the catarrhal stage.

Illness presents with coryza (catarrhal stage) and is followed in about 2–5 days by a paroxysmal cough (paroxysmal phase). A deep inspiratory gasp or whoop is taken at the end of a paroxysm of coughing and at this stage vomiting may occur. Attacks may be precipitated by feeding or pressure on the trachea. Young infants may not whoop, but may become cyanosed from hypoxia and repeated paroxysms may be associated with apnoea. Early complications include pneumonia and pertussis encephalopathy associated with convulsions. Death is almost entirely confined to infants with infections during the first few months of life and before immunization has been performed (see below). The paroxysmal phase generally lasts for about 6 weeks but may persist for 3 months.

The diagnosis is a clinical one and is normally straightforward, but paroxysmal cough may also occur during viral (adenovirus or respiratory syncytial virus) and *Chlamydia trachomatis* infections. Pneumonia may occur, more often bronchopneumonia than lobar. Chest X-ray may also reveal areas of pulmonary collapse. Pertussis is a notifiable disease in Britain. Notification should proceed following a clinical diagnosis even in the absence of a positive culture.

The organism can be cultured on Bordet Genou medium following collection of a nasopharyngeal swab (cotton wool bud on a thin flexible wire wand). The isolation rate is highest during the catarrhal stage with its non-specific symptoms and isolation rates during the early paroxysmal phase are less than 50%. Such cultures should be taken on all children with suspected pertussis. A total white blood cell count of $>20 \times 10^9/1$ with predominant lymphocytes suggests infection.

Young infants will almost certainly require hospital admission; this is recommended for those with cyanotic episodes. Treatment with erythromycin during the catarrhal stage shortens the course of illness. This antibiotic is recommended during the infectious period to reduce the risk of transmission to other infants. Phenobarbitone or salbutamol have been claimed to lessen the severity of the paroxysms and are recommended in young infants. In severe cases mechanical ventilation may be required and adequate sedation with an opiate is recommended. Tube feeding is often necessary during the early paroxysmal phase. Rarely bronchiectasis may develop as the result of pertussis.

Pertussis is a preventable infection. To reduce the risk of infection during early infancy it is essential that older siblings are immunized.

BRUCELLOSIS

Brucellosis is named after Bruce, a British medical officer, who isolated *Micrococcus mellitensis* from four individuals with Undulant or 'Malta Fever'. The generic name of the causative agent which is a Gram-negative aerobe was later changed to Brucella. There are three species causing disease in humans; *melitensis*, *abortus* and *suis*. The infection is found world-wide and is primarily a disease of animals, especially goats, sheep and pigs, producing abortion and reduced lactation. Humans become infected following direct contact with animals, or ingestion of unpasteurized milk and products derived from infected animals. Rarely infection follows blood transfusion.

The incubation period is about 1–3 weeks and infection may be subclinical. The disease may have either a gradual or acute onset with fever, sweats, weakness, backache and arthralgia. Clinical signs include lymphadenopathy, but splenomegaly is clinically obvious in only 50% of children with bacteraemia. Complications are uncommon and include meningoencephalitis, endocarditis and osteomyelitis. The total white blood cell count may be reduced and a lymphocytosis may be present.

Ideally, the diagnosis should be made by culture of lymph node, blood or other body fluid, but large amounts of such material may be required and isolation methods are not routinely available. A standard agglutination test is available which detects infection caused by *Brucella* sp. causing disease in humans.

Early treatment reduces the risk of complications and tetracycline is recommended for 3 weeks. A longer course of trimethoprim/sulphamethoxazole is recommended in children under the age of 10 years because of the risk of staining of the teeth when tetracycline is given.

SALMONELLA

Salmonella infections present in a number of different ways, as gastroenteritis, enteric fever (see below under typhoid fever), bacteraemia and focal infection such as osteomyelitis. Salmonella is a Gram-negative rod. The major reservoirs of infection are animals, especially poultry, as well as contaminted water supplies. Many species produce gastro-enteritis alone, although these may produce invasive infection such as meningitis or osteomyelitis during early infancy, in the immunosuppressed and in children with haemoglobinopathies such as sickle cell disease. The incubation period for gastro-enteritis is 6–72 hours and there is an acute onset of nausea, vomiting, diarrhoea and abdominal pain. The stools may be bloody and purulent. There is a risk of dehydration in early childhood; protracted diarrhoea may be a feature of such infections. Diagnosis of infection is made by culture of stool and blood but serology is unhelpful. There is no place for antibiotics in the treatment of uncomplicated Salmonella gastro-enteritis: these agents do not shorten the course of the illness. Attention should be paid to correction of dehydration where this occurs. Salmonella bacteraemia may occur as part of enteric fever or alone, and treatment with antibiotics such as chloramphenicol or ampicillin are recommended. All Salmonella infections are notifiable in Britain and carriers attending nurseries or schools are normally excluded until three stool specimens have been negative.

TYPHOID FEVER

This is 'enteric fever' caused by *Salmonella typhi*; *S. paratyphi* infection results in paratyphoid fever. The onset of enteric fever may be gradual with headache, and a slow stepwise increase in temperature over a few days which may persist for several weeks. The pulse rate is lower than that expected from the degree of fever. Diarrhoea or constipation may occur and abdominal pain is usual. Gastrointestinal symptoms may be absent in children infected in the first 2 years of life. Clinical signs include rose-coloured spots on the abdomen and splenomegaly. Investigations show a leucopenia in older children and leucocytosis during infancy. Definitive diagnosis is by isolation of *S. typhi* from blood, and stool should also be cultured. Serology may be difficult to interpret but can provide supportive evidence of infection.

Children with typhoid fever may require intravenous fluids, and all should receive antibiotics; chloramphenicol, ampicillin or trimethoprim/ sulphamethoxazole depending on the sensitivity of the organism. Children should be barrier-nursed during their hospital stay and excluded from school or nurseries if the carrier state persists. The persistent carrier may need treatment with high-dose ampicillin or even cholecystectomy.

Typhoid immunization does not give complete protection to infection, but should be given to travellers to areas where the disease is endemic and to close contacts of carriers.

FOOD POISONING

This describes illness following the ingestion of food contaminated with bacteria which produce toxins that are absorbed when the food is eaten, or from toxins synthesized following replication of bacteria in the host. The absence of fever in children with food poisoning may be useful in differentiating these cases from salmonellosis, shigellosis and viral gastro-enteritis where fever is common.

C. perfringens may be isolated from meats and if such foods are ingested uncooked, diarrhoea and abdominal pain develop in 8–12 hours. Toxin is produced by organisms within the bowel.

Staphylococcal food poisoning follows ingestion of enterotoxin produced by *Staphylococcus aureus* found in dairy products and meat. The illness has a sudden onset 1–6 hours after ingestion of contaminated food and is characterized by vomiting, profuse diarrhoea and abdominal pain. *Bacillus cereus* spores may be present in foods such as fried rice, vegetables and meat and are able to withstand short periods of boiling. Ingestion of an enterotoxin or the bacteria which elaborate a toxin *in vivo* results in diarrhoea, vomiting and abdominal pain. Treatment of food poisoning is supportive and antibiotics are not required.

Botulism

Clostridia botulinum poisoning has been reported during infancy, acquired from ingestion of toxin in honey used to flavour dummies. In botulism there is gradual onset of hypotonia, constipation and respiratory failure. Such infection may be a rare cause of the sudden infant death syndrome (SIDS).

LEPTOSPIROSIS

This is caused by the spirochaete Leptospira, but in Britain the disease is normally caused by *L. icterohaemorrhagica*. The infection is transmitted from the secretions of infected animals, an example being children bathing in streams may drink water contaminated by rat urine. The incubation period is from 1 to 4 weeks. The illness has an abrupt onset with fever, headache, conjunctival suffusion and general malaise (septicaemic phase). After about 4 days the fever subsides and leptospirochaetes disappear from blood and cerebrospinal fluid. The second stage of the illness (immune phase) is characterized by meningitis and uveitis: in about 10% of patients hepatic and renal failure may develop. Diagnosis in the early stage of illness is by culture of blood and CSF. Children should be treated with penicillin but this is ineffective after the onset of the immune stage.

MENINGOCOCCAL DISEASE

Neisseria meningitidis is the commonest cause of bacterial meningitis in Britain with a peak incidence during the pre-school years. There were 582 notified cases of meningococcal meningitis in England and Wales in 1986. The organism is a Gram-negative diplococcus. There are nine serotypes of which B and C are the most prevalent in Britain. Transmission occurs from person to person and acquired from respiratory tract secretions. Although the incubation period may be as little as 1 day, this may be considerably longer as infection may occur in children colonized with the meningococcus. Most infections in children result in meningitis which is not always associated with septicaemia. There may be a short history of coryzal symptoms followed by fever, malaise and in children with septicaemia a maculo-papular rash which may precede a petechial eruption. The petechial rash is a more consistent feature and lesions do not blanch on pressure. Children with meningitis may complain of headache and have a reduced level of consciousness. Infants may be irritable and refuse feeds. Neck stiffness may not be present in children under the age of 18 months; during infancy neck retraction may sometimes be seen. Meningococcal septicaemia (meningococcaemia) may be present in the child with meningitis but is associated with a rapidly progressive fulminant infection with disseminated intravascular coagulation resulting in adrenal failure (Waterhouse–Friderichsen syndrome). Infections may be complicated by arthritis, myocarditis and pneumonia.

Mortality is high, particularly in meningococcaemia, but whenever meningococcal infection is suspected, whether septicaemia or meningitis, investigation and treatment should be initiated urgently. The clinical diagnosis should be confirmed by examination of a Gram stain of cerebrospinal fluid for Gram-negative diplococci which should then be cultured. Blood cultures should also be performed. Antigen detection tests (latex agglutination) may be useful where antibiotics have been given previously. When a clinical diagnosis of meningococcal infection has been made and the journey to hospital will take anything more than a few minutes, then treatment should be given immediately. Ideally a blood culture should be taken followed by an intravenous injection of benzyl-penicillin. Both procedures may be difficult and intramuscular injection is acceptable. Investigation can be completed on admission to hospital and further supportive treatment given. The close contacts of children with meningococcal infection are at increased risk of infection. Family members and children who have been in close contact in nurseries and school should be given antibiotic prophylaxis in the form of a 2-day course of rifampicin. It is recommended that the child with meningococcal infection is given this antibiotic because the carrier state may persist in spite of treatment with penicillin. Immunization may be indicated where several cases occur in an institution, but vaccine is only available for serotypes A and C. These serotypes predominate in the 'meningitis belt' in Africa but B serotypes are most common in Britain.

Other infections

TOXOPLASMOSIS

About half the population have antibodies to the protozoan *Toxoplasma gondii* by middle age. Most infections are acquired postnatally but infection acquired by the mother during pregnancy may lead to congenital toxoplasmosis. Transmission may occur from ingestion of cysts which survive in undercooked meat, particularly lamb, or from the ingestion of cysts which are shed by cats commonly infected with this organism. Infection is asymptomatic in most children, although an illness like glandular fever with fever and lymphadenopathy may develop. Congenital toxoplasmosis is discussed on p. 369.

HISTOPLASMOSIS

This is caused by the fungus *Histoplasma capsulatum*. Infection does not occur in Britain but is encountered in many parts of the world. Infection is acquired through inhalation of airborne spores from soil contaminated by bird or bat droppings. The incubation period is several weeks. Disease may present in a number of ways; acute disseminated histoplasmosis is seen in the first few years of life and may present with fever, rash, cough and diarrhoea. Clinical findings include generalized lymphadenopathy and hepatosplenomegaly: a pancytopenia is common. Acute pulmonary histoplasmosis is seen in older children who develop an influenza-like illness and in whom chest X-ray shows evidence of pulmonary infiltrates and hilar lymphadenopathy. In most children infections are asymptomatic. Diagnosis is by microscopic identification of yeasts in stained specimens of bone marrow, lymph nodes, liver or spleen. These specimens should be cultured as should blood and sputum. The histoplasmin skin test can also be used in diagnosis although it may be negative during acute infection. Acute disseminated disease should be treated with amphotericin B or ketoconazole.

Congenital infections

A number of organisms have a relatively mild effect on babies and children, but may be devastating if acquired in early embryonic or fetal life during the stage of rapid organ development. The most important are discussed here.

RUBELLA

The congenital rubella syndrome (CRS) follows maternal rubella infection when it occurs during the first 18 weeks of gestation. Infection during the first 12 weeks results in the most severe abnormalities which affect the heart, eye and central nervous system. Congenital heart defects include patent ductus arteriosus or pulmonary arterial or valvar stenosis. The most common eye manifestation is a retinopathy with typical discrete black patchy pigmentation and which for this reason is described as 'pepper and salt'. Cataracts may occur in up to 25% of infants infected during the first trimester. CRS is associated with intrauterine growth retardation and microcephaly with mental retardation and cerebral palsy. Some infants with CRS have thrombocytopenic purpura from birth and develop neonatal hepatitis and among this group there is a high mortality. Infection between the thirteenth and eighteenth week

of gestation results in sensorineural hearing impairment alone and this is often bilateral. Children with congenital rubella account for up to 30% of children with sensorineural deafness. Termination of pregnancy is advised for maternal infection up to the eighteenth week of gestation. It is hoped that the introduction of MMR will lead to a fall in the incidence of congenital infection.

CYTOMEGALOVIRUS

Congenital infection with CMV occurs in about 3:1000 live births in Britain. In most cases this follows primary infection in the mother but reactivation of a previous infection may occur. About 5% of infants with congenital infection present at birth with an acute illness known as cytomegalic inclusion disease associated with petechiae, thrombocytopenia, conjugated hyperbilirubinaemia, chorioretinitis, microcephaly and cerebral calcifications. This has a high mortality and many survivors are severely handicapped. Another 5% of infants with congenital CMV have sensorineural hearing impairment as the only manifestation of infection and the remaining 90% are normal. It is important to perform tests of hearing at the earliest opportunity when congenital CMV infection has been identified so that hearing aids can be fitted if necessary. Deafness does not occur following acquired infection.

Diagnosis of infection is most easily made by culture of urine or throat secretions on cell monolayers. Isolation on specimens collected before 3 weeks of age suggests congenital infection. Measurement of CMV IgM antibody may be helpful in confirming infection. There is no satisfactory antiviral agent available for CMV infection and although a vaccine would be desirable, as yet, none is available.

HIV INFECTION

Infants delivered to HIV-infected mothers may not become infected, but transplacentally acquired HIV antibody may persist in the infant until about 15 months. These infants are referred to as having indeterminate status. Other infants may become infected, that is they are HIV positive beyond 15

Infection	Investigation
Bacterial infection	
Endocarditis (p. 238)	Multiple blood cultures
Pelvic, perinephric abscess	Observation, laparotomy
Pyelonephritis (p. 257)	Urine culture
Osteomyelitis (p. 481)	Blood culture; bone aspirate
Meningococcaemia (p. 366)	Blood culture
Tuberculosis (p. 555)	Tuberculin test, lymph node biopsy, sputum culture
Typhoid fever (p. 365)	Blood culture
Brucellosis (p. 364)	Serology, culture
Leptospirosis (p. 365)	Culture, serology
Tularaemia	Culture, serology
Viral	
Cytomegalovirus infection	Culture, serology
Infectious mononucleosis	Serology
Hepatitis (p. 209)	Serology
Human immunodeficiency virus infection	Serology
Fungal	
Histoplasmosis	Histoplasmin test; serology
Protozoal	
Malaria (p. 572)	Thick blood film
Toxoplasmosis	Serology
Unknown aetiology ? an infection	
Kawasaki disease (p. 478)	No diagnostic test
Collagen vascular disease	
Juvenile chronic arthritis (Still's disease (p. 475))	No diagnostic test
Systemic lupus erythematosus (p. 478)	Antinuclear antibody; LE cells
Polyarteritis nodosa	Biopsy
Malignancy	
Acute lymphoblastic leukaemia	Blood film; bone marrow
Hodgkin's and non-Hodgkin's lymphoma (p. 456)	Histology (e.g. lymph nodes)
Fever of neutropenia	Blood culture
Miscellaneous	
Ulcerative colitis (p. 203) and Crohn's disease (p. 202)	Histology
Central and nephrogenic diabetes insipidus (p. 408)	Electrolytes
Drug fever	Withdrawal of drug
Ectodermal dysplasia	—

Table 21.3 Causes of fever of unknown origin with relevant investigations.

months, but remain asymptomatic. Symptomatic infection associated with immunological abnormality and following vertical transmission may develop after the age of 4 months. This can be acquired immune deficiency syndrome (AIDS), or the AIDS related complex (ARC), which may progress to AIDS with the development of opportunistic infection.

Clinical features of ARC during infancy include failure to thrive, diarrhoea, persistent candidiasis, atopic eczema and interstitial pneumonitis. Diagnosis of AIDS is described on p. 361.

TOXOPLASMOSIS

Congenital infection is uncommon in Britain; perhaps 200–300 cases per year. Signs include microcephaly and/or chorioretinitis, but in most cases infection is not diagnosed at birth but only when visual problems become apparent in later childhood. Diagnosis of congenital infection is by serological means, and where there is strong suspicion of infection, several samples may be needed during the first few months of life. Postnatally acquired infection does not result in ophthalmological abnormalities. The antibiotics normally used during infancy, pyrimethamine and sulphadiazin or spiramycin are of only limited efficacy and no adequate control trials have been performed.

SYPHILIS

Infection caused by the spirochaete *Treponema pallidum*, if untreated during pregnancy, may be transmitted to the fetus through the placenta. Sequelae include spontaneous abortion or hydrops fetalis. An infant suffering from congenital syphilis may present with nephrotic syndrome and unexplained jaundice or neonatal hepatitis. 'Snuffles' associated with a profuse nasal discharge may develop in early infancy and inflammation of the nasal cartilage results in the classical 'saddle nose deformity'. Other clinical features include meningitis, chorioretinitis, and osteitis. Congenital syphilis although rare (approximately 10 cases per year in Britain) is a preventable condition. A serological test for syphilis should be performed in the first

trimester of pregnancy in all women and later in those at high risk of infection. The test offered commonly is the Venereal Disease Research Laboratory (VDRL) slide test which detects antibodies to the cardiolipin antigen in the bacteria. Infection is confined by a more specific treponemal antibody test such as the fluorescent treponemal antibody absorption (FTA–ABS). Infection detected in the mother during pregnancy should be treated with penicillin as should the infant if treatment was in the last month of pregnancy or if an inadequate course of penicillin was given. The prognosis of infants born to women with syphilis and treated during pregnancy is good.

Fever of unknown origin (FUO)

Although the original definition of fever or pyrexia of unknown origin was applied to fever persisting for 3 weeks or more with a temperature of >38.4°C (101°F) recorded on several occasions, it is acceptable to apply this term where fever has persisted for more than 1 week. The most common causes of FUO in childhood are infectious and collagen diseases. There is a long list of causes (Table 21.3) and although this may appear daunting many of these can be excluded by taking a good history. Particularly important points include:

1 Foreign travel which might suggest malaria or brucellosis.

2 Bowel symptoms; a pelvic abscess, Crohn's disease and salmonellosis.

3 Rash and joint pain (juvenile rheumatoid arthritis).

The physical examination is equally important; for instance, the detection of a cardiac murmur and splinter haemorrhages is suggestive of infective endocarditis (p. 238); rose spots and splenomegaly of typhoid fever (p. 365). Investigations depend on the differential diagnosis and are listed in Table 21.3.

Further reading

Nicoll A, Rudd P. (Eds) *British Paediatric Association Manual on Infections and Immunizations in Children.* Oxford University Press, Oxford 1989.

22
METABOLIC DISORDERS

Metabolic disorders are an extremely diverse group of conditions which are usually genetically determined and may present at almost any age. They are all rare and may be difficult to diagnose. This chapter does not attempt to discuss all the disorders of metabolism but will highlight those which are relatively more common, or where the presentation may cause diagnostic confusion.

Disorders of carbohydrate metabolism

Sugars form a major part of the infant diet, particularly the milk sugar, lactose. Sucrose and maltose are disaccharides more commonly found in the diets of older children. These disaccharides are digested in the bowel by specific disaccharidases to the monosaccharide sugars, glucose, fructose and galactose which are then absorbed through the bowel mucosa. Absence of disaccharidases may lead to diarrhoea (see Chapter 12). Galactose and fructose must be metabolized through a number of enzyme steps to glucose. Absence of these enzymes causes severe disease often presenting with hypoglycaemia. Hypoglycaemia is an important feature of many illnesses of children and is discussed in detail in Chapter 23.

GALACTOSAEMIA

This condition results from a deficiency of the enzyme galactose-1-phosphate uridyl transferase which is required for the conversion of galactose-1-phosphate into glucose-1-phosphate. An accu-
mulation of galactose-1-phosphate occurs which has a toxic action on the brain, lens, liver and kidney by inhibiting cell metabolism in these organs. The inhibition of carbohydrate metabolism in the liver leads to hypoglycaemia. The clinical features result from damage to these organs and from hypoglycaemia. Lactase digests lactose in milk to galactose, which is toxic for patients with galactosaemia.

Clinical features. The baby is normal at birth but within a few days of starting milk begins to vomit and to have diarrhoea, leading to progressive wasting. Jaundice develops at the end of the first week or during the second week; this should not be confused with the more common causes of neonatal jaundice (p. 106) which occur sooner after birth. There is progressive enlargement of the liver, this being the most striking physical sign (Fig. 22.1). Hypoglycaemia causes lethargy, refusal to suck and may lead to convulsions.

Death may occur early. If the baby survives and is untreated, cataracts develop within a few weeks. There is also progressive mental retardation associated with retardation of growth.

Proteinuria and generalized amino-aciduria result from renal tubular damage. A reducing substance is present in the urine, shown by chromatography to be galactose.

The condition is inherited as an autosomal recessive characteristic. The homozygous state is manifest clinically as galactosaemia, while the heterozygous state can be detected by an abnormal galactose tolerance curve. The enzyme defect

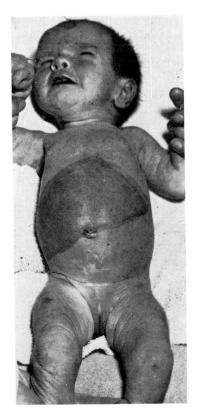

Fig. 22.1 Galactosaemia in a baby aged 2 weeks. The child was jaundiced and the liver, whose outline has been drawn in, much enlarged.

can be demonstrated at birth in families at risk by assaying the enzyme level in cord blood.

Treatment. The child must immediately be placed on a diet from which lactose and galactose are excluded. Special milk substitutes are available.

Prognosis. With treatment, the acute symptoms from hypoglycaemia and the accumulation of galactose-1-phosphate, such as vomiting, diarrhoea, anorexia and lethargy disappear. Proteinuria and amino-aciduria also disappear at once, but mental retardation and cataract are irreversible and, for this reason, immediate diagnosis and treatment are essential if these complications are to be prevented.

FRUCTOSAEMIA

This is due to deficiency of the enzyme fructose-1-phosphate aldolase. When such patients are fed food containing fructose or sucrose they develop severe hypoglycaemia. The disorder is inherited as an autosomal recessive condition.

The newborn infant remains perfectly well so long as he is fed lactose in breast milk only. When weaned and fructose or sucrose are introduced, symptoms of acute hypoglycaemia develop and may be severe enough to cause loss of consciousness or convulsions. The child fails to thrive and has poor appetite associated with vomiting, hypotonia and hepatomegaly. Recurrent episodes of hypoglycaemia may cause mental retardation. Older patients, who are usually found among the relatives of affected infants, have a strong aversion to sweet foods. By avoiding these they are able to remain well. Ingestion of fructose also causes renal tubular dysfunction with renal tubular acidosis, and loss of phosphate and amino acids in the urine.

Investigations. Diagnosis is confirmed by an intravenous or oral fructose tolerance test which causes a fall in blood glucose. Care should be taken immediately to treat symptomatic hypoglycaemia arising as a result of the test.

Management. The patient must be placed on a life-long fructose- and sucrose-free diet.

Fructosuria

This should not be confused with fructosaemia. Fructose is excreted in the urine but the patient remains asymptomatic and thrives. There is no hypoglycaemia.

THE GLYCOGEN STORAGE DISEASES

Glucose is stored in the body as glycogen and is synthesized and degraded by a series of enzyme steps. A variety of enzyme defects in liver and muscle lead to the glycogen storage diseases. Only two occur in children.

Type I glycogen storage disease (von Gierke's)

This is an autosomal recessive condition and is due to a deficiency of glucose-6-phosphatase. The child presents in the first 2 years of life with failure to thrive, abdominal pain and progressive hepatomegaly which may be present from birth. Episodes of hypoglycaemia occur during periods of stress, causing vomiting, convulsions and sometimes loss of consciousness. Hyperglycaemia may occur after meals because the liver cells are so filled with glycogen that they cannot absorb a sudden intake of glucose. The children tend to be short but obese. Xanthomata are commonly seen over the extensor surfaces of hands and feet. A bleeding tendency is common due to the liver dysfunction.

Investigations. The fasting blood glucose is low and there is no response to an injection of adrenalin or glucagon. The glucose tolerance curve is persistently high. Liver biopsy shows an increase in the amount of glycogen and is also used to demonstrate the specific enzyme defect.

Management. Symptomatic improvement can be achieved by adjusting the diet in order to maintain a reasonably constant blood sugar. Small frequent meals are helpful.

Type II glycogen storage disease (Pompe's)

This is a rare autosomal recessive disorder involving lack of acid maltase in the heart and skeletal muscles. The presentation is with hypotonia in infancy and cardiomegaly which may be massive. Cardiac failure in the first year is common. Hypoglycaemia does not occur but the prognosis is hopeless.

Disorders of lipid metabolism

Lipid metabolism is extremely complex and its disorders are still being unravelled. Disorders of lipid metabolism can be grouped into various major categories.

LIPOPROTEIN DEFICIENCIES

Lipoproteins are the molecular complexes by which lipids are transported in the blood. Chylomicrons are the largest particles and resemble minute globules of fat in the blood. Other lipoproteins are described on the basis of their density as very low- (VLDL), low- (LDL) and high-density lipoproteins (HDL).

Abetalipoproteinaemia

Patients with this disorder cannot synthesize normal lipoproteins. It is inherited as an autosomal recessive condition. The main features initially are gastrointestinal (malabsorption), and neurological. The red cells show a typically crenated appearance and are referred to as acanthocytes. Later the children show progressive neurological abnormality with ataxia, peripheral neuropathy and later retinal degeneration.

Diagnosis is made on lipoprotein electrophoresis as there is absence of low-density lipoproteins. Management includes giving fat-soluble vitamins (including vitamin E) which are likely to be deficient due to the steatorrhoea.

Hyperlipoproteinaemias

This is a group of inherited disorders characterized by high levels of a variety of lipoproteins.

Type I. This is characterized by very high levels of chylomicrons. The main clinical features are extensive eruptive xanthomata at any site, abdominal pain and hepatomegaly. Treatment is by dietary restriction of fat, and the prognosis is relatively good.

Type II. This is associated with extremely high levels of cholesterol in the affected homozygotes who go on to develop very severe arterial disease in their early twenties. Extensive xanthomata are seen in both homozygotes and heterozygotes. The heterozygotes also have high levels of cholesterol and premature arterial disease. The importance of this condition is that dietary treatment from early childhood will modify the severity of the vascular disease. Low saturated fat and cholesterol diets must be rigidly applied and clofibrate potentiates the cholesterol lowering effect.

Sphingolipidoses

The sphingolipids are a complex group of substances which are important in neural function. The gangliosides are one group of sphingolipids and the best-known disorder of this compound is Tay–Sachs disease (see below). Enzyme defects involving the sphingolipids cause accumulation of these compounds within the brain and other organs and are associated with severe dysfunction of the central nervous system and extensive demyelination of cerebral white matter.

G_{M2} gangliosidosis (Tay–Sachs disease)

This autosomal recessive condition is due to a deficiency in hexosaminidase A which can be detected in the serum of heterozygote carriers as well as affected cases and is therefore important for genetic counselling. Although a rare condition, Tay–Sachs disease is particularly common in Jews. The infant is normal for the first 3–6 months of life; progressive mental retardation then develops, followed by spasticity, convulsions and blindness. A cherry-red spot at the macula is the characteristic feature. Hyperacusis is an early feature, causing an increased startle reflex; this sign precedes the development of the cherry-red spot. The degree of disturbance of the white matter is sufficient to cause the brain to increase in size so that enlargement of the head is detectable in the majority of cases. There is no effective treatment.

Generalized G_{M1} gangliosidosis (Pseudo-Hurler's disease)

This autosomal recessive condition, due to absent β-galactosidase enzyme, is less common than the G_{M2} form. Affected children exhibit failure to thrive, hepatosplenomegaly, developmental delay and kyphosis. Their coarse features have been likened to Hurler's disease (p. 375) hence the term 'pseudo-Hurler's'. The diagnosis is confirmed by detecting low enzyme levels in leukocytes.

Gaucher's disease

This probably represents a group of conditions due to a defect in the enzyme β-glucosidase which causes accumulation of glucosyl ceramide in various tissues, particularly the reticulo-endothelial system. Two forms of the disease occur:

Acute infantile Gaucher's disease. Deposition of the cerebroside occurs in the brain as well as in the reticulo-endothelial system. The infant appears normal at birth but soon becomes apathetic, feeds poorly and there is progressive physical and mental retardation. Death occurs within the first year of life.

Chronic Gaucher's disease. About half the cases present in older children, the rest during adult life. The child becomes wasted but there is no mental retardation as the brain is not involved. The abdomen enlarges from hepatomegaly and splenomegaly.

In both types there is anaemia from marrow involvement (leucoerythroblastic anaemia), the bones fracturing easily. Thrombocytopenia may occur early, causing haemorrhagic manifestations. The typical Gaucher cells are striped, being found in the bone marrow or on rectal biopsy.

Niemann–Pick disease

In this condition there is an accumulation of sphingomyelin in the nervous system and elsewhere. The child, who is often Jewish, is normal at birth but during the first year of life there is a steady mental and physical deterioration; death from progressive anaemia and wasting occurs within the first 3 years of life. The liver and spleen enlarge, the skin becomes discoloured and lymph nodes are palpable. A cherry-red spot at the macula may appear as in Tay–Sachs disease. The abnormal cells can be seen on marrow or rectal biopsy; these are foamy as opposed to the striped cells seen in Gaucher's disease. This disease is inherited as an autosomal recessive disorder.

Batten's disease

This is another rare autosomal recessive condition with deposition of abnormal lipid material in the brain. The biochemical defect is not well understood. Clinically it presents in a number of forms:

Infantile or late infantile. Regression of learned skills occurs in the first or second year of life followed by seizures and dementia. The child is reduced to a vegetative state and dies at between 6 and 7 years of age.

Juvenile form. The initial feature is visual failure in 5–8-year-old children associated with optic atrophy. Later fits develop and eventually the child shows signs of dementia.

Diagnosis is difficult as there is no measurable enzyme defect. Tissue biopsy (including brain) shows abnormal deposits of lipids. There is no treatment.

THE LEUKODYSTROPHIES

This group of conditions describes a pathological appearance of abnormal cerebral white matter. Myelination may initially develop normally, but becomes destroyed by the disease; or the nature of the myelin may be abnormal from the onset.

Metachromatic leukodystrophy

This is distinguished by the accumulation of metachromatically staining material in the areas of dysmyelination. The content of this material is cerebroside sulphate resulting from a deficiency of the enzyme cerebroside sulphatase. Similar staining material is also found in the liver and kidney.

Clinical features. The disease presents in three forms:
1 Infantile – neonatal development being normal and symptoms commencing between 12 and 18 months.

2 Juvenile – the onset being between 5 and 10 years.
3 Adult – the onset particularly occurring in the second decade.

There is slow development of weakness and ataxia, and loss of tendon reflexes. Speech becomes impaired, vision lost and eventually there is complete dementia followed by death. Cranial nerve palsies often occur. The fundus usually shows optic atrophy, but a cherry-red spot as seen in Tay–Sachs disease (see p. 373) has been reported. The protein in the cerebrospinal fluid is raised.

Diagnosis can be made by an examination of the urinary deposit which may show desquamated renal cells containing metachromatic material. Renal and rectal biopsy may show the same material. The nerve cells remain normal but the metachromatic material in the nerve fibres may extend right down the peripheral nerves, so that a skin biopsy can be used to show the material in myelinated nerves of the skin. Involvement of the peripheral nerves causes prolonged conduction time.

Krabbe's disease

This form of leukodystrophy is a disease of infants resulting from a deficiency of the lysosomal enzyme galactocerebroside-β-glucosidase. It is characterized by the presence of 'globoid' cells in the white matter, these being large multi-nucleated phagocytic cells surrounding the small blood vessels. The infant is normal at birth, but at about 3 months becomes irritable and vomits. This is followed by increasing rigidity associated with convulsions, blindness and deafness. Death usually occurs within 1 year of the onset. There is a rise of protein in the cerebrospinal fluid and nerve conduction velocity is decreased.

THE MUCOPOLYSACCHARIDOSES

A group of complicated compounds, referred to as mucopolysaccharides, are important substances for normal connective tissue. Disorders of these molecules are collectively known as the mucopolysaccharidoses and are genetically determined and progressive in nature. Only some present in childhood and these are briefly discussed here. Diagnosis is made on the basis of either dermatan or heparan sulphate in the urine.

Type I mucopolysaccharidosis (Hurler's syndrome)

This is an autosomal recessive condition due to an overproduction of certain acid mucopolysaccharides which are then stored in the body. No physical abnormalities are present at birth, the diagnosis seldom being made before the age of 6 months. A grotesque facial appearance, previously labelled 'gargoylism', associated with mental defect and dwarfism, gradually develops. The corneas are clouded (Fig. 22.2), the liver and spleen enlarge and an umbilical hernia is common. The umbilical hernia has not usually been present from birth and may be the reason for which the child is brought to the doctor. Lateral X-ray of the spine shows a beak-shaped deformity of one or two vertebrae, causing an angular kyphosis. Large quantities of dermatan sulphate are found in the urine. Scheie's syndrome is now included in this group.

Type II mucopolysaccharidosis (Hunter's syndrome)

The less frequent Type II condition is inherited as a sex-linked recessive trait so that only boys are affected. The affected boys have coarse features and kyphosis but no clouding of the corneas (Fig. 22.3). About half are deaf, whereas deafness seldom occurs in the other types of mucopolysaccharidosis. Dermatan or heparan sulphate may be found in the urine. There is no known treatment for the condition.

Type III mucopolysaccharidosis (Sanfilippo syndrome)

This is probably the commonest type, comprising 30% of the patients. They suffer severe progressive mental retardation, but show few of the facial features seen in some of the other types of mucopolysaccharidosis.

The skeletal changes do not appear until after the first year. The neck becomes short, the chest barrel-shaped, the spine kyphotic and there is flattening of the lumbar vertebrae. This causes a semi-crouching stance and a waddling gait. The facial appearance is characteristic, the mouth being broad and the teeth widely spaced; the nose is short and the maxilla prominent. The wrists are enlarged and the fingers misshapen.

Type IV mucopolysaccharidosis (Morquio's syndrome)

This type differs from the others in that skeletal deformities predominate and intelligence is normal. It is inherited as an autosomal recessive trait

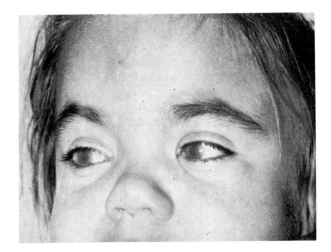

Fig. 22.2 Hurler's syndrome. Clouding of the cornea is visible.

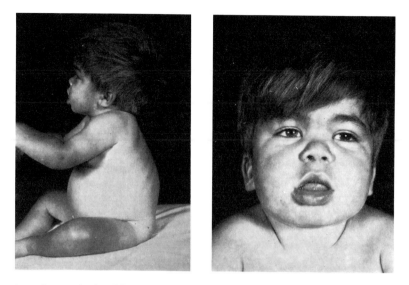

Fig. 22.3 Hunter's syndrome. The facial features are coarse and an angular kyphosis is present in the lower thoracic spine. There is no clouding of the corneas.

and is associated with the urinary excretion of keratan sulphate.

Type VI mucopolysaccharidosis (Maroteaux–Lamy syndrome)

Patients with this type have severe skeletal changes and short stature. The facies are not as severely changed as in Hurler's syndrome and intelligence is normal.

Disorders of amino acid metabolism

Amino acids are the building blocks of proteins and an enzyme is necessary in order for each step in the elaboration of complicated protein molecules. There are many clinically important disorders of amino acid metabolism; the commoner ones will be discussed here.

PHENYLKETONURIA

In these patients an absence of phenylalanine hydroxylase prevents the conversion of phenylalanine to tyrosine. A rise of phenylalanine occurs in the blood, its breakdown products, phenyl-

pyruvic, phenyllactic and phenylacetic acids appearing in the urine. Mental deficiency results, either from the toxic effect of the excess phenylalanine or, more probably, from the accumulation of some phenylalanine metabolite. The incidence in the UK is 1:12 000 births and the disease is inherited as an autosomal recessive condition.

The babies seem normal at birth, but progressive mental deterioration occurs from the age of a few weeks. Vomiting, irritability and convulsions result from the accumulation of toxic metabolites. The children usually have fair hair, since tyrosine is required for melanin production, and blue eyes. Eczema is common. The incisors are widely spaced and the urine gives a musty smell from phenylacetic acid.

Diagnosis. Early diagnosis is essential in order to prevent mental retardation. All newborn babies should be screened on the sixth day of life using the Guthrie inhibition test which detects a rise in serum phenylalanine. In this method, blood from a heel prick is cultured with *B. subtilis* in media containing a growth inhibitor which is suppressed by phenylalanine; a positive test is therefore indicated by growth of the organism. A false negative result can arise if the infant is on an antibiotic which inhibits growth of the organism, or if the child is not being fed milk. The level of phenylalanine must be estimated quantitatively on all suspected cases and on the siblings of known cases.

Treatment. The child is given a low phenylalanine diet, the exact amount being determined by serial phenylalanine blood levels. Since this amino acid is essential for growth it cannot be excluded completely but its level should be kept at 25–100 µmol/l. Escape from dietary control may occur during bouts of infection when a particular check on blood levels must be kept.

The duration of dietary control is still under investigation. It is probably reasonable to stop the diet when brain growth has been completed at about 10 years of age but the diet must be reinstituted prior to a woman becoming pregnant in order to avoid damage to the fetal brain.

MAPLE SYRUP DISEASE

The characteristic smell of the urine accounts for the name of this form of mental deficiency. The children develop fits in the first week of life and if untreated become severely mentally handicapped and spastic, dying young. There is a multiple but patterned amino-aciduria involving valine, leucine and isoleucine. A special diet comprising synthetic amino acids is required. This is more complicated than in phenylketonuria because each patient requires individual adjustment of the diet according to his metabolic pattern. The disease is inherited on an autosomal recessive basis.

HARTNUP DISEASE

This form of mental defect is named after the first family with the condition to be described. The defect is in tryptophan metabolism, appearing to be due to a specific defect in the transport of amino acids in the cells of the jejunum and proximal renal tubules. The amino-aciduria is multiple but patterned. The mental defect comes on slowly, is not severe and in some patients the intellect may be normal. In addition, there is photosensitivity which results in a pellagra-like rash, and cerebellar ataxia. Treatment with nicotinamide and a diet low in tryptophan may cause symptomatic improvement, although it does not alter the amino-aciduria.

HOMOCYSTINURIA

This is a more recently discovered inborn error of metabolism which, like the others, is also inherited on an autosomal recessive basis. The defect involves the metabolism of the essential amino acid methionine leading to the urinary excretion of homocystine.

Children with this disorder are usually moderately mentally handicapped and often suffer from convulsions. They are fair skinned with a malar flush. Many of the features of Marfan's syndrome (p. 485) are present; ocular defects, especially dislocation of the lens associated with iridodonesis, skeletal defects, especially arachnodactyly, chest deformities and a high arched palate. Thrombotic episodes, which do not occur in Marfan's syndrome, are a particular feature resulting from greatly increased platelet stickiness.

Since homocystinuria is a steadily progressive disease with the constant threat of thrombosis, treatment is worthwhile at any age. Early diagnosis is essential since a low-methionine diet with added L-cystine will prevent symptoms. Pyridoxine and folate supplements should also be given.

TYROSINAEMIA

This autosomal recessive inborn error usually presents with failure to thrive, vomiting, hepatomegaly and rickets. Mental retardation is unusual. A prominent feature is impairment of renal tubular function with glycosuria and amino-aciduria. Renal rickets occurs in all cases. In the later stages of the illness, liver cirrhosis and jaundice occur.

Dietary treatment is usually successful in modifying the course of the disease. Restriction in dietary phenylalanine and tyrosine is important.

UREA CYCLE DISORDERS

The urea cycle detoxifies ammonia derived from urea. There are a number of metabolic steps in this process and consequently a number of inborn errors are possible. They usually present in the newborn period with vomiting, lethargy and failure to thrive. The serum ammonia level is always high and it is this that causes the neurological toxicity. Treatment is by means of a low-protein diet but these children are very susceptible to intercurrent infection which may cause severe metabolic compromise. Prognosis for normal development in those presenting in the neonatal period is poor.

Transient hyperammonaemia, without a recognizable biochemical defect, is seen in infants, particularly those born prematurely. It is usually a self-limiting condition.

ORGANIC ACIDAEMIAS

This is due to a group of inborn errors involving particular amino or organic acids. Presentation is as diverse as the biochemical abnormalities and a variety of presenting symptoms occur including fits, mental retardation and hypotonia, failure to thrive and severe metabolic acidosis. The child may present in the neonatal period or later in childhood depending on the defect.

The diagnosis is made on the basis of abnormal plasma and urinary chromatography. Some are treatable by dietary manipulation but the prognosis is often poor.

Disorders of mineral and bone metabolism

RICKETS

Rickets is a disease of growing bone and is due to impaired mineralization. Nutritional rickets, common in the developing world, is rarely seen in Europe or USA, and is discussed fully in Chapter 29. Neonatal rickets is described on p. 114. Vitamin D consumed in the diet is stored in the liver as ergocalciferol (vitamin D_2). Cholecalciferol (vitamin D_3) is produced in the skin by the action

of ultraviolet light, but neither form is biologically active. Vitamin D is converted in the liver to 25-hydroxyvitamin D and then transported, bound to protein, to the kidney to be hydroxylated further to 1,25-dihydroxyvitamin D. This final hydroxylation occurs when the active form of vitamin D is required. When needs are less, it is converted to the inactive 24,25-dihydroxyvitamin D form. It is interesting that 1,25-dihydroxy D_3 behaves more like a hormone than a vitamin in that it is secreted by the kidney and is transported by the blood to have its effects on other organs; mainly the bones and the bowel.

The action of the renal form of vitamin D is to enhance calcium and phosphate absorption from the bowel, and together with parathormone liberate calcium from the bone. It also acts on the reabsorption of calcium through the renal tubules. Hypophosphataemia stimulates 1,25-dihydroxyvitamin D_3 production which causes increased phosphate and calcium absorption from the bowel.

There are clearly a number of possible causes of rickets based on the complicated metabolism of vitamin D. These are summarized in Table 22.1. Some anticonvulsant drugs such as phenobarbitone and phenytoin may induce rickets by interfering with vitamin D absorption or metabolism.

Renal rickets

Rickets may occur in association with renal disorders which do not respond to the ordinary curative doses of vitamin D. This disorder may be glomerular or tubular in origin and, to prevent confusion, it is preferable to speak of 'glomerular rickets' and 'tubular rickets' rather than 'renal rickets'. Normal renal function is required for

Table 22.1 Causes of rickets in children.

Nutritional rickets (see p. 549)
Malabsorption
Renal rickets
Glomerular
Tubular
Drug induced

hydroxylation of cholecalciferol (D₃) which converts it to the active agent.

Glomerular rickets

This form is often referred to as 'renal rickets' or renal osteodystrophy and results from chronic glomerular insufficiency. It may be due to congenital malformations such as bilateral renal hypoplasia, severe renal infections or chronic glomerulonephritis. The impaired glomerular function causes retention of urea, phosphate and creatinine. Lowering of the blood calcium occurs secondarily to the raised phosphate which induces secondary hyperparathyroidism; an important diagnostic difference from tubular rickets.

Treatment. The rickets can be cured only if successful treatment of the primary renal condition is possible. If this is impossible high doses of vitamin D may effect an improvement. Recently a very effective synthetic vitamin D compound, 1-alpha-hydroxy D₃, has been introduced to treat bone disease of renal origin. This compound is rapidly metabolized to 1,25-dihydroxy D₃, the active agent, whose function is to increase calcium absorption. The compound has a short biological effect so that the hazard of inducing hypercalcaemia is small; it is therefore safer than giving massive doses of vitamin D. Aluminium hydroxide given orally helps to reduce the high level of serum phosphate.

Tubular rickets (Fanconi syndrome)

This may be due to an inborn error of metabolism affecting the renal tubules. There are a number of causes listed in Table 22.2.

There is a leak of phosphate into the urine due to failure of tubular reabsorption. In addition, amino-aciduria and glycosuria are commonly seen. The ensuing hypophosphataemia leads to rickets. Bicarbonate loss may also occur leading to renal tubular acidosis. This is a genetically determined, usually X-linked condition, and it is not responsive to physiological amounts of vitamin D. It is sometimes referred to as 'vitamin D resistant rickets'. The children usually present between 1 and 2 years with anorexia and failure to gain weight. The child is irritable and develops vomiting, thirst and constipation followed by the appearance of rickets. Polyuria may be found and is due to an associated failure of water reabsorption. There may be bouts of fever for which no infective cause can be found and which are probably due to dehydration. Episodes of weakness, lethargy and even coma may occur.

The condition responds to massive doses of vitamin D since this is able to increase the reabsorption of phosphate by the tubules.

Renal tubular acidosis

This describes a group of disorders due to renal tubular dysfunction. It may be seen with tubular rickets (see above) and many of the causes are similar. It usually presents with failure to thrive, weakness or dehydration.

The disorder may be due to either proximal or distal tubular abnormalities. The proximal form is due to reduction in the absorption of bicarbonate in the proximal tubules. Potassium is often lost along with the bicarbonate which causes weakness. The distal form is due to failure of the tubule to excrete acid. In both conditions there is a metabolic acidosis usually with an alkaline urine. The serum chloride levels are always high and the plasma phosphate is usually low leading to tubular rickets. Nephrocalcinosis may occur.

Table 22.2 Causes of tubular rickets.

Hereditary tubular hypophosphataemia
Galactosaemia
Renal tubular acidosis
Cystinosis
Tyrosinaemia

Cystinosis

This is a rare metabolic disorder which is usually inherited as a recessive characteristic. Cystine is deposited in the reticulo-endothelial system, especially in the liver, spleen, lymph glands and bone marrow. It is also deposited in the renal tubules; when this occurs the tubular damage causes the identical features of the De Toni–Fabre–Fanconi syndrome. Cystine crystals can be demonstrated in the cornea by slit lamp and in the bone marrow samples. Most patients die before the age of 10 years.

Cystinuria

This must be differentiated from cystinosis. The only abnormality is the presence of cystine and other characteristic amino acids in the urine, with the subsequent chance of forming cystine stones in the urinary tract. Cystine is not deposited in other tissues so that, apart from the problem of stones, there is no risk to life.

Hypercalcaemia

The definition of hypercalcaemia is a sustained elevation in serum calcium above 2.5 mmol/l. Table 22.3 lists the commoner causes of hypercalcaemia in infants and children. Unlike the majority of metabolic disorders discussed in this chapter, hypercalcaemia is not an inborn error and is not genetically determined in the majority of cases. Hyperparathyroidism is an important cause and is discussed in Chapter 23. Hypercalcaemia may cause nephrocalcinosis with gradual impairment of renal function.

HYPERVITAMINOSIS D

Overdosage of vitamin D should no longer occur. It has been suggested that some infants who deve-

Table 22.3 Causes of hypercalcaemia.

Hypervitaminosis D
Infantile hypercalcaemia
Primary hyperparathyroidism (p. 421)
Chronic renal failure
Hypophosphatasia
Hyperthyroidism
Immobilization
Malignancies

lop hypercalcaemia are unusually sensitive to the effects of vitamin D.

Infants with hypercalcaemia become anorexic, irritable and start to refuse milk but continue to drink water. The serum calcium is raised, but the phosphorus level is normal. Nephrocalcinosis may be apparent in abdominal X-ray or ultrasound examination.

The infants should be given a low-calcium diet; special low-calcium milk and cereal preparations are available. No additional vitamin D should be given. On this regime the serum calcium gradually falls and the nephrocalcinosis may regress.

INFANTILE HYPERCALCAEMIA (WILLIAM'S SYNDROME)

These children present with severe hypercalcaemia and have characteristic 'elfin-like' facies, including exaggerated epicanthic folds and a *retroussé* nose. A squint is common and the lower lip hangs loosely. Supravalvular aortic stenosis is a common feature, often accompanied by hypertension. X-rays show osteosclerosis with an increase in bone density at the base of the skull and ends of the long bones. The children are very irritable and show mental retardation. The cause of this disorder is not known.

Management. A low-calcium diet together with corticosteroids reduces the plasma calcium levels but the prognosis for normal development is poor. Surgery to correct the aortic stenosis is usually necessary.

HYPOPHOSPHATASIA

This is a rare disease due to an inborn error of metabolism which is inherited as a recessive characteristic. The essential biochemical abnormality is low or even absent alkaline phosphatase.

Clinical features. The majority of patients present in infancy and the bone lesions may be present at birth. Failure to thrive is the essential feature. There is anorexia, vomiting, irritability and intermittent fever. The skeletal lesions resemble rickets and X-rays show grossly defective calcification so that the zone of provisional calcification disappears, irregular calcification only occurring in the metaphysis. Irregular formation of new bone may occur under the periosteum. The teeth are hypoplastic, often being lost early. Renal impairment may result from hypercalcaemia.

Treatment and prognosis. A low-calcium diet should be given, but there is no definitive treatment.

ENDOCRINE DISORDERS

An intact endocrine system is of fundamental importance for the growth and development of the fetus, infant and child. All cells and tissues are influenced by the activities of the peripheral endocrine glands whose secretions are orchestrated by complex rhythmic messages from the pituitary.

The pituitary gland has neuronal and vascular connections with the hypothalamus and higher brain centres. The relationship between the brain and endocrine system is exemplified by the neurohypophyseal circuit, in which cells of the supra-optic and para-ventricular nuclei of the anterior hypothalamus synthesize antidiuretic hormone (ADH) and oxytocin which migrate along axons to be stored in nerve terminals in the posterior pituitary. Osmoreceptors close to, or within, the supra-optic nucleus regulate secretion of ADH and complex neural mechanisms regulate oxytocin secretion during lactation (see p. 65).

In recent years hypothalamic-releasing hormones responsible for anterior pituitary stimulation have been identified and are in clinical use. These include thyrotrophin-releasing hormone (TRH), gonadotrophin-releasing hormone (GnRH), growth-hormone-releasing hormone (GHRH), and corticotrophin-releasing hormone (CRH). These short peptides are released in pulses into the hypophyseal portal blood vessels and stimulate specific anterior pituitary cells to synthesize and store the trophic hormones which include luteinising hormone (LH), follicle-stimulating hormone (FSH), growth hormone (GH), and adrenocorticotrophic hormone (ACTH).

It is vital to recognize the pulsatile character of some secretions (e.g. LH, FSH, GH) and circadian variations (e.g. ACTH) so that appropriate blood sampling or provocation testing can be performed. For this reason, random growth hormone assays in a paediatric clinic are an expensive waste of time. In contrast, the more steady-state secretions of the peripheral glands (e.g. thyroid hormones, sex steroids) often allow evaluation without specific testing procedures. Figure 23.1 illustrates the anatomy and physiology of the endocrine system. Investigations will be dealt with under individual disorders.

Growth

Optimal growth is an important index of child health. Although suboptimal growth is often a sign of ill health or disease, its accurate assessment in the community is difficult because of inadequate measuring equipment and techniques. Consequently children with treatable causes of short stature frequently suffer because of delayed diagnosis.

By definition, 3% of the population lie on or below the third centile. Most of these small children are normal and should not be subjected to special investigations. Growth screening methods must attempt to distinguish children who are pathologically short or growing at an abnormal velocity, as shown in Figure 23.2.

Techniques of measurement

In the first year after birth serial weight measurements are commonly used to assess growth because supine length measurements are difficult,

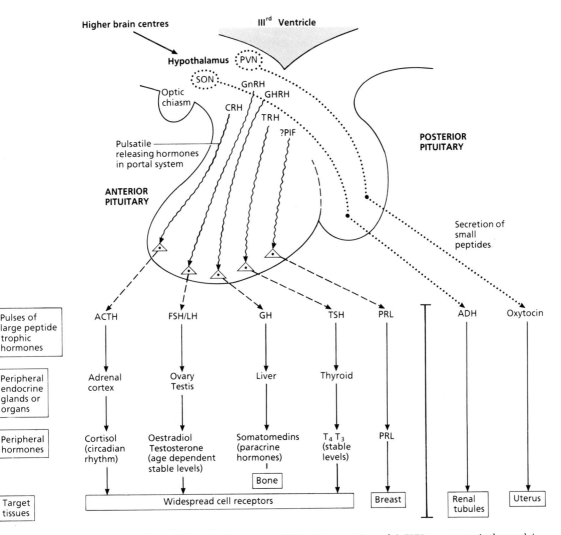

Fig. 23.1 Anatomy and physiology of the endocrine system. SON – Supra-optic nuclei, PVN – paraventricular nuclei, GnRH – gonadotrophin-releasing hormone, GHRH – growth-hormone-releasing factor, CRH – corticotrophin-releasing hormone, TRH – thyrotrophin-releasing hormone, PIF – prolactin-inhibiting factor, PRL – prolactin, ADH – antidiuretic hormone.

but inexpensive and accurate infant measuring mats are now available (see Fig. 23.3). When children are old enough to stand, their heights should be measured as part of health surveillance screening programmes (p. 39). Measurement of height can only be accurate if some form of fixed ruler is available to measure the exact distance between the ground and a flat object brought down on to the vertex of the head at right angles to a back-board or wall (see Fig. 23.4). Even in paediatric clinics with expensive stadiometers, serious inaccuracies occur unless a consistent technique is used.

PLOTTING GROWTH

Single measurements of height, weight or head circumference give limited information because

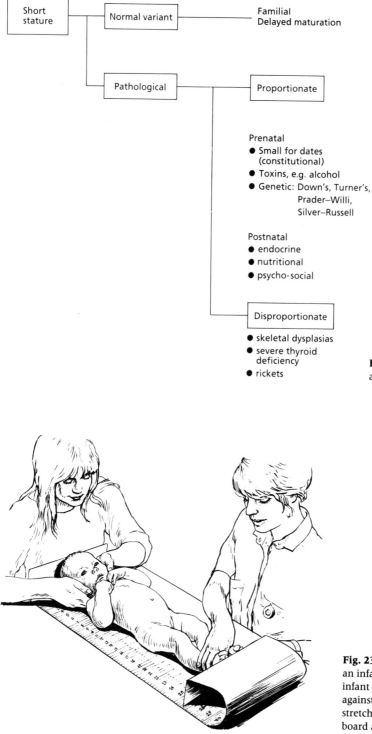

Fig. 23.2 An approach to diagnosis in a child of short stature.

Fig. 23.3 Method for measuring length in an infant accurately. One person holds the infant under the mandible with the vertex against the head board, whilst the other stretches the extended legs with the foot board against the soles of the infant's feet.

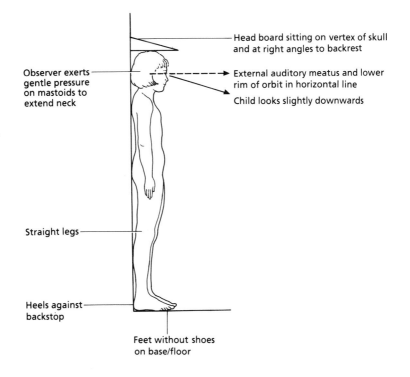

Head board sitting on vertex of skull and at right angles to backrest

Observer exerts gentle pressure on mastoids to extend neck

External auditory meatus and lower rim of orbit in horizontal line

Child looks slightly downwards

Straight legs

Heels against backstop

Feet without shoes on base/floor

Fig. 23.4 Technique for measuring standing height.

growth is a dynamic process. Nevertheless, the first measurement acts as a baseline and should be plotted precisely on a standard height centile chart. If the child's measurement causes concern, a second height measurement should be performed after a gap of at least 3 months. When the line of growth deviates away from the centile channels, this indicates an abnormal growth pattern and further investigation should be considered.

Growth velocity

This is the height gained over a period of 12 months, or if measured for a fraction of a year (e.g. 6 months) the height gained multiplied accordingly (e.g. × 2). A growth velocity chart is illustrated in Figure 23.5.

WHO TO MEASURE AND WHEN

1 *Infancy*
● All infants at some time during their first 2 years.

● Selected infants:
   those born of low birth weight (less than 2500 g),
   sick children,
   children who are failing to thrive,
   any young child whose health or well being is causing concern.

2 *Pre-school*
● When old enough to stand (18−24 month screen).
● 3.5 year screen.

3 *School*
● 5, 7, 10−11-year screen.

WHEN TO RE-MEASURE

This is essential in the following children.
● Those less than the third centile
● Those thought to be growing slowly
● Those with worrying symptoms or signs (see below)
Remeasurement should be performed at intervals of not less than 3 months.

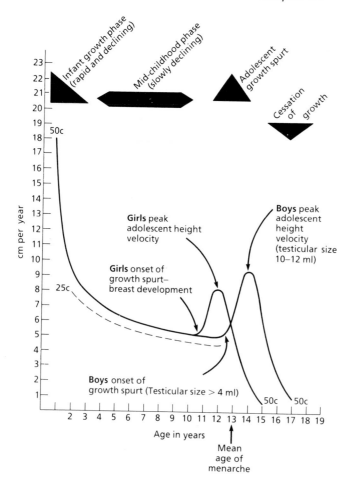

Fig. 23.5 Height velocity chart for boys and girls showing the influence of stages of puberty. If the velocity remains below the twenty-fifth centile in mid-childhood, then the height will deviate downwards away from the normal centile channels.

REFERRAL FOR FURTHER GROWTH ASSESSMENT

Screening of height will detect a group of children who require further expert assessment. Indications for referral include:

1 Those more than three standard deviations below the mean (approximately 5 cm below the third centile).

2 Growth pattern deviating away from centile lines.

3 Growth velocity over a 1-year period of less than the twenty-fifth centile.

4 With worrying symptoms (see below).

5 Children of moderately short stature (less than the tenth centile) with obesity. Primary obesity in children should stimulate prepubertal growth. Conditions with secondary obesity such as Cushing's syndrome or Prader–Willi syndrome inhibit growth.

6 Children who are moderately short (less than the tenth centile) with tall parents.

The short child

CLINICAL ASSESSMENT

The history is important, including family history of short stature and the elucidation of worrying symptoms such as:

• Headaches
• Visual disturbances
• Diarrhoea
• Anaemia
• Polydipsia

The examination should evaluate carefully the facial appearance, the limb length, disproportionate or dysmorphic appearance, blood pressure, thyroid size, elbow carrying angle and posterior hairline, retinal fundi and visual fields to confrontation.

The signs and symptoms will provide clues about diagnoses such as the osteodystrophies, Silver–Russell syndrome, Turner's syndrome, renal disease, malnutrition, malabsorption (e.g. coeliac disease) and the possibility of intracranial tumours.

Parental heights

These should be measured whenever possible and target height for the child ascribed as follows (see Fig. 23.6).

1 On a girl's height chart plot the mother's height (M).

2 Subtract 12 cm from the father's height (F) and plot his corrected centile (FCC). On a boy's height chart add 12 cm to the mother's height.

3 Mid-point between M and FCC is the mean parental centile (MPC).

4 MPC ± 8.5 cm gives the child's predicted or target height with 95% confidence limits. It is often reassuring to describe these limits to anxious parents.

INVESTIGATIONS

In most cases when there are no clues suggesting pathological short stature, the only action taken should be a further accurate height measurement after a gap of 3 or 4 months to recalculate growth velocity.

Children whose height, history or examination are causing concern should have basic screening tests performed, including full blood count, urea and electrolytes, creatinine, calcium, alkaline phosphatase, bicarbonate, thyroid function, midstream urine for culture, karyotype in girls, and a radiograph of the left-hand and wrist for bone age (p. 38).

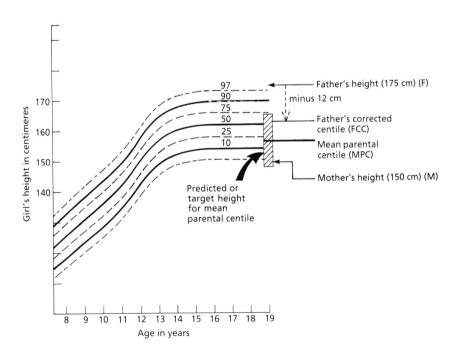

Fig. 23.6 Calculation of a target (or predicted) height for a child when the parents' heights are known.

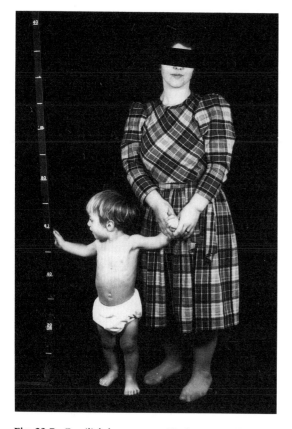

Fig. 23.7 Familial short stature. The boy was referred with short stature, but the mother, who was also short (140 cm), was noted to have short upper limbs and other bony abnormalities of the wrist. They both had a previously unrecognized syndrome of dyschondrosteosis which is dominantly inherited.

CAUSES OF SHORT STATURE

Familial short stature

This is probably the commonest type of referral. Measure and observe the parents whenever possible as the parents may be of short stature because of an unrecognized syndrome (see Fig. 23.7), or they may have lived in deprived circumstances as children. In these circumstances, target heights are not applicable and the child might have significant pathology.

Plot the parental centiles and ascribe a target height for the child. Reassure the parents that the child is healthy and normal. In familial short stature, the bone age is usually similar to the chronological age.

Short stature with delayed maturation

This is another common type of referral. Characteristically the child will be 4 or 5 cm below the third centile, have a growth curve deviating slightly away from the centile channel, and growth velocity just below the twenty-fifth centile. The bone age is usually 2 or 3 years behind the chronological age and there is often delayed puberty.

It is in the early years of secondary school that boys in particular are teased because of their short stature and immaturity. There is often a familial history of delayed maturation and the prognosis is usually excellent.

Most of these children have normal growth hormone provocation tests, although studies of 24-hour secretory profiles suggest smaller growth hormone pulses and it seems that additional growth hormone in some cases may accelerate growth. Ethical and financial considerations will clearly limit such treatment to a few children who are severely disturbed by their slow growth progress.

When puberty is delayed in boys beyond 15 years, depot testosterone for 3 or 4 months or oxandrolone may enhance growth and cause a marked psychological uplift without advancing bone age adversely. In girls, ethinyl oestradiol in a very low dose may be similarly beneficial.

Thyroid deficiency

All cases of short stature and low growth velocity ought to have thyroid function tests because at the time of presentation clinical signs may be absent or minimal (p. 411).

Growth hormone deficiency

The incidence of this condition remains uncertain with estimates for severe deficiency ranging from 1:5000 to 1:30 000 children. Partial deficiency states are becoming more frequently recognized.

The causes of growth hormone (GH) deficiency include:

1 *Primary*
idiopathic isolated growth hormone deficiency, multiple congenital hypothalamic pituitary deficiencies.

2 *Secondary*
associated with congenital disorders, e.g. septo-optic dysplasia, hydrocephalus, cleft lip and palate, intra-uterine rubella, empty sella syndrome,
tumours: craniopharyngioma, Langerhans' cell histiocytosis (p. 472),
irradiation, trauma, meningoencephalitis.

Investigations. Growth hormone assays are expensive and difficult. Special tests are therefore only justified in children who have been assessed by careful height measurements and who have one or more of the following characteristics:
1 Height more than three standard deviations below the mean.
2 A growth velocity below the twenty-fifth centile over the course of a whole year.
3 Have physical features or history suggestive of idiopathic growth hormone deficiency (e.g. males, breech delivery, weight centile more than height centile, retarded bone age, crowded mid-facial features).
4 Features of multiple hormone deficiencies, e.g. hypoglycaemia, micropenis ($\pm$ undescended testis), antidiuretic hormone deficiency.
5 History compatible with secondary pituitary deficiency.

Few departments are able to assess physiological 24-hour pulsatile secretion and a post-exercise growth hormone level not infrequently gives falsely low levels. Traditionally pharmacological provocation tests have been used to stimulate GH secretion, the most standardized being insulin-induced hypoglycaemia, but this has inherent dangers and requires careful supervision. In younger children, especially those with suspected cortisol deficiency, glucagon stimulation may be used. In older children oral clonidine or an arginine infusion are more commonly used.

All growth hormone provocation tests have at least a 15% failure rate in normal children and as it is traumatic to repeat a provocation test, investigators have often performed a second provocation test after the insulin hypoglycaemia using substances such as GHRH, arginine infusion, clonidine or l-DOPA. Perhaps now that growth hormone treatment is more readily available, multiple growth hormone provocation tests will be less commonly employed. Other hypothalamic pituitary provocation tests may be performed in conjunction with the growth hormone tests, such as TRH, GnRH tests as well as associated assays of cortisol and prolactin. If the bone age is greater than 10 years, the child should be primed with sex steroids before growth hormone testing. For details of tests see reference texts.

Management. In 1985, cases of the lethal Creutzfeldt–Jakob disease transmitted by slow-virus infection were described in young adults who had received pituitary-derived growth hormone 10–15 years previously. Synthetic recombinant human DNA growth hormone rapidly became available. The mode of its administration and therapeutic indications are being explored. For severe growth hormone deficiency thrice weekly or daily subcutaneous injections of growth hormone are prescribed. A trial of growth hormone injections is indicated in children with partial growth hormone deficiency and in other syndromes associated with short stature and slow growth velocity, but should be discontinued if there is no worthwhile acceleration of velocity.

Constitutional short stature

Characteristically in this condition there is a history of intra-uterine growth retardation and continuing growth below the third centile. In addition, the children may show either a retarded or normal bone age, or a poor pubertal growth spurt with eventual short stature. The Silver–Russell syndrome falls into this category. In some cases a

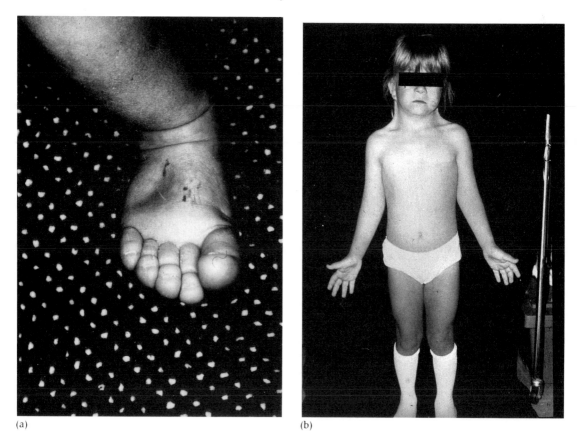

(a)   (b)

Fig. 23.8 Turner's syndrome. (a) Lymphoedema of the foot in a newborn. (b) Webbing of the neck and wide carrying angle of the elbows in a 6-year-old girl.

trial of growth hormone injections will be indicated but advancement of bone age must be watched carefully.

Short stature due to emotional deprivation

There is no doubt that some children with markedly suboptimal growth and poor hypothalamic function (including low growth hormone levels) are suffering from emotional and social deprivation (see Chapter 28). In extreme cases, there are bizarre compulsive eating and drinking habits, disturbed sleep patterns and educational problems. Many less severe cases are not brought to the attention of doctors; hence the importance of community growth screening programmes.

Turner's syndrome

Turner's syndrome is found in 1:3000 girls and this is discussed in detail on p. 123. In virtually all cases there is a combination of short stature, absent puberty and infertility.

These girls may be recognized at birth by the typical combination of peripheral lymphoedema (Fig. 23.8a), dysplastic nails, and coarctation of the aorta. In later childhood they may present with short stature, weight on a higher centile than height, a wide carrying angle at the elbow (Fig. 23.8b) and low posterior hairline. Those not diagnosed in childhood present at adolescence with delayed puberty and primary amenorrhoea.

There is a progressive decline in growth velocity

and despite oestrogen and other therapy the height prognosis has remained poor with a mean adult height of 143 cm.

Management. Parents who learn of the diagnosis early in the child's life require careful explanations and reassurance, particularly that mental development is likely to be within the normal range. Anomalies of the cardiovascular system and renal tract should be excluded or treated if present. When the growth velocity falls to a low level at the age of about 5 years, consideration should be given to treatment with growth hormone injections, low-dose oestrogens and perhaps oxandrolone to increase growth velocity. It remains to be seen whether ultimate adult height is significantly enhanced.

The child should be taken through puberty at a time similar to her peer group, with gradually increasing doses of oestrogens until breakthrough bleeding occurs when a low-dose combination pill is introduced to regularize menstruation.

Discussions about infertility are best left until the adolescent girl seems maturely receptive.

Coeliac disease

Children with coeliac disease (p. 196) may present only with short stature or suboptimal growth velocity and without other obvious clinical manifestations. Small bowel biopsy must be considered if a slowly growing child also has anaemia or gastrointestinal symptoms. A gluten-free diet will allow catch-up growth.

Complex syndromes presenting as short stature

These are summarized in Table 23.1.

The tall child

Most tall children are tall because their parents are tall. The parents of a few very tall girls who have a height prediction above about 180 cm become disturbed by the prospect of their daughter's extreme eventual height and request treatment. Ethinyl oestradiol has been used in high dosage starting

Table 23.1 Complex conditions associated with short stature.

Down's syndrome
Bony dysplasias
Prader–Willi syndrome
Pseudo-hypoparathyroidism
Silver–Russell syndrome
Fetal alcohol syndrome
Fanconi's anaemia
Septo-optic dysplasia

when the height is more than 165 cm. The usual effect is a brief acceleration of growth followed by growth inhibition, bone maturation and rapid epiphyseal fusion. Although reductions in final height of 3.5–7.3 cm may be achieved, many paediatricians feel uncomfortable prescribing high-dose oestrogens for this indication.

Obese children tend to be tall, have an accelerated puberty, finish the adolescent growth spurt early and may have a compromised final adult height. Obese pre-pubertal children who are of short stature ought to be investigated to rule out conditions such as hypothyroidism, Cushing's syndrome and bony dysplasias.

All causes of pathological tall stature are uncommon but their features need recognition.

1 *Endocrine causes*
(a) Precocious puberty (see p. 395).
(b) Gigantism. This is exceedingly rare. It is caused by a pituitary growth hormone secreting adenoma which occasionally enlarges enough to damage other pituitary functions. The secretions of the adenoma may not respond to endocrine therapy, but require a combination of pituitary surgery and irradiation.

2 *Dysmorphic syndromes*
(a) Marfan's syndrome. This is discussed on p. 485. Oestrogen therapy before puberty has been used to reduce the pubertal growth spurt and final height.
(b) Homocystinuria. Marfan-like habitus but with mental retardation, dislocating lens, stiff joints and recessive inheritance.

(c) Karyotype XXX. These girls have Marfan-like habitus with mild mental retardation and this has been referred to as the 'super-female' syndrome.

(d) Soto's syndrome (cerebral gigantism). Characteristic facies with down-slanted palpebral fissures, high prominent forehead, recessed frontal hairline and prognanthism. These infants are large for dates at birth and show accelerated growth and skeletal maturation but exhibit marked delay in psychomotor development. They have early but normal puberty and usually normal adult height.

(e) Klinefelter's syndrome (see p. 126). Testicular hypoplasia causes delayed incomplete puberty with a tall, slim eunuchoid appearance and gynaecomastia. These changes can be avoided by the use of testosterone therapy. Many individuals with Klinefelter's syndrome have intelligence well within the normal range and behavioural difficulties are not as common as was previously thought.

The fat child

Obesity can be diagnosed visually but more objectively by skin-fold thickness measurements for which centile charts are available. A further definition of obesity is when the weight exceeds the expected weight for height by more than 20%.

By this definition, the prevalence of obesity is 25% in the first year, less than 5% at 5 years, about 9% at 15 years, and 12% at 25 years. Thirty per cent of older adults are said to be overweight.

The metabolic causes of obesity are poorly understood. Some obese children and adults eat excessively but many do not. Psychological problems often stimulate overeating and obesity causes secondary behavioural difficulties. Obesity stimulates early childhood growth and bone maturation. Obese pre-pubertal children who are of below average height should be investigated (see section on short stature).

Several statements can be made about the prognosis:

1 Most fat babies do not become fat children.

2 Obese 5-year-olds are more likely to become obese adolescents.

3 Obese adolescents are very likely to become obese adults.

The outlook for obese children is gloomy. Calorie restriction and behaviour modification appears successful in the short-term, but 80% relapse. Prevention of obesity from an early age must be the aim of family, school and community education programmes.

Prader–Willi syndrome

This is a rare syndrome involving hypotonia in the neonatal period, short stature and severe obesity developing in the first 6 years of life. In addition, there is often low IQ (<80) together with small penis and maldescended testicles. Some cases show a specific deletion on the number 15 chromosome.

Disorders of the gonads

The testis

The major endocrine function of the testis resides in the Leydig cells which secrete testosterone. Testosterone promotes male fetal sexual differentiation and the development and maintenance of pubertal and adult secondary sexual characteristics. The fetal testis also produces anti-Mullerian hormone responsible for the regression of the Mullerian structures and inhibin which helps to regulate follicle-stimulating hormone secretion.

The seminiferous tubules represent 75% of testicular volume and contain germ cells, spermatogonia and Sertoli cells. High local concentrations of testosterone and other testicular hormones are required for normal maturation of spermatogonia to spermatozoa.

Sperm maturation and fertility are more sensitive to damage than testosterone production.

TESTICULAR MALDESCENT

During the third month of gestation Leydig cell hyperplasia occurs with high fetal testosterone production and male differentiation. The fetal testes then begin their descent from the posterior abdomen towards the internal inguinal ring.

Leydig cells continue to produce testosterone

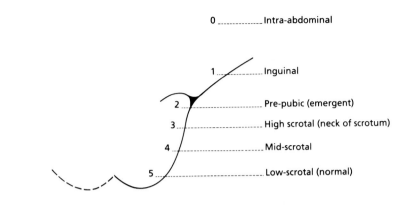

0 .... Intra-abdominal

1 .... Inguinal

2 .... Pre-pubic (emergent)

3 .... High scrotal (neck of scrotum)

4 .... Mid-scrotal

5 .... Low-scrotal (normal)

Fig. 23.9 Positions and descriptions of testicular descent and maldescent.

into the early neonatal period, but they then de-differentiate into mesenchymal cells until pubertal gonadotrophins stimulate the return of Leydig cell activity.

During the third trimester of pregnancy the testes continue their descent towards the scrotum. Recent reports from the Oxford Cryptorchidism Study Group have shown that the incidence of incomplete descent of the testis in babies of birth weight less than 2000 g (or less than 32 weeks gestation) is 50%, diminishing to 20% of those weighing 2000–2499 g (approximately 32–34 weeks gestation) and 5% of those weighing more than 2500 g. At full-term birth Scorer's classic studies showed 2.5% of infants had incomplete testicular descent. By 3 and 12 months after expected date of delivery 1.6 and 0.75% of infants, respectively, are still cryptorchid. The higher the position of the testis at birth the less likely is spontaneous descent. Further descent occurs during puberty so that 0.3% of adults are said to have an incompletely descended testis.

Studies of schoolchildren and hospital statistics of orchidopexies in Britain suggests that the incidence of incomplete descent of the testis at mid-childhood is four or five times higher than the prevalence described at 1 year. The reasons for this are not fully understood. Some testes migrate back upwards due to contraction of spermatic cord tissues and the development of the cremasteric reflex. Undoubtedly testosterone is the most likely candidate to influence the tension of supratesticular tissues and promote descent.

Clinical features

In the infant and pre-school child the position of the incompletely descended testis may be difficult to determine. The testis should be 'milked' downwards from above to its lowest position along the normal line of descent. The child should be as relaxed as possible and the examiner's hands warm. After examination in the supine position it is often useful for the older boy to be in a crouching posture to relax the cremasteric reflex. The possible malpositions of the testis may be classified as in Figure 23.9. Those testes which can be manipulated into positions 4 or 5, and remain there for a few seconds but then move upwards to positions 3, 2 or 1 by cremasteric reflex should be classified as retractile.

Management

It is extremely important to re-examine infants who have an undescended testis at birth. Treatment before 2 years may reduce the likelihood of infertility.

Hormonal treatment. Human chorionic gonadotrophin (HCG) has been used for many years to stimulate testosterone production and hence provoke testicular descent. The treatment has never been subjected to controlled trial.

More recently the administration of GnRH by injection or intranasal spray has been used under strictly controlled trial conditions with variable results. Hormonal therapy is not effective when the testis is impalpable, but in cases where the testis is just emerging from the inguinal canal or is at the scrotal neck, treatment with two 4-week courses of intranasal GnRH (200 µg t.d.s.) may be effective. This therapy may help to decide whether surgical treatment is necessary in about 30% of cases.

Orchidopexy. If a gonad cannot be located, preoperative ultrasound examination may be helpful. Testes in abdominal or inguinal canal positions require surgery. There are often associated anatomical abnormalities, such as congenital hernias and fascial or fibrous adhesions. The operation aims to secure an adequate length of vas deferens and blood vessels in the cord to permit placement of the testis in the scrotum, to ensure the testis remains in the scrotum and to repair an associated hernia. The testis is usually fixed in the lower scrotum within a Dartos muscle 'pouch'. In some cases this is difficult and the testis may be secured in an upper scrotal position which may improve spontaneously at puberty. The testis can also be examined in that position for possible complications, such as neoplasia.

Complications

Impaired fertility. There is histological evidence to show that after the age of 2 years the undescended testis shows a decrease in seminiferous tubal size and spermatogonia with an increase in fibrous tissue. Clinical studies confirm that fertility is impaired in bilateral cryptorchidism.

Impaired Leydig cell function. Usually testosterone production is unimpaired but with different degrees of testicular non-descent there will be varying degrees of primary testicular abnormality and secondary damage, including Leydig cell dysfunction in severe cases of bilateral non-descent.

Malignancy. The undescended testis with or without orchidopexy has a 35 times greater risk of malignancy than the descended testis. Testicular tumours are discussed in Chapter 25.

Torsion of the testis. This is more likely to occur in a maldescended testicle, but more frequently occurs in a normal testis. If a testis twists on its stalk, or spermatic cord, the blood supply to the gland may be endangered. Early diagnosis is essential to avoid irreversible infarction. The peak incidence is during puberty, occurring with equal frequency on each side, but if one side is affected there is a 30% chance of torsion later on the opposite side.

In the older child if the torsion is seen within 6 hours it is tender, swollen and firm. The testis is drawn up into the scrotal neck and the thickened or twisted cord can be felt. After this time the scrotum becomes red and oedematous resembling an inflammatory mass. The differential diagnosis includes epididymitis, orchitis, strangulated hernia, trauma or tumour. If there are no urinary leukocytes or symptoms and the boy is at or before puberty, the diagnosis of a tender, painful testis should be torsion until proved otherwise. Another diagnostic clue is finding that the other testis lies in a somewhat horizontal position making it more likely to twist.

Surgical exploration to untwist the testis should be performed as an emergency and the other side fixed at the same time.

Neonatal torsion presents at birth as a painless, blue–red, firm, swollen scrotum which is sometimes difficult to distinguish from a scrotal haematoma in a breech baby or a strangulated hernia. Unfortunately, unless immediate exploration is performed the testis will be non-viable.

Male gonadal insufficiency. Absence of testicular development or bilateral torsion may render a boy anorchic. He will require testosterone therapy in puberty and the insertion of prosthetic testes when the scrotum is mature.

The ovary

The fetus and neonate secrete high levels of gonadotrophins to stimulate ovarian activity and oestrogen levels are similar to those of early puberty. The stimulated fetal and neonatal ovary is often found to have follicular cysts which later regress and then the ovary remains quiescent until the end of the first decade.

Ovarian cysts detected prenatally by ultrasound may decompress spontaneously but those that are large (more than 4 cm in diameter) often require operative removal because of torsion or destruction of the rest of the ovary. Large oestrogen-secreting ovarian cysts are a rare cause of precocious pseudo-puberty. Benign and malignant ovarian tumours may secrete either oestrogens or androgens and require urgent removal.

Ovarian dysgenesis

This is most commonly associated with Turner's syndrome (p. 123), but may occur without chromosomal anomaly. In the latter cases, treatment with oestrogens should allow normal pubertal growth, but infertility will be irreversible.

Puberty

NORMAL PUBERTY

The age of onset of puberty varies greatly between individuals and the triggering mechanisms remain unclear. Puberty results from pulsatile hypothalamic secretions of gonadotrophin-releasing hormone causing a progressive rise in gonadotrophins as puberty advances.

In girls, from the age of 8.5 years, ultrasound examination of the ovaries shows increasing numbers of growing follicles more than 4 mm in diameter indicating normal ovarian maturation. Puberty is not usually established until the ovary has a volume of 3 ml. The earliest clinical sign of female puberty is breast bud development. In boys the earliest signs are an increase in testicular size; above 3 ml volume or >2.0 cm long, with thinning and softening of the scrotal sac. The subsequent stages and centiles of puberty are described on the Tanner growth charts, but it is important to remember that 3% of girls already show signs of puberty by 9 years (boys 10 years) and 97% of all children have signs of puberty by their fourteenth birthday.

The usual sequence (and mean ages in years) of pubertal development in girls is:
- breast enlargement (11.2)
- pubic hair (11.4)
- peak height velocity (12)
- menarche (13)
- cessation of growth (16)

In boys the sequence is:
- testicular growth (12)
- public hair (12.5)
- peak height velocity (14)
- slowing of growth (then voice breaking and later facial beard) with cessation of growth (18)

The height increment in puberty also varies between individuals and can only be predicted approximately on the basis of target parental height and bone age. In girls it amounts to about 21 cm (13 cm before and 8 cm after menarche) and in boys 27 cm. In order to achieve the mean pubertal peak height velocity at 8.5 cm per year in girls or 9.5 cm per year in boys, endocrine contributions are required from both the sex steroids and growth hormone; the former particularly enhancing spinal growth and the latter limb growth.

PRECOCIOUS PUBERTY

Signs of secondary sexual development in girls before 8 years or in boys before 9 years usually warrant investigation. True puberty caused by activation of the hypothalamic–pituitary–gonadal axis must be differentiated from pseudo-puberty provoked by the peripheral production or administration of sex steroids. Table 23.2 lists the causes of true precocious puberty and pseudo-puberty.

Clinical features

Precocious puberty presents five times more commonly in females, when it is likely to be idiopathic, than in boys when a central nervous system lesion should be sought.

Secondary sexual characteristics will be evident, often accompanied by distressing emotional upset, especially in girls with early menstruation. In boys with true precocious puberty the testicular size will be in the pubertal range but in pseudo-

Table 23.2 Causes of true precocious puberty and pseudo-puberty.

True precocious puberty (central or complete)	Pseudo-puberty (peripheral or incomplete)
Constitutional/idiopathic Intracranial lesions with hypothalamic activation Associated with syndromes such as Silver–Russell, Albright hypothyroidism	Congenital adrenal hyperplasia Sex steroid administration (e.g. contraceptive pill) Tumours Oestrogen producing Androgen producing (arising from ovary, adrenal, testicle or interstitial cell)

puberty they remain pre-pubertal in size. The children will be tall with rapid growth velocity, advanced bone age and if left untreated there will be early epiphyseal closure and stunted adult height.

Examination should concentrate on accurate pubertal staging, virilization in a girl, measurement of blood pressure, fundoscopy, abdominal and rectal examinations to rule out tumours, a search for skin and neurological abnormalities and palpation for a goitre (hypothyroid precocious puberty).

Investigations

Initially girls may be watched carefully to see if there is progression or regression of signs. The most useful investigation is ultrasound scanning of the abdomen to rule out adrenal, ovarian or other tumours, as well as to measure ovarian follicular development and uterine size. Measurement of serum luteinizing hormone (LH), follicle–stimulating hormone (FSH) and oestradiol levels may help to confirm true pubertal progression. If a girl is virilized an urgent search for the source of androgens is required, concentrating on the ultrasound scan, urine and blood androgens and 17-hydroxy-progesterone levels. Thyroid function, and bone age estimation should be performed and CT head scan considered.

In boys an initial CT brain scan is the most important investigation because of the distinct possibility of intracranial pathology. Other investigations include serum TSH, LH, FSH, testosterone, 17-hydroxy-progesterone levels and urinary androgen assays.

Management

Specific treatment will be required for intracranial lesions, congenital adrenal hyperplasia and all the other various abdominal tumours. Many girls with idiopathic precocious puberty may not require drug therapy but will be helped by expert psychological support because of the discordant physical and emotional development.

Drug therapy is indicated if sexual development, particularly early menstruation, is imposing extreme difficulties on the child or if skeletal maturation accelerates rapidly. In these cases cyproterone acetate, which has superseded medroxy-progesterone acetate is used. It may be logical to give a larger dose in the evening to suppress nocturnal gonadotrophin release.

More recently intranasal and subcutaneous depot preparations of gonadotrophin-releasing hormone analogues have been used to block pituitary receptors, inducing more complete and long-acting gonadotrophin suppression with improved inhibition of both sexual development and skeletal advancement.

DELAYED PUBERTY

Complete absence of secondary sexual characteristics in a girl of 14 years or a boy of 15 years usually warrants investigation.

Causes

1 Idiopathic or familial.
2 Gonadal insufficiency:
 (a) Agenesis or dysgenesis (idiopathic, Turner's syndrome, Klinefelter's syndrome).
 (b) Inflammation, cystic disease, maldescent, torsion, post-chemotherapy or irradiation (p. 445).
 (c) Steroid biosynthetic defects.
3 Hypothalamic-pituitary disorders:

(a) Multiple pituitary hormone deficiency syndromes.

(b) Inflammation, tumours (e.g. craniopharyngioma, prolactinoma), post-chemotherapy or irradiation.

(c) Systemic or nutritional disorders (asthma, coeliac, anorexia nervosa).

(d) Specific syndromes (Kallmann, Prader–Willi).

Clinical features

Most commonly, delayed puberty presents as short stature with delayed maturation. Often when first examined after referral, signs of puberty are apparent and the growth rate spontaneously increases. There is often a familial history of late development but general clinical clues to pathology must be sought, as in the cases of short stature (see above). More specifically, it is important to check on previous general health, school achievements (poor in Klinefelter's syndrome), anosmia (Kallmann's syndrome), poor nutrition (malabsorption or anorexia) and genital ambiguity (see p. 418).

Investigations

Baseline tests should include full blood count, renal, liver, thyroid function, chromosomes and bone age assessment. Gonads which are not palpable should be sought by ultrasound scanning. If these tests are normal or negative an LHRH provocation test may help to show if the pituitary is responsive but will not predict spontaneous puberty. Pituitary function tests in delayed puberty are notoriously difficult to interpret. In boys, an HCG test may help to show testosterone production.

Management

If spontaneous puberty does not occur by 15 years in girls or 16 years in boys there is often a psychological need to induce puberty by giving oestradiol or testosterone (see sections on short stature and delayed maturation) and this will be essential if there is gonadal or pituitary insufficiency. Gona-dotrophin therapy by means of pulsatile infusion or injections may well help to induce fertility in cases of hypogonadotrophic hypogonadism.

Disorders in the control of blood sugar

Diabetes mellitus

Diabetes in childhood is a serious life-long fluctuating disorder requiring disciplined and dedicated care by parents and professionals. Children who adapt successfully to cope with its management live healthy, active lives at normal schools with few restrictions.

The onset of childhood diabetes may occur at any age and its incidence is reported to be increasing in many countries. In Britain it affects 2:1000 children below the age of 16 years. The long-term prognosis remains of great concern with a 25% reduction in life span and significant morbidity due to vascular complications affecting the retinae, kidneys, heart and peripheral nerves.

Controversy still surrounds the debate about how tight the diabetic control needs to be to delay or prevent long-term vascular complications. What is certain is that very poor control is associated with suboptimal growth, delayed maturation, reduced well-being and the onset within 10–15 years of significant retinopathy and nephropathy. The challenge to the paediatrician is to develop a diabetes education and support service capable of motivating families towards the goal of tight control without inducing negative behavioural reactions. Several major developments in diabetic management in the past decade have made these objectives more attainable for many children.

AETIOLOGY

Only 1:10 children who develop diabetes have a first degree relative with diabetes. In contrast there are many families where both insulin-dependent (IDDM) and non-insulin-dependent (NIDDM) diabetes seem to occur frequently. Genetic susceptibility to IDDM exists and approximately 60 or 70% of this susceptibility resides in the HLA region on chromosome 6, the strongest association being HLA–DR 3/4 heterozygosity. Siblings of a child with diabetes have a 5% chance of becoming diabetic by the age of 20 and surprisingly even HLA identical siblings carry only a 10–15% risk.

Factors other than inheritance must play a part in the development of IDDM although specific environmental factors including diet, viral infections (particularly Coxsackie B), stress and toxins have not been clearly identified. Before the acute onset of symptoms there may be a long latent period of 3 or more years during which time 90% or more of the pancreatic beta cells are destroyed or damaged. During this process the majority of cases have significant serum titres of islet cell antibodies. It is not known whether islet cell antibodies are causing cell damage or are markers of a destructive process.

CLINICAL FEATURES

The characteristic symptoms are excessive thirst, polyuria and nocturia. Rapid weight loss, unexpected enuresis, lethargy, loss of appetite and, in girls, perineal irritation and candidal infection are commonly experienced. The length of history is often only 2–6 weeks. Infants are more difficult to diagnose, rapidly deteriorating with dehydration and acidotic tachypnoea often wrongly labelled as pneumonia. Severe diabetic ketoacidosis is accompanied by vomiting, acute abdominal pain and deteriorating consciousness.

A family doctor will only diagnose diabetes in one or two children in a professional lifetime. The complaint of polyuria with polydipsia (p. 407) should always be investigated and the diagnosis made with a urinary glucose dipstick which shows marked glycosuria.

Confirmation of hyperglycaemia is obtained using a capillary blood glucose indicator stick. Even if the child seems well, immediate referral for specialist advice should be made because metabolic decompensation may occur rapidly.

MANAGEMENT

Most children are ketotic but not markedly acidotic at the time of diagnosis. They can be reassured that their extreme thirst and nocturia will disappear almost immediately following the first injection of insulin and the fear of metabolic decompensation is removed.

From the first point of contact with the diabetic team the parents and the child should be provided with consistent, uncomplicated information about diabetes and a plan of action should be discussed. This is best given by a small number of experienced personnel, including a doctor who will be providing ongoing support, a senior nurse (sister, liaison diabetes nurse) and a dietitian. More than three voices cause confusion.

Initiating insulin therapy

A quick-acting insulin (0.3–0.5 U/kg) is given subcutaneously. If the child is outside the infant stage the person giving the first injection should sit beside the child who can assist in holding the

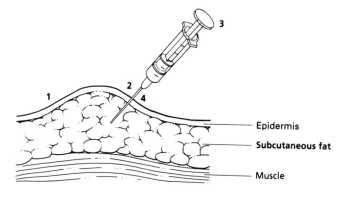

Fig. 23.10 Technique for subcutaneous insulin injection. The same technique can be used for growth hormone injection.
1 Gently pinch skin.
2 Push needle in vertically at least 1 cm.
3 *Do not* pull back plunger – push inwards only.
4 When removing the needle quickly cover site with a tissue or cotton wooland massage gently.

Epidermis
Subcutaneous fat
Muscle

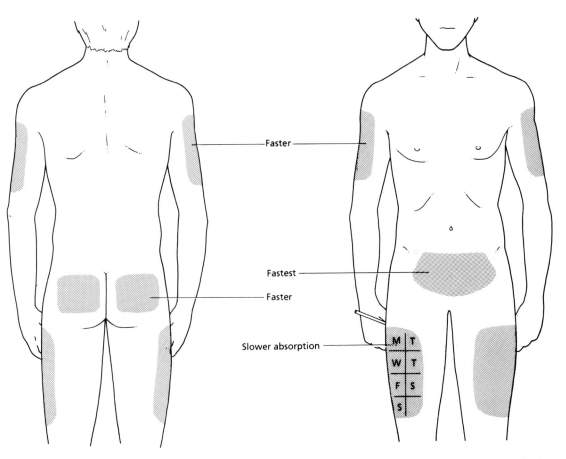

Fig. 23.11 Suggested grid pattern of subcutaneous insulin injections with differential speeds of insulin absorption.

hand of the injector. This encourages any child of school age to help with the injections from an early stage. The injection technique is standardized and rotation of sites is essential (Figs. 23.10 and 23.11) to prevent lipohypertrophic lumps causing erratic insulin absorption. Quick-acting insulin may be continued twice daily for several days or weeks at a dose which reduces the pre-prandial blood glucose towards normality over the first 7–10 days. No long-term benefit is gained from a rapid return to normoglycaemia and although an early switch to longer acting insulins is often made, it may precipitate confidence-shattering hypoglycaemia just as the child becomes more mobile.

Early supervision

Most children who develop diabetes are admitted to hospital so that the initiation of therapy can be closely supervised. It is equally possible to conduct this process in the child's home so long as supporting staff are able to visit regularly in the first few days and telephone contact is readily available 24 hours a day. Indeed, parents and children gain great comfort and confidence in realizing that they can cope with the management in their home environment.

Whether in hospital or in the home the topics listed in Table 23.3 should be discussed and the equipment made available.

Table 23.3 Topics to be covered with the family before discharging a new diabetic child from hospital, together with the equipment and support necessary to provide adequate care at home.

Topic	Equipment and support
Injections (see above)	Disposable plastic syringes
Urine testing	Glucose test dipsticks
Home blood glucose monitoring	Capillary BG indicator sticks Finger-stabbing device, lancets Monitoring book
Diet	Diet sheet, carbohydrate exchange list and food plan
Hypoglycaemia	Dextrosol, glucagon, 'Hypostop'
Childhood illnesses	Advice – never stop insulin
Return to school	BDA school pack Liaison with school
Exercise and sport	Advice and encouragement
Identity bracelets or necklets	Addresses
Meeting other parents	Addresses, diabetes books, etc.
Information about joining the British Diabetic Association	

Diet

A dietitian should assess the child's usual total daily carbohydrate and calorie intake and suggest a meal plan based on the following principles:

Carbohydrate intake. This should be higher than in the usual British diet. Aim at more than 45% energy intake as carbohydrate with regular eating spaced across the day as three main meals and three snacks. An increase in the fibre content of the carbohydrate will help to delay and prolong the absorption of sugars. A marked reduction in sweets and sugars is advised except before strenuous exercise. Most dietitians recommend count-

ing the carbohydrate intake as 10-g portions or exchanges which helps in maintaining some consistency of intake. Regular review of carbohydrate intake is essential to keep pace with the child's growth.

Fat intake. This should be reduced to less than 35% of total energy, balanced by the increase in carbohydrate. A reduction in saturated fats may have long-term advantages.

These healthy eating recommendations should be seen as being positively beneficial for the whole family.

Later insulin therapy

For 1 or 2 weeks after the start of insulin treatment the child often eats voraciously to replace the lost weight. Thereafter the sugar control quickly improves as the pancreas continues to secrete endogenous insulin. During this 'honeymoon period' insulin dosages are greatly reduced to avoid hypoglycaemia.

Total daily insulin dosages range from <0.5 U/kg/day during the 'honeymoon period' to approximately 1 U/kg/day until the adolescent growth spurt when 2 U/kg/day (or more) are often necessary to maintain good control. There remains some controversy over the choice of either one or two daily injections of insulin. There is no strong evidence that twice-daily injections allow better control in the first few years after diagnosis, but if one injection is started it may be difficult to switch to two during adolescence. Of more importance is to assess whether a chosen insulin regime is providing good 24-hour control and is well tolerated by the child.

There are many different insulins available, administered according to different schedules. Clinicians will choose insulin regimes of which they have experience and which can be adapted to individual needs. Often children are instructed in the mixing of the soluble, clear, quick-acting insulin with a medium-acting cloudy insulin. Mixtures of insulins are often given in the proportion of 66% of the total dose in the morning and 33%

in the evening. Both injections should consist of a ratio of quick:medium insulin of 1:2.

A number of fixed mixtures of insulin in ratios of quick:medium (30:70 or 50:50, etc.) are available. Evidence from adult studies show that they are not associated with poorer control and they may be particularly acceptable to small children and in families where compliance is a problem.

Multiple injection regimes using quick-acting insulin given by pen injectors before the three main meals (20% of the total dose prior to each meal) with a long- or medium-acting insulin before bed (40% of the total insulin dose) are becoming popular with teenagers. Greater flexibility of meal times, leaving out snacks and more variability of food intake are possible, but improved diabetic control is not necessarily obtained.

Insulin infusion pumps have a limited role in paediatrics due to non-acceptance, hazards of sudden ketoacidosis and skin infections.

Monitoring control

Every child must be encouraged to learn that testing urine or blood is done for the positive reasons of knowing how much insulin to give, preventing hypoglycaemia and avoiding long-term diabetes-related damage. Monitoring should not be performed as a threat to children to catch them out when they cheat on their diet.

Urinary glucose testing by dipstick has superseded the tedious test tube methods. The aim is to keep as many urine tests as possible clear of glucose. It is dangerous to accept regular mild glycosuria because this only occurs in association with significant hyperglycaemia.

Most diabetic infants and children accept capillary blood glucose monitoring and it is best to negotiate the number to be performed. Suggested times of monitoring are shown in Figure 23.12. The aim is to adjust the evening insulin and diet so

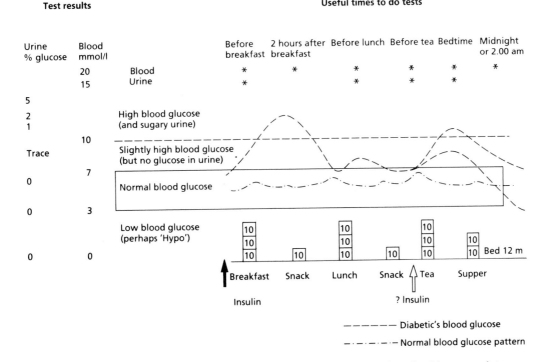

Fig. 23.12 Diabetic control. Relationship between blood sugars, insulin dosage and meals with suggested times to perform blood and urine tests to monitor control.

that the pre-breakfast blood glucose is as near to normality as possible without nocturnal hypoglycaemia. Fine-tuning of daytime blood glucose levels can then be attempted by adjustments of morning insulin, diet and exercise.

Glycosylated haemoglobin (HbA₁) is a naturally occurring haemoglobin fraction which has a glucose molecule attached to the globin chain. HbA₁ measurement in diabetic children has contributed enormously to the assessment of control because it reflects prevailing blood glucose levels over several preceding weeks. It is possible to achieve near normal levels (5–8%) in well-motivated children.

Children with diabetes should be seen if possible in a designated children's diabetic clinic three or four times each year, by consistent, experienced personnel, to monitor control and to assess growth and development. When growth is suboptimal, consider associated disorders such as coeliac disease and hypothyroidism.

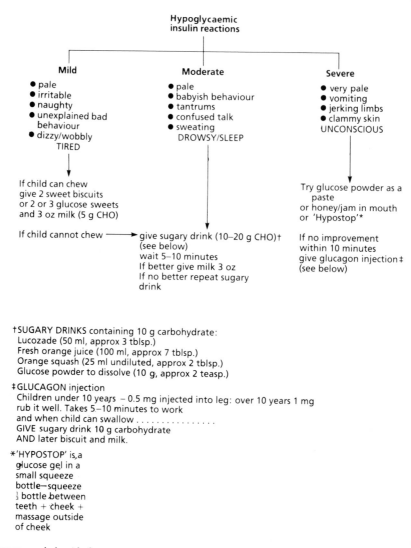

Fig. 23.13 Recommended guide for parents to recognize hypoglycaemia and its treatment.

MANAGEMENT PROBLEMS·

Hypoglycaemia

Attempting to manufacture a hypoglycaemia reaction in hospital is frustratingly impractical. The parents and child should be taught how to recognize and cope with different grades of hypoglycaemia (Fig. 23.13).

Intercurrent illness

If a diabetic child is ill, nauseated or vomiting it is important to observe the following rules:
- always give the insulin
- stop solid foods
- give clear fluids in small volumes frequently. The fluids should contain sugar (e.g. Lucozade, lemonade, fruit juice)
- monitor blood glucose levels
- gradually revert back to easily digested food as the stomach settles

Parents must know that persistent vomiting should precipitate hospital admission.

DIABETIC KETOACIDOSIS (DKA)

Less than 25% of children nowadays present with DKA. A few children thereafter have recurrent hospital admissions in DKA, nearly always due to emotional non-acceptance of diabetes and non-compliance.

DKA is a grave illness with a significant mortality. It requires emergency treatment and obsessional care. The major causes of morbidity and mortality in drowsy diabetic children are vomiting with aspiration, iatrogenic hypoglycaemia, electrolyte disturbances (particularly hypokalaemia) and cerebral oedema.

Management

On admission:
1 Take a careful, quick history. The length of history and severity of symptoms are important.

2 Assess the degree of dehydration as discussed on p. 274.
3 Look for infection. It is rarely bacterial, but this may be impossible to evaluate in the severely ill child.
4 Take note of other diseases.
5 Record level of consciousness and vital signs including blood pressure. Attach the child to an ECG monitor to assess the height of the T-wave as a quick guide to hyperkalaemia. Examine retinal discs.
6 Measure blood sodium, potassium, urea, and glucose. Record blood gases and a full blood count and blood culture at the same time.
7 Mid-stream urine (MSU) specimen and swabs for culture.
8 If the child is drowsy pass a naso-gastric tube to empty the stomach and drain continuously.

IV fluids:
1 Set up a 0.9% saline infusion through an adequate-sized cannula.
2 If there is shock give 10−20 ml/kg of plasma in the first hour.
3 The 24-hour fluid requirement is estimated and started before giving insulin. Add the deficit (dehydration) to the maintenance, but supplemental fluid for fever, polyuria and vomiting is not needed in the first calculation. Infuse the calculated fluid volume evenly over 24 hours. It is most important to remember that over-enthusiastic fluid infusion with rapid reduction in osmolality may contribute to irreversible cerebral oedema.
4 Potassium chloride is added to the infusion at a rate of 3 mmol/kg/24 hours, providing that the ECG shows no evidence of hyperkalaemia.

Insulin. There are several different insulin regimes possible. A continuous low-dose insulin infusion is recommended because large boluses of insulin are rapidly degraded by the liver, much is insulin are rapidly degraded by the liver, much is lost via the kidneys and the plasma half-life of insulin is a matter of minutes. The insulin is given through a syringe pump to give an initial insulin dosage of 0.06 U/kg/hour.

Antibiotics. These are not given routinely unless a source of bacterial infection is found or septicaemia is suspected.

Bicarbonate treatment. This is rarely necessary. The arguments against it are that sufficient insulin should prevent ketogenesis, a rapid infusion of bicarbonate causes a fall in plasma potassium, bicarbonate increases plasma pH but the CSF pH often falls because of the rapid diffusion of CO_2 across the blood–brain barrier.

Bicarbonate therapy may be considered if hyperventilation is distressingly prolonged, if cardiac function is impaired or lactic acidosis is present.

Oxygen. Oxygen is administered to comatose or semi-conscious patients as their PO_2 is often low.

Blood glucose. The fluid and insulin infusions should result in a linear decrease of blood glucose levels checked hourly with capillary blood glucose recordings, but also every 2 hours in the laboratory because capillary tests are occasionally misleading in the presence of dehydration. If the rate of fall of blood glucose is >5 mmol/l/hour the rate of insulin infusion should be reduced.

When the blood glucose falls to 13 mmol/l the infusion should be changed from normal saline to 0.18% saline (with 4% dextrose). The blood glucose should continue to be monitored and the insulin infusion should be adjusted according to the glucose level in the blood.

Electrolytes. These should be checked 2 hours and 6 hours after starting treatment. If plasma Na^+ rises above 143 mmol/l change to the more dilute saline infusion.

Oral intake. The dehydrated child may demand oral fluids, but initially (whilst drowsy) it is safer to restrict this to sips of cold water. When better hydrated, small drinks may be tried and within 12–24 hours most children will be able to drink safely.

When this point is reached, giving subcutaneous insulin can be considered. This should be started 1 hour before stopping the continuous insulin infusion to avoid a rebound hyperglycaemia. Quick-acting human insulin (2 U/kg/24 hours in three divided doses) should be given. The following day a similar dose may be required but from then on a twice-daily insulin regime may be started at about 1–1.5 U/kg/day.

Continuing ketonuria or considerable variations in glycaemia or glycosuria will occur in the first few days and should not cause worry as long as the child is clinically well. Adjustments should be made according to pre-meal capillary blood glucose tests; the results of which may serve as a good educational exercise to the child and parents.

Complications of DKA

1 Vomiting and aspiration. Avoid this by the use of a naso-gastric tube.
2 Very severe acidosis (pH <7.05); use bicarbonate cautiously.
3 Incipient cerebral oedema suspected because of a decrease in conscious level 4–9 hours after initiating therapy. Signs of papilloedema occur with brain swelling. Early use of mannitol infusion is vital to reverse this dangerous complication.
4 Hyperosmolality due to raised Na^+ and very high blood glucose. If this occurs then more cautious fluid replacement with 0.45% saline is recommended.

LONG-TERM COMPLICATIONS

After 5–10 years of diabetes, the paediatrician should remain vigilant in the search for tissue damage by examining the retinae, measuring urinary albumin and renal function. Adverse emotional reactions, often in families unable to cope with diabetes, are the commonest cause of poor diabetic control. Efforts should be made to recognize these disturbances in the child and family and to some degree they may be prevented by good education, continuing constant support, the organization of parent groups and diabetic holiday camps.

It should be recognized that all children with diabetes have phases of serious non-compliance and rebellion; some become deceitful and fabricate results and a few even provoke episodes of hypoglycaemia or DKA. In the most serious cases the help of personnel skilled in child and family psychology who also understand diabetes may be helpful, but the most important factor in preventing complications is for the parent and child to maintain contact with, and retain confidence in, the diabetes management team.

Transient diabetes mellitus in infancy

Very rarely in the first 6 weeks after birth an infant becomes severely hyperglycaemic (blood glucose up to 110 mmol/l), mildly ketotic and severely glycosuric. This causes dehydration, fever and weight loss. Most such babies are born at full-term, but are severely growth-retarded and insulin levels are found to be lower than expected. After a few weeks or months of treatment with insulin the infant recovers and glucose tolerance returns to normal. This suggests that there has been a delayed maturation of islet cell function. A number of these infants do develop IDDM later in life so careful instruction of parents is important.

Hypoglycaemia

Hypoglycaemia is the commonest serious metabolic crisis occurring throughout infancy and childhood. It has the potential not only to cause brain damage but also, when associated with an endocrine abnormality such as cortisol deficiency, to be life threatening.

Glucose is of central importance in the metabolic pathways being the vital immediate energy substrate for cellular metabolism. Immediate sources of glucose to maintain normoglycaemia are from the diet and liver glycogen (via glycogenolysis). Less immediate mechanisms resulting in an increase in blood glucose (the process of gluconeogenesis) are:
1 Conversion of protein to form glucogenic amino acids.
2 Conversion of fats to form glycerol from which glucose is produced.

Table 23.4   Causes of hypoglycaemia.

Glucocorticoid deficiency
Seen in association with endocrine disorders, e.g.
  Adrenomedullary deficiency
  Growth hormone deficiency
  ACTH deficiency

Hyperinsulinaemia
Newborn and infant
  Infants of diabetic mothers
  Nesidioblastosis
  Rh incompatability
  Wiedemann–Beckwith syndrome
Older children
  Islet cell adenoma (insulinoma)
  Massive non-pancreatic tumour
  Leucine sensitivity

Others
Intra-uterine growth retardation
Starvation
Liver disease
  Glycogen storage diseases
  Galactosaemia
  Reye's syndrome
Inborn error of amino acid metabolism
  e.g. maple syrup urine disease

During periods of starvation or hypoglycaemia metabolic pathways are activated by endocrine responses to maintain normoglycaemia. One of the essential features is the suppression of insulin secretion allowing lipolysis to produce ketone bodies as an alternative energy source.

Aetiology

Hypoglycaemia may be due to unavailability of substrate or to hyperinsulinism. Neonatal hypoglycaemia is discussed in Chapter 7. The causes of hypoglycaemia are listed in Table 23.4 and the individual conditions are discussed at the end of this section.

Clinical features

Hypoglycaemic symptoms in older children are described in the section on diabetes mellitus. In infants hypoglycaemia may present as apathy, unusual episodes of drowsiness, irritability, abnormal cry, pallor, myoclonic jerking episodes, frank convulsions or episodes of coma. Any children with unexplained convulsions or coma must have an immediate capillary blood glucose measurement. Outside the neonatal period hypoglycaemia has been defined as a blood glucose of <2.2 mmol/l, but recent studies suggest that a blood glucose of <2.6 mmol/l causes measurable neurological change and therefore should be treated.

Investigations

Investigations must be pursued with urgency and reversal of hypoglycaemia achieved without delay. An investigation plan is shown in Figure 23.14.

Management

At the time of taking the critical first blood sample an intravenous 10% glucose solution should be set up to give a rapid bolus of 0.5 g/kg glucose

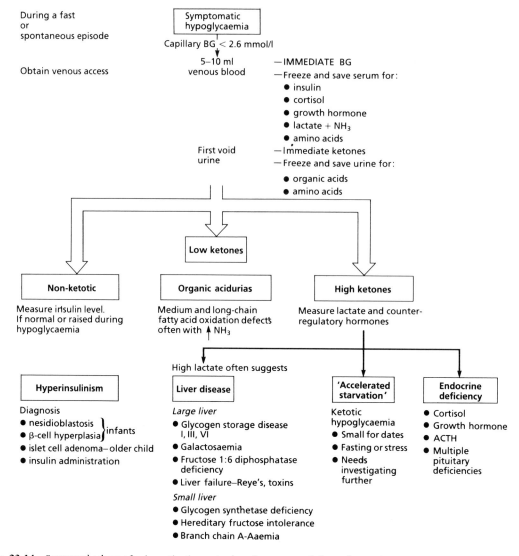

Fig. 23.14 Suggested scheme for investigating episodes of symptomatic hypoglycaemia.

followed by an infusion of about 0.5 mg/kg/hour glucose to maintain normoglycaemia. Later treatment depends on the cause.

NESIDIOBLASTOSIS

This is the commonest cause of persistent intractable hypoglycaemia in the newborn or in early infancy. The severity of the hypoglycaemia makes it potentially extremely damaging. It is due to a disorganized increase in pancreatic endocrine cells, particularly the insulin-producing beta cells.

Diagnosis is based on the following features:

1 Severe hypoglycaemia with no ketonuria.
2 Hypoglycaemia requiring a glucose infusion of more than 10 mg/kg/minute to maintain normoglycaemia.
3 During hypoglycaemia, insulin in the blood is measurable (>5 IU/l) or high (>40 IU/l).

There are no sensitive methods of distinguishing between nesidioblastosis and a discrete insulinoma.

Management. In addition to high-concentration glucose infusion, drugs such as hydrocortisone, diazoxide or chlorothiazide may be given to try and maintain blood glucose in the normal range. If the level remains low despite these agents, surgical intervention aiming to remove 85–90% of the pancreas is then urgently indicated. Whilst awaiting surgery the long-acting somatostatin analogue, octreotide, administered by multiple injections or infusion, is the drug most likely to inhibit insulin release.

ISLET CELL ADENOMA (INSULINOMA)

This does occur in the newborn period, but is much more rare than diffuse nesidioblastosis, whereas the reverse would be true in later childhood. The diagnosis is made during pancreatic surgery performed for hyperinsulinaemic hypoglycaemia.

LEUCINE SENSITIVITY HYPOGLYCAEMIA

The amino acid leucine provokes insulin secretion in all individuals. A few infants and children are particularly sensitive to leucine and most are eventually found to have islet cell hyperplasia or forms of nesidioblastosis. They may be treated with a low-leucine (low protein, low milk) diet and/or diazoxide.

GLUCOCORTICOID DEFICIENCY

All the causes of glucocorticoid deficiency (especially in conjunction with adrenomedullary and growth hormone deficiency) are likely to be associated with hypoglycaemia at times of stress. This also applies to cases of isolated growth hormone deficiency and adrenocorticotrophic hormone (ACTH) deficiency. All these conditions are associated with the production of ketones during the hypoglycaemic episodes and insulin levels are unrecordably low.

KETOTIC HYPOGLYCAEMIA

All causes of hypoglycaemia, except hyperinsulinism, are associated with some degree of ketogenesis. The term 'ketotic hypoglycaemia' is, therefore, a description rather than a diagnosis. Many children given a label of 'ketotic hypoglycaemia' are found subsequently to have an endocrine or metabolic disorder. However, despite investigation a group of young infants remain; often they are males, born small for dates, remain underweight, and during periods of stress, exercise or starvation rapidly become hypoglycaemic with convulsions (so-called 'accelerated starvation').

The cause of this syndrome may be a small liver, poor glycogen reserves and uninhibited high peripheral glucose uptake despite caloric deprivation. The syndrome demonstrates the liability of young children to become hypoglycaemic during prolonged starvation. All young children, and this group in particular, should have a regular consistent calorie intake to prevent ketonuria. Ketotic hypoglycaemia often improves before the age of 7 years.

Polyuria and polydipsia

Polyuria (passing large volumes of urine, usually by day and night) must be distinguished in the

Table 23.5 Causes of polyuria and polydipsia with appropriate investigations.

Condition	Investigations
Diabetes mellitus	Urine dipstick for glucose
Diabetes insipidus	Urine osmolality low and relatively raised serum osmolality
Chronic renal failure	Hypertension Uraemia and raised serum creatinine Reduced glomerular filtration rate Abnormality of the upper renal tracts seen on imaging techniques
Hypercalcaemia (and hypercalciuria)	Raised serum calcium
Habit drinking	Exclude other causes first Concentrates urine with fluid deprivation

clinical history from frequency (passing urine frequently but usually of small volume). Pathological polyuria will be accompanied by polydipsia. These two symptoms should always be investigated. Table 23.5 lists the most important causes.

Although habit drinking is the most common cause of polyuria and polydipsia, particularly in infants, fluid deprivation at home should not be suggested until the other serious pathologies, such as diabetes insipidus, have been excluded.

DIABETES INSIPIDUS (DI)

In severe forms of DI the urine cannot be concentrated above the osmolality of serum (295 mosmol/l); in less severe forms it may be concentrated up to 600–700 mosmol/l but not above.

There are a number of causes of DI:

1 Renal (vasopressin insensitivity):
  • Hereditary X-linked
  • Renal (chronic renal failure, cystinosis, sickle cell disease)
  • Severe potassium depletion
2 Central (vasopressin deficiency):

• Familial dominantly inherited
• Hypothalamic or pituitary trauma
• Intracranial tumours and deposits (e.g. craniopharyngioma, germinoma, Langerhans' cell histiocytic disorders (p. 472))
• Post-meningitic (tuberculosis, etc.)
• Syndromes (e.g. DIDMOAD)

In anterior pituitary diseases with cortisol deficiency, water excretion is poor but is suddenly enhanced by steroid replacement. Space-occupying lesions occasionally destroy not only the vasopressin-producing nuclei but also the thirst centre with the danger of severe hyperosmolar dehydration. All cases of DI with a history of headaches or visual disturbances must have urgent neuro-radiological investigation.

Investigation. DI may be further characterized by determining the relationship between urine osmolality (U_{osm}) and plasma osmolality (P_{osm}) during free access to water (see Fig. 23.15). When the U_{osm}–P_{osm} values fall within the normal ellipse (A) no further tests for DI are required, but if the child is relatively over-hydrated and the results fall within ellipse (B), a short period of fluid deprivation will demonstrate a shift to the right of both ellipses (towards area C in cases of DI). Intra-

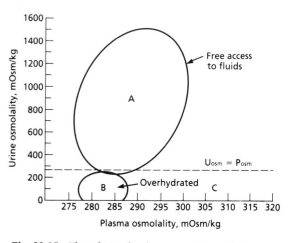

Fig. 23.15 The relationship between urine and plasma osmolality. Area A – normal child with free access to fluids. Area B – normal, but over-hydrated child. Area C – child with diabetes insipidus before or after a short (3 hour) period of fluid restriction.

DDAVP 10–20 µg will differentiate between central and renal DI.

Management. Central DI is readily treated with the vasopressin analogue desmopressin (DDAVP), given intranasally in doses of 5–20 µg two or three times daily. Renal DI is difficult to manage, but occasionally salt restriction and diuretics help.

Thyroid disorders

The thyroid hormones, thyroxine (T_4) and tri-iodothyronine (T_3) are formed by iodination of the amino acid tyrosine and have a fundamental role in metabolism. T_3 is the most metabolically active thyroid hormone. It stimulates both protein synthesis and turnover and has a direct effect on mitochondrial function. T_3 is principally formed from T_4 by mono-deiodination outside the thyroid gland. Thyroid hormones circulate in blood bound to thyroid-binding proteins, but free unbound T_3 is biologically most important.

Although thyroid hormones are essential for normal postnatal growth, the situation in fetal life is less clear. Active T_3 is not found in the human fetus until about 30 weeks gestation whereas its analogue reverse-T_3, which is inactive in adults, is present in the fetus. Paradoxically, although the newborn with thyroid aplasia might have mild skeletal immaturity, fetal growth appears normal, despite the fact that maternal thyroid hormones do not traverse the placenta in significant amounts. Thus the role of thyroid hormones in fetal growth remains a subject of speculation.

During the stress of birth there is normally an acute rise in thyroid-stimulating hormone (TSH) followed within hours by increases in T_3 and T_4. TSH falls to <10 mU/l by 4 days postnatally. Apart from diabetes mellitus, thyroid hormone deficiency is the commonest endocrine disorder in childhood.

The causes of thyroid disease can be divided into congenital and acquired disorders summarized in Table 23.6.

Table 23.6 Causes of hypothyroidism.

Congenital	Acquired

Developmental abnormalities of the thyroid gland (aplasia, hypoplasia or ectopia) (80%; sporadic)	Thyroiditis
	  Hashimoto's
	  Post-viral
	  Subacute

Inborn errors of thyroxine synthesis (10–15%)
  Iodine trapping defect
  Iodination defect
	Hypothalamic pituitary disorders
	  Trauma
	  Post-irradiation
	  Tumours

Iodine deficiency (endemic cretinism)	Iodine deficiency

Maternal goitrogens
  Carbimazole
  Iodine
	Post-thyroidectomy

Hypothalamic pituitary disorders
  Septo-optic dysplasia
  Isolated TRH deficiency
  Cleft lip and palate midline syndromes
	Drugs
	  Carbimazole

	Associated syndromes
	  Down's
	  Diabetes mellitus
	  Pendred's

Hypothyroidism

Congenital hypothyroidism is either a *primary* abnormality of the thyroid gland or a thyroid deficiency *secondary* to hypothalamic/pituitary abnormalities.

CONGENITAL PRIMARY HYPOTHYROIDISM

Retrospective studies indicate an incidence of this condition in the order of 1:7000 children with females being affected four times more commonly than males. Newborn screening programmes introduced in many countries have revealed a prevalence of 1:3500 because screening allows early detection of infants with compensated hypothyroidism who may not have presented later in childhood with overt hypothyroidism. The screening test usually performed is by measurement of TSH 5 or 6 days after birth using heel-prick blood spots collected on filter paper.

Clinical features. Most newborn hypothyroid infants do not have signs or symptoms but the diagnosis may be suggested by:
- Hypothermia
- Prolonged jaundice
- Lethargy and slow feeding
- Prominent tongue and coarse facial features

- Umbilical hernia
- Large posterior fontanelle
- Goitre (in inborn errors of thyroxine synthesis)

In areas where screening tests are not available these clinical features become more obvious (see Fig. 23.16) and the infant may also become constipated and show progressively more delay in development and growth.

If the screening TSH is significantly raised (>40 mU/l) the diagnosis should be confirmed as soon as possible by definitive thyroid function tests and a knee X-ray which shows delay in epiphyseal maturation. In equivocal cases a radio-isotope thyroid scan (see Fig. 23.17) should be considered. Other congenital abnormalities should be looked for, such as cardiac defects which have a higher incidence in hypothyroid infants.

Management. Thyroxine therapy should be instituted without delay. The aim being to increase thyroid hormone levels to the high/normal range with suppression of TSH into the normal range. Growth and bone age should be monitored regularly. Thyroxine is given as a single daily dose according to the child's age:

Age	Dose/day	Dose/kg/day
0–9 months	25–37.5 µg	8–10 µg
9 months–3 years	50 µg	4–6 µg
3–12 years	75–150 µg	3.75 µg

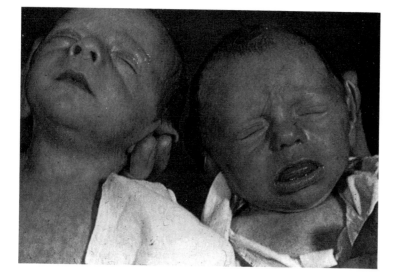

Fig. 23.16 Congenital hypothyroidism in one twin (infant on right) showing slight coarsening of the facial features and macroglossia.

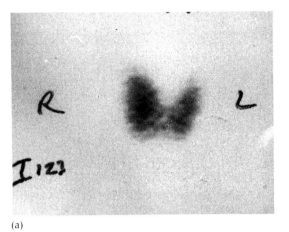

(a)

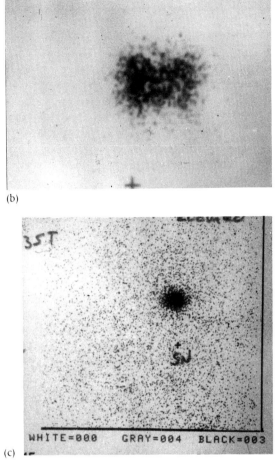

(b)

(c)

Fig. 23.17 Examples of ^{123}I-radio-isotope scans. (a) Adolescent girl with goitre showing the isthmus and bilobed thyroid structure. (b) Neonate without goitre, but with compensated congenital hypothyroidism showing a small bilobed thyroid gland. (c) Neonate with high TSH and low T_4 and T_3 showing midline ectopic or dysplastic thyroid gland (SN: suprasternal notch).

If there is any doubt about the initial diagnosis, treatment with thyroxine may be discontinued between the ages of 1 and 2 years for 4 weeks, the infant put on T_3 10 μg b.d. for 21 days and the thyroid function repeated after 28 days. A rise in TSH will confirm permanent hypothyroidism.

Prognosis. Before screening tests became available, infants gradually developed symptoms of 'cretinism'. The treatment was commenced several weeks or months after birth and this was commonly associated with mental retardation and cerebellar dysfunction.

Parents of infants with positive neonatal screening tests should be reassured that although treat-ment is for life, when it is started before 4 weeks and compliance is good, the developmental prognosis is excellent. Even when the neonatal test have indicated severe thyroid deficiency, psychometric testing of children at school entry has revealed a range of IQs no different from control children without hypothyroidism.

CONGENITAL SECONDARY HYPOTHYROIDISM

Isolated hypothalamic or pituitary hypothyroidism is very rare but it occurs more frequently in association with multiple pituitary deficiency syndromes. Neonatal screening by detection of raised TSH for primary congenital hypothyroidism will miss cases of secondary hypothyroidism so that they may present clinically as cases of prolonged neonatal jaundice or growth failure. Fortunately these infants seem to escape neurological damage even though the diagnosis may be delayed and there is marked retardation of bone maturation.

Diagnosis is confirmed by low T_4 and T_3 levels with low TSH or levels within the normal range, but which fail to rise adequately during a TRH test. Treatment is with thyroxine (see above) with monitoring of thyroid hormone levels (not TSH), growth and bone maturation.

ACQUIRED CHILDHOOD OR JUVENILE HYPOTHYROIDISM

An estimated 1–2% of children have measurable anti-thyroid antibodies and of these perhaps 10% become hypothyroid. The commonest type of childhood hypothyroidism is *Hashimoto's chronic lymphocytic thyroiditis* with an estimated incidence of between 1:1000 and 1:5000 in children between 5 and 15 years of age. Females predominate and a firm goitre may be present. There may be other family members affected and there are clear associations with other syndromes or disorders (diabetes, arthritis, Addison's disease, Down's, Turner's, or Noonan's syndromes).

Clinical features. The presentation of juvenile hypothyroidism is often slow and subtle in onset and therefore overlooked. The child may exhibit poor growth, increased weight gain, cold or dry skin, constipation, goitre and may develop anaemia and bradycardia. School performance is usually not adversely affected. Primary juvenile hypothyroidism occasionally presents as advanced puberty due to TRH stimulation of gonadotrophins.

Investigations. As overt clinical signs may be absent, it is important to measure thyroid function in children with goitre, short stature, slow growth velocity or whenever a diagnosis of hypothyroidism is suggested. Many children with goitre and positive anti-thyroid antibodies remain euthyroid and a number of children with goitre become hypothyroid without detectable anti-thyroid antibodies.

Management. This is with thyroxine according to age and size (see p. 410).

Hyperthyroidism and thyrotoxicosis

NEONATAL THYROTOXICOSIS

If a mother has Graves' disease (active or inactive) associated with high levels of thyroid-stimulating immunoglobulins (TSI) there is a risk of thyrotoxicosis in the newborn infant. It is a rare but serious condition presenting as irritability, vomiting, diarrhoea, failure to thrive, tachycardia and heart failure.

Prevention may take the form of treatment of active maternal Graves' disease, but if neonatal thyrotoxicosis occurs it may be treated with a combination of potassium iodide, propranolol, or carbimazole. The thyrotoxicosis subsides within 3–6 months as the TSI levels fall.

JUVENILE THYROTOXICOSIS

Classical Graves' disease is rare in childhood. It usually occurs in girls with a combination of goitre, sweating, weight loss, nervousness, tremor, irritability, palpitations, staring eyes, fatigue, muscle weakness and deterioration of school performance. Clinical diagnosis is often straightforward although children with anxiety states are sometimes difficult to differentiate. Biochemically either the T_4 or T_3 or both will be raised two or three times above mean normal levels. Sensitive TSH assays reveal suppressed levels and if there is any doubt a TRH test will confirm TSH suppression. Thyroid auto-antibodies are nearly always present.

Management. An anti-thyroid drug (e.g. carbimazole) will be needed to suppress thyroid hormones into the normal range and thereafter the dose should be titrated carefully to avoid induced hypothyroidism. The child may also need propranolol if symptoms of tachycardia and tremor are extreme.

Prognosis. The majority of children relapse on cessation of treatment. In a few centres, therefore, thyroidectomy is the treatment of choice, but in most units subtotal thyroidectomy is advised following relapses of thyrotoxicosis after 2–4 years of medical treatment. Although radio-iodine is effective in suppressing Graves' disease the inherent dangers of irradiation to the immature thyroid tissue preclude its widespread use.

Adrenal disorders

The full functional role of the fetal adrenal cortex is uncertain but it is an essential part of the feto–placental biosynthetic pathway of the major pregnancy steroid oestriol. The 'adult' adrenal supersedes the fetal cortex soon after birth but the three anatomical zones of the adult cortex are not distinct until adolescence.

The causes of adrenal disorders may be either congenital or acquired and can be subdivided further as either primary or secondary (Table 23.7). ary (Table 23.7).

Congenital adrenal hyperplasia (CAH)

Several enzyme defects of the adrenal cortex are associated with low cortisol production, inadequate feedback to the hypothalamus and raised ACTH. This enhances the growth of the adrenal gland and stimulates excessive activity in the other biosynthetic pathways (see Table 23.7).

21 HYDROXYLASE DEFICIENCY

This causes 95% of cases of CAH formerly called adreno-genital syndrome. In Britain it occurs in 1:5000–10 000 infants although there is worldwide variability. The position of the enzyme deficiency (see Fig. 23.18) leads to variable deficiencies in the production of both cortisol and aldosterone and an increase in precursor 17-OH-progesterone which is preferentially metabolized to androstenedione.

Clinical features

1. Effects of mineralocorticoid deficiency. One-half of European cases present at between 1 and 3 weeks

	Congenital	Acquired

Table 23.7 A classification of adrenal disorders.	**Primary**
	Inborn errors (enzyme deficiencies)
	  Congenital adrenal hyperplasia
	  Glucocorticoid deficiency
	  Mineralocorticoid deficiency
	Structural abnormalities
	  Congenital adrenal hypoplasia
		Primary
		Adreno-cortical insufficiency
		  Acute haemorrhage, infection,
		    steroid suppression
		  Chronic – 'Addison's' syndrome
		Adreno-cortical excess
		  Glucocorticoids – Cushing's
		    syndrome
		  Androgens – premature
		    adrenarche, adenoma, carcinoma
		  Mineralocorticoids – Conn's
		    syndrome
		Adreno-medullary excess
		  Phaeochromocytoma

	Secondary
	Hypothalamic–pituitary insufficiency
		Secondary
		Hypothalamic–pituitary disease
		  Insufficiency
		  Excess – Cushing's syndrome

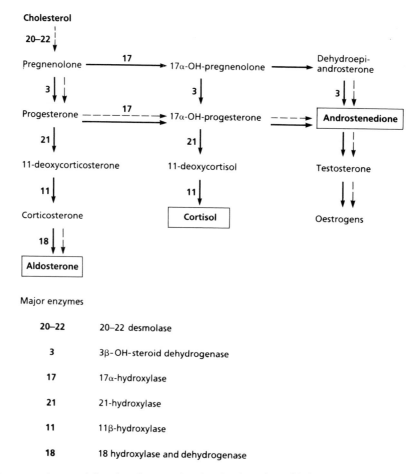

Major enzymes

20–22	20–22 desmolase
3	3β-OH-steroid dehydrogenase
17	17α-hydroxylase
21	21-hydroxylase
11	11β-hydroxylase
18	18 hydroxylase and dehydrogenase

Fig. 23.18 Enzyme pathways of the adrenal cortex showing the sites of possible biochemical defects.

after birth with weight loss, prolonged jaundice, vomiting, severe salt depletion, hypotension and dehydration. Some babies die from this serious condition. Before the development of a salt-losing crisis, females should be recognized by their ambiguous genitalia.

2. Non-salt-losing CAH. Half the cases do not show significant salt loss because the enzyme deficiency does not express itself along the mineralocorticoid pathway. These cases exhibit variable degrees of androgenization and present later. Males show rapid growth, advanced bone age and signs of early pseudo-puberty. Females show similarly advanced growth with clitoromegaly, labial fusion, pubic hair and hirsutism.

3. Effects of excess androgens. In the first trimester of pregnancy the female fetus will be virilized to a variable degree. Severe forms result in ambiguous genitalia (severe clitoromegaly and dense labial fusion). Milder forms may only cause noticeable clitoromegaly later in childhood. The male infant with CAH cannot be distinguished from normal. Occasionally high ACTH/MSH levels cause increased genital and breast pigmentation. For surgical correction of genital abnormalities see the section on ambiguous genitalia (p. 418).

Investigations

In the non-salt-losing condition, the serum electrolytes are normal, but there are high serum

Table 23.8 Biochemical and clinical abnormalities in the varieties of congenital adrenal hyperplasia.

Enzyme defect	Hormone status				Genitalia		Salt balance	BP
	ACTH	17-OH-prog.	Cortisol	Aldo.	Male	Female		
20–22	↑	↓	↓	↓	Amb	N	Loss ++	↓
3	↑	↓	↓	↓	Amb	± Viril	Loss +	↓
17	↑	↓	N or ↓	↑	Amb	N	Retention	↑
21	↑	↑	N or ↓	N or ↓	N	Viril	N or Loss ++	No or ↓
11	↑	↑	↓	↓	N	Viril	Retention	↑
18	N	N	N	↓	N	N	Loss +	↑

Amb: ambiguous, Viril: virilized, N: normal.

levels of 17-hydroxy-progesterone, androstenedione and testosterone. Urinary pregnanetriol and androgen derivatives will be raised.

In the salt-losing group, measurements of serum electrolytes will show low serum sodium chloride, raised potassium and urea with high renal salt loss. Urinary and serum steroid estimations take days or weeks to be reported and are often difficult to interpret but the most important findings are markedly raised serum 17-OH-progesterone and androstenedione with raised urinary metabolites, pregnanetriol and androgen derivatives. More sophisticated investigation would reveal high ACTH, low aldosterone and high serum renin. Table 23.8 summarizes these biochemical abnormalities.

Management

The salt-losing crisis in the newborn must be reversed by intravenous normal saline. The shocked infant may require plasma. Parenteral aldosterone can be given but is rarely available. Alternatively, long-acting depot deoxycortolone pivalate may be used, or a suspension of fludrocortisone, but these are of secondary importance to adequate saline. Careful monitoring of the electrolytes and blood pressure is essential. Hydrocortisone 25 mg 6-hourly intravenously initially covers the period of resuscitation and will suppress ACTH production. Thereafter the steroid management of CAH is delicate, particularly in infancy and puberty

and should be undertaken by an experienced paediatrician.

Optimal steroid therapy is best assessed by regular clinical examination, growth assessment, bone age measurements and may be supplemented by serum electrolytes, 17-OH-progesterone, androstenedione, testosterone levels and urinary steroid output. Some units are able to assess ACTH and renin levels and studies show that the availability of salivary or blood spot 17-OH-progesterone profiles may optimize difficult control.

Prognosis

Parents must be reassured that with careful management children with CAH should grow normally and girls will maintain femininity and have normal sexual function. Height prognosis remains a worry particularly when steroid dosage is excessive in infancy or inadequate in puberty. Enzyme deficiencies of the adrenal cortex are autosomally recessively inherited. Although it is not often requested it is possible to predict the likelihood of a subsequent affected fetus by HLA-typing of family members and the fetus in early pregnancy. Recent reports have shown that treatment with dexamethasone from the early weeks of pregnancy may prevent virilization of the affected female fetus.

Congenital adrenal hypoplasia

Hypoadrenalism occurring in the neonate or infant due to hypoplasia, malformation or absence of the adrenals is uncommon but not rare. There is an estimated incidence of 1:12 500 births and 1:600 infant deaths. There is an association with severe maternal pre-eclampsia. Oestriol formation during pregnancy is dependent upon the synthesis of specific sulphated steroid precursors by the fetal adrenals and being supplied to the placenta for cleavage of the sulphate side chain. If placental sulphatase activity is present, an unrecordably low oestriol level in pregnancy suggests primary or secondary fetal adrenal hypoplasia.

The fetal adrenal may not grow adequately because of hypothalamic or pituitary insufficiency. Many cases, however, are primary developmental anomalies, some of which have an hereditary or familial aetiology.

Clinical features. Adrenal insufficiency with sudden collapse, apnoea, hypoglycaemia or sudden death may occur in the neonatal period. Occasionally hyperpigmentation may be present and in some milder cases, adrenal insufficiency only becomes apparent later in infancy during times of stress.

Investigations. An early Synacthen test in babies born to mothers with very low oestriol levels will sometimes, but not always, help in the diagnosis. Such infants must be watched with vigilance until unequivocally normal cortisol secretion is confirmed and there is no evidence of characteristic hyponatraemia, acidosis or hypoglycaemia with rising potassium levels.

Management. Infants need hydrocortisone and many will also require fludrocortisone although a few have isolated glucocorticoid deficiency.

ACUTE ADRENAL INSUFFICIENCY

Acute adrenal insufficiency is a life-threatening event presenting as shock, salt loss and hypoglycaemia often precipitated by stress, such as infections (particularly meningococcal septicaemia (p. 366)), severe neonatal crises (with adrenal haemorrhage) and certain malignancies. Children particularly at risk are those with already existing adrenal or pituitary disorders or those previously treated with high-dose steroids. Treatment is directed at hypoglycaemia, cortisol deficiency, shock and salt depletion.

CHRONIC ADRENAL INSUFFICIENCY

The classical disease described by Addison was caused by tuberculous destruction of the adrenal gland. This is now rare in Britain as is autoimmune adrenalitis which may occur in association with other immune disorders. More often chronic adrenal insufficiency is associated with hypothalamic–pituitary disorders, calcified adrenals and a variety of rare syndromes.

Clinical features. The presentation is often insidious in primary adrenal insufficiency with lethargy, weakness, weight loss and increased melanin pigmentation, particularly in the skin creases and scars. Occasionally the disorder presents as an adrenal crisis (see above).

Investigations. Haemoglobin, serum sodium chloride, glucose and cortisol levels are low. Serum potassium, urea, calcium and ACTH are likely to be raised. The diagnosis is confirmed by a Synacthen test which shows an inadequate (<200 nmol) rise in serum cortisol 30 or 60 minutes after Synacthen. Partial adrenal insufficiency is difficult to diagnose because of equivocal biochemical results.

Management. Hydrocortisone should be given to maintain good health and normal growth velocity. After starting hydrocortisone, urinary salt losses, serum electrolytes and blood pressure should be measured to assess whether mineralocorticoid replacement is necessary.

Adrenal disorders – special precautions

Children who have primary or secondary adrenal disorders and all children taking long-term steroids should carry or wear identification of their steroid dosage. Parents must be warned of the possibility of adrenal crises at times of stress such as feverish illnesses, vomiting episodes or surgery. Advice to parents should include doubling or trebling steroid dosage during these episodes and carrying a supply of hydrocortisone semi-succinate for injection if vomiting or collapse occurs.

Adrenal cortical over-activity

CUSHING'S SYNDROME

Glucocorticoid excess causes growth failure, obesity, hirsutes and hypertension. Other features include a change in facial appearance, mood swings, plethora, striae, bruising, osteoporosis and muscle weakness. The cushingoid appearance has been common in the past due to steroid medication, but the disease described by Cushing of pituitary adenoma with bilateral adrenal hyperplasia is rare in childhood.

The younger the child and the more prominent the androgenic features the more likely that there is primary adrenal disease (e.g. adenoma, carcinoma) rather than secondary ACTH dependent disease.

Investigations. Urinary free cortisol, urinary 17-oxogenic steroids and diurnal estimations of serum cortisol are the most frequent baseline investigations. A morning cortisol of 200–600 nmol/l should fall in an unstressed child by more than 50% by 11 pm. In conditions of cortisol excess the haemoglobin, haematocrit and bicarbonate levels tend to be high and eosinophil, lymphocyte and potassium levels are low. Adrenal androgens should also be estimated. If steroid levels suggest Cushing's syndrome a pathological diagnosis must be attempted by pituitary fossa X-rays, ultrasound of the adrenals, IVP, CT or MRI scan of the pituitary and possibly arteriography and adrenal isotope scans.

Dexamethasone suppression tests may not clearly differentiate pituitary dependent or primary adrenal Cushing's syndrome in children. Plasma ACTH measurements are often unhelpful although an elevated 11-pm ACTH level strongly suggests pituitary-dependent disease.

Management. Adrenal tumours should be removed surgically but only when electrolyte disturbances have been corrected and excess cortisol production has been suppressed by steroid administration (e.g. dexamethasone) or metyrapone. Post-operative steroid cover is necessary. If a pituitary adenoma is confirmed the optimal treatment is transphenoidal microadenoma resection. External pituitary irradiation has been used successfully in children without significant early damage to other pituitary functions. Local irradiation with yttrium seeds has also been used with success.

Failing all else bilateral adrenalectomy will rapidly reverse seriously incapacitating Cushing's syndrome but subsequent growth of an ACTH-secreting pituitary adenoma will occur in up to 70% of children.

Whatever the treatment, careful long-term follow-up of endocrine function is essential.

VIRILIZING ADRENAL TUMOURS

These are rare. In infants they are more likely to be due to adenoma but in adolescence to malignant carcinoma.

They may present with a mixture of Cushing's syndrome and virilization. Ultrasound, CT or radio-isotope scans of the adrenals should reveal the diagnosis which will be confirmed biochemically with raised serum androgens and excess urinary oxosteroids.

Treatment is surgical with pre- and post-operative steroid cover. Large tumours often metastasize. Carcinomas are not usually sensitive to radiotherapy or antimitotics.

Adrenal medullary disorders

ADRENAL MEDULLARY INSUFFICIENCY

A lack of catecholamine response to stress usually presenting with hypoglycaemia has been suspected in a few children, but is difficult to substantiate. These cases may well have other more fundamental metabolic abnormalities. Even after bilateral adrenalectomy most individuals do not show signs of catecholamine insufficiency.

ADRENAL MEDULLARY EXCESS

Neural crest tumours (neuroblastoma, ganglioneuroma)

These tumours may have their origins in the sympathetic chain or the adrenal gland (see Chapter 25). They may secrete excess catecholamines and metabolites and occasionally they are associated with profuse watery diarrhoea caused by secretion of the gut hormone vasoactive intestinal peptide (VIP). Symptoms remit when the tumour is resected.

Phaeochromocytomas

Occasionally children present with profuse sweating, pallor, palpitations weakness, headache and vomiting due to excess catecholamine release. Hypertension is often present. Increased urinary excretion of noradrenaline and sometimes adrenaline with their metabolite vanillyl mandelic acid (VMA) are found. The tumour is best localized by radio-isotope adrenal scan. Treatment is by operative removal of the usually benign tumour or tumours.

The child with ambiguous genitalia

Humans, like most mammals, with XX sex chromosome constitution are female and those with XY sex chromosome constitution are male because the Y chromosome switches on a succession of male-determining genes. Male-determining appears to be synonymous with 'testis-determining' because if the testis is absent or severely dysplastic the fetus retains a female phenotype. At about 7 weeks gestation the first male-specific gonad cells to differentiate are Sertoli cells which surround and nurture germ cells. The first identifiable Sertoli gene product, anti-Mullerian hormone, inhibits the development of Mullerian structures which in the female become the fallopian tubes, uterus and upper part of the vagina. It was thought that a male-specific H–Y antigen expression on the long arm of the Y chromosome acted as the testis inducer but it is now known that the testis-

determining factor maps to the short arm of the Y chromosome.

Androgen-secreting Leydig cells are also under Sertoli cell influence and during the next critical period in fetal life (10–12 weeks) testicular testosterone influences the development of the male internal genitalia (vas deferens, epididymis and seminal vesicles) from the Wolffian ducts. Testosterone must be converted by 5-alpha-reductase to dihydrotestosterone before masculinization of the external genitalia occurs.

Aberrations of this complex male-determining process cause incomplete differentiation of the male genitalia. In contrast, genetic females who appear masculine must have been influenced by excessive androgens from endogenous or exogenous sources.

An approach to diagnosis

The child born with ambiguous genitalia often presents a difficult clinical problem demanding expert, sensitive and urgent attention. The differential diagnosis of ambiguous genitalia is shown in Figure 23.19.

If ambiguity is recognized at birth the staff of the maternity unit must not attempt to assign gender. The parents should be told immediately that there is uncertainty and urgent tests will be carried out to clarify the situation. Before rapid karyotyping became available gender was often assigned as female if the phallus appeared so small that it was deemed unlikely ever to be functional. With modern cytogenetics the dilemma may be approached along different more scientific lines.

GENETIC SEX DETERMINATION

Buccal smear techniques are inaccurate. Results of sex chromosome karyotyping can be obtained within 3–5 days and should be transmitted to the parents with a careful proviso that the infant is XY, but perhaps 'maleness' is so incomplete that it seems that the Y chromosome is not functioning and that the child is more female than male. This will allow discussion on gender assignment. If the result is XX there should be no problem of gender

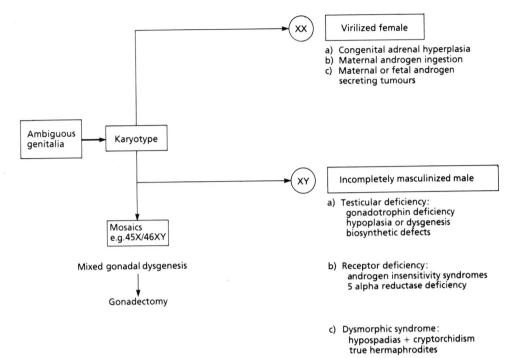

Fig. 23.19 Differential diagnosis of ambiguous genitalia.

assignment but a search for the cause of masculinization will be necessary.

GONADAL SEX

The initial assessment should pose the following questions.

1 Is there a family history? (e.g. female with CAH, androgen insensitivity syndromes, enzyme disorders).

2 Has the mother ingested drugs likely to cause virilization?

3 Is there a history of neonatal deaths? (e.g. CAH with salt loss).

4 Is a gonad palpable at birth? (If yes, it can be assumed to have testicular tissue, although in later neonatal life a prolapsing ovary into an inguinal hernia is not rare).

5 Is there excessive pigmentation of genital or breast skin? (e.g. CAH).

Ultrasound scanning may locate and identify the gonads and the other intra-abdominal organs

(e.g. female internal genitalia, grossly hypertrophied adrenals, adrenal or gonadal tumours). The anatomy of the urethral and vaginal openings may be clarified by contrast media radiography.

GENDER ASSIGNMENT

In *genetic females* gender assignment is female and the most likely diagnosis will be congenital adrenal hyperplasia (p. 413) but the possibility of maternal drug ingestion and androgen-secreting tumours must be investigated.

In *genetic males* gender assignment will be problematic if the phallus is very small with no palpable erectile tissue or if Mullerian structures are identifiable. Infants with *mosaicism* of the sex chromosomes often have dysgenetic gonads secreting inadequate amounts of androgen and anti-Mullerian hormone.

If anatomically the XY or mosaic infant has a vagina and uterus with a tiny phallus and dysgenetic gonads the suggested gender assignment should be female and the abnormal gonads removed in infancy because of the later risk of neoplastic transformation.

If no Mullerian structures are discernible the causes of poor androgenization may be elucidated by:

1 A LHRH test to detect gonadotrophin deficiency or hypergonadotrophic hypogonadism.

2 An HCG test with measurement of both testosterone and dihydrotestosterone to assess testicular responsiveness and the possibility of 5-alpha-reductase deficiency.

3 Urinary steroid analysis (in specialized laboratories) to detect biosynthetic defects.

4 A testosterone sensitivity test. Whilst awaiting the results of investigations, two intramuscular injections of depot testosterone at monthly intervals should be given with measurement of the phallic size. If the response is equivocal a third, larger injection is given. Appreciable phallic growth indicates that further enlargement is likely during puberty or with exogenous testosterone and male gender assignment is possible. The induced phallic enlargement also facilitates surgery.

Testicular feminization syndrome (TFS)

If there is no measurable phallic response to testosterone and the HCG test shows a normal or supra-normal secretion of testosterone and dihydrotestosterone, the most likely diagnosis is some form of androgen insensitivity syndrome (e.g. testicular feminization syndrome) and the infant would be best reared as a girl. TFS is usually a sex-linked disorder and testes should be left *in situ* until after the development of breast tissue.

GENDER IDENTIFICATION

When gender is assigned there may be a need for corrective surgical procedures such as clitoral reduction, vaginoplasty, or primary hypospadias repair. This is best performed before the child becomes aware of the genital anomalies; if possible before 18 months and certainly before starting school.

It is important for the paediatrician and some-times a genetic counsellor to support the child and parents through the uncertainties of gender assignment, sexual identification and corrective surgery.

SECONDARY SEXUAL MATURATION

The spontaneous production of endogenous sex steroids or introduction of exogenous therapy will allow pubertal maturation. The child who has previously required genital surgery may need further cosmetic correction but it must be remembered that considerable spontaneous changes occur (e.g. vaginal enlargement) during sexual maturation.

During puberty, emotional problems arise in this group of children if they are not carefully prepared for, and reassured about, the changes to be expected at a time appropriate to each individual's maturity.

Disorders of the parathyroid glands

Calcium balance is maintained by a complex interaction between dietary intake, renal and gastrointestinal excretion, the effects of parathyroid hormone (PTH) and calcitonin hormones and the metabolites of vitamin D. The main actions of PTH are to promote the release of calcium from bone and to stimulate renal reabsorption of calcium and tubular excretion of phosphate.

Hypoparathyroidism

PRIMARY HYPOPARATHYROIDISM

Failure of secretion of PTH results in hypocalcaemia and hyperphosphataemia and may manifest acutely as convulsions, tetany, cramps, paraesthesiae, laryngeal stridor and neuromuscular excitability (positive Chvostek or Trousseau signs).

The neonate may exhibit transient hypocalcaemia with suppression of neonatal PTH due to maternal hyperparathyroidism. Persistent infantile hypocalcaemia with hypoparathyroidism is occasionally associated with cardiovascular anomalies, thymic aplasia, or impaired immunity (diGeorge syndrome).

Later in childhood idiopathic hypoparathyroidism (IHP) may occur sporadically or be familial. Boys and girls are equally affected and onset is most commonly in the second decade.

Chronic hypocalcaemia may result in cataract formation, epilepsy and ectopic deposition of calcium in the skin or basal ganglia.

SECONDARY HYPOPARATHYROIDISM

This occurs most commonly after thyroid surgery but may occur after multiple transfusions for chronic haemolytic anaemias with iron deposition in the parathyroid and other endocrine glands.

PSEUDO-HYPOPARATHYROIDISM

Clinical manifestations of hypocalcaemia occasionally occur in children with normal PTH levels. This indicates PTH insensitivity or resistance. Many such children have characteristic physical features including short stature, round facies, metacarpal shortening and sometimes mild to moderate mental retardation. This syndrome, also known as Albright's osteodystrophy, is more common in girls and is usually diagnosed in the first decade of life.

PSEUDO-PSEUDO-HYPOPARATHYROIDISM

A further group of children may have all the physical features of Albright's osteodystrophy but show no hypocalcaemia and have low/normal PTH levels.

Pseudo-hypoparathyroidism appears to be genetically linked to pseudo-pseudo-hypoparathyroidism because several kindreds have been described where the characteristic features have been associated with both syndromes. Autosomal dominant inheritance is the most likely pattern although X-linked dominance has been suggested in some families.

Occasionally children with these syndromes have hypothalamic or primary thyroid dysfunction with thyroxine and growth hormone insufficiency.

Management. Severe, acute hypocalcaemia is treated by a slow intravenous infusion of 10% calcium gluconate with ECG monitoring. When tetany, fits or muscle spasm are reversed, oral calcium may be used. In the past the various forms of hypoparathyroidism and hypocalcaemia have been treated with pharmacological doses of calciferol (vitamin D_2), but this has a very long half-life and was liable to induce persistent hypercalcaemia and renal damage. The preferred treatment is now the vitamin D_3 analogue 1α-hydroxycholecalciferol which has a much shorter half-life. Hypercalcaemic episodes are more short-lived but careful monitoring of serum calcium and titration of doses is essential.

Prognosis

The cause of the mental retardation which sometimes occurs with hypoparathyroidism is not known and there is no certainty that earlier treatment of hypocalcaemia prevents this or the ectopic calcification in the lens or the brain.

Hyperparathyroidism

PRIMARY HYPERPARATHYROIDISM

Although this is not uncommon in adults it is very rare in childhood. In infancy there may be parathyroid hyperplasia but as age increases adenoma formation becomes more likely. It is usually sporadic, but familial cases have been described, sometimes as part of multiple endocrine adenomatosis (e.g. pancreatic, adrenal, gastrin-producing adenomas). Increased PTH secretion causes hypercalcaemia, increased renal phosphate clearance, and hypophosphataemia associated with hyperchloraemic acidosis.

Symptoms of hypercalcaemia include lethargy, hypotonia, anorexia, vomiting, abdominal discomfort and constipation. Hypercalciuria causes polyuria and polydipsia and a tendency towards renal stone formation and bone decalcification.

Primary hyperparathyroidism must be distinguished from benign familial hypercalcaemia (low calcium excretion in the urine with normal PTH levels) or other serious disorders, such as malignancies which may elevate the serum calcium with suppression of PTH levels.

The treatment is exploration of parathyroids with removal of hyperplastic or adenomatous glands.

SECONDARY HYPERPARATHYROIDISM

Maternal hypoparathyroidism with chronic hypocalcaemia may induce fetal and neonatal hyperparathyroidism causing transient symptoms of hypercalcaemia.

When rickets is severe enough to cause hypocalcaemia, secondary hyperparathyroidism is induced and skeletal demineralization is increased.

In end-stage renal failure phosphate retention causes a fall in serum calcium stimulating hyper-parathyroidism. The high PTH levels increase calcium resorption from the bones. This exacerbates the osteodystrophy of renal failure which is also associated with impaired vitamin D metabolism.

Further reading

Brook CGD. (Ed.) *Clinical Paediatric Endocrinology*, 2nd Edn. Blackwell Scientific Publications, Oxford 1989.

Kaplan SA. *Clinical Pediatric and Adolescent Endocrinology*. WB Saunders Co., Philadelphia 1982.

Hughes IA. *Handbook of Endocrine Tests in Children*. Wright, Bristol 1986.

Baum JD., Kinmouth A-L. (Eds) *Care of the Child with Diabetes*. Churchill Livingstone, Edinburgh 1985.

Drash AL. *Clinical Care of the Diabetic Child*. Year Book Publications Inc., Chicago 1987.

Aynsley-Green A., Soltesz G. *Hypoglycaemia in Infancy and Childhood*. Churchill Livingstone, Edinburgh 1985.

24
HAEMATOLOGICAL DISORDERS

In order to recognize the haematological changes seen in disease states, it is important to understand the normal haemopoietic system, and to be aware of the changes that occur throughout the period of fetal development, infancy and childhood. Figure 24.1 shows sites of blood production in fetal and postnatal life.

Haemoglobin is formed by the pairing of globin chains, so each molecule contains two globin chain pairs. During fetal life, different globin chains are produced, the resulting haemoglobin differing from adult haemoglobin. Embryonal haemoglobins ε_4 and $\alpha_2\varepsilon_2$, are replaced by fetal haemoglobin, HbF ($\alpha_2\gamma_2$), which is the major haemoglobin found in the fetus, produced from 6 weeks gestation until birth. Beta chains are produced in small amounts from a similar age, but production greatly increases at the time of birth, as gamma chain production falls. HbA ($\alpha_2\beta_2$) is the main haemoglobin of postnatal life, with small amounts of HbA$_2$ ($\alpha_2\delta_2$) also found from late gestation throughout life (Fig. 24.2). HbF has a high affinity for oxygen (p. 53), so transplacental oxygenation is good, the high haemoglobin concentration ensuring adequate tissue oxygenation. At birth, with lung expansion, appropriate oxygenation of the blood can occur readily, and tissue uptake then becomes a priority. HbF production is switched off, beta chain production increases, resulting in rising HbA levels, which with its lower oxygen affinity and better release of oxygen to tissues, is more suited to postnatal life. Abnormalities and imbalances of globin chain synthesis result in the thalassaemia syndromes, and these are discussed later. Neonatal red cells not only contain a different haemoglobin from adult cells, but they are also less deformable, have a shorter life span, lower red cell enzyme activity levels, and weak expression of red cell antigens that determine blood groups.

Normal haemoglobin ranges vary during infancy and childhood, as shown in Table 24.1. Platelet counts and total white cell counts do not vary greatly, but the white cell differential in infancy shows a reversal of the normal neutrophil : lymphocyte ratio. Iron stores in infancy are primarily in the red cells present at birth, so early cord clamping, preventing the return of placental blood to the baby, may result in reduced iron stores.

The anaemic child

Symptoms of anaemia are more likely if anaemia develops acutely, and may include pallor, tiredness, general misery, poor appetite, lack of energy and weakness, or breathlessness on climbing stairs. Initial assessment should include a full evaluation of age, race, background family details, dietary assessment and medical history. Bruises and petechiae, telangiectasia and cavernous haemangiomata should be looked for, the sclera should be inspected for jaundice, and the child examined to detect lymphadenopathy and/or hepatosplenomegaly. Failure to thrive and weight loss are important features, and skeletal abnormalities may point to a specific marrow hypoplasia syndrome.

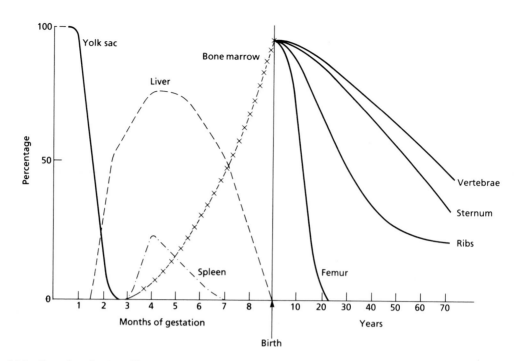

Fig. 24.1 Sites of production of haemopoietic tissue throughout life. (Reproduced with permission from Hoffbrand AV, Lewis SM. (Eds) *Post-Graduate Haematology*, 2nd Edn. 1981. Heinemann, London.)

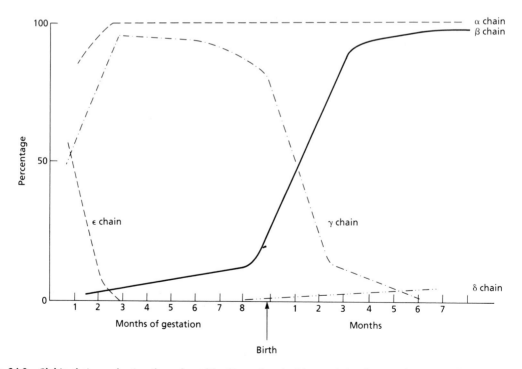

Fig. 24.2 Globin chain production throughout life. (Reproduced with permission from Nathan DG, Oski FA. (Eds) *Haematology of Infancy and Childhood*, 3rd Edn. 1987. WB Saunders, Philadelphia.)

Table 24.1 Normal haematological values in childhood.

	Newborn	3 months	1 year	3–6 years	10–12 years	Adult ♂	Adult ♀
Hb (g/dl)	13–19	9.5–13.5	10.5–13.5	12–14	11.5–14.5	13–18	11.5–16.5
MCV (fl)	106	95	70–86	73–89	77–91	76–96	
WBC ($\times 10^9$/l)	10–26	6–18	6–18	5–15	4.5–13.5	4.5–13.5	
N (%)	60	30	30	50	60	60	
L (%)	40	70	70	50	40	40	
Pl ($\times 10^9$/l)	150–400	150–400	150–400	150–400	150–400	150–400	
Retics (%)	2–6	0.2–2	0.2–2	0.2–2	0.2–2	0.2–2	

(Adapted from Dacie JV, Lewis SM. (Eds) *Practical Haematology*, 6th Edn. 1984. Churchill Livingstone, Edinburgh.)

Classic signs of iron deficiency described in adults, such as koilonychia, cheilitis and dysphagia are rare in childhood, although pica (eating mouthfuls of earth) is seen.

A convenient classification of anaemia is based on the physiological mechanisms underlying the anaemia, including causes of reduced or ineffective red cell production, shortened red cell life span, and red cell loss (Table 24.2). The aetiology, particularly in a complex multi-system disease, may be multi-factoral.

Investigations. Investigation should include a full blood count, mean corpuscular volume (MCV), white cell differential, blood film comment, and reticulocytes. These tests can be performed rapidly,

Table 24.2 Classification of anaemia.

Reduced red cell production
Aplastic anaemia
Red cell aplasia
    Congenital, e.g. Diamond–Blackfan anaemia
    Acquired, e.g. transient erythroblastopenia, parvovirus
    infection
Marrow replacement
    Leukaemia
    Solid tumour infiltration, e.g. neuroblastoma
    Myelosclerosis or fibrosis
Reduced erythropoetin production
    Renal disease
    Chronic inflammation
    Protein malnutrition
    Low oxygen affinity haemoglobinopathies
    Hypopituitarism, hypothyroidism

Ineffective red cell production
Cytoplasmic maturation defect
    Iron deficiency
    Thalassaemia
Nuclear maturation defect
    B_{12} or folate deficiency
    Metabolic defect
Congenital dyserythropoietic anaemias
Sideroblastic anaemia

Short red cell life span
Haemoglobin defects
    Structural, e.g. sickle cell anaemia
    Synthetic, e.g. thalassaemia
Membrane defects
    Congenital, e.g. hereditary spherocytosis
    Acquired, e.g. liver disease
Metabolic defects
    Glycolytic pathway, e.g. pyruvate kinase deficiency
    Pentose phosphate pathway, e.g. G6PD deficiency
Immune mediated
    Iso-immune, e.g. Rh or ABO incompatability
    Auto-immune, e.g. drug- or viral-induced, connective
    tissue disorder
Others
    Mechanical, e.g. microangiopathic haemolytic
    anaemia, haemolytic uraemic syndrome, DIC
    Thermal, e.g. burns
    Drugs, e.g. oxidant drugs
    Infections, e.g. malaria, Gram-negative septicaemia
    Environmental pH, e.g. paroxysmal nocturnal
    haemoglobinuria

Blood loss
Frank loss, e.g. trauma, surgery, epistaxis
Occult, e.g. gastrointestinal bleeding

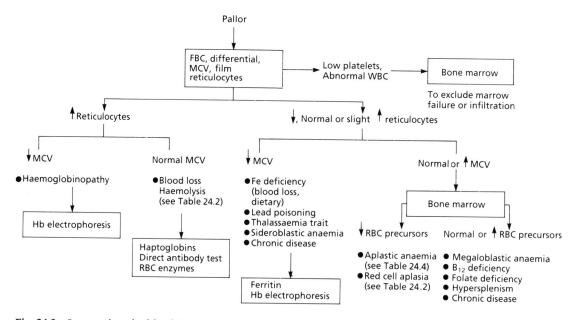

Fig. 24.3   Suggested method for the investigation of anaemia.

and only require a small volume of blood such as can be obtained from a finger stab (Fig. 24.3). In severe, poorly compensated anaemia, it may be necessary to complete the investigations in as short a time as possible, so treatment can be started. As blood transfusions affect serum B12 and red cell folate analysis, haemoglobinopathy screening, and tests for haemolysis, particularly red cell enzyme assays, these samples should be taken before transfusion commences. Well-compensated, chronic anaemia may not require transfusion, but should correct steadily once appropriate therapy is instituted.

Blood transfusions may have considerable unwanted effects on the recipient, including red and white cell antibody production, and transfusion-related viral infections such as hepatitis B and HIV. All blood transfusions should be carefully considered and only given if an adequate response cannot be obtained with other therapeutic measures.

Iron-deficiency anaemia

In health, 5–10% of dietary iron is absorbed, although up to 20% of dietary iron can be absorbed in deficiency states. The limitation of absorption can prevent compensation in states of excessive iron loss and result in low iron stores and anaemia. Iron stores exist in the form of ferritin, or haemosiderin in macrophages of the reticuloendothelial system. Most body iron is in the form of haemoglobin. At birth, all the body iron is maternal in origin, but by 1 year, approximately 70% is maternal, and this figure has fallen to 30% by 2 years of age. A pre-term baby will have reduced iron stores, as most trans-placental transfer of iron occurs in the last trimester of pregnancy.

Consideration of daily iron requirements at different ages will identify times when iron deficiency is common (Table 24.3). Excessive iron loss will exacerbate the tendency to iron deficiency. Inorganic dietary iron is mainly in the ferric form, which is converted to the ferrous form by gastric acid, and absorbed in the duodenum. Decreased gastric acid, or duodenal abnormalities, will reduce absorption, as will iron overload, chronic inflammation, alkalis and dietary phytates. Absorption is increased in pregnancy by vitamin C, and in chronic erythroid hyperplasia states.

Table 24.3 Iron losses and requirements throughout childhood. (From *WHO Technical Reports Series*, No. 452.)

	Urine, faeces (mg)	Daily loss Skin, menses	Requirement for growth	Total loss (= requirement)
Infant (0–4 months)	0.5			0.5
(5–12 months)	0.5		0.5	1.0
Child	0.5		0.5	1.0
Adolescent ♂	0.9		0.9	1.8
Adolescent ♀	0.9	1.0	0.9	2.8
Adult ♂	0.9			0.9
Menstruating ♀	0.9	1.9		2.8
Post-menopausal ♀	0.9			0.9

Clinical features. Presentation is with anaemia, koilonychia, stomatitis, but glossitis is rarely seen. A careful history should be taken of details of birth (term or pre-term, or multiple birth), and dietary intake. Blood loss may be overt or occult, as in gastrointestinal bleeding, and malabsorption may be present.

Investigations. Iron deficiency is diagnosed by examination of the blood film, and from the serum ferritin, and increased stainable iron is capacity are less accurate measures, as the capacity to bind iron fluctuates in various disease states, and results may be difficult to interpret. Blood film features include hypochromia, microcytosis, pencil cells, elliptocytes, and occasional target cells. Apparent iron deficiency may result from disordered iron metabolism, as in chronic inflammation or sideroblastic anaemia. This latter condition causes a typical blood picture, but with raised serum ferritin, and increased stainable iron is found. It is rare for a bone marrow examination to be required in the diagnosis of iron deficiency.

Management. The underlying cause, if identified, should be treated and iron supplements given in the sulphate, gluconate or fumarate form. These are easily absorbed, but may cause nausea, diarrhoea, or constipation, and stools will become very dark. The expected increase in haemoglobin is approximately 1 g per week, with reticulocytes appearing first and remaining at a level of approximately 5–10% until the haemoglobin has risen.

Rarely, parenteral iron is required, given as an intravenous infusion if oral medication is impossible. Treatment should continue for at least 3 months after the haemoglobin has returned to normal to build up iron stores, and may need to be continued long-term if there is an ongoing, unavoidable source of iron loss.

Haemosiderosis

Occasionally, the control of iron absorption is deranged resulting in iron overload. This may be primary or secondary. The primary form is called haemochromatosis and is an inherited disorder, with uncontrolled iron absorption and increasing iron stores leading to skin pigmentation, endocrine disorders, cirrhosis and cardiac failure in adult life. If diagnosed in childhood, because of a family history, the sequelae of iron overload may be prevented or delayed by a programme of venesection to reduce iron stores.

Secondary haemosiderosis is usually iatrogenic, from repeated blood transfusions for dyserythropoietic anaemias such as thalassaemia. Each unit of blood transfused adds 200–250 mg of iron to the stores, with potential severe long-term toxicity.

Folate deficiency

Folate is found in most foods, particularly liver, green vegetables and nuts, but is easily destroyed by heating, making dietary deficiency common.

Body stores are sufficient for only 3–4 months. Requirements in infancy are high, and as many infants are fed sterilized milk, folate supplements are necessary. Goat's milk is very low in folate. Absorption of folate is rapid and efficient, occurring in the small intestine. Tropical sprue and coeliac disease may cause folate deficiency, but surgery to the small bowel, unless massive, will not cause malabsorption. Defective metabolism of folate is reported, as is defective transport across the intestinal mucosa, but both are extremely rare.

Diagnosis. Folate deficiency is diagnosed by the finding of a macrocytic anaemia, with megaloblastic bone marrow changes. Neutrophils may be hypersegmented, and in severe deficiency, leucopenia and thrombocytopenia are found. Serum folate and B_{12} levels should be checked; the red cell folate which reflects body stores being more useful than the serum folate which fluctuates depending on recent dietary intake. The underlying cause should be treated, and oral supplements given until the haemoglobin is normal; or if a chronic extra requirement is identified, long-term supplements are indicated.

B_{12} deficiency

Although rarer than folate deficiency, this can present a major diagnostic problem. Body stores are adequate for 3–4 years, and as trans-placental passage occurs preferentially to the fetus, even infants of B_{12}-deficient mothers usually have adequate B_{12} stores for the first few years of life. B_{12} is in all foods of animal origin. Intrinsic factor is secreted by the gastric mucosa, and binds to B_{12}, the resulting complex is absorbed in the terminal ileum. B_{12} is then bound to plasma transport proteins, called Transcobalamin I, II and III (TCI, TCII, TCIII). The B_{12}/TCI and TCIII complex is tightly bound, and B_{12} is not easily released to the tissues. B_{12}/TCII, however, releases B_{12} to the tissues easily. Vitamin B_{12} assays measure total bound B_{12}.

Clinical features. Presentation is as discussed for folate deficiency, with no differentiating haematological features. Severe B_{12} deficiency is, however,

associated with neuropathy and treatment is essential to prevent permanent neurological damage, and to ensure normal development of the neurological system in those patients who present in infancy. Low B_{12} levels may be due to malabsorption of B_{12}, but juvenile onset of adult-type pernicious anaemia is rare. Absence of intrinsic factor, without antibody formation, is also rare, and presents at 2–4 years of age, when maternal B_{12} stores are depleted. This is an autosomal recessive condition.

Partial gastrectomy, or resection of the terminal ileum results in B_{12} malabsorption, and anaemia develops once stores are depleted. Coeliac disease and tropical sprue can affect absorption at the terminal ileum.

Management. Treatment of B_{12} malabsorption is by parenteral B_{12}, 1000 μg once a month providing adequate amounts for needs and stores. A reticulocyte response should be seen by 7 days after the start of treatment.

Transcobalamin II deficiency

In TCII deficiency, an autosomal recessive condition, B_{12} is not available for metabolism. Presentation is within a few weeks of birth, with anaemia, failure to thrive, diarrhoea and vomiting, and a megaloblastic bone marrow. The diagnosis can be suspected from the early presentation, and rapid confirmation by TCII assay permits early treatment, which is essential for normal neurological development.

Management. TCII deficiency requires massive doses of parenteral B_{12}, life-long, to overcome the lack of a suitable transport protein.

Aplastic anaemias

These are defined as pancytopenia with absent or reduced marrow precursors of all three cell lineages. The classification of aplastic anaemia is in Table 24.4. Approximately one-third of cases are due to drugs or toxins, and one-third are idiopathic. Severe aplastic anaemia is defined by three

Table 24.4 Classification of aplastic anaemia.

Acquired
Idiopathic
Drug-induced: dose-related, or idiosyncratic
Toxins and chemicals
Radiation
Infection: bacterial, or viral
Pregnancy
Thymoma
Paroxysmal nocturnal haemoglobinuria

Constitutional
Fanconi's anaemia
Schwachman–Diamond syndrome

---

criteria neutrophils $<1.0 \times 10^9/l$, platelets $<20 \times 10^9/l$ and reticulocytes $<1\%$ (corrected for haematocrit). Milder forms, termed hypoplastic anaemia, may progress to the severe form, or remit spontaneously.

Diagnosis. The history may be acute, requiring differentiation from acute leukaemia, or prolonged, with recurrent infections, bleeding and pallor. Pancytopenia is found and examination of the bone marrow shows a hypocellular picture. Severe aplastic anaemia, of any aetiology, is a serious disorder, the majority of patients dying within the first year of diagnosis from infection or bleeding, although spontaneous complete recoveries are recognized.

Management. Treatment is by removal of the cause if exposure to a drug or toxin is implicated, and supportive care with blood products and antibiotics as required. Bone marrow transplantation from an HLA-compatible sibling has the best chance of success, especially if performed early in the course of the disease, but a suitable donor is found in only 25% of patients. Mismatched, or matched, unrelated donor transplants carry the risk of graft rejection, and graft-versus-host disease. If no compatible donor is available, a course of intravenous anti-lymphocyte globulin (ALG) is given, which is believed to act on those patients who have auto-immune-mediated aplasia, with excess T cell suppressor activity. Severe allergic

reactions, defibrination, and serum sickness characterized by rash and arthralgia may be seen. Response may be delayed for 4–6 months, but a second course is indicated if there is no observed response after this time. Thirty per cent of patients will have a satisfactory partial or complete response. Steroids or androgens may stimulate the marrow into production, but this treatment has limited success and considerable side-effects, particularly infections, and hepatic damage.

Treatment of moderate aplasia is best judged on the merits of each individual case; life-threatening treatment should not be offered if symptoms are mild. However, if deterioration occurs over a period of months, during which aggressive blood product support is required, and infections with antibiotic-resistant organisms become established, the chances of successful bone marrow transplant are reduced.

FANCONI'S ANAEMIA

Fanconi's anaemia is a constitutional anaemia, that may not present with pancytopenia until late childhood or adulthood. Classically, it is described as an autosomal recessive condition, associated with congenital anomalies such as skin hyperpigmentation, thumb anomalies, low birth weight, microcephaly, renal anomalies, microphthalmia and mental retardation. It has now been shown that in cell culture specific chromosomal breaks occur, and this abnormality may be found in family members with no other stigmata of Fanconi's anaemia. Although aplasia may develop at any age, it usually appears in the first 3–5 years of life, affecting platelets initially, and gradually progressing to pancytopenia. Steroids or androgens may induce partial response for variable periods. Bone marrow transplantation should be considered on its merits for each patient, depending on the severity of the pancytopenia, and the presence of other defects.

DIAMOND–BLACKFAN ANAEMIA

Constitutional pure red cell aplasia is known as Diamond–Blackfan anaemia, and presents as anaemia within the first year of life. The inheritance is autosomal dominant, but with variable penetrance. Sixty-five per cent of patients are diagnosed in the first 6 months of life, some being anaemic at birth. Ninety-five per cent have presented by 1 year of age. Approximately 25% of patients have associated congenital abnormalities, short stature unresponsive to growth hormone; renal and cardiac abnormalities have been reported. Anomalies of the thumb are also noted, but less frequently than in Fanconi's anaemia. There is a macrocytic blood film, HbF is higher than expected for age, and the red cells retain fetal characteristics. Erythroid precursors in the marrow are reduced.

Management. Treatment initially is by high-dose steroids, reducing slowly when a response is noted. Blood transfusions are given to maintain a haemoglobin level compatible with normal growth and development, together with iron chelation therapy to prevent excessive iron overload. The natural history of the disease is variable, up to 20% of patients having a spontaneous or steroid-induced remission, although some become transfusion-dependent again later in life. A second trial of steroids may be successful, even if no response was seen initially. Survival is reduced in those patients who are transfusion-dependent, as a result of iron overload and other transfusion-related problems.

Transient erythroblastopenia of childhood (TEC)

This form of acquired pure red cell aplasia differs from Diamond–Blackfan in that the age at presentation is older (1–3 years), the anaemia is not macrocytic, and HbF is normal. Bone marrow erythroid precursors are reduced. It is believed to be viral-induced although no single causative virus has been isolated. The erythroid aplasia is temporary, followed by erythroid hyperplasia, reticulocytosis, and rising haemoglobin. Recovery is spontaneous, but blood transfusion is indicated for symptomatic anaemia. Recurrence of aplasia is extremely rare, and TEC is not the prelude to other more serious marrow disorders.

Haemolytic anaemias

THALASSAEMIA

Thalassaemia is an inherited haemolytic anaemia, caused by abnormal synthesis of a globin chain in the haemoglobin molecule, resulting in accumulation and excess of the other normal chains in the red cell. Thalassaemia is not a single disease state, but a collection of disorders involving different globin chains, many different molecular defects, and greatly varied clinical patterns. It occurs in high frequency in populations originating from the Middle East, Mediterranean regions, India and the Far East.

Types

Beta thalassaemia major is the disorder with the greatest clinical importance, and will be discussed in detail. Beta chain synthesis is absent (β^0), or reduced (β^+), with accumulation of free alpha chains in the red cells. Fetal haemoglobin ($\alpha_2\gamma_2$) is normally produced, but HbA ($\alpha_2\beta_2$) is absent or reduced. The clinical picture depends on the genes inherited, the severest form, called Cooley's anaemia, is caused by homozygosity of the β^0 gene (β^0/β^0). The heterozygote or carrier state (β/β^0 or β/β^+) is termed thalassaemia minor, and inheritance of β^0/β^+ or β^+/β^+ results in thalassaemia intermedia.

Thalassaemia minor is not a condition that requires therapy, but recognition is important for genetic counselling. It is characterized by low-normal haemoglobin, low MCV, raised HbF and A_2, but normal ferritin. Thalassaemia intermedia has a varied clinical picture and course, and each patient needs full investigation and review to determine the optimal therapy. Anaemia, splenomegaly and marrow hyperplasia are present, but if growth and development are normal, folic acid supplements are the only treatment required. Massive splenomegaly leads to splenectomy, and some patients become transfusion-dependent.

Clinical features. In beta thalassaemia major (β^0/β^0, or severely affected β^0/β^+) the haemolgobin continues to fall in infancy as HbF is reduced. Diagnosis is made between 6 and 12 months of age, by which time the child may be profoundly anaemic with very bizarre hypochromic, microcytic red cells, and nucleated red cells in the peripheral blood. Without transfusion, death would ensue. Transfusion given only when anaemia becomes symptomatic results in skeletal deformities from marrow hypertrophy and massive splenomegly with a poor quality of life.

Management. Treatment now consists of hyper-transfusion regimes, designed to suppress marrow activity by keeping the haemoglobin above 12 g/dl. Splenic enlargement is delayed until later in childhood, and growth and development is normal. Transfusions can be planned for 4-weekly intervals, and can be given overnight so as to avoid missing school, or be given in a day unit with schooling continuing. However, iron is not lost from the body, and as each unit of blood contains approximately 0.25 g of iron, considerable iron overload with cardiac and endocrine sequelae results. Subcutaneous desferrioxamine, given over 12 hours by continuous infusion, 5 or 7 nights a week, chelates iron and promotes iron excretion. Parents and patients are taught to assemble the syringe pump and insert the needle. With education, and good compliance, iron overload problems are delayed. Vitamin C helps the urinary excretion of iron, but should not be given in excess as it may increase cardiac toxicity. Even with good compliance, death from iron overload will occur in early adult life.

Thalassaemia can be cured by bone marrow transplantation, and in those with a compatible sibling this option should be offered between 2 and 8 years of age. Risks of graft-versus-host disease, or infection-related deaths, particularly from cytomegalovirus, must be weighed against risks of long-term transfusions and eventual death from iron overload.

Iron overload results in liver, endocrine and exo-crine gland, skin and cardiac muscle damage. Growth is poor, puberty is delayed, and diabetes may develop. Arrhythmias and cardiomyopathy are serious complications, and cardiac failure the usual cause of death. High-dose desferrioxamine can be given for short periods to reduce iron load rapidly, but has retinal and auditory toxicity. At present, there is no alternative to long-term sub-cutaneous injections.

Ante-natal diagnosis is possible if family studies have been done prior to pregnancy to identify the gene defect responsible. Chorionic villus biopsy in the first trimester will identify a homozygous fetus, and termination can be offered early.

SICKLE CELL ANAEMIA

Sickle cell anaemia (HbSS) is an autosomal recessively inherited haemolytic anaemia resulting from a structural defect of the beta haemoglobin chain. Deoxygenated HbS is relatively insoluble, and distorts red cells into a sickle shape, which sludge in small vessels, become irreversibly sickled, and are removed from the circulation. Incidence is high in West and Central Africa, Cyprus, Greece, the Middle East, India and in the black populations of the USA and West Indies. The carrier rate is as high as 20% in some areas of Central Africa.

Clinical features. The children show features of chronic haemolytic anaemia, with added features typical of red cell sickling. Anaemia is severe (haemoglobin 6−8 g/dl) with reticulocytosis of 10−20%, with occasional sickle cells seen on the blood film. Hepatosplenomegaly is not unusual in young patients, but by 5 years of age splenic infarcts occur and the spleen disappears as 'auto-splenectomy' takes place. HbF is raised to 2−5%, but particularly in Middle East populations may reach levels of 20−30% due to the high incidence of a gene for hereditary persistence of fetal haemoglobin, resulting in a milder clinical course with less sickling crises. Despite the low haemoglobin, children lead active lives, partly because they have become accustomed to the low haemoglobin, but also because HbS is a low-affinity haemoglobin and readily gives up O_2 to the tissues. Features of sickling crises include severe pain caused by infarction in bones, lungs or spleen, often triggered by viral infections, or exposure to cold. Profound anaemia may be due to an episode of acute haemolysis, a viral-induced aplastic crisis (usually parvovirus infection is identified), or folate deficiency. Acute hypovolaemia follows splenic sequestration in young patients, and cerebrovascular accidents are a serious consequence of sickling in cerebral vessels.

Management. Treatment consists of analgesia and plentiful fluids to reduce sickling. Infection is common in infarcted areas, and antibiotics may be required. Transfusions are reserved for severe lung infarction and following cerebral sickling, to keep HbS levels low, and prevent further problems. Regular folic acid is needed and prophylactic penicillin is given to older children.

All members of at-risk populations should be screened and the diagnosis confirmed by haemoglobin electrophoresis. The carrier state has genetic implications and also increases anaesthetic risks. It is essential to maintain adequate oxygenation and hydration during anaesthesia and recovery to prevent sickling. Early diagnosis has been found to reduce morbidity in childhood as parent education is improved. Ante-natal screening of families will identify infants at risk of inheriting HbSS. Cord blood electrophoresis on these babies will show HbF and a small amount of HbS in the affected infant, instead of the expected HbA. By 6 months of age, when significant HbA should be present, only HbF and S are found. HbF protects the infant from sickling and other crises which start to appear in late infancy as the proportion of HbF falls.

HAEMOLYTIC DISEASE OF THE NEWBORN

A Rhesus (Rh) negative mother will produce anti-D in response to fetal Rh-positive red cells that cross the placenta, usually at the time of delivery. The antibody will affect subsequent Rh-positive pregnancies. Fetal cells are coated with antibody and haemolysed, resulting in anaemia and erythroid hyperplasia with outpouring of nucleated red cells. Increasing anaemia leads to oedema, cardiac failure and pre-term delivery or fetal death. The clinical implications of this condition are discussed in Chapter 7.

Institution of anti-D prophylaxis has reduced the incidence of Rh haemolytic disease of the newborn, and improvements in intra-uterine transfusion techniques and neonatal care for the pre-term has greatly improved the outlook for those affected. Other red cell antigens, such as Kell, Duffy and C and E of the Rh complex, cause the same clinical picture, but their incidence is low. ABO incompatibility rarely causes severe fetal haemolysis, but may be a cause of neonatal jaundice (see p. 106).

HEREDITARY SPHEROCYTOSIS

Hereditary spherocytosis (HS) is a structural abnormality of the red cell membrane inherited as an autosomal dominant condition. It is the commonest form of inherited haemolytic anaemia in Northern Europeans, with a family history present in at least 75% of cases. Presentation is in childhood, although diagnosis may be delayed until adulthood. Episodes of mild anaemia and jaundice, often following a viral infection, may be noted and investigations reveal the characteristic blood film features of anaemia, with reticulocytosis and microspherocytes. Red cell osmotic fragility is increased. More unusually, a child will present with profound anaemia, but with normal white cells and platelets. This is caused by an 'aplastic crisis' following parvovirus infection. In late teenage or adult life, pigment gallstones may form. HS is a cause of prolonged neonatal jaundice.

Management. The definitive treatment for HS is splenectomy, which does not cure the defect, but as abnormal red cells are no longer trapped in the splenic vessels, haemolysis is reduced and the red cell life span is lengthened. Splenectomy should be deferred until the early teens when the benefits outweigh the risk of infection. Pneumococcal vaccination (Pneumovax) and prophylactic penicillin are needed. Occasionally, severe haemolytic episodes lead to early splenectomy, but most patients can be managed conservatively with long-term folic acid supplements. HS is a mild disease, compatible with normal activities throughout life and a normal life span.

GLUCOSE-6-PHOSPHATE DEHYDROGENASE DEFICIENCY

Glucose-6-phosphate dehydrogenase (G6PD) deficiency is an inherited red cell enzyme deficiency affecting the pentose phosphate pathway. It is common in West Africa, the Mediterranean, the Middle East, Thailand and China, but very rare in Northern Europeans. Inheritance is X-linked recessive, so the disease is seen in males, with heterozygote females having approximately 50% of normal enzyme levels, but no clinical manifestations. The condition presents as one of four clinical patterns:

Acute drug-induced haemolysis

Oxidant drugs result in NADP accumulation in the red cell, and G6PD is required to reduce this back to NADPH. Deficiency results in irreversibly oxidized red cells and haemolysis. Drugs implicated are anti-malarials, sulphonamides, some antibiotics, and some analgesics. These drugs should be avoided as their use will result in acute intravascular haemolysis, with anaemia, jaundice, and haemoglobinuria, typically starting 2–3 days after exposure. If use of the drug cannot be avoided, adequate hydration, prevention of hypotension and transfusion should prevent the major renal complications of intravascular haemolysis.

Favism

Mediterranean or Middle Eastern type G6PD-deficient patients are sensitive to the fava bean or the pollen of the fava plant, and severe haemolysis occurs soon after contact. Not all episodes of contact result in haemolysis and the patient is also at risk from oxidant drugs and infections.

Chronic haemolysis

The rare North European type causes low-grade haemolysis, particularly after infections which may also cause haemolysis in other G6PD-deficient patients.

Neonatal jaundice

Seen particularly in the Mediterranean form of G6PD deficiency, jaundice develops 2–5 days after birth and reaches high levels, so that exchange transfusion to prevent kernicterus may be indicated. Often no exposure to oxidant drugs is identified.

Clinical features. G6PD deficiency should be suspected in male patients of the appropriate ethnic background with acute haemolysis. The blood film will be normal when not haemolysing, but will show irregular, fragmented red cells, reticulocytosis, and apparent haemoglobin separation from the red cell membrane during haemolytic episodes. The diagnosis is confirmed by G6PD assay, but as the enzyme level is higher in immature red cells, it may appear normal in active haemolytic states with reticulocytosis. The test should be repeated when the haemolytic episode is over.

Management. Treatment is by long-term folate supplements together with education and prevention of contact with oxidant drugs and fava beans. Parents should carry a list of drugs to avoid and this list would be displayed prominently in hospital notes and sent to GPs. There is no place for splenectomy.

Coagulation disorders

NORMAL HAEMOSTASIS

Haemostasis is maintained by a complex system of activators and inhibitors of clotting with positive and negative feedback mechanisms, which are capable of preventing massive blood loss from minor vessel wall lesions, and yet can be self-limiting to the damaged area, ensuring continued circulation of the blood. Congenital or acquired defects within this complex system will result in clinical syndromes of bleeding or a thrombotic tendency. The major components of this haemo-

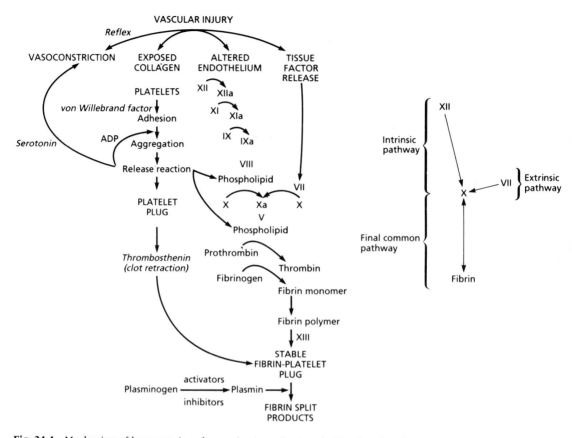

Fig. 24.4 Mechanism of haemostasis and screening investigations for bleeding disorders. (Adapted from Nathan DG, Oski FA. (Eds) *Haematology of Infancy and Childhood*, 3rd Edn. 1987.)

static system are the blood vessels, platelets, and circulating coagulation and fibrinolytic factors.

Figure 24.4 shows the response to vascular injury leading to formation of a stable clot, and the basic investigations to identify the abnormality. Factor assays will be required to confirm a diagnosis. The investigation of bleeding in childhood is shown in Figure 24.5.

Bruises (ecchymoses) and mucocutaneous bleeding may result from vessel wall abnormalities, such as hereditary haemorrhagic telangiectasia or Ehlers–Danlos syndrome. Scurvy (p. 547) presents with a vasculitic peri-follicular haemorrhagic rash. Henoch–Schönlein purpura (p. 261) is also a vasculitic rash, with normal platelets and coagulation. Platelet disorders result in bruises, mucocutaneous bleeding and petechiae, which are pin-point sub-

cutaneous haemorrhagic spots that do not blanch on pressure. Platelets may be quantitatively defective following reduced production or increased destruction, or functionally abnormal with either inherited or acquired defects (Table 24.5). Significant bleeding is unlikely to occur until counts fall below $50 \times 10^9/l$, unless there has been surgery or trauma. In patients with platelet levels between 20 and $50 \times 10^9/l$, bruises will appear in response to minor trauma and epistaxis may be a problem. In patients with platelets below $20 \times 10^9/l$, severe spontaneous bleeding may occur, and petechiae will be present. Severe coagulation factor deficiencies result in spontaneous muscle and joint bleeds, particularly from late infancy onwards. Surprisingly little bleeding occurs in early infancy, although there may be bleeding at separation of

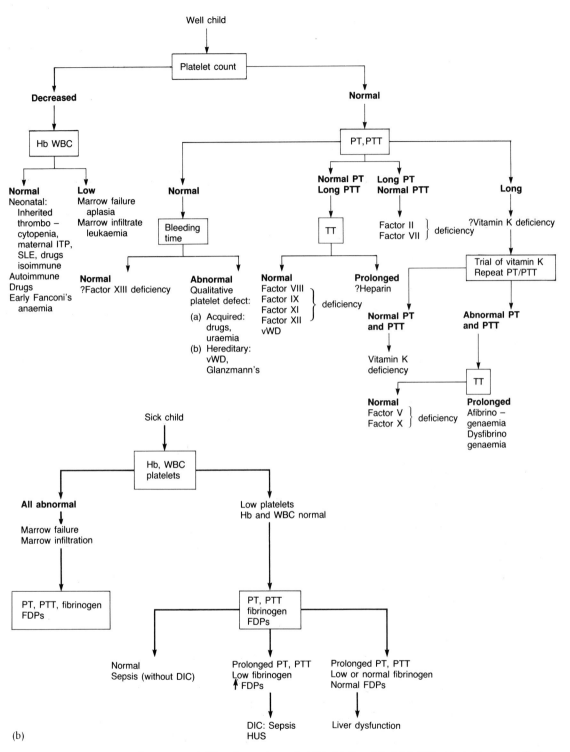

Fig. 24.5 Investigations of bleeding in childhood. (a) The well child. (b) The sick child. PTT tests: intrinsic and final common pathways; PT tests: extrinsic and final common pathways; and TT tests: final common pathways. (Adapted from Gross SJ, Stuart MJ. (1977) *Clin Perinatol* **4**: 259)

Table 24.5 Classification of platelet abnormalities.

Functional defects
Inherited
  von Willebrand's disease
  Storage pool disorders
  Glanzmann's thrombasthenia
  Bernard–Soulier syndrome
Acquired
  Drugs, e.g. aspirin
  Uraemia
  Myeloproliferative disorders

Quantitative defects

Reduced production
Congenital
  TAR
  Fanconi's anaemia
  Bernard–Soulier syndrome
  Wiscott–Aldrich syndrome
Acquired
  Marrow infiltrate, e.g. leukaemia, solid tumours
  Severe aplastic anaemia
  Toxins, drugs

Reduced survival
Immune mediated
  Auto-immune (SLE, ITP)
  Iso-immune (neonatal)
  Drug-induced
DIC
Microangiopathic haemolytic anaemia, e.g. HUS
Giant haemangiomata (Kasabach–Merritt syndrome)
Splenomegaly
Massive or exchange transfusions
Extracorporeal circulation

the umbilical cord (classically factor XIII deficiency, but also others), or if circumcision is performed. Mild degrees of factor deficiency may not be detected until later in childhood, after dental extractions or other minor operations. A very sick child, with acute onset of massive bruising and haemorrhage, is most likely to have disseminated intravascular coagulation (DIC), although leukaemia and solid tumours with marrow infiltration may also present with acute onset haemorrhagic manifestations.

Platelets are detected in the fetus from the eleventh week of gestation, and by 28 weeks are at normal levels. Factor VIII is within the normal range from as early as the twentieth week of gestation, rising to above 'normal' levels at delivery. Vitamin K dependent factors (factors II, VII, IX and X) are low in the term newborn, approximately 50% of the adult level, and even lower in pre-term infants. Antithrombin III and protein C, both coagulation inhibitors, are also low; overall, a neonate has a tendency to thrombosis rather than haemorrhage. Factors XI and XII are low at birth, which produces no clinical abnormality, but has an *in-vitro* effect, prolonging the PTT. Breast milk is low in vitamin K, and a completely breast-fed baby may be at risk of vitamin K deficiency, particularly if other risk factors, such as prematurity or antibiotic therapy, are present. Prophylactic vitamin K given soon after birth reduces the risk of haemorrhagic disease of the newborn.

Inherited bleeding disorders

Inherited bleeding disorders occur in approximately 1 : 10 000 births, with haemophilia A accounting for 80% of these disorders. The most important of these disorders are discussed here.

HAEMOPHILIA A

This is a sex-linked, recessive disorder, in which the bleeding tendency is due to a partial or complete factor VIII deficiency. Normal factor VIII levels are 0.5–1.5 IU/ml of plasma; severe haemophilia is defined as <0.01 IU/ml factor VIII, moderate as 0.01–0.05 IU/ml, and mild as 0.05–0.5 IU/ml. Within a kinship, the severity of haemophilia remains constant. The factor VIII molecule consists of a small coagulant portion, termed FVIIIC, attached to a large portion which is essential in platelet function, the von Willebrand factor, or FVIII : vWF. In haemophilia, FVIIIC is reduced, but FVIII : vWF is normal and platelet function is intact.

Clinical features. A family history is present in more than 50% of cases, others are spontaneous mutations. The diagnosis is made by a history of bruising, spontaneous muscle and joint bleeds, or secondary haemorrhage following surgery. A bleed is heralded by joint stiffening, followed by severe pain, and if no treatment is given, the joint becomes swollen and immobile with a large haemarthrosis. With conservative treatment the pain and swelling will slowly resolve, but will leave a chronically damaged joint, with muscle wasting, and an inflamed and swollen synovium, which bleeds repeatedly. Eventually bone damage and joint ankylosis occurs. Affected joints are usually large, weight-bearing joints, such as knees and ankles, with elbows next most commonly affected. Small joints, such as fingers and wrists, are rarely sites of spontaneous bleeding. Full blood count, platelets and bleeding time are normal, but the PTT is prolonged. A low FVIIIC level confirms the diagnosis.

Management. Treatment is by replacement of the missing factor, as cryoprecipitate or factor VIII concentrate. Rest and adequate analgesia are essential, with mobilization once the pain has settled to prevent muscle weakness and joint instability. Haemarthroses should not be aspirated. Early treatment prevents the sequence of events leading to joint damage, but delayed or inadequate treatment may result in a bleed taking weeks to resolve. Parents are taught to administer factor VIII intravenously and keep supplies at home. By 8–10 years of age, some patients will give their own therapy. Haemophiliacs should lead as normal a life as possible and not be restricted from any activities except body contact sports. Moderate and mild haemophiliacs have few spontaneous bleeds, but may have joint bleeds in response to trauma, or bleed following dental extraction. The same principles of early, adequate treatment apply.

Intravenous DDAVP will raise factor VIII levels by approximately 20% in moderate and mild haemophiliacs, an effect that can be repeated for 2–3 days, thereby allowing a bleed or dental extractions to be treated without the use of blood products. External bleeding should be treated with the clot-stabilizing drug, tranexamic acid which is an anti-fibrinolytic agent, until the risk of secondary haemorrhage is past. Aggressive use of blood products, despite careful donor selection and screening, carries a risk of transfusion-derived viral infections. Hepatitis B vaccine should be given to all newly diagnosed haemophiliacs and heat-treated factor VIII concentrates used in preference to cryoprecipitate.

Carriers are detected by measuring the FVIIIC/FVIII : vWF ratio, or with specific gene probes identified by analysis of index patient DNA if available. Ante-natal diagnosis is then possible by chorion villus biopsy at 10–12 weeks gestation. If an affected male fetus is identified by gene probes, early termination can be offered. If no informative probe is available, fetal factor VIII can be measured by fetal blood sampling at 16–18 weeks gestation, and late termination is possible if levels are undetectable. Termination of pregnancy may not be acceptable to the family, in which case ante-natal diagnosis is inappropriate, but an atraumatic delivery should be planned.

HAEMOPHILIA B (CHRISTMAS DISEASE)

This is a sex-linked recessive bleeding disorder, due to absent or reduced factor IX. It accounts for 10% of all inherited bleeding disorders. Presentation and diagnosis is as haemophilia A, but with a low factor IX assay and normal factor VIII assay. Principles of treatment are identical to haemophilia A, but using factor IX concentrates.

The carrier state is hard to define, as it is based on factor IX levels only and carriers may have normal factor IX levels. The normal fetus has a low factor IX, so fetal blood sampling is open to interpretive error. Reliable gene probes have not yet been identified for the majority of haemophilia B kinships.

VON WILLEBRAND'S DISEASE

This is a very pleomorphic disorder, but essentially it is a defect of the entire FVIIIC/FVIII : vWF molecule, resulting in low FVIIIC, and abnormal platelet function. It is inherited as an autosomal dominant condition. Heterozygotes are partially deficient, with a relatively mild clinical course characterized by epistaxis, gastrointestinal bleeds, and in females, menorrhagia. Homozygotes, with

<0.01 IU/ml FVIIIC, have a clinical picture more like severe haemophilia A, although spontaneous joint bleeds are unusual. Investigations show a moderately prolonged PTT, normal PT, TT and platelet count, but prolonged bleeding time, and abnormal platelet aggregation with ristocetin. Treatment is with cryoprecipitate or factor VIII concentrate which contain both FVIIIC and FVIII : vWF. DDAVP also produces a rise in FVIIIC.

Acquired bleeding disorders

ACUTE IDIOPATHIC THROMBOCYTOPENIC PURPURA (ITP)

This is defined as thrombocytopenic purpura in the absence of drug toxicity, or other disease. Normal or increased numbers of megakaryocytes are present in the bone marrow. It is the commonest cause of thrombocytopenia in childhood, and usually follows a brief, self-limiting course. Diagnostic distinction from leukaemia and aplastic anaemia, which require early active intervention, is necessary. The peak age incidence is between 3 and 6 years, although it may occur throughout childhood. The sex ratio is equal.

Acute ITP in childhood is believed to result from interaction with viral antigen/antibody complexes, which cause partial aggregation of platelets, and their subsequent removal by the spleen. Marrow production is increased, but is unable to compensate for the greatly decreased platelet half-life. Once viral antigen/antibody complexes are cleared from the body, the process is 'switched-off', and counts return to normal.

The chronic relapsing form, seen in adults and adolescents is an auto-immune process, and IgG may be demonstrated bound to platelet membranes. The condition may occur in conjunction with other auto-immune conditions, such as systemic lupus erythematosis, auto-immune haemolytic anaemia, and some lymphoproliferative disorders.

Clinical features. Onset is acute, often 2–3 weeks after an acute viral infection, with bruising and petechiae and sometimes mucus membrane bleed-

ing. Gross gastrointestinal or urinary tract bleeding is rare.

Investigations. The blood count is normal apart from thrombocytopenia, generally $<20 \times 10^9/l$. Bone marrow examination shows increased megakaryocytes.

Management. Recovery is spontaneous in >80% of cases, the natural history of the condition from presentation to recovery being from 2 to 4 weeks. Most patients, therefore, do not require treatment, but should be observed until spontaneous recovery occurs. Treatment is indicated if significant mucus membrane bleeding is present, or if no recovery is observed. Intravenous immunoglobulin, given daily for 3–5 days, acts by reticuloendothelial blockade, preventing splenic clearance of platelets. Response is within a few days, and side-effects are rare. High-dose steroids may be used, but recovery takes 7–10 days, and considerable side-effects such as hypertension, gastrointestinal bleeding and glycosuria can complicate the treatment course. The risk of intracranial bleeding, estimated at 1%, should be weighed against side-effects of treatment by steroids or immunoglobulin.

Ten to twenty per cent of patients follow a chronic relapsing course, and may require long-term, low-dose steroids to maintain safe platelet levels, or splenectomy if significant bleeding is observed. Prophylactic penicillin and pneumococcal vaccine should be given if splenectomy is performed.

DISSEMINATED INTRAVASCULAR COAGULATION

Disseminated intravascular coagulation (DIC) is a process triggered by many varied stimuli, in which there is activation of the coagulation cascade leading to fibrin deposition, followed by fibrinolysis and eventual depletion of coagulation factors, fibrinogen and platelets. The net result is bleeding. It is an uncontrolled exaggeration of normal haemostatic mechanisms.

DIC may be compensated, with evidence of increased fibrin degradation products (FDPs), but coagulation tests are normal and there is no haemorrhage. Uncompensated DIC is characterized by prolonged coagulation tests, due to falling fibrinogen, platelets, and coagulation factors, particularly factors V, VIII and XIII together with increased FDPs, but no haemorrhage. Clinical DIC has the above features, with haemorrhage in addition. Despite the intravascular coagulation, evidence of fibrin deposition is rarely found at autospy. DIC may be triggered by infections, trauma, intravascular haemolysis, or tumour lysis.

Clinical features. Presentation may be acute, with a shocked, hypotensive child admitted to the hospital. Purpuric areas may be present, or appear rapidly, and oozing from puncture sites or frank haemorrhage is seen. This florid picture is typical of DIC caused by bacterial endotoxin, commonly meningococcal.

Management. This involves treatment of the underlying cause, when identified. Hypotension should be corrected and appropriate antibiotics given in adequate doses. Correction of the coagulation abnormality is essential, including the use of fresh frozen plasma (FFP), cryoprecipitate, and platelet transfusions. FFP should be used for correction of both hypotension and coagulation defects prior to laboratory results being available. Blood counts and coagulation tests should be repeated every few hours to determine the need for blood products. Massive platelet and FFP transfusion may be required if consumption is continuing and rapid changes in clinical and laboratory findings may be observed. Once the underlying disorder is controlled, the requirement for supportive blood products reduces and gradually bleeding stops and tests return to normal. Severe areas of gangrene and necrosis, particularly of the periphery, may result.

The use of heparin in the treatment of DIC is limited to situations in which compensated DIC is likely to worsen as a result of treatment for the underlying disorder, such as the start of treatment for acute promyelocytic leukaemia. Heparin has no place in the treatment of established, uncompensated DIC.

Granulocyte abnormalities

Defective granulocytes result in recurrent severe bacterial infections such as pneumonia, septicaemia, or local abscess formation. If neutrophil numbers are reduced, bone marrow examination is required to assess myeloid precursors, their growth characteristics in culture, and to rule out marrow infiltration. A functional defect is suspected if the count is normal, and further tests will assess the ability of neutrophils to migrate to the site of infection, engulf and kill bacteria.

NEUTROPENIA

Low numbers of circulating neutrophils (neutropenia) may be acquired as a result of marrow hypoplasia from drugs or infections, or infiltration, auto-immune states, and hypersplenism. In cyclical neutropenia, the neutrophils swing from undetectable to normal levels in peripheral blood, following a 21-day cycle. Mouth ulcers and skin infections occur when the counts are at the nadir. Marrow myeloid precursors are reduced cyclically. In benign idiopathic neutropenia, marrow precursors appear normal, and infections are rarely severe.

Kostmann's disease. In this condition, infants are born with absent neutrophils and myeloid precursors. It is probably autosomal recessive in inheritance and the mortality in infancy is high.

DEFECTIVE NEUTROPHIL FUNCTION

This can either be an acquired disorder, as in chronic malnutrition, or be inherited, as in chronic granulomatous disease.

Chronic granulomatous disease

This is an X-linked recessive disorder in which neutrophils have markedly impaired bacteriocidal ability, especially for *Staph. aureus*, serratia species, and fungi. Affected boys have chronic recurrent infections with granuloma and abscess formation, resulting in hepatosplenomegaly, destructive lung lesions, and osteomyelitis. Treatment consists of close surveillance, prompt institution of adequate antibiotics, and prolonged therapy to ensure eradication of infection. Despite these measures, the disease is usually fatal in childhood. Bone marrow transplantation should be considered early, before intractable infection is present.

Immunodeficiency

hThe immune response is discussed in detail in Chapter 21. In summary, B lymphocytes produce immunoglobulins which are responsible for humoral immunity. T cells are responsible for cellular immunity. An adequate immune response depends on an interaction between T and B lymphocytes.

Immunodeficiency may be primary and caused by a genetic defect or secondary to other conditions such as nephrotic syndrome, malnutrition, cytotoxic drugs or AIDS following infection with human immunodeficiency virus infection (p. 361).

Primary immunodeficiencies are rare, but a number of different types have been recognized.

TRANSIENT HYPOGAMMAGLOBULINAEMIA OF INFANCY

This occurs as a result of delayed maturation of the immune system. The normal fetus can produce IgM in response to infection by the twentieth gestational week. At birth, maternal IgG is present in the neonatal circulation as the result of transplacental passage, and the infant does not start production of IgG until 3 months of age. Some infants, presenting with chest infection and wheeze, are found to have lower than expected IgG and IgA, although B-cell numbers are normal. Normal immunoglobulin production starts by 3 years of age, but antibiotics and immunoglobulin infusions may be required in the interim.

X-LINKED AGAMMAGLOBULINAEMIA (BRUTON'S DISEASE)

This is characterized by a decrease in all immunoglobulin subtypes, and absent circulating B cells.

Repeated severe bacterial infections occur from late infancy, maternal IgG giving some protection in early infancy. A family history of death from overwhelming infection in maternal male relatives may be obtained. Treatment is by vigorous antibiotic therapy for infections, and regular injections of immunoglobulin. The prognosis is good, although by adolescence, long-term complications may appear.

SEVERE COMBINED IMMUNODEFICIENCY (SCID, SWISS TYPE)

This is characterized by absent B and T lymphocytes, absent lymph nodes and thymus tissue, and severe bacterial, viral and fungal infections. It is inherited as an autosomal or X-linked recessive. Affected children rarely survive the first 2 years of life despite intensive supportive care. Bone marrow transplantation from an HLA-matched sibling is curative, but if there is no compatible donor, mismatched transplants, despite considerable morbidity from graft-versus-host disease, are giving some hope in an otherwise uniformly fatal disease.

OTHERS

Other conditions may be associated with immunodeficiency including ataxia telangiectasia, Wiscott–Aldrich syndrome (thrombocytopenia and eczema), and Di George syndrome (absent thymus with cardiac and great vessel anomalies). Partial defects affecting only one antibody class are also seen.

Generalized lymphadenopathy

During childhood, the lymph nodes and thymus are larger than in adult life, and will fluctuate in size in response to local infections, or generalized infections, usually viral. At puberty, the lymphatic tissue in the body regresses, although nodal enlargement will still occur in response to infection. Table 24.6 lists the causes of generalized lymphadenopathy.

Generalized lymphadenopathy should be investigated with a chest X-ray, full blood count, and a search for a causative agent, including EBV

Table 24.6 Causes of generalized lymphadenopathy in children.

Infection
Viral
  Infectious mononucleosis
  Cytomegalovirus
Bacterial
  M. tuberculosis
  Brucella
Others
  Toxoplasma gondii

Malignant disease
Leukaemias
Lymphomas

Disorders of the immune system
Chronic granulomatous disease
Agammaglobulinaemia
Kawasaki's disease (p. 478)

and tuberculosis. A trial of antibiotics may be indicated; persistently enlarged, or craggy, matted nodes should be biopsied.

Recurrent infections may be a normal feature of young children, or reflect granulocyte dysfunction, or an immune-deficiency disorder. Baseline investigations should include a full blood count with differential, serum immunoglobulins, chest X-ray, and careful examination for lymph nodes. Failure to thrive suggests a significant defect warranting neutrophil and lymphocyte function tests.

Further reading

Nathan DG, Oski FA. (Eds) *Haematology of Infancy and Childhood*, 3rd Edn. 1987 WB Saunders, Philadelphia.
Hoffbrand AV, Lewis SM. (Eds) *Postgraduate Haematology*, 2nd Edn. 1981 Heinemann, London.
Dacie JV, Lewis SM. (Eds) *Practical Haematology*, 6th Edn. 1984 Churchill Livingstone, Edinburgh.

25
CANCER IN CHILDREN

Malignant disease is rare in children under the age of 15 years and has an annual incidence of approximately 1:10 000. A general practitioner would therefore see only one or two cases in a career, and the general paediatrician a handful of cases every decade. Nevertheless, it is the second commonest cause of non-accidental death in children. Because cancer is unexpected, children are often referred to specialist units after treatment for other more common disorders whose symptoms have been mimicked by the malignancy. It is important, therefore, that paediatricians are aware of the spectrum of presenting symptoms of malignancy and that these are borne in mind when conditions behave in an atypical manner. In this chapter some aspects of the aetiology, presentation, investigation and management of paediatric malignancy are considered.

Aetiological factors

Only very rarely can an answer be provided to the inevitable question posed by the parents of a newly diagnosed child with cancer, 'What could have caused the disease?'. With the exception of retinoblastoma, where the genetic basis has now been clearly defined, the response usually given is that cancer develops as a result of a combination of factors, including individual predisposition, viral and environmental factors.

FAMILIAL

For practical purposes, the likelihood of a sibling developing cancer is negligible and, in general,

parents should be reassured that there is no need for any special vigilance or screening tests. Statistically, the risk is increased to about three times that of the normal population, and this relates in particular to brain tumours, sarcomas and lymphomas.

There are a number of relatively rare inherited diseases which are associated with an increased risk of malignancy and some of these are listed in Table 25.1.

Genetic factors. Detectable abnormalities include:
1 Defects in the somatic cell karyotype which are associated with the development of cancer in certain tissues, such as deletion of chromosome 13 and retinoblastoma.
2 Chromosomal abnormalities found in the tumour cell karyotype such as the t(4:11) translocation associated with lymphoblastic leukaemia.
3 Alterations in genes on individual chromosomes which may be related to malignant transformation of that cell such as c-myc amplification seen in Burkitt's lymphoma.

Somatic chromosomal abnormality. Retinoblastoma (p. 470) is a rare example of a tumour which is clearly inheritable and for which the mechanism of inheritance and chromosomal location have been extensively studied. Forty per cent of retinoblastomas are familial. About 5% of cases have a visible deletion of a variable portion of chromosome 13 and this is the site of the retinoblastoma gene.

Patients with small deletions of chromosome 13

Table 25.1 Inherited diseases which are associated with an increased incidence of malignancy.

Primary disease	Inheritance	Predisposed tumour
Neurofibromatosis	AD	Sarcoma, neuroma, meningioma, glioma, phaeochromocytoma, leukaemia
Tuberous sclerosis	AD	Fibroma, cardiac rhabdomyosarcoma
Familial polyposis coli	AD	Colonic carcinoma
Peutz–Jegher	AD	Ovarian granulosa cell sarcoma
Haemachromatosis	AD/AR	Hepatic carcinoma
Multiple exostosis	AD	Osteosarcoma, chondrosarcoma
Bruton's disease, Wiskott–Aldrich syndrome	XR	Leukaemia, lymphoma
Ataxia–telangiectasia	AR	Leukaemia, lymphoma, glioma
Bloom's syndrome	AR	Leukaemia, gastrointestinal
Fanconi's disease	AR	Acute myeloid leukaemia, hepatic
Beckwith's syndrome	AR	Adrenal carcinoma, Wilms' tumour
Tyrosinemia, galactosemia, Wilson's syndrome, alpha 1-antitrypsin deficiency	AR	Hepatic carcinoma

AD = Autosomal dominant.
AR = Autosomal recessive.
XR = X-linked recessive.

also have a reduction in esterase D activity, a gene which is close to the retinoblastoma gene. This provides a convenient way to screen large numbers of retinoblastoma patients for the presence of chromosome 13 deletion. DNA probes, detecting polymorphism within the gene, have been developed and predict the likelihood of retinoblastoma in asymptomatic children.

Predisposition to carcinogenesis due to a defect in the repair of DNA may be inherited. Following injury by X-irradiation, ultraviolet (UV) light or chemotherapy, the damaged genetic material cannot be correctly reconstituted. This is important in patients with Fanconi's anaemia (p. 429) and ataxia–telangiectasia (p. 293).

Karyotype abnormalities in tumour cells. With more refined analysis, an increasing number of chromosomal abnormalities are detected which appear consistently in certain tumours and probably have a direct role in initial malignant transformation. These include the translocations in myeloid leukaemia and some forms of lymphoblastic leukaemia. Monosomy 7 is found in a pre-leukaemic myelodysplastic syndrome. Some cases of Wilms tumour are associated with deletion of chromosome 11.

ONCOGENES AND MALIGNANCY

An 'oncogene' may be defined as a base sequence which is found in the genome of certain retro-viruses, which when transferred into animal host cells or cell lines, causes malignant transformation. Identical sequences have been found in the human genome and are called 'proto-oncogenes' or often 'oncogenes' for short. Many of these proto-oncogenes encode proteins which are important in the normal control of cell division and maturation. The viral genes are not subject to the same controlling influences as the normal mammalian genes, and this is thought to be the mechanism by which the oncogenic retro-viruses induce malignancy.

Conditions where chromosome translocations appear to be involved in oncogene over-activity are B cell lymphoma and chronic granulocytic leukaemia (CGL).

VIRAL FACTORS

The influences of viruses may be either direct or indirect. In African Burkitt's lymphoma, the role of Epstein–Barr virus (EBV) has been studied extensively. A high percentage of lymphoma cells are shown to carry the EBV genome, whereas in the European or sporadic form, less than 10% are shown to be EBV positive. EBV has the ability to 'transform' or 'immortalize' an abnormal B cell clone which has appeared due to random chromosomal alteration. In Africa, the likelihood of the latter may be increased due to B-cell stimulation by endemic malaria.

Human immunodeficiency virus (HIV) may exert an indirect effect by inducing immunodepression leading to the development of lymphomas or Kaposi's sarcoma.

ENVIRONMENTAL FACTORS

It is well known that accidental or deliberate exposure to radiation leads to an increased risk of leukaemia. In the past, prenatal exposure to low-dose irradiation during pelvimetry resulted in various types of malignancy, the incidence of which was directly proportional to the dose received. Children may be more prone than adults to radio-induced tumours mainly affecting the thyroid and parathyroid glands, bone, soft tissue and brain.

The controversy regarding leukaemic clusters adjacent to nuclear energy installations remains unresolved. It is likely that a firm conclusion will only be reached once the number of children involved and time of follow-up are sufficient to allow adequate statistical analysis of disease incidence. Whether the current circumstantial evidence will halt the expansion of the nuclear energy programme remains to be seen, but if so, a definitive answer may never be reached.

Exposure to UV light in susceptible genotypes, such as xeroderma pigmentosa, may lead to skin cancer. In the normal adult there is a clear link between sun exposure and squamous cell carcinoma, but the incidence of skin cancer in children is very low.

CHEMICALS

Prolonged treatment with androgens for conditions such as Fanconi's anaemia is associated with an increased incidence of hepatic carcinoma. The prenatal administration of diethylstilboestrol is associated with clear cell adenocarcinoma of the vagina in offspring. Cytotoxic agents, in particular the alkylating agents, are associated with an increased incidence of malignancy, especially myelogenous leukaemia. This risk is, however, small and usually occurs in heavily pre-treated patients, often those who have had extensive irradiation, for example in relapsed Hodgkin's disease.

Principles of treatment

SURGERY

Surgery is the oldest therapy for malignant disease and continues to have an important role. Complete excision alone will cure about 30% of localized osteosarcoma and 70% of Stage I Wilms' tumour, but the high incidence of covert metastases in most tumours means that cure also requires systemic chemotherapy.

Attempts to resect tumour completely at presentation are now made less frequently due to effective pre-operative chemotherapy. This makes the surgery simpler and less extensive, with consequently fewer sequelae. It may also increase the likelihood of complete surgical excision, removing the need for radiotherapy to residual disease.

Another use of surgery is the 'second look' procedure following chemotherapy. With certain tumours, e.g. rhabdomyosarcoma and germ cell tumours, this may have an important role in confirming remission status and helping to decide the need for local irradiation or further chemotherapy.

CHEMOTHERAPY

Cytotoxic drugs are essentially cell poisons for which the therapeutic ratio (the proportion of tumour cells killed to normal cells killed) is high. The level of 'acceptable toxicity' depends on the prognosis of the particular tumour, and with many regimens the threshold between toxic and therapeutic dose is low. At one extreme, localized Wilms' tumour may be curable with 10 weeks' out-patient treatment using a single drug, vincristine, with minimal complications. At the other extreme, multi-agent regimens for metastatic neuroblastoma require frequent hospital admission for supportive care, followed by toxic high-dose chemo-radiotherapy with bone marrow rescue.

For some localized diseases only one or two drugs are used, but in most regimens for leukaemia and solid tumours several active agents are combined. The methods of drug scheduling may be the result of proven synergistic activity but are usually somewhat empirical. Often agents without overlapping toxicity are combined to enable maximal doses to be given. As a general principle, the most effective way of giving chemotherapy is to give as much as possible over a short period of time. The previous philosophy of 'maintenance therapy' giving relatively low drug doses over a prolonged period has lost favour. Regimens are becoming shorter, but often at the expense of considerable early morbidity.

RADIOTHERAPY

The problems of the late effects of irradiation on growing bone and soft tissues have led to the increasing tendency to avoid irradiation where possible, or to reduce the dose to a level which spares normal tissue without compromising anti-tumour activity. Irradiation is rarely used at presentation. An exception is when there is spinal cord or optic nerve compression where a short course may be appropriate. However, chemotherapy may be equally effective under these circumstances, particularly with lymphoma or neuroblastoma. The other exception is in the management of brain tumours, where the role of chemotherapy is still under evaluation, and radiotherapy is the mainstay of treatment for inoperable lesions. With many solid tumours, irradiation is used to consolidate local control after chemotherapy and surgery.

Late effects

As more than half of all children with cancer are now expected to be cured, considerable attention is being paid to the concept of 'cure at least cost'.

With improved pre-operative chemotherapy, mutilating surgical procedures can now be avoided in the majority of patients and major surgical sequelae should be a thing of the past. Long-term complications from chemotherapy and irradiation are often due to an interaction of the two.

GROWTH ARREST

Radiation-related growth defects may be due to a direct effect on bone and soft tissue. For example, following treatment of an orbital rhabdomyosarcoma in the younger child there will be considerable facial asymmetry due to underdevelopment of the orbit and its contents. Normal growth of the spine and hip may be seriously impaired by radiotherapy to adjacent tissues. Inclusion of the long bone epiphyses in younger children will lead to growth arrest and limb asymmetry, and irradiation to the diaphyseal region may lead to abnormal bone modelling.

Linear growth will also be affected indirectly by the influence of radiation on hormonal function. Abnormal growth of children with cancer is often multi-factorial, involving subtle abnormalities in function of the pituitary gland or on hypothalamic production of growth hormone releasing factor.

In general, any child who has had cranial irradiation must be closely followed at a growth clinic, jointly by oncologists and paediatric endocrinologists. Any suggestions of reduced growth velocity indicates evaluation of hypothalamo-pituitary function. If this is abnormal, growth hormone replacement therapy should be considered.

DEVELOPMENTAL IMPAIRMENT

Whole brain irradiation for leukaemia has been shown to have a small but significant effect on reducing IQ and causing subtle deficits in areas of learning such as numeracy. This has been used as an argument for replacing irradiation with more intensive intrathecal and CNS-directed chemotherapy. Adverse effects are dose- and age-dependent and are most marked in young children with brain tumours who receive higher dose treatment.

INFERTILITY

Treatment-related infertility is an issue frequently raised by parents. Irradiation of ovaries and testes, even at small doses, will produce infertility, but there are rarely indications for this form of treatment. Some drugs, in particular, alkylating agents such as cyclophosphamide, will almost invariably cause sterility in boys but the ovary is considerably more resistant and long-term follow-up studies have shown that most girls retain fertility.

SECOND TUMOURS

It is a cruel fact that between 1 and 5% of cancer patients will develop a second tumour as a result of their treatment. Moreover, recent intensification of treatment regimens may increase the likelihood of this further. In general, the complication is dose-related, as in the case of second bone tumours following irradiation for soft tissue sarcoma or retinoblastoma. There is a clear link between second tumours and the administration of alkylating agents. The highest incidence being in Hodgkin's disease where a combination of alkylating agents plus irradiation is involved. Acute myeloid leukaemia is the commonest haematological second tumour, although acute lymphoblastic leukaemia and Hodgkin's disease have also been reported. Soft tissue sarcomas are the usual second solid tumours, apart from those affecting irradiated bone.

Supportive care

COMPLICATIONS OF CHEMOTHERAPY

Sepsis

The source of bacterial sepsis in the immuno-suppressed child is usually endogenous, e.g. gut, skin, oronasopharynx. For this reason, strict isola-tion is not necessary in specialized centres where children with common infectious diseases are not usually managed. In contrast, if the oncology patient is receiving treatment in a unit where there is frequent turnover of general paediatric cases, it is advisable that the child be nursed in a separate cubicle.

Major pathogens vary between hospitals, but the common bacteria are the Gram-negatives (*E. coli*, pseudomonas, and klebsiella) or Gram-positives (*Staphylococcus epidermidis*, *Staph. aureus*, or *Staph. enterococci*). *Staph. epidermidis* has become an increasing problem with widespread use of indwelling central catheters.

The single most important factor in the management of suspected sepsis in immunocompromised patients is the *early* parental administration of appropriate broad-spectrum antibiotics. In the severely neutropenic child deterioration is rapid and the results of blood cultures should not be awaited. If there is significant fever (over 38.5°C) or if the child is clinically unwell, it is preferable to give a short course of intravenous antibiotics and then stop after 3–5 days if the cultures are negative and there has been a rapid resolution of fever. Tachycardia, hypotension or poor peripheral perfusion in the absence of fever should be presumed to be sepsis-related and treated.

It is important that in the child with a persistent fever, regular (at least daily) blood cultures are done. Yeasts and fungi such as *Candida albicans* or aspergillosis are an increasing problem with the more intensive and profoundly immunosuppressive treatment regimens. Early use of intravenous amphotericin has reduced the mortality in children with leukaemia. Viral agents such as herpes simplex, herpes zoster and cytomegalovirus (CMV) are also potential problems. Acyclovir has had a dramatic effect on the management of herpetic lesions. Anti-CMV agents are under investigation.

Use of blood products

Bone marrow suppression may cause thrombo-cytopenia, anaemia and granulocytopenia. Platelet transfusions are readily available and should be used to prevent serious bleeding in thrombocytopenic children. Packed red cells are generally given if the haemoglobin drops below 8 g/dl or if there is symptomatic anaemia. The value of granulocyte transfusion is unproven and these are rarely given.

Intestinal toxicity

After severe myelosuppression, intestinal toxicity is the most common and important acute side-effect of chemotherapy. The rapid cell turnover rate in oral and intestinal mucosa makes these tissues particularly susceptible. Mucositis is commonly seen and although usually of short duration may be extremely painful and distressing.

Severe diarrhoea can occur after intensive chemotherapy and consequent fluid and electrolyte abnormalities require close surveillance and active replacement therapy. On occasions parenteral nutrition is needed. Severe abdominal pain may respond to antispasmodics such as Buscopan but parenteral opiates are often required. In severe cases clinical signs can mimic an acute 'surgical abdomen'.

Central venous catheters

With the increased intensity of chemotherapeutic regimens a high percentage of patients have central venous catheters placed shortly after the diagnosis. The Hickman or Broviac catheter is inserted most commonly in the right atrium, usually via the subclavian or internal jugular vein, using an open surgical approach or percutaneous insertion. The lines are tunnelled for several inches under the skin, emerging on the anterior chest wall. Catheter-related infection usually involves Gram-positive cocci (*Staph. epidermis* or *Staph. aureus*) but the incidence of catheter infection during non-neutropenic periods should be less than 5%.

Tumour lysis syndrome

This results from a rapid breakdown of tumour cells associated with initial chemotherapy for leukaemia or lymphoma. If there is either a high presenting white cell count or extensive nodal disease, even steroids or vincristine will lead to rapid tumour breakdown with release of potassium and uric acid. For this reason it is essential that such patients receive allopurinol and are hydrated with dextrose–saline during the induction period to prevent renal failure, with at least 8-hourly monitoring of electrolytes.

Nausea and vomiting

One of the major difficulties for the child undergoing chemotherapy is the emetic effect of most treatment regimens. Once the child has experienced persistent nausea and vomiting, anticipatory symptoms become a prominent and often intractable problem. A variety of anti-emetic agents exist but few produce a reliable effect and in most patients a variety of cocktails have to be tried. The price of effectiveness may, however, be severe sedation precluding out-patient drug administration. Commonly used drugs include metochlopramide, dexamethasone and lorazepam.

PSYCHO-SOCIAL SUPPORT

Cancer in a child is obviously devastating for the family and the impact on relationships is far reaching and may be irreversible. Specialist social workers are now attached to most units and provide an important link between the medical and nursing team and the families. They may also play a role in liaising with GPs and schools, helping to inform and to clarify the frequent misconceptions concerning children with cancer. In general the children themselves show remarkable resilience, but overt psychological problems can arise and require formal attention by a paediatric psychologist and psychiatrist.

The area of psycho-social support is potentially a very broad one and is often at risk of being neglected in the face of increasing demands on medical and nursing staff time for other aspects of supportive care.

ANALGESIA

Achieving rapid, adequate analgesia for pain at initial presentation, during treatment or during terminal illness is of great importance. Disease-related pain does not usually respond well to non-opiate analgesics and rapid escalations to morphine and diamorphine are recommended. These are often only needed for short periods and potential dependence is of no significance. At presentation, severe bone pain will respond rapidly to effective chemotherapy and opiates can rapidly be tailed off. Steroids may also be of some help with bone pain.

OUT-PATIENT CARE

Many regimens are given as out-patient treatment, during which the patient may be only moderately neutropenic but is always, to some extent, immunocompromised. Under these circumstances, the local paediatrician or the GP may be involved. A low threshold for contacting the specialist centre is essential, but often there are simple anxieties which can be dealt with locally. Contact with infectious diseases is a common problem, particularly with regard to chickenpox and measles. Contact with other children who are in the infectious period either before or after the appearance of a rash is an indication for prophylactic hyper-immune globulin in the case of measles, or zoster immunoglobulin in the case of chickenpox. There is, however, no point in the administration of either of these if more than 72 hours have elapsed since the time of contact. The morbidity of chickenpox has dramatically reduced with the introduction of intravenous acyclovir which should be given at the first sign of the rash. The intravenous route should be used initially although one may change to the oral route if there is a rapid response. Recrudescence of both herpes simplex and zoster lesions should actively be treated with oral or intravenous acyclovir. Although these lesions may initially seem innocuous they can rapidly become progressive.

Contact with other infectious diseases such as mumps or rubella is of little significance and reassurance of the patients is all that is necessary. Whether or not to keep children away from school for prolonged periods because infectious diseases are 'going round' is a difficult problem. In general,

this is undesirable as it is important to try and treat these children as normally as possible.

Septrin prophylaxis is given to children on continuing therapy for acute leukaemia to prevent *Pneumocystis carinii* pneumonia. Despite this, any child on chemotherapy with a dry persistent cough or tachypnoea should immediately be referred back to the specialist centre for assessment and advice.

TERMINAL CARE

Although half of all children with cancer will be cured, there remains the other half where treatment fails and it is important that as much effort is put into permitting a dignified and pain-free death as was expended in the initial aggressive therapy. There is an increasing trend towards the use of specialist home care nurses who provide a high level of support for families caring for dying children at home. The GP, however, plays an important role in the care of such children. It is essential that during the management of the child the local physicians are informed so that in the event of treatment failure they are in a position to be optimally involved.

The use of slow-release morphine (MST) which needs to be given only two to three times a day has helped in the long-term maintenance of analgesia for such patients. Elective insertion of central lines for the terminal care period may be justified in some cases for administration of analgesia, anti-emetics or even blood products. Subcutaneous infusion of diamorphine using a 'butterfly' needle and a portable pump is a useful technique. It is important that the likely nature of the child's death is explained clearly to the parents as the major fears of pain or haemorrhage can usually be allayed.

Clinical and pathological assessment of malignancy

PRESENTATION

Patients may have been investigated extensively for more common disorders and have often received therapy for presumed infectious or inflammatory conditions. A typical example is the late diagnosis of leukaemia, where there has been several weeks history of general malaise and lethargy, diagnosed as a viral infection or nutritional anaemia. Similarly, bone or joint pains caused by leukaemia or metastatic disease such as neuroblastoma may initially be treated as osteomyelitis or osteochondritis before an accurate diagnosis is made. Unusual neurological signs such as transient diplopia or focal headaches may be the initial presenting feature of an intracranial neoplasm. As in the adult, cancer in children is a great mimic and should always be considered

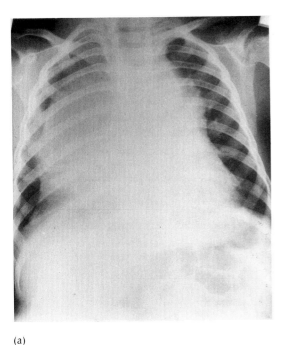

(a)

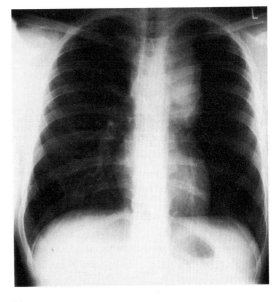

(b)

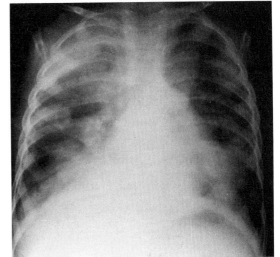

(c)

Fig. 25.1 Radiological appearances of malignant disease involving the chest. (a) Large mediastinal mass due to a T cell lymphoma. (b) Mediastinal and hilar glands of Hodgkin's lymphoma. (c) Pulmonary metastases in Wilms' tumour.

where symptoms are atypical or unexpectedly persistent.

IMAGING

Plain radiographs remain an important component of any diagnostic work-up. In some cases these may be almost pathognomic, such as the large anterior mediastinal mass of T cell non-Hodgkin's lymphoma, or the calcified abdominal mass of neuroblastoma. Plain films of painful limbs may show features of Ewing's sarcoma or osteosarcoma, or may reveal the osteolytic lesions characteristic of neuroblastoma or sarcoma. Routine chest X-ray remains part of the initial staging of any tumour that has potential for pulmonary metastases (Fig. 25.1). If possible, negative findings on chest X-ray should be confirmed by CT scan. Table 25.2 lists the differential diagnosis of a thoracic mass detected on chest X-ray. It is important to localize the tumour to the anterior or posterior mediastinum by both PA and lateral X-rays.

The development of high-resolution ultrasound has simplified the initial evaluation of abdominal disease, demonstrating the origin of a tumour and also providing useful information about regional infiltration or nodal involvement. The use of ultrasound is often the first step and subsequent diagnostic procedures stem from this.

CT scanning is essential for clarifying the anatomical origin of a primary tumour and also determines whether there are lung, liver or nodal metastases. For brain tumours, CT scanning has almost completely replaced angiography or ventriculography. The role of magnetic resonance imaging (MRI) is still under evaluation, but it already has an important use in spinal tumours, either primary or secondary, often avoiding the need for invasive myelography.

Technetium bone scanning is a prerequisite for excluding bony metastases and will often detect lesions not evident on a skeletal survey. One problem with the bone scan for evaluating disease response is that it remains abnormal during healing and a persistently abnormal scan does not necessarily mean persisting disease.

PRINCIPLES OF STAGING

Because of the high cure rates in localized tumours compared with disseminated disease, it is essential that treatment regimens are defined by the extent of disease. For example, localized Wilms' tumour which is completely resected at presentation will be 90% curable with several doses of a single agent, whereas with metastatic disease at presentation at least three drugs must be used to achieve a cure rate of around 60%. Even more striking is neuroblastoma, where completely resected disease will be curable in 80% with no chemotherapy, whereas disseminated disease has only a 10–20% cure rate despite very intensive multi-agent treatment. The imaging techniques discussed above provide information on the extent of local infiltration, indicating resectability of the lesion. Nodal involvement and metastatic disease in lung, liver, bone or brain can be readily detected. Routine assessment of bone marrow in

	Anterior mediastinal	Posterior mediastinal
Malignant	Non-Hodgkin's lymphoma Hodgkin's lymphoma Malignant germ cell tumour Rhabdomyosarcoma, Ewing's sarcoma Thymoma	Neuroblastoma Ganglioneuroblastoma Sarcoma Phaeochromocytoma
Benign	Teratoma Cystic hygroma Haemangioma Thymic cyst	Ganglioneuroma Schwann cell tumour Neurofibroma Bronchogenic cyst

Table 25.2 Differential diagnosis of thoracic mass evaluated by PA and lateral chest X-ray.

Table 25.3 General outline of 'staging' system for solid tumours. Details will vary between diseases, depending on the metastatic pattern and specific prognostic factors.

Stage I	Localized tumour that has been completely resected at presentation
Stage II	Localized tumour where there is microscopic residue after initial surgery, either in primary lesion or local lymph nodes
Stage III	Regional disease, often with extensive infiltration of adjacent tissue and lymph nodes, where initial resection is not possible
Stage IV	Metastatic disease with spread to lung, bone, liver, bone marrow or CNS

conditions such as neuroblastoma, where there is a high incidence of marrow metastases, will complete staging and is essential before the commencement of chemotherapy. Although these procedures may necessitate an anxious waiting period for the parents it is important that the treatment programme embarked on is of appropriate intensity from the outset. Table 25.3 outlines the principle of staging tumour extent at presentation.

PATHOLOGICAL DIAGNOSIS

Accurate pathological diagnosis is obviously essential prior to starting treatment in the majority of cases. A rare exception to this rule is T cell non-Hodgkin's lymphoma with massive mediastinal tumour and upper airway obstruction where an anaesthetic for biopsy might be life threatening. Chemotherapy induces rapid reduction in tumour size and a biopsy can then be performed within 24 or 48 hours once the anaesthetic hazard has passed. Similarly, in neuroblastoma, where there is an elevation of catecholamines and classical radiological features, biopsy may be felt to be hazardous.

At biopsy it is essential that an adequate amount of tissue is taken for detailed histological study. Haematoxylin and eosin preparations alone are no longer adequate and the use of special stains may be relevant, as well as immunohistochemical studies for lymphoid or neuroblastoma cell surface markers.

Bone marrow evaluation depends on the disease suspected. If there are circulating leukaemic blast cells, then a single aspirate is sufficient for detailed analysis. If the diagnosis is unclear, trephine biopsy should be performed and may be a prerequisite with aplastic anaemia or metastatic disease. With many solid tumours, secondary deposits may be patchy, and bilateral aspirate and trephine biopsies are recommended. Although a single aspirate may be done under local anaethesia in the older child, general anaesthesia is preferable for the majority and is usually mandatory for a trephine biopsy.

Specific malignancies

The leukaemias

Leukaemia is the malignant transformation of haemopoietic precursor cells in the bone marrow. The stage of cell differentiation at which this transformation occurs determines the cell lineage involved and thus the morphological and immunological characteristics of the leukaemic cell clone. Subclassification is based on the clinical behaviour of the disease (acute progressive or chronic indolent) and on the cell lineage (myeloblastic, lymphoblastic, megakaryocytic and erythroblastic). Finally, with lymphoblastic and myelocytic leukaemias there are further subgroups determined by morphological features, cytochemical staining and immunological 'markers' (Fig. 25.2). The latter are antigens expressed on the cell membrane or in the cytoplasm which can be detected by immunofluorescent techniques using monoclonal antibodies raised against these antigens.

Aetiological factors in leukaemia remain obscure. To date no viral agent has been implicated in childhood leukaemia. Evidence of environmental factors remains speculative and controversy about clustering at the site of nuclear power plants, nuclear disposal sites or high-tension electricity installations continues. Because of the relative rarity of leukaemia in childhood it is difficult to obtain statistically meaningful data on this issue.

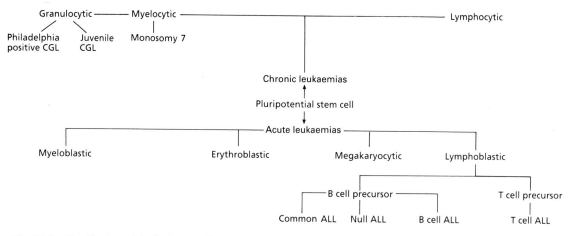

Fig. 25.2 Classification of the leukaemias based on cellular origin.

ACUTE LYMPHOBLASTIC LEUKAEMIA (ALL)

Diagnosis. The presenting features of acute lymphoblastic leukaemia (ALL) reflect either the suppression of normal myelopoiesis due to marrow infiltration or are related to the involvement of lymph nodes. Symptoms may be subtle and resemble other common disorders (Table 25.4). The diagnosis can be made in some patients by examination of the peripheral blood film which may contain circulating leukaemic blast cells. A bone marrow aspirate is, however, mandatory for confirmation of diagnosis and subclassification of the leukaemia. Standard cytochemical and immuno-

logical tests currently done are shown in Table 25.5. Occasionally transient marrow hypoplasia precedes ALL and may mimic aplastic anaemia. Reactive lymphocytosis due to viral infections may cause diagnostic difficulty, but the other clinical signs are usually helpful. If in doubt it is advisable to repeat the marrow aspirate as the disease will eventually declare itself. Examination of spinal fluid is normally done at presentation, although if the peripheral blast cell count is very high this may be delayed for several days to avoid the theoretical risk of contaminating the central nervous system with blast cells, as well as to avoid confusion in the interpretation of CSF findings

Table 25.4 Childhood disorders presenting with features similar to acute leukaemia.

Presenting features	Differential diagnosis
Anaemia, general malaise	Nutritional anaemia, aplastic anaemia, viral illness
Easy bruising	Constitutional, trauma, non-accidental injury, idiopathic thrombocytopenia, aplastic anaemia
Bone and/or joint pain	Rheumatoid arthritis, septic arthritis, osteomyelitis, irritable hip, osteochondritis
Lymphadenopathy	Bacterial infection, mumps, infectious mononucleosis
Liver and spleen enlargement	Viral infection

Table 25.5 Routine evaluation of bone marrow and CSF in suspected leukaemia.

Bone marrow aspirate
Morphology
Cytochemistry
FAB classification (L$_1$, L$_2$, etc.)
Immunological surface markers
Blast cell karyotype

CSF analysis
Cell count
Cytospin examination

in the event of a traumatic tap. X-rays should be performed routinely to determine if there is mediastinal enlargement, which in the case of T-cell leukaemia may produce significant tracheal compression. Abdominal ultrasound should also be performed to exclude infiltration of the kidneys, particularly in patients with a high presenting white cell count, as this is of importance in avoiding renal complications during induction chemotherapy.

Management. The management of ALL follows the sequence summarized in Table 25.6. The aim of initial treatment in ALL is to achieve remission with intensive chemotherapy. At the end of this 'induction' period the bone marrow should be clear of all detectable disease. Most current regimens include vincristine, prednisolone, daunorubicin and asparaginase. Severe pancytopenia is

usually seen for 7–14 days after the onset of treatment and it is during this period that the maximum morbidity occurs. In patients with bulky disease (massive lymphadenopathy, liver and spleen involvement or white cell count over 100 $\times$ 10^9/l), very careful attention must be given to electrolyte imbalance and renal function due to the risk of tumour lysis syndrome. Intensive supportive care may be required during induction and the patient should remain in hospital until the blood count has recovered. The need for further intensive chemotherapy after achieving remission remains unclear and is currently under investigation.

The second phase of treatment is directed toward the central nervous system (CNS). Prior to the development of 'prophylactic' or CNS-directed therapy, up to 60% of patients had disease relapse in the central nervous system. Cranio-spinal irradiation or cranial irradiation with several injections of intrathecal methotrexate reduces the incidence of CNS relapse to less than 10%. Concern about the effect of irradiation on endocrine function, such as growth hormone deficiency and premature puberty, and on intellectual development, has led to attempts to replace this form of treatment modality with chemotherapy alone. This consists of more intensive and prolonged intrathecal chemotherapy, possibly including cytarabine and hydrocortisone. High-dose intravenous methotrexate will effectively penetrate the central nervous system.

Table 25.6 Phases of treatment for acute childhood leukaemias.

Type of leukaemia	Induction	CNS-directed treatment	Consolidation	Continuation
Acute lymphoblastic	Vincristine Prednisolone Asparaginase Daunorubicin	Cranial irradiation or high-dose i.v. methotrexate Intrathecal methotrexate	Cytarabine Etoposide Thioguanine Daunorubicin	Methotrexate 6-mercaptopurine Vincristine Prednisolone
Acute myeloblastic	Daunorubicin Cytarabine Thioguanine Etoposide Amsacrine	Intrathecal methotrexate	Repeat induction-type combination Or high-dose chemoradiotherapy with bone marrow rescue	

The third phase of treatment is 'maintenance' or 'continuing therapy'. This consists of low-dose out-patient treatment with pulses of intravenous chemotherapy and is generally continued for 2 years. The duration of continuing treatment has been progressively reduced from 4 to 2 years in prospective randomized studies which showed no advantage from more prolonged treatment. It is conceivable that the duration could be reduced further in the future, particularly in the context of more intensive initial treatment. During continuing treatment, despite the fact that the blood count is kept above 1×10^9 neutrophils per litre, the patient is immunosuppressed to a significant degree and although bacterial infections are less of a problem there is an important risk from *P. carinii* and viral infections such as chickenpox and measles. To prevent the former, prophylactic Septrin is given throughout the period of treatment, and for the latter, immunoglobulin and acyclovir should be given without hesitation when indicated.

Prognosis. Prognostic features in ALL tend to vary depending upon the intensity of treatment, but in general, adverse factors include: age less than 1 year or more than 10 years at presentation, male sex, a presenting white cell count greater than 50×10^9/l, central nervous system leukaemia at presentation and a persistence of blast cells in the marrow aspirate 2 weeks into induction treatment.

The B ALL subtype has done very badly in the past on standard regimens, but the outlook for this has been improved by the use of intensive non-Hodgkin's lymphoma-type regimens. Leukaemias with hypodiploid chromosome abnormalities such as t(4:11) or Ph+ are associated with a poor prognosis.

It is possible to identify particularly high-risk patients for whom experimental regimens are justified. These include young infants, especially those with high white cell counts and chromosome abnormalities, or any patient with greater than 100×10^9 white cells per litre at presentation. Elective high-dose therapy with allogenic bone marrow transplantation or autologous bone marrow rescue are currently under evaluation for such patients.

Most relapses occur within 1–3 years (Fig. 25.3) but children are generally not considered cured until they reach 5 years of continued remission and even then very late relapses beyond 10 years can occur. Bone marrow relapse is the most common event, but relapse into the CNS or the testis also occurs. The time after treatment at which relapse occurs is of importance and in the past, disease recurring during continuing chemotherapy was unlikely to be curable, whereas relapse occurring years after cessation of treatment had a

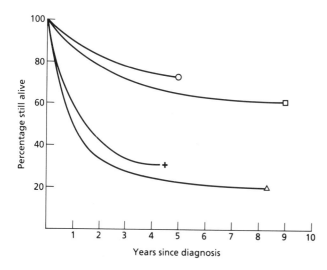

Fig. 25.3 Actuarial survival curves for leukaemia based on the data from the United Kingdom Children's Cancer Study Group (UKCCSG). The two top lines refer to acute lymphoblastic leukaemia and the two bottom to acute myeloblastic leukaemia. Shorter lines refer to the period 1984–87 and the longer line to 1980–83.

small chance of salvage with alternative chemotherapy. This distinction is, however, less clear with some recent intensive regimens using allogenic marrow transplant. A second remission may be achieved in the majority of patients, but is usually of short duration. One group of patients who do particularly well are those with an isolated testicular relapse occurring off treatment. After either orchidectomy or testicular irradiation and systemic re-induction chemotherapy, the majority of patients will remain in remission. Treatment of isolated CNS relapse remains unsatisfactory as there is a high incidence of subsequent bone marrow relapse despite systemic re-treatment. Repeat irradiation including the spine is usually necessary, but total body irradiation with bone marrow transplant is under evaluation.

ACUTE MYELOID LEUKAEMIA (AML)

There are few specific clinical signs of acute myeloid leukaemia (AML). Lymphadenopathy tends to occur less commonly than in ALL and characteristic skin rashes or solid leukaemia deposits may occur. The diagnosis is made on morphological, cytochemical and surface marker characteristics. Disseminated intravascular coagulation is a particular problem in some forms of AML. The risk of CNS involvement is similar to ALL and between 5 and 10% have blast cells in the CSF at presentation. Other extramedullary manifestations such as testicular involvement are unusual.

Management. With recent very intensive induction regimens, remission rates of over 80% are achieved. However, subsequent disease relapse remains a major problem. It seems unlikely that conventional continuing treatment as used in ALL is appropriate in AML and most regimens involve a short period of intensive pulsed or semi-continuous treatment. Intrathecal methotrexate alone appears to be effective as CNS-directed treatment.

High-dose therapy with allogenic bone marrow transplant has an important role. Patients who have HLA-matched sibling donors are generally treated in this way in first remission, an approach which currently leads to the lowest relapse rate.

CHRONIC LEUKAEMIAS

Chronic leukaemias are very uncommon in children. Chronic granulocytic leukaemia (CGL) accounts for only 2–5% of all cases and chronic lymphocytic leukaemia is rarely if ever seen. CGL in childhood may resemble the adult disease or be of the more chemoresistant juvenile form, which lacks the characteristic Philadelphia chromosome.

Lymphoma

Lymphoma are divided on the basis of histological features, immune markers and natural history into two broad groups: Hodgkin's lymphoma and non-Hodgkin's lymphoma. Prognosis and treatment differ widely and therefore accurate initial diagnosis is essential.

HODGKIN'S DISEASE

Hodgkin's disease is a tumour predominantly involving lymph nodes with infiltration by a mixed population containing both the neoplastic component and a reactive inflammatory or stromal cell component. The precise origin of the Hodgkin's cell remains unclear. Although these cells lack positivity for almost all histochemical and immunological markers for lymphoid or histiocytic origin, it seems likely that it is of haemopoietic rather than connective tissue origin. The 'Rye' pathological classification is based upon both the predominant cell type and microscopic structure. The nodular sclerosing form is characterized by bands of collagenous connective tissue encircling nodular areas of lymphoid tissue which contain an infiltrate of Hodgkin's cells. This is the commonest form in adolescence. In the younger child the 'mixed cellularity' form predominates. Here there is a diffuse cellular infiltrate composed of a mixture of histiocytes, neutrophils, eosinophils, plasma cells and Hodgkin's cells. The 'lymphocyte-predominant' subgroup is composed almost entirely of lymphocytes and histiocytes. Small clusters of Hodgkin's cells are seen. This form is associated with a particularly good prognosis and it has been suggested that the heavy lymphocytic infiltration may reflect an intense immunological response by the host correlating with the good outcome.

By contrast, the 'lymphocyte-depleted' form, with predominant fibrosis and little reactive cellular infiltrate, has a poor prognosis. It should be emphasized that the prognostic importance of this pathological subclassification has been reduced somewhat by the impact of highly effective chemotherapy.

The incidence of Hodgkin's disease is 5:1 000 000 children under 15 and the majority of cases present over 10 years of age. A point of epidemiological interest is that in 'under-developed' African countries younger children are affected and tend to have mixed cellularity or lymphocyte-depleted Hodgkin's disease. In the more socioeconomically 'advanced' populations the age of onset is later and the more favourable histological types predominate. It has been suggested that this reflects acquired immune tolerance to a pathogen, and such immunity is lacking in the former group. Moreover, in 'developed' countries the disease is less common in children from large families or where there has been a high incidence of minor viral infections, suggesting that early exposure to a pathogen may reduce the severity of the subsequent disease. To date, however, no specific viral agent has been isolated.

Diagnosis. Eighty per cent of patients present with disease on one or both sides of the neck and 60% have mediastinal disease. Innocent lymphadeno-pathy (p. 440) in the cervical and submandibular regions frequently occurs with upper respiratory tract infections, but nodes in the lower neck and supraclavicular region are more suspicious. Nodes in Hodgkin's disease are typically pain-free, of rubbery consistency and may have been present for several weeks, often spontaneously varying in size. Associated symptoms reflecting systemic disease should be carefully sought, such as weight loss, night sweats, unexplained fever, or persistent

pruritis. These symptoms are indicative of the systemic spread of the disease. Initial investigations should include chest X-rays and ESR. Diagnosis rests on tissue biopsy which should be of sufficient size to exclude reactive or infected nodes. An accessible lymph node is usually possible to find, but occasionally with isolated mediastinal disease open biopsy is required.

Staging investigations include CT scan of the abdomen and thorax. Routine lymphangiography is no longer standard practice in children as it may be a technically difficult and unpleasant procedure. The diagnostic yield over a CT scan alone is minimal. As most patients now receive chemotherapy, precise delineation of nodes is of less importance than previously when involved nodal groups were selectively irradiated. Similarly, staging splenectomy, although the most accurate way of defining involvement of the spleen, is no longer performed. A CT scan will provide information regarding this organ and, moreover, isolated splenic involvement in the absence of nodal disease elsewhere is uncommon. There is a not insignificant operative morbidity and the risk of pneumococcal sepsis following splenectomy has been a problem in the past. Bone marrow trephine biopsy should be performed in patients with non-localized disease. Aspirate is inadequate due to patchy infiltration.

The disease is staged using the Ann Arbor classification:

Stage I and II disease are, respectively, localized to a single node or multiple nodes above the diaphragm;

Stage III involvement of the nodes above and below the diaphragm or spleen involvement;

Stage IV dissemination to the bone, marrow, liver, lung.

Management. Treatment strategies may have varying emphasis on the relative roles of radiotherapy and chemotherapy. Although high cure rates are achieved with extended field irradiation, even in patients with Stage III disease, the sequelae in growing children are unacceptable and the trend is therefore towards chemotherapy alone for most patients. The current UK regimen in-

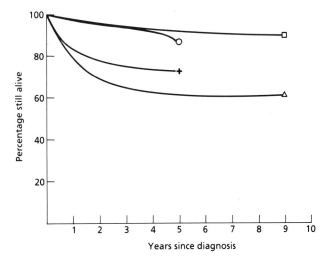

Percentage still alive

Years since diagnosis

Fig. 25.4 Actuarial survival curves for cases of lymphoma. The two top lines refer to Hodgkin's disease and the two bottom lines to non-Hodgkin's lymphoma. The periods of treatment are given in Fig. 25.3.

volves radiotherapy alone only in patients with Stage I disease in whom staging is particularly important. All other stages receive chemotherapy. Conventional chemotherapy includes a number of alkylating agents, but in order to avoid subsequent infertility and other late effects, drugs such as adriamycin and etoposide are now used.

Additional irradiation is only given to patients with initially bulky mediastinal disease. With this approach, up to one-fifth of patients with Stage I disease will relapse but the majority, if not all, are curable with subsequent chemotherapy.

Late relapses may occur in Hodgkin's disease and therefore prolonged follow-up is required before one can say that the patient is cured (Fig. 25.4).

NON-HODGKIN'S LYMPHOMA (NHL)

This malignant proliferation of lymphoid precursor cells has the same cellular origin as leukaemia. The lymph nodes are usually the predominant site of disease with, in some cases, secondary involvement of the bone marrow, CNS and other organs. Thus, unlike the leukaemias, nodal excision or local irradiation were in the past curative in a small number of cases. However, with the advent of highly effective chemotherapy these two modalities have little place.

In children four main categories of disease have

been described: diffuse lymphoblastic (T cell), diffuse undifferentiated (B cell), diffuse lymphoblastic non-B non-T, and diffuse histiocytic. As with ALL, the aetiology is unknown.

Diagnosis. The presentation of NHL depends on the site involved. T cell NHL can present as a medical emergency with rapidly progressive upper airway obstruction and superior vena caval obstruction (Fig. 25.1a). There may be extensive cervical lymphadenopathy. B cell NHL in the abdomen presents as abdominal pain or a palpable mass. Nodal involvement in the ileum may lead to intussusception and intestinal obstruction. With advanced disease there may be ascites and marked weight loss. Liver, spleen and kidney infiltration may also occur. Marrow and CSF involvement are seen in both T and B forms of NHL. Traditionally, cases with greater than 25% tumour infiltration of bone marrow are classified as 'leukaemia' and in the case of B cell leukaemia there is a particularly high incidence of CNS disease. Less than 25% marrow involvement is classified as Stage IV disease.

Routine staging investigations should include defining the extent of nodal involvement with chest X-ray and abdominal ultrasound or CT body scan. As chemotherapy is given to all patients, precise definition of nodal involvement is less important than in Hodgkin's disease. Bone marrow aspirate and spinal fluid cytology are evaluated as in leukaemia.

The disease is staged using the Murphy classification. Localized disease (Stage I and II) is uncommon; Stage III disease involves multiple sites above and below the diaphragm and includes any thoracic primary or extensive abdominal disease. Stage IV is distant extranodal metastases.

Management. In the case of tracheal compression, obstruction can rapidly be relieved with chemotherapy. Irradiation of initial bulk nodal disease following chemotherapy has no value. Cranial irradiation is at present used for early CNS treatment in T cell disease, but in B cell NHL, intrathecal chemotherapy alone is sufficient unless there is CNS involvement at presentation.

Surgery should only be used to obtain a tissue diagnosis although bone marrow, ascitic fluid or pleural effusion cytology often provides the diagnosis. Chemotherapy for NHL should be selected on the basis of histological and immunological subtype. T cell disease is treated in the same way as acute leukaemia. By contrast, B cell NHL is treated with a short pulsed multi-drug regime, including cyclophosphamide, adriamycin and methotrexate, for between 6 and 9 months. With this approach survival rates are high (see Fig. 25.4).

AFRICAN BURKITT'S LYMPHOMA

This condition, although sharing a common B-cell origin and probably some aetiological features, is a separate clinical entity from European B cell non-Hodgkin's lymphoma. The former typically affects males between 6 and 8 years and involves the jaw, abdomen and CNS. There is a very clear association with EBV and the tumour is highly chemosensitive.

Neuroblastoma

Neuroblastoma arises from fetal neural cells (neuroblasts) which normally migrate from the neural crest to the sympathetic ganglia and adrenal gland. The tumour may thus arise at any site where sympathetic nerve tissue is found. The usual site is the adrenal gland, but it may also arise from sympathetic ganglia in the neck, chest, abdomen and pelvis. Rarely, ectopic forms arise in the kidney.

This is the commonest intra-abdominal tumour in children and the incidence is approximately 1:100 000 children under 15 years. The median age of presentation is 2 years, but it is occasionally seen in adolescents or even adults. Primitive neuroblastic tissue, indistinguishable from the tumour, is found in up to 2% of autopsies performed on children under 3 months of age, suggesting a high spontaneous regression rate of 'neuroblastoma *in situ*'.

Diagnosis. Neuroblastoma most frequently presents as an abdominal mass with associated systemic features due to metastatic disease. The latter include weight loss, general malaise, bone and joint pain, anaemia and fever. Focal neurological signs may be present if there is primary intraspinal disease, extension of para-vertebral disease into the spinal canal, or if there is compression of the pelvic nerves. Intracranial metastases occur but are very rare. Hypertension at presentation is due to either catecholamine release or renal vascular compression. Diarrhoea can result from the release of vasoactive intestinal peptides by the tumour. A specific subgroup presenting with cerebellar ataxia and nystagmus (the 'dancing eyes' syndrome) is associated with a well-differentiated intrathoracic primary and has a particularly good prognosis.

Frequently there is a long history of persistent or recurrent abdominal pain ascribed to other more common causes until the systemic features develop. Subtle radiological abnormalities may be missed and the child with pelvic or femoral pain may be mistakenly treated for 'irritable hip' before the correct diagnosis is reached. With advanced disease, exophthalmos and periorbital discolouration due to disease infiltration may occur.

Thoracic tumours are rarely symptomatic and may be detected at the time of chest X-ray for another cause. These are usually well-differentiated tumours with a favourable outcome.

Investigations. Diagnosis may be confirmed on CT scan (Fig. 25.5a). Catecholamine levels are almost

Fig. 25.5 Imaging in neuroblastoma. (a) Abdominal CT scan (enhanced with niopam) showing a large mass on the left side behind the stomach (S). (b) MIBG scan showing significantly increased uptake of isotope in a child with extensive abdominal and bilateral cervical node involvement (arrowed). The normal faint uptake by liver and parotids is also seen. (c) MRI scan in a child with extensive marrow involvement. Abnormal signal is seen in both femora, pelvis and spine.

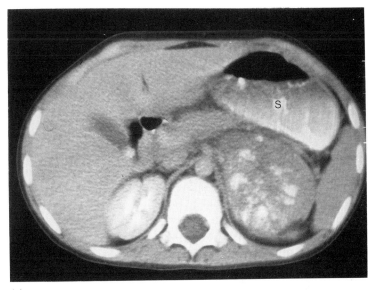

(a)

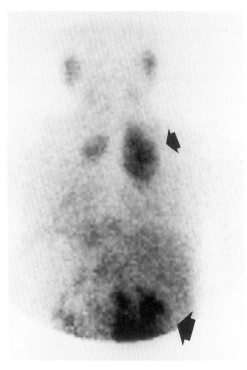

(b)

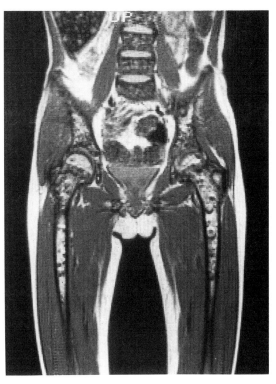

(c)

invariably elevated. The urine metabolites, homo-vanillic acid (HVA) and vanillylmandelic acid (VMA) are raised in about 85% of patients and dopamine is raised in about 90% of patients. In the past, 24-hour urine collections have been recommended in order to avoid false negative results due to the episodic nature of catechol-aminic release from the tumour. With recent advances in chromatography the sensitivity of assays has improved and a random urine sample in which the catecholemine metabolites are quantified in relation to the creatinine content is sufficient. Around 10% of patients will, however, be metabolite-negative.

Skeletal surveys are now rarely used as technetium bone scan is more accurate for detecting bony metastases. Meta-iodobenzylguanidine (MIBG) is taken up specifically by the tumour and is increasingly used as an accurate tool for both diagnosis and assessment of treatment response (Fig. 25.5b). MRI can also be used to demonstrate marrow disease (Fig. 25.5c). Because of the patchy nature of bone marrow involvement in neuroblastoma a single aspirate is inadequate for documenting marrow metastases. Trephine biopsies are essential.

Pathological subgroups in neuroblastoma have been devised in an attempt to assess prognosis more accurately. Most classifications are based on the degree of differentation. This ranges from the benign, highly differentiated form with a high percentage of mature ganglion cells, through the intermediate ganglioneuroblastoma containing a mixture of cell types, to the highly undifferentiated malignant small round cell neuroblastoma. The latter is associated with early metastatic spread and bad prognosis.

Management. Using the International Neuroblastoma Staging System, Stage I and II (completely resected or microscopic residue) are usually well-differentiated tumours with few adverse prognostic features and are curable by surgery alone. It is likely that some such tumours remain quiescent and may even resolve spontaneously. The decision to remove asymptomatic, localized, thoracic ganglioneuroma is based more on grounds of allaying anxiety than hard evidence that such a tumour will progress or metastasize. There is clear evidence that microscopic residue after resection of such lesions does not lead to recurrence in the majority of patients. Neither radiation nor chemotherapy is necessary unless there is nodal involvement when a short course of chemotherapy should be given. Survival at 5 years is approximately 90%.

Stage III disease is unresectable at presentation, but pre-operative chemotherapy will usually shrink the mass sufficiently to permit complete resection. Improvements in the efficacy of chemotherapy and in surgical technique have led to

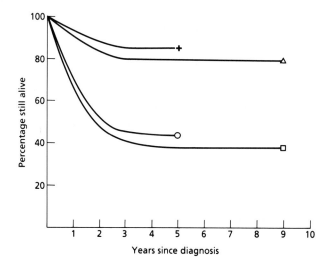

Fig. 25.6 Actuarial survival curves for Wilms' tumour (upper two lines) and neuroblastoma (lower two lines). The periods of treatment are given in Fig. 25.3.

improved survival in such patients (about 60% at 5 years).

Stage IV disease with metastases to bone, bone marrow, nodes, liver or skin has been widely regarded as virtually incurable. There is, however, increasing evidence that with intensive chemotherapy up to 20% of such patients will be long-term survivors. To some extent the site of metastatic disease influences prognosis, being better for those with only distant nodal involvement and worse for those with extensive multiple bony metastases. Age is, however, the strongest prognostic feature in Stage IV disease and patients under 18 months do significantly better than older children. Figure 25.6 summarizes the prognosis for neuroblastoma.

Management of Stage IV neuroblastoma involves a combination of chemotherapy, surgery and radiotherapy. In about two-thirds of patients there will be complete clearance of metastatic disease and surgical resection of the primary is usually recommended. Complete resection or resection with only microscopic residue is achieved in about half the patients. As in Stage III tumours local irradiation may have a role in treating residual disease.

STAGE IVS NEUROBLASTOMA

This is a separate disease entity, occurring almost invariably in infants under 1 year of age. The behaviour of this 'cancer' is unique. Despite extensive infiltration of bone marrow, liver, and skin the disease will usually resolve spontaneously over several months. The primary site is generally supra-renal and is of small volume. The clinical features which distinguish Stage IVS from Stage IV in young infants are the presence of bony metastases or distant nodal metastases. The latter are true Stage IV patients and require intensive chemotherapy but their outlook is comparatively good.

Although Stage IVS is self-limiting, early morbidity is not insignificant. This is predominantly due to the massive hepatomegaly with splinting of the diaphragm and consequent respiratory distress. The resultant mortality may be as high as 20% from respiratory insufficiency combined with sepsis or complications of therapeutic manoeuvres. The initial 'wait and watch' policy is appropriate, but at the first sign of significant respiratory embarrassment low-dose radiation should be given to the liver, or small doses of chemotherapy. This usually produces tumour shrinkage and resolution of symptoms. Progression to true Stage IV disease occurs in less than 10% of patients.

Wilms' tumour (nephroblastoma)

The incidence of Wilms' tumour is approximately 6:1 000 000 children under 15 years of age. The median age at diagnosis is 3.5 years, but occasionally older children or even adults are affected. There is a characteristic association between Wilms' tumour, aniridia and hemihypertrophy of trunk and limbs. The deletion of part of chromosome 11 in Wilms' tumour may indicate loss of a regulatory gene and be of importance in the malignant transformation of nephroblasts.

A pathological subclassification divides tumours into two broad groups; 'favourable' and 'unfavourable'. The favourable group comprises about 90% of patients, in whom there is usually evidence of tubular or glomerular differentiation. The unfavourable subgroup is either anaplastic or sarcomatous.

Diagnosis. Wilms' tumour usually presents as an abdominal mass. A baby sitter or grandparent may notice the swelling which, because of its slow evolution and the general well being of the child, has been missed by the parents. In most cases there are few or no systemic symptoms. About one-fifth of patients show a low-grade intermittent fever. Haematuria occurs in only 10–15% of patients. Hypertension is seen in approximately 10% and may be due to either renal vascular compression leading to ischaemia or ectopic renin or ACTH production by the tumour.

Management. Initial clinical examination gives a clue to operability as a mobile well-circumscribed mass without nodal or retroperitoneal extension is often resectable despite its size. An initial IVP may be done to demonstrate the presence of a

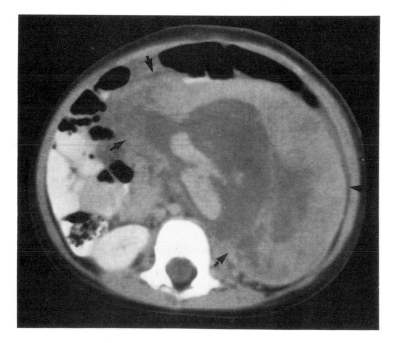

Fig. 25.7 Wilms' tumour. CT scan of the abdomen showing a very large non-calcified renal tumour (arrowed).

normal contralateral kidney although ultrasound has largely superseded this. The ultrasound is initially used to confirm the organ of origin and also gives information on nodal and vena caval involvement. CT scan is, however, desirable for accurate pre-operative assessment (Fig. 25.7). The contraindications to any initial surgery include an infiltrating tumour, inferior vena cava involvement or any distant metastases. There is a recent trend toward more frequent use of pre-operative chemotherapy because rapid tumour shrinkage leads to simpler surgical procedures and a lower risk of tumour rupture into the peritoneal cavity. Although clinical diagnosis is correct in 95% of cases, it is current policy in the UK that if there is not to be an initial nephrectomy, all tumours are biopsied rather than confirming the diagnosis at later surgery.

In Stage I disease (completely resected at diagnosis) a short course of vincristine is given and for other stages combination chemotherapy is used, adding adriamycin and actinomycin D. Irradiation to the tumour bed is limited to those with initially unresectable disease and some patients with unfavourable histology.

Cure rates with Stage II disease (minor residual disease at initial surgery) exceed 80%. Even with initially unresectable tumours 5-year survival is around 75%. With metastatic disease, usually in the lung (Fig. 25.1c), this is reduced to approximately 60%. Lung irradiation may be used in the latter group if the response to chemotherapy is slow.

In about 5% of cases, there is bilateral disease at presentation. This can be successfully treated with a combination of initial chemotherapy and subsequent bilateral partial nephrectomies. Cure rates are in the order of 75%. Survival figures for Wilms' tumour are shown in Figure 25.6.

Brain tumours

Intracranial neoplasms are the commonest solid tumours in childhood with an overall incidence of approximately 1:50 000 children under 15 years old. There are several histological subgroups comprising both embryonal tumours such as medulloblastoma or germinoma and adult-type glioma and astrocytoma. Lesions such as neuroma, meningioma and pituitary tumours are less fre-

Table 25.7 Classification of brain tumours based on primary site.

Supratentorial
Cerebral astrocytoma
    Frontal
    Temporal
    Parietal
Lateral ventricle ependymoma
Craniopharyngioma
Primitive neuroectodermal tumour ⎫
Choroid plexus papilloma   ⎬ Especially <1 year
Meningioma
Teratoma ⎭

Infratentorial
Astrocytoma
Medulloblastoma
Brain stem glioma
3rd ventricle ependymoma

Intraspinal
Extradural
    Neuroblastoma
    Sarcoma
    Lymphoma
Intradural
    Neurofibromatosis
    Dermoid
    Lipomata
Intramedullary
    Astrocytoma

quently seen in children than in adults. The anatomical origin and tumour subtypes are listed in Table 25.7.

Diagnosis. Presenting features reflect either raised intracranial pressure or mass effect due to a space-occupying lesion. Severe recurrent or persisting headaches are relatively rare in children and these should be viewed with a high index of suspicion (see p. 291). Symptoms include early morning vomiting and nausea or subtle alterations in behaviour. Focal third or sixth nerve palsies can occur. In small infants there may be rapid or slowly progressive development of macrocephaly with a prominent anterior fontanelle. With the more indolent low-grade gliomas a large head or wide fontanelle may be detected at routine checks.

The signs due to a space-occupying lesion depend on the site. Medulloblastomas will often produce cerebellar ataxia and nystagmus; parietal tumours may be associated with focal weakness and suprachiasmal lesions cause visual disturbance often with nystagmus. Brain stem lesions usually present with multiple cranial nerve palsies.

Clinical evaluation will assist with localization of the lesion, but the mainstay of diagnostic studies is the CT scan. This has almost completely replaced the need for invasive procedures such as cerebral arterial angiography or air ventriculography. For children under 4 years old, a general anaesthetic is usually necessary for satisfactory imaging. The use of intravenous contrast is essential and may aid both the detection of small lesions and delineation of the tumour extent. MRI has few proven advantages over CT scan although the clarity of anatomical detail is striking (Fig. 25.8). MRI may, however, be superior with brain stem tumours and some posterior fossa lesions where bone artefact impinges on CT resolution. It is also an invaluable tool for evaluation of spinal masses.

Management. Surgery plays an important role. Insertion of a ventriculo-peritoneal shunt may produce a dramatic improvement in symptoms by relieving raised intracranial pressure. Wherever possible, initial complete resection should be performed and in the past the extent of initial surgery has been a major factor in the likelihood of cure. If complete resection is impossible, debulking may have a role in relieving local compression. An important function of surgery is to provide tissue for histological diagnosis. In the past, radiotherapy has been standard treatment for the majority of lesions irrespective of histology and therefore pathological subtype may have been of major importance. With attempts to refine radiotherapy techniques together with the development of new chemotherapy strategies it is important that good histological information is available in patients wherever possible. In small children with deep inaccessible tumours (thalamus, mid-brain, pineal region and brain stem) this is often difficult but stereotactic techniques may be useful.

After surgery a course of radiotherapy is almost invariably given over several weeks. With inoper-

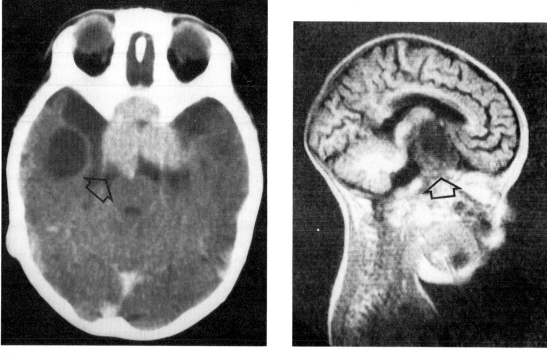

(a)   (b)

Fig. 25.8 Imaging techniques for tumour in the supra-chiasmal region (arrowed). (a) CT scan with contrast enhancement. (b) Lateral MRI scan.

able lesions this may be the sole therapy. Because of the disappointing cure rates in patients with high-grade gliomas and incompletely resected medulloblastomas there is increasing interest in the use of more aggressive chemotherapy. There is also major concern about neurological sequelae in the small infants, in whom irradiation of a bulky tumour involves overlap with considerable volumes of normal brain tissue.

ASTROCYTOMAS

These can be divided on the basis of their histological appearances into low grade and high grade. A cure rate of 60% is expected with low-grade tumours but the prognosis is very poor in high-grade astrocytomas.

NEUROECTODERMAL TUMOURS

These are primitive highly malignant tumours which occur above the tentorium in younger chil-

dren. They may be histologically indistinguishable from medulloblastomas and have a tendency to spread through the CSF pathways. They are usually highly chemosensitive.

EPENDYMOMAS

These account for 10% of brain tumours and arise from the ventricular lining. Histologically they often appear relatively benign but may spread through the CSF and occasionally into the upper spinal cord. Radiotherapy is the major form of treatment and survival at 10-year follow-up is around 40%.

MEDULLOBLASTOMAS

These are the commonest tumours occuring below the tentorium. The tumour is usually in the midline of the cerebellum and tends to seed early to CSF. Management is by surgical resection, followed by chemotherapy and radiotherapy. Vincristine and CCNU are the standard drugs used. Current 5-year survival is around 50% and bad prognostic features include: age less than 5 years at presentation, male sex, incomplete resection, and involvement of the brain stem, cerebellar vermis or CSF.

CEREBELLAR ASTROCYTOMA

These are relatively benign and usually cystic. Where surgically resectable there is a 90% chance of cure.

BRAIN STEM GLIOMA

Although these are also relatively benign they are extremely difficult to treat in view of their anatomical position as most of these tumours arise in the pons. Radiotherapy remains the mainstay of treatment but cure rates are generally less than 20%.

OPTIC GLIOMA

These are low-grade astrocytomas presenting with a mass at the optic chiasma or along the optic nerve (see Fig. 25.8). About 25% are associated with neurofibromatosis. They are often very slow growing and in older children may be treated by radiotherapy with over 70% survival. In small infants a 'wait and watch' policy is sometimes followed.

CRANIO-PHARYNGIOMA

These are benign slow-growing tumours, but complete surgical resection is usually impossible. Aspiration alone may be appropriate followed by irradiation, and cure rates in the region of 80% can be expected.

INTRASPINAL TUMOURS

Intraspinal tumours are uncommon. These rarely arise within the spinal cord and more commonly develop from the dura or extradural structures. The presenting symptoms are due to pressure on the spinal cord and depend on the level involved and the rapidity of tumour growth. Motor weakness with limp or abnormality of gait are seen and back or root pain may occur. Sacral lesions lead to bladder or bowel dysfunction. With very slow-growing lesions musculo-skeletal abnormalities may develop. Investigation should include plain X-ray, CT scan and MRI.

Management. Occasionally, treatment is with chemotherapy alone, in the cases of lymphoma or neuroblastoma for example, where the diagnosis may be made without biopsy. More often initial surgery is indicated and resection may be possible. The use of radiotherapy or adjuvant chemotherapy depends on the tumour type.

Soft tissue sarcomas

The commonest soft tissue sarcoma in childhood is the rhabdomyosarcoma. This arises from embryonal striated muscle precursor cells. On the basis of cell morphology and stromal features, rhabdomyomas are divided into two histological groups, the embryonal and the alveolar types.

Diagnosis. About half the cases of rhabdomyosarcoma are found in the head and neck region at sites such as the orbit, naso-pharynx, middle ear and face (Fig. 25.9). One-quarter affect the genito-urinary system, involving the bladder, prostate, vagina, uterus or para-testicular region. The remainder involve the extremities, trunk or retroperitoneum. Presentation depends on the site of the primary tumour. Lesions of the head and neck can present as superficial swellings, but may extend into the facial bones, causing extensive bony and cartilaginous destruction. There may be intracranial extension or involvement of the base of the skull, producing cranial nerve palsies. Nasopharyngeal lesions often present with nasal obstruction or a blood-stained mucous-like discharge. Orbital tumours cause proptosis, strabismus and occasionally are localized to the conjunctiva. Orbital lesions may be misdiagnosed as cysts, orbital cellulitis or an idiopathic squint. Bladder tumours can cause dysuria, haematuria, strangury or present as an abdominal mass. Blood-

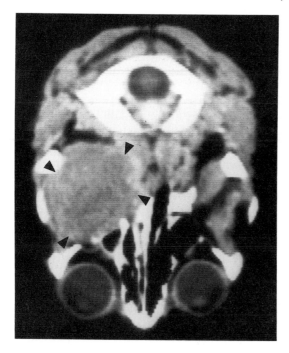

Fig. 25.9 CT scan showing a large rhabdomyosarcoma (arrowed) arising in the left maxillary fossa and extending from the retro-orbital region to the posterior nasal space.

stained vaginal discharge is usually the first sign of a vaginal tumour which is often of loose, fleshy character (botryoid tumour). Limb lesions are usually painless and have variable rapidity of growth.

Management. Staging investigations should include chest X-ray and CT scan of the primary site. Technetium bone scan and bone marrow aspirate and biopsy should also be performed. The extent of tumour, i.e. regional with infiltration of adjacent tissues or localized to the site of origin, is of major prognostic significance. In general, localized disease can be completely resected either at presentation or following chemotherapy. With regional disease non-mutilating initial surgery is impossible and there is often microscopic residue following surgery even after chemotherapy. Sites with a particularly good prognosis are the orbit, para-testicular region, vagina and bladder. The

poorest prognostic groups remain those with para-meningeal lesions (nasopharynx, para-nasal sinuses, middle ear and base of skull) in whom local surgical control is particularly difficult and there are high rates of local recurrence, sometimes with meningeal involvement. Patients with metastatic disease also do badly, in particular those with bone marrow involvement. Unless the primary tumour is localized and readily resectable initial surgery is limited to biopsy alone. Chemotherapy is then given for 4–6 months to achieve maximal tumour shrinkage. If complete remission is achieved by this approach and where possible proven by second-look surgery, then irradiation is probably unnecessary. In certain sites, such as the nasopharynx or orbit, it is particularly difficult to prove complete remission following chemotherapy, and in these cases if there is any suspect lesion on CT scan, irradiation should be given.

With most treatment regimens the 5-year survival for completely resected, localized disease should exceed 80%. For regional disease, where complete remission is achieved with chemotherapy alone or combined with surgery or radiotherapy for minimal residual disease, cure rates approach 70% with the exception of high-risk para-meningeal primaries. For metastatic disease, long-term survival remains less than 25%.

Bone tumours

Bone tumours in children are usually primary rather than secondary deposits. The two commonest primary bone tumours are osteosarcoma and Ewing's sarcoma and each tend to have a prediliction for different parts of the skeleton.

OSTEOSARCOMA

Osteogenic sarcoma is the commonest primary bone tumour in children. The incidence is about 2:1 000 000 children under 15 years of age, with a median onset of 12 years. The age distribution suggests an association with a period of rapid growth and the high incidence in weight-bearing lower limb bones may be of significance. Osteosarcomas may follow radiotherapy for soft tissue sarcoma or retinoblastoma.

By definition an osteogenic sarcoma must have a sarcomatous stroma and direct formation of osteoid or bone. Pathological subdivisions reflect the predominant cell type, i.e. fibroblastic, chrondroblastic or osteoblastic. There is a rare, highly undifferentiated small cell osteosarcoma which may be difficult to distinguish from other small cell tumours. Subgroups are also based on radiological features with medullary, osteolytic (telangiectatic), periosteal and paraosteal forms. The latter are relatively benign with minimal metastatic potential.

Diagnosis. The commonest presenting feature of a bone tumour is localized pain, with or without swelling. Occasionally the latter may be quite marked in the absence of any significant pain. There is usually some reduction in normal function and pathological fractures may occur. The commonest sites for osteosarcoma are femur (50%), tibia (30%) and humerus (10%). Plain X-ray shows evidence of soft tissue involvement in three-quarters of patients. There is usually a mixed lytic/osteoblastic component, but in 20% it is purely lytic or blastic (Fig. 25.10). A characteristic feature is the 'sunburst' appearance due to elevation of periosteum and new bone formation. Differential diagnosis includes osteomyelitis, traumatic fracture, eosinophilic granuloma, other neoplasms such as Ewing's sarcoma and metastatic lesions (neuroblastoma or lymphoma). Benign lesions such as osteoma and chrondroma generally have more clearly defined edges on X-ray.

Management. Biopsy is essential and this should be done through a skin site which can be excised at the time of definitive surgery. Routine staging studies include chest X-ray and CT scan. Technetium bone scan may detect bony metastases or the rare polyostotic form. CT and/or MRI scans of the involved bones will delineate the extent both of soft tissue involvement and of intramedullary extension. As is the case in Ewing's sarcoma the MRI may be particularly useful in this role (Fig. 25.11).

Management requires close co-operation between the oncologist and the orthopaedic surgeon so that the timing and type of surgery is optimal, both in terms of cancer control and functional outcome.

In the pre-chemotherapy era, amputation, with or without local irradiation, produced long-term relapse-free survival of 20% at best. Recent figures as high as 50% with surgery alone have been claimed, but this improvement over historical controls is unexplained and may reflect patient selection. Randomized trials have demonstrated that both relapse-free survival and overall survival are significantly improved by chemotherapy, with adriamycin, cisplatin and high-dose methotrexate regimens, following amputation. Pre-operative chemotherapy is now widely used and has the advantage of achieving tumour reduction prior

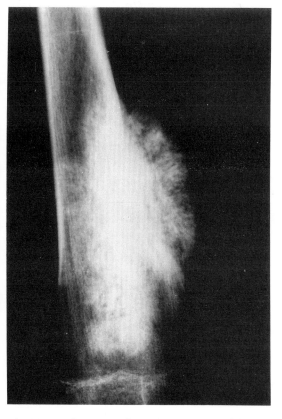

Fig. 25.10 Plain X-ray of osteogenic sarcoma of the tibia. Disruption of the cortex with radial 'sunburst' appearance due to spicules of new bone formation is seen.

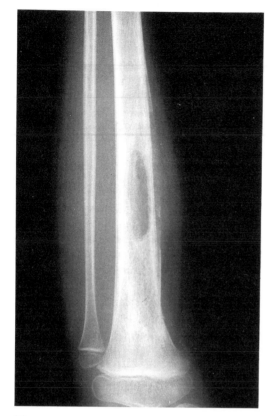

(a)

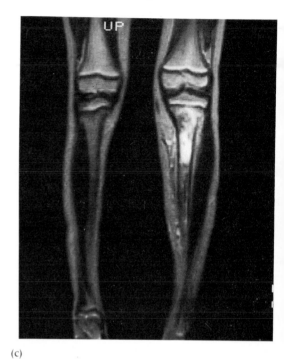

(c)

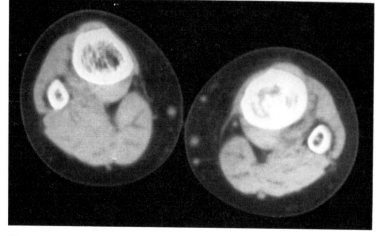

(b)

Fig. 25.11 Ewing's sarcoma of the tibia. (a) Plain X-ray showing a localized lytic lesion with overlying periosteal reaction. (b) CT scan of the same patient showing the intramedullary tumour mass and some soft tissue infiltration. (c) MRI scan of same tumour. Disease can be seen extending up to the epiphyseal plate and into soft tissue. This was not apparent on plain X-ray or CT scan.

to surgery, thus facilitating conservative limb-preserving procedures.

Amputation at the level of the bone above that involved with disease was the traditional surgical approach in the past, but with effective pre-operative chemotherapy, there is an increasing trend towards *en bloc* resection of the tumour, with limb preservation. Amputation at presentation remains, however, the treatment of choice for a very large lesion, particularly if there is infection or a pathological fracture.

It is important to select which patients are suitable for limb preservation carefully and early cosmetic results should not be the sole end-point. In children who still have several centimetres of growth, the long-term result may be poor due to marked limb shortening. If this is only a few centimetres then adjustable prostheses which may be lengthened are suitable. Alternatively the epiphysis on the contralateral leg may be stapled to prevent growth of the normal limb. With extensive tibial tumours, where most of the distal bone must be resected, there may be difficulty in finding attachment for the femoral musculature, which results in poor function. For these reasons, amputation with early mobilization may be the treatment of choice. Children quickly adapt to detachable limb prostheses and after a short period acquire remarkable agility.

Where a limb-preserving approach is suitable, a number of options are available. These include: metal prostheses for knee, shoulder or elbow joints; autologous bone grafts, e.g. fibula replacing part of the humerus and allogenic bone grafts from cadavers, where insertion of long sections of bone may be possible. Bone grafting often requires prolonged immobilization and, moreover, there remains a significant risk of the patient ultimately requiring amputation. An unusual but effective approach for lower femur or upper tibial lesions is the rotationplasty. Here nerves and vessels to the foot are preserved and the distal limb is re-grafted on to the stump, facing posteriorly. Inserted in a detachable limb prothesis, this provides greater control than a conventional stump.

The single most important adverse prognostic feature is metastatic disease at presentation. This most commonly involves lung or bone and the latter has a particularly poor outlook. Lung irradiation plays no role in the management of lung metastases and has no prophylactic value.

Osteosarcoma is an unusual tumour in that surgery has an important role in the management of pulmonary metastases. Resection of secondary deposits which have shrunk but remain present after chemotherapy may improve survival and, similarly, in the case of isolated pulmonary relapse, resection of the lesions may be curative. It is, however, normal practice to give second-line chemotherapy, if possible, in addition to surgery.

EWING'S SARCOMA

The incidence of Ewing's sarcoma is similar to osteosarcoma and it also affects the older age group. The tumour is composed of a diffuse, structureless infiltration of small round cells with irregular, rounded or oval nuclei and slightly granular cytoplasm. Because of the lack of specific pathological features, the diagnosis is largely based on the tumour site, and by exclusion of other small round cell tumours such as neuroblastoma, lymphoma or rhabdomyosarcoma.

Diagnosis. Typically, the disease presents with local bone pain, swelling or soft tissue extension. Fever occurs in about a third of patients. The diaphyseal region is typically involved in contrast to osteosarcoma where the lesion is usually epiphyseal. Bone sites most commonly involved are the pelvis (25%), femur (15%), rib (15%) and humerus (5%). Iliac primaries may be associated with an extensive soft tissue mass presenting as an abdominal mass. Para-vertebral lesions may present with focal weakness. About 25% of patients have metastatic disease at presentation involving lung, pleura, bone marrow or other bones.

On plain X-ray (see Fig. 25.11a) the lesion can be lytic or mixed lytic/sclerctic and may be lamellated with new bone formation. Cortical penetration is less common than with osteosarcoma. About two-thirds have a soft tissue mass (see Fig. 25.11b) and pathological fractures are sometimes seen.

Management. Initial staging investigations concentrate on detection of metastatic disease using technetium bone scan and chest X-ray or CT scan of the lungs. Bone marrow aspirate and trephine should be done in all patients with bulky primary disease. CT scan of primary disease in long bones gives valuable information about the degree of soft tissue involvement and the extension of disease in the medullary cavity. Recently, MRI has been used to evaluate disease at these sites (see Fig. 25.11c). This is of particular importance in planning limb-preserving surgery as the margins of excision must be well clear of any residual tumour.

With surgery or radiotherapy alone overall survival used to be around 15%. Combined with effective systemic chemotherapy, cure rates for lesions of small volume and particularly at distal sites are now over 60%. With large-volume lesions, the outcome remains poor with a 10–20% long-term survival. The presence of metastases at diagnosis and the degree of soft tissue extension also influence prognosis. Treatment strategy depends upon site and size of tumour. An expendable bone, such as a metatarsal or a fibula can be resected as a primary procedure. In general, however, chemotherapy with adriamycin, cyclophosphamide or ifosfamide is given initially. Once tumour shrinkage has been achieved, local treatment with non-deforming surgery or radiotherapy is carried out. Due to the high incidence of local recurrence much emphasis is laid on the latter procedures.

Retinoblastoma

Retinoblastoma is a tumour of neuroectodermal origin arising in retinal tissue. It is a rare tumour affecting about 1:16 000 live births. In about 60% of cases only one eye is affected, in the remaining cases the lesion is bilateral. The relationship between retinoblastoma and deletions on chromosome 13 has already been discussed and as in the case of Wilms' tumour may involve loss of a regulatory gene.

Diagnosis. Clinical presentation usually occurs before 3 years of age and rarely later than 5 years.

Tumour is usually confined to the eye and loss of the normal red reflex (p. 57) indicates the presence of a space-occupying lesion behind the lens. Small masses arising in the macular region may disturb vision and lead to strabismus. With multiple lesions there may be secondary glaucoma. Spread of the tumour is initially along the optic nerve and into the spinal fluid. Rarely marrow or bone metastases are found.

Differential diagnosis from infective lesions such as *toxocara canis* can usually be made by an experienced paediatric ophthalmologist.

Management. The treatment of retinoblastoma depends on the extent of the tumour and in general is as conservative as possible. If the optic disc is involved more radical surgery is required. Focal treatment involves a variety of forms of carefully focused radiation therapy using either external beams or cobalt sources applied locally to the globe.

Enucleation of the eye is now relatively uncommon but where necessary as much of the orbital portion of the optic nerve must be excised with the eye to obtain histological confirmation regarding tumour infiltration. Adjuvant chemotherapy is used in the presence of optic nerve or heavy choroidal involvement.

Where the tumour is solitary and there is no family history, recurrence in the same eye or the contra-lateral eye is unlikely, but close follow-up is none the less necessary. Examination under anaesthesia should be done every 3–4 months for 2 years, then 6-monthly up to 5 years of age. These patients should be looked after in specialized units where survival should approach 100% in patients with localized disease. Only about 30% survive where there is optic nerve involvement and 75% with choroidal invasion.

Where there is no previous family history and one affected child, siblings incur about a 5% risk of being affected. By contrast, the offspring of a parent with bilateral disease have a 50% chance of being affected. Similarly where a parent has had a unilateral retinoblastoma and a child has been affected, there is again a 50% chance of subsequent children being involved.

Liver tumours

Primary liver tumours in childhood account for about 2% of all malignancies and are usually either hepatic carcinoma or hepatoblastoma although rarely sarcomas occur. Benign lesions include haemangioma, hamartoma and adenoma.

Hepatoblastoma is an embryonal tumour arising in primitive hepatocytes. It usually presents in infancy and is rare over 5 years of age. The tumour cells of hepatic carcinoma resemble those seen in adult disease.

Diagnosis. The presenting sign is usually an abdominal mass, often with marked distension. Pain is unusual but there may be a history of anorexia and vomiting. Plain X-ray may show calcification and ultrasound reveals the liver to be the site of origin. A CT scan is usually sufficent to delineate the extent of the primary tumour which is of major importance when deciding on initial therapy. Liver function tests are generally within the normal limits, although occasionally there may be obstructive jaundice due to biliary tract involvement.

Elevation of serum alpha fetoprotein (AFP) is an invaluable marker for hepatoblastoma and is also elevated in about half the patients with hepatic carcinoma. A characteristic feature of hepatoblastoma is a marked thrombocytosis possibly due to tumour production of thrombopoietin. Although the diagnosis is almost certain with raised AFP levels and an intrahepatic tumour, histological confirmation should be obtained with either open or closed liver biopsy if pre-operative chemotherapy is to be given. If complete resection of the lesion is possible needle biopsy should not be performed but rather definitive surgery.

Management. Completeness of surgical excision is the most important single prognostic factor, but operative mortality may be as high as 15%. Lesions which are localized to a single lobe may be amenable to initial surgery but larger lesions extending into both lobes or involving the porta hepatis will initially be inoperable and require chemotherapy. About 60% of patients with localized, resectable hepatoblastoma will be cured. This is, however, a highly chemosensitive tumour and therefore adjuvant chemotherapy with adriamycin alone is given to patients with completely resected disease. Where the primary is considered unresectable, more intensive chemotherapy, usually including cisplatin, is given and surgery delayed until the AFP is normal and CT scan indicates operability. At this time angiography may have a useful role in planning surgery.

Germ cell tumours

Germ cell tumours arise in the pluripotential germ cell which normally migrates in fetal life from the yolk sac endoderm to the genital ridge. Tumours therefore occur in the testis, ovary or in sites of aberrant migration, namely the sacrococcygeal area, retroperitoneum, mediastinum and pineal region. Dysgerminomas or seminomas are derived from the primitive, undifferentiated germ cell. The more differentiated cell population which contributes to the embryo gives rise to teratomas, and trophoblastic or yolk sac tumours arise from extraembryonal precursor cells. Malignant germ cell tumours in children tend to have histological features which reflect this range of cell populations; the yolk sac tumour produces AFP and the trophoblastic tumour produces beta human chorionic gonadotrophin (HCG). Pure teratomas are usually benign, although they may contain sub-populations of yolk sac or trophoblastic cells.

TESTICULAR TERATOMA

These usually present as a painless swelling, or if there is extensive nodal involvement, with abdominal pain and a palpable mass. Surgical exploration should never be through the scrotal skin as this carries a risk of tumour contamination and may result in inadequate excision of involved cord. The testis should be removed through an inguinal excision following high ligation of the cord. These tumours are normally predominantly of yolk sac origin and therefore produce AFP.

If there is no evidence of metastatic disease in lung, bone or liver, surgical excision is likely to be curative. AFP levels should be followed weekly until normal and provided the elimination half-life is not prolonged (normally less than 5–7 days) no further action is required. A slow half-life or a failure to reach normal levels necessitates further re-evaluation to look for persistent or recurring disease. In remission the patient should be followed with monthly AFP measurements for 12 months and then 3-monthly for 2 years, beyond which time the risk of relapse is minimal.

For tumours which do not produce AFP, a similar approach may be followed with close clinical and ultrasound or CT examination. In the event of relapse or metastatic disease at presentation these patients are highly curable with chemotherapy usually containing cisplatin and etoposide.

OVARIAN TUMOURS

These present with abdominal pain, and an abdominal or pelvic mass. Occasionally there may be vaginal bleeding. Dysgerminomas or yolk sac tumours are commonest and up to 15% will be bilateral at presentation. Staging investigations are as for testicular tumours, and with localized disease, unilateral salpingo-oophorectomy without post-operative radiation or chemotherapy will be curative in the majority of patients. With more extensive disease, chemotherapy is usually the primary treatment modality rather than extensive mutilating surgery. This is a highly chemosensitive tumour and may be cured by chemotherapy alone.

SACROCOCCYGEAL TERATOMA

Sacrococcygeal teratomas present in the neonatal period and are usually highly differentiated and benign. Complete resection including excision of the coccyx is curative in most cases. In a minority, usually those with extensive intra-abdominal disease or the older child, the pathology may be more malignant. In such cases there may be dysuria, difficulty with defaecation or neurological symptoms. Chemotherapy is effective and the overall prognosis is good. In general radiotherapy is not needed.

Histiocytic disorders

Histiocytes are part of the monocyte phagocytic cell system which, interacting with other components of the immune response, play an important role in defence against infection and foreign particles. The main pathological entities involving the histiocyte are Langerhans' cell histiocytosis (previously known as histiocytosis X), malignant histiocytosis, and the virus-associated haemophagocytic syndrome.

Langerhans' cell histiocytosis (LCH) covers a broad range of clinical syndromes which used to be known as eosinophilic granuloma of bone, Letterer–Siwe disease of skin and lung, and Hand–Schuller–Christian disease with multi-system involvement. Because these entities all involve the same cellular abnormality and are spectrums of the same disease they are no longer separated in this way. The pathognomic feature of LCH is the presence of the typical Langerhans' cell with its grooved, lobulated nucleus. The cell itself does not have any phagocytic capacity, although haemophagocytosis is commonly associated with the disease when extensive.

It is important to stress that LCH is an immunological abnormality and not cancer, but it is frequently managed by paediatric oncologists because when treatment is necessary cytotoxic agents are often used.

Diagnosis. LCH may be considered in two broad groups; localized and generalized disease. Localized disease usually involves bone and may present with pain or a tender mass. Often asymptomatic lesions are found on routine X-ray for other reasons. An irregular lytic lesion with clearly defined borders is characteristic and although the radiological features are almost pathognomic, biopsy confirmation is usually sought. This in itself may induce spontaneous remission of the lesion. A skeletal survey, which is more accurate than bone scan for defining lesions, should be done to determine the extent of the disease. If there is no clinical evidence of other system involvement, i.e. no skin lesions, anaemia or hepatosplenomegaly, further staging investigations are unnecessary. No therapeutic intervention is usually required and although lesions were irradiated in the past, the only indications for this are where pain is persistent despite curettage or if there is partial collapse of a vertebral body with neurological symptoms. Complete vertebral collapse, if asymptomatic, does not benefit from irradiation.

Diabetes insipidus can result from disease involvement of the pituitary gland or hypothalamic involvement secondary to lesions arising in the orbit, sphenoid or mastoid. Chemotherapy or radiotherapy may be necessary.

Generalized disease can involve skin, nodes, lung, bone, liver, spleen and bone marrow. The subgroup with the worst prognosis is infants with liver, spleen and marrow involvement, often associated with extensive skin disease. Skin lesions may resemble severe flexural eczema but are distinguished by a purpuric component. Maculopapular rashes occur and there may be extensive yellow crusting on the scalp. Otorrhoea due to mastoid involvement can be an intractable problem.

Extensive involvement of the skull leads to large boggy soft tissue swellings with alarmingly large lytic lesions in the underlying bone. Lung involvement presents with diffuse pulmonary infiltration or honeycomb appearance.

Management. Management of multi-system LCH depends on the extent of the disease and the symptoms caused. The condition may be relatively indolent and little intervention is required, but with severe skin involvement or mastoid disease prednisolone and vincristine are usually first-line agents. Topical mustine may also be effective. With refractory disease or the extensive multi-organ involvement of infants, more aggressive chemotherapy, e.g. etoposide, is necessary. With infant multi-system LCH there remains significant septic mortality due to myelosuppression from marrow involvement or generalized debility.

Malignant histiocytosis

This is a rare malignant proliferation of histiocytic cells which presents with lymphadenopathy and systemic malaise, such as recurring fever and weight loss. Bone marrow involvement also occurs and this condition is usually treated as high-grade lymphoma.

Further reading

Altman AJ, Schwartz AD. In: Schaffer AJ, Markowitz M. (Eds) *Malignant Diseases of Infancy, Childhood and Adolescence.* WB Saunders Co., Philadelphia 1983.

Finegold M. (Ed.) *Pathology of Neoplasia in Children and Adolescents.* WB Saunders Co., Philadelphia 1986.

Pizzo PA, Poplack DG. (Eds) *Principles and Practice of Paediatric Oncology.* Lippincott, Philadelphia 1989.

Riehm H. (Ed.) *Malignant Neoplasms in Childhood and Adolescence.* Karger, Basel 1986.

Voute PA, Barrett A, Bloom HJG, Lemerle J, Neidhardt MK. (Eds) *Cancer in Children.* Springer-Verlag, Berlin 1986.

26
DISORDERS OF THE BONES AND JOINTS

Most bones are cartilaginous and are formed by the deposition of bone mineral into a pre-formed cartilaginous structure at epiphyses. The cartilage is formed and modelled by chondroblasts and chondroclasts while bone is formed and modelled by osteoblasts and osteoclasts. Growth occurs at the growth plate; the epiphyseal cartilage. The metaphysis is the weakest part of the bone and lies between the growth plate and the centre of a bone, called the diaphysis. The bones of the vault of the skull and the clavicle are membranous bones, being formed by the deposition of mineral into the membrane without being preformed in cartilage. Bone requires an initial protein matrix into which the bone minerals can be deposited. Defects in bone can affect the protein (e.g. osteogenesis imperfecta) or mineral content (e.g. rickets). The transfer of minerals into the fetus is maximal in the last month of fetal life. The infant continues to have a great nutritional need for calcium, phosphorus and vitamin D.

As bone matures, growth proceeds and is maximal in the long bones but significant growth occurs in the spine too. As a direct result of this, the long bones have an increased blood supply predisposing them to the spread of haematogenous infection, e.g. osteomyelitis.

Growth hormone affects activity at the growth plate while vitamin D and parathormone affect the mineralization of bone. Steroids affect the protein matrix content and can cause osteoporosis. Genetic disorders can primarily affect the epiphysis (e.g. epiphyseal dysplasia), the growth plate (e.g. achondroplasia), the metaphysis (e.g. metaphyseal

dysostosis) or the diaphysis, as in osteogenesis imperfecta. Cranio-synostosis syndromes primarily affect the membranous bones of the skull but often have associated abnormalities in other bones, such as syndactally.

Diseases of bones and joints can be acute or chronic in onset, but usually cause pain, swelling, limitation of use or deformity. The child will usually present because of a limp, pain or swelling or because of the deformity. Pain can be referred so that pain from a hip joint can often be felt in the thigh or even the knee and it is therefore always necessary to examine the whole limb to include, in an X-ray, the next adjacent long bone and joint. Look also for signs of systemic disease which may suggest a generalized disease process or infection.

Arthritis in childhood

Arthritis in childhood has a different pattern to that seen in the adult where crippling destructive disease is common. In the child, acute arthritis is not uncommon, often occurring after viral diseases or trauma, but chronic disease lasting more than 3 months only affects 1:1000 children before the age of 16 years. The prognosis for the majority is good with destructive disease being uncommon. One of the hallmarks of arthritis is early morning stiffness. If on waking the child is stiff and takes a few minutes or more to loosen up and be fully mobile, then the disease is often a chronic arthritis. The duration of early morning stiffness is a good indicator of the activity of the disease and this will vary as the disease activity changes.

Terminology is a problem. In Britain, disease recognized as being chronic is usually called juvenile chronic arthritis (JCA). In the USA it is usually called juvenile rheumatoid arthritis (JRA); a term which in Britain is reserved for the very rare patients, usually female, who have developed adult-type rheumatoid arthritis whilst a child. It is only these latter patients who have a positive rheumatoid factor in the blood. There is a trend on both sides of the Atlantic to consider the term juvenile arthritis instead of JCA or JRA to avoid further confusion.

PAUCIARTICULAR ARTHRITIS

The most common type of chronic arthritis in childhood is pauciarticular JCA. This disease affects only a few joints, up to four, and most often affects medium-sized joints such as the knees, ankles or elbows. Occasionally small joints are also affected.

Clinical features. Pain in the joint, swelling or a limp are the most common presenting features causing limitation of movement. This can lead to contractures when the joint is kept still, often in a position of flexion, to avoid pain. On examination, the joint is often swollen, warm and flexed with surrounding muscle wasting. The swelling can be due to synovial thickening as well as an effusion (Fig. 26.1). The joint usually shows limitation of movement due to pain.

Up to 50% of children will develop a chronic iridocyclitis. This condition involves inflammation of the anterior chamber of the eye which is often asymptomatic and can cause severe eye disease. The children should therefore be examined regularly by slit-lamp for evidence of inflammation.

Blood tests may show a raised ESR with, usually, a normal blood count. Between 10 and 50% of the children will have a positive antinuclear factor.

Management. There is no curative treatment but pain relief and physiotherapy are essential to maintain muscle strength and a full range of joint

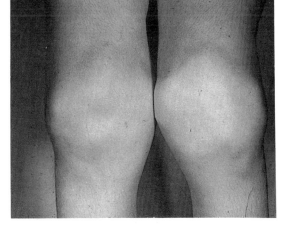

Fig. 26.1 Juvenile chronic arthritis affecting the knees. There is marked synovial thickening as well as joint effusion.

movements. Then, when the disease does resolve, as usually occurs, the child will be left with a fully functioning joint. Pain relief is usually obtained with non-steroidal anti-inflammatory agents such as naproxen. Aspirin is very useful but may predispose to Reye's syndrome. Indomethacin is also useful and if given at night will reduce early morning stiffness. If the joint does not have a full range of movement, a splint can be used at night to encourage the joint back to full mobility, but this usually requires straightening a flexed joint. A wrist is splinted in the slightly extended position of function. If muscle strength is maintained, this will help to protect the joint from trauma. The muscles are an essential part of the protection for any joint, without which damage easily and frequently occurs. Swimming, being non-weight bearing, is excellent exercise for this purpose. Bicycle or tricycle riding is also excellent for lower limb disease with the body weight supported by the saddle. Occasionally when a joint is persistently troublesome an intra-articular injection of steroid, with drainage of any effusion, can lead to substantial relief for some months.

Long-term joint disease is rare if contractures are avoided and usually occurs in girls who go on to develop a true polyarthritis.

POLYARTICULAR DISEASE

Polyarticular disease affects 15% of children with JCA, traditionally affecting five or more joints. Any joint can be affected and girls are more often polyarthritic than boys. The neck is often affected and a full range of neck movements must be vigorously maintained. Restriction causes serious morbidity, including an inability to drive a car when grown up.

Treatment is as described for pauciarticular disease. Second-line drugs such as gold, penicillamine and hydroxychloroquine may be required to modify the course of the disease, especially if erosions are seen on X-ray. In general, the prognosis is good but one-third of patients have erosive disease 5 years after onset.

SYSTEMIC DISEASE

Systemic onset disease presents in pre-school children; the younger the child the worse the prognosis. Frequently the children present with a fever of unknown origin, but within 3 months a diagnosis of systemic arthritis has been made in one-half of these children. Hepatosplenomegaly and anaemia can occur and a fleeting macular rash is characteristic.

If non-steroidal anti-inflammatory drugs fail to suppress the disease, steroids and later gold, penicillamine and hydroxychloroquine may be required. Steroids cause rapid osteoporosis in these immobile patients and are best given as an alternate day regime.

OTHER TYPES

Spondiloarthritis, occurring predominantly in boys who are HLA B27-positive, frequently presents with peripheral joint disease at onset. The hips are most often affected and enthesopathy (inflammation at the insertion of tendons) often occurs at the heel. Some patients have a family history of acute iritis or ankylosing spondilitis. This disease is referred to as juvenile onset ankylosing spondilitis.

Psoriatic arthritis and Reiter's disease, as well as reactive arthropathy, can occur in childhood.

Rheumatic fever

This is a connective tissue disease which follow infection with Group A, beta haemolytic streptococcus, often of the throat or skin. It is rare in Britain but remains common in many parts of the world where infection and poverty are found. Its importance rests with the serious cardiac sequelae which can occur.

Clinical features. The child may have a history of a preceding sore throat and usually presents with arthralgia most commonly in the knees, ankles, elbows and wrists. The pain stays in one joint for 1–2 days before moving to the next. A mild fever, pallor and sweating are common and erythema marginatum occurs in 10%. This is a pinkish-red ring-like macular rash affecting the trunk. Rheumatic nodules occur in 10% of cases, but are rarely seen within 2 weeks of the onset. They are painless and are found on the elbow, the ulnar border of the forearm, the dorsum of the hands and the occiput. Their size varies from 0.5 to 2.5 cm and their presence is strongly correlated with moderate to severe carditis.

Carditis is common and tachycardia is the most significant sign (p. 569). A systolic murmur is almost invariable, but most soft mid-systolic murmurs are innocent. In 60%, however, the murmur represents significant valvular disease with a diastolic murmur being heard in the majority. Pericarditis is seen in some cases and if heart failure occurs it is due to myocarditis.

Chorea can also occur, being more common in females and older children (p. 293). The involuntary, purposeless movements are non-repetitive and increase when the child is asked to perform a task requiring concentration. They cannot be reproduced on request. Associated muscle weakness can be severe. The chorea can last for weeks, but eventually subsides completely.

Investigations show a mild anaemia, leucocytosis and raised ESR. A raised anti-streptolysin O (ASO) titre is found in 80% of cases. The ECG shows a prolonged PR interval in 85%.

The diagnosis is often easy when a number of features are present, particularly carditis and

Table 26.1 Diagnostic criteria for rheumatic fever.

Major	Minor
Carditis	Evidence for streptococcal infection
Chorea	Previous rheumatic fever
Arthritis	Arthralgia
Subcutaneous nodules	Fever
Erythema marginatum	Prolonged PR interval
	Elevated acute phase reactants

chorea, but mild cases occur and a confident diagnosis cannot always be made, and for this reason diagnostic criteria for rheumatic fever have been described and these are listed in Table 26.1. The presence of either two major or one major and two minor criteria make the diagnosis very probable, but in current UK practice doubt still often exists. Emphasis should certainly be placed on demonstrating evidence for preceding streptococcal infection and when in doubt careful repeated assessment of the CVS with follow-up is important.

Management. Treatment requires bed-rest usually for some weeks and while acute signs last. Penicillin is essential to eliminate any remaining streptococci and it should be continued as a single daily dose until after puberty to prevent recurrent attacks. Aspirin, 100–120 mg/kg/day in four divided doses is given for 2 weeks followed by 60–70 mg/kg/day until active disease has ceased, usually within 4–6 weeks of onset. Watch for evidence of salicylate toxicity in the form of vomiting, headache, tinnitus, deafness and hyperpnoea. Aspirin reduces fever and arthralgia but does not affect the long-term outcome. Steroids are not thought to affect the long-term outcome either, but can help curtail acute carditis. This is useful since aspirin can cause heart failure in those with cardiomegaly.

Prognosis. Rheumatic carditis is the only potentially lethal complication of the acute phase of rheumatic fever and it is also the only carditis which results in long-term sequelae. One-third of children with rheumatic fever will develop rheumatic heart disease, most commonly pure mitral stenosis, mitral regurgitation with mitral stenosis or aortic regurgitation. In Britain this rarely causes symptoms in childhood. The signs of mitral regurgitation disappear in 70% for up to 8 years after the illness.

Auto-immune disorders

DERMATOMYOSITIS

Dermatomyositis is a rare chronic inflammatory disease predominantly affecting the skin and muscles. In childhood, dermatomyositis is not associated with underlying malignancy.

Clinical features. Onset is usually with insidious weakness, muscle tenderness and misery. The rash is characteristic, consisting of a violaceous hue around the eyelids, over the bridge of the nose and often on the flexor surface of the thigh or back of the hand (see Plate 10). The affected muscles can be firm and thickened and in some patients hard calcified nodules develop in the subcutaneous tissue. These can rupture through the skin exuding calcified material and may become infected (Plate 11). The diagnosis can often be made clinically. A raised creatinine phosphokinase (CPK) level in the blood reflects muscle damage and is often, but not invariably, found in this condition. The level is not a reliable indicator of disease activity. A muscle biopsy may be helpful in showing inflammation of the muscle, and confirms the diagnosis.

Management. Treatment is with steroids, initially daily but with a rapid reduction and change to a single dose on alternate days when the disease is under control. Without steroids one-third of patients die and another third are left severely crippled, but this can be reduced to 10% mortality and 10% severely crippled with the careful use of steroids. The skin disease can be exacerbated by sunlight. Physiotherapy is essential to prevent contractures and to maintain muscle strength.

SCLERODERMA

This is a rare disorder which is usually generalized and primarily affects collagen in the skin and occasionally in the oesophagus. Induration and contracture within the skin cause a taut shiny skin particularly on the hands and face. Raynaud's phenomenon can occur. The pattern is characteristic and the diagnosis can be made clinically. Penicillamine and steroids are both used with limited success.

Morphoea

An unusual localized form of scleroderma is called morphoea. Initially, linear erythematous oedematous streaks change to atrophic yellow shiny areas around which the whole of the affected limb or face may fail to grow.

SYSTEMIC LUPUS ERYTHEMATOSIS (SLE)

This disorder is rare in the first decade but then becomes more common, with the onset of one-fifth of all cases beginning in childhood. In girls, only 30% of cases present prior to puberty and it is found more frequently in blacks compared to other races. It is caused by auto-antibodies to DNA

Table 26.2 Common symptoms and signs of SLE.

Common symptoms
Arthralgia or arthritis
Rash
Fever
also
Fatigue and weight loss
Raynaud's phenomenon

Common findings
Fever and raised ESR
Thrombocytopenia and purpura
Haemolytic anaemia
Lymphadenopathy
Splenomegaly and occasionally hepatomegaly
Nephrotic syndrome or acute nephritic syndrome
Peripheral neuropathy
Epilepsy or psychosis
Pleurisy
Pericarditis

which usually occur spontaneously but which can be drug-induced, in which case withdrawal of the drug results in resolution of the disease.

Clinical features. The disease is very variable because it affects many tissues, any one of which can result in the presenting symptoms (see Table 26.2). The onset can be insidious or acute, but most often includes fever, malaise, arthralgia and a characteristic rash. The rash is usually scaly and erythematous, develops over the bridge of the nose in a 'butterfly' distribution (Plate 12) and is sensitive to light. This can affect the whole body and vasculitic changes may be seen especially on the palmar surface of fingers and the nails.

Arthralgia is common, but actual arthritis occurs less frequently and joint deformity is rare. Pleurisy, pericarditis, hepatosplenomegaly and lymphadenopathy are common and neurological problems occur in 50% of cases. Kidney disease, which has the greatest morbidity, occurs in 80% and usually presents with acute nephritis (p. 262) which can progress rapidly; nephrotic syndrome is less common. The prognosis is worse if a renal biopsy shows a proliferative or membranous nephritis.

Management. Treatment is with steroids. Initially large doses are required, but these are reduced when the disease is under control. Immunosuppression with azathioprine, cyclophosphamide, plasmaphoresis and anti-malarials is also sometimes required.

Death and serious complications are frequently due to the side-effects of treatment, especially infection. Severe infective episodes will occur in 20% at some time. Before the use of steroids, the disease was usually fatal in childhood, but now there is a 90% 5-year survival. Few survivors go into complete remission and relapses are common.

KAWASAKI'S DISEASE

This disease, first recognized in Japan where it is quite common, and also found in the USA, is less common in Europe. It is not often seen in developing countries.

Clinical features. It is an acute febrile illness most common in children under 5 years. The fever is moderately severe and usually lasts for more than 5 days. During this time the child is irritable and often has signs of conjunctivitis without a purulent discharge, a sore throat, cracked lips and occasionally a 'strawberry' tongue. As the acute phase subsides, erythema and oedema of the extremities occurs and generalized lymphadenopathy is found. At this stage, desquamation occurs which is characteristic and which affects the palms of the hand and soles of the feet (see Plate 13). In view of the clinical presentation, the disease was called the muco-cutaneous lymph node syndrome.

Up to 50% of affected individuals develop coronary artery aneurysms which may be detected on ultrasound examination. These usually regress over months, but 2–3% of all affected children die, usually in the first 3 months, from coronary thrombosis or aneurysmal rupture. The risk is highest in those who develop a platelet count of more than 1000×10^9/l. Because of this, aspirin therapy is recommended at 120 mg/kg/day reducing to 20 mg/kg/day when acute symptoms subside. Aspirin should be maintained at least until the platelet count has returned to normal or until ultrasound evidence of coronary disease has resolved.

The painful hip

Pain in the hip or sudden onset of limp in a child should always be taken seriously and the child referred for a hospital opinion. There are a number of important causes to consider.

IRRITABLE HIP

Irritable hip is also sometimes called transient synovitis of the hip or even observation hip. The child is afebrile and presents with a limp due to pain which also causes restricted movement of the hip joint. Rotation in flexion is most often restricted. It is important to remember that referred pain from the hip is often felt in the thigh or knee and to examine the hips carefully in all cases where the child complains of knee pain.

It is most common in boys and the peak age incidence is 4–10 years. It is the commonest cause of hip pain in childhood, accounting for 90% of children presenting with a limp due to a painful hip. The cause is not known but most cases settle within a week if bed rest is maintained until a full range of movement is obtained. Recurrences occur in 15% of cases usually within a year.

Since the child presents with a limp and pain on moving the hip joint, other diseases must be excluded by careful clinical examination as well as X-rays and blood tests if necessary.

The diagnosis is distinguished from septic arthritis, which causes a fever, and Perthe's disease which can have a normal X-ray initially, but symptoms are usually insidious in onset and slow to resolve. In older children, slipped femoral epiphysis is more common, and this group should have their hip X-rayed. A tumour in the femur can be overlooked and all persistent or recurrent cases should have an X-ray of the hip joint as well as the whole length of the femur.

PERTHE'S DISEASE

Perthe's disease affects 1 : 2000 children between the ages of 4 and 10 years. Boys are four times more commonly affected than girls. It occurs in relatives more often than expected by chance and involves both hips in 15% of those affected. The aetiology is not known but the pathology begins with avascular necrosis of the femoral head which is usually painless initially. The subchondral or crush fractures which result from Perthe's disease are painful and it is usually at this stage that the child presents with a limp. Pain, limp and restriction of joint movement are usually mild.

Investigations. Investigations are required in all suspected cases. Although an X-ray can be normal in 30% initially, after a few weeks the femoral head may increase in opacity and begin to deform, becoming flattened or mushroom-shaped (Fig. 26.2). Loss of more than 2 mm of femoral head height (from the base of the femoral head to the roof of the acetabulum compared to the normal side) is a bad prognostic sign. Subluxation of the femoral

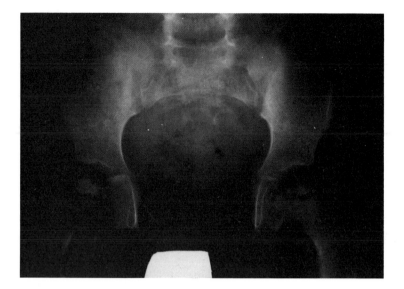

Fig. 26.2 Severe Perthe's disease of both hips which has left the femoral heads grossly distorted. A normal hip can be seen on the right side of Figure 26.3.

head causes unequal weight distribution and excessive femoral head deformity.

Management. Treatment is controversial. It is symptomatic only (pain relief with restricted activity) in about 50%. In the remainder there is no consensus view apart from the need to prevent subluxation of the femoral head. Bed rest with traction is required for those with the worst symptoms and X-ray appearances. The hip is often kept in abduction, sometimes in a plaster cast to allow the child to go home. If necessary, an osteotomy of the femoral neck allows the femoral head to be repositioned within the acetabulum.

Prognosis. The younger the child, the better the prognosis regardless of X-ray appearance. Girls have a worse prognosis. In the long-term, 40% will have normal hips, 40% will have minor symptoms and 20% will require hip replacement as adults.

SLIPPED FEMORAL EPIPHYSIS

This disorder of unknown aetiology occurs in those over the age of 10 years and around the time of puberty when growth is at its maximum. Occasionally there is a history of recent trauma. It is more common in boys and is bilateral in 25%. Pain often develops suddenly, but can develop slowly and cause the child to limp. On examination, the leg is held externally rotated and there is limitation of abduction and internal rotation. X-rays should be taken in the frog position (the hips abducted and internally rotated) when the femoral head can be seen to have moved medially (see Fig. 26.3).

Treatment consists of immediate bed rest followed by the insertion of metal pins through the epiphysis into the femoral head to prevent further slipping.

Infection

SEPTIC ARTHRITIS

Acute septic arthritis occurs most commonly in the large weight-bearing joints; the hip, knee and ankle. In 10% of cases, more than one joint is affected. The infection is blood-borne. In 50% of all cases the pathogen is *Staphylococcus aureus* which is almost invariably the pathogen when this condition occurs in the newborn. In a further 25% of cases *Haemophilus influenzae* is the cause. This organism is particularly likely to affect children under the age of 4 years and is a considerably commoner cause of septic arthritis in these

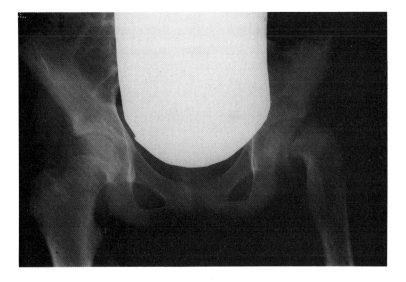

Fig. 26.3 Slipped femoral epiphysis. The femoral epiphysis on the left side has slipped along the line of the growth plate. The right side is normal.

young children than other organisms. Haemolytic streptococci can also cause septic arthritis but Gram-negative organisms are rare except in the newborn or the immunocompromised child.

Clinical features. The child is usually febrile (except the newborn) and is in pain. The infant frequently immobilizes the limb leading the parents to believe that the child is unable to move it. The natural puffiness of a well-nourished infant may disguise a swollen joint and care must be taken to examine each joint through its full range of movement. Older children complain of pain in the joint. The white blood count is usually raised with a polymorphonuclear leucocytosis. A blood culture frequently identifies the pathogen.

Management. Early diagnosis and treatment are essential to prevent the rapid destruction of articular cartilage which can occur. Aspiration of the joint is useful both diagnostically (a Gram stain may help to identify the organism) and therapeutically. Antibiotics can be injected into the joint but should be give intravenously for a minimum of 24 hours. Most children will hold the joint immobile because of pain, but splints or traction can give further pain relief. As soon as the pain has subsided a full range of joint mobility should be encouraged with physiotherapy.

Acute septic arthritis of the hip requires special consideration since frequently the pus has gained access to the joint from an underlying osteomyelitis of the femoral neck. The capsule of the hip joint is unique in that it encloses the epiphyseal growth plate where osteomyelitis in the child usually develops. Longer antibiotic treatment is therefore required, usually for 6 weeks. Aspiration of pus from the hip joint improves the prognosis and should always be performed.

Chronic septic arthritis

This usually presents with an effusion, with or without pain, and frequently affects the knee. Tuberculosis is the causal agent and it is, therefore, rare in developed countries except in immigrants (p. 555). There may be signs of disseminated tuberculosis, but frequently a synovial biopsy is required for diagnosis. A Heaf test is usually positive. Rifampicin and isoniazid are a suitable combination of antibiotics. Complete recovery of joint function is uncommon unless proper treatment begins early.

ACUTE OSTEOMYELITIS

This disease, like acute septic arthritis, is due to blood-borne infection and in 75% of cases is due

to *Staph. aureus* while in 15% it is due to streptococci. The remainder are due to Gram-negative
organisms and occasionally *Haemophilus influenzae*.
Any bone can be affected, but the long bones
(especially femur and tibia) and the bones of the
foot are most often involved. In a few children,
more than one site will be affected. Within the
bone, the site affected will depend on age since the
blood supply to the bone will be maximal in different areas at different ages. In the neonate, the
blood supply is maximal to the main epiphysis. In
the older child, the blood supply is maximal to the
growth plate, while in mature bone the blood supply is maximal in the diaphysis. Since the femur is
most frequently affected, in the neonate infection
will spread to the joint causing septic arthritis of
the hip. The hip joint capsule encloses the epiphysis
of the femoral head which is often destroyed (Fig.
26.4). In the older child the growth plate is infected
with resultant diminished growth. In the adult the
diaphysis is infected with few sequelae.

Clinical features. Newborns present with an immobile limb, as in septic arthritis, and the parents
often believe the limb is paralysed. They are often
ill and septic but rarely febrile. Older children
complain of severe pain in the affected bone. The
bone is very painful to touch although the area of
tenderness can be quite localized. The older child
will be febrile with a raised white blood count and
a blood culture will often allow a bacteriological
diagnosis to be made. X-rays do not help in the
acute phase except to exclude other causes of
pain, such as a fracture or tumour. Usually 10 days
will pass before periosteal new bone formation is
seen in the bone itself. The periosteal new bone is
formed by the periostium which has been stripped
off the cortex by pus (Fig. 26.4). Osteomyelitis can
be mistaken for cellulitis but this latter condition is
rare unless secondary to visible trauma to the skin
or secondary to an underlying osteomyelitis.

Management. Treatment, if begun within 24–48
hours of diagnosis, is with antibiotics alone which
must include large doses of anti-staphylococcal
drugs. These are best given intravenously for 2–3
days. If the symptoms have not settled by 48–72

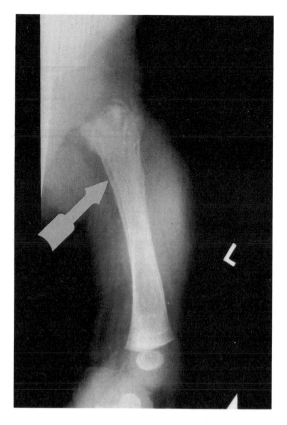

Fig. 26.4 Osteomyelitis in a neonate following
staphylococcal septicaemia. Because of the young age
the femoral head and upper femoral growth plate have
been destroyed. The arrow shows typical new periosteal
bone formation in the healing stage.

hours or if the diagnosis is made after 2–3 days of
symptoms, then surgical drainage is indicated.
Antibiotics are given for at least 6 weeks. However, 90% of children can be cured without surgery.
Chronic osteomyelitis is rare with early prompt
treatment and is usually complicated by a sequestrum of dead bone within the area of infection;
surgery is essential in these cases.

Unusual organisms are found in the immunocompromised patient, in children with compound
fractures, and in those with sickle cell anaemia
where salmonella is often the cause (p. 431).
Ampicillin with flucloxacillin is the treatment of
choice in a child with sickle cell anaemia, while
in the immunocompromised and those with

compound fractures, pus as well as blood should be obtained for culture. Broad spectrum antibiotics are modified in the light of culture results.

Spinal deformities

SCOLIOSIS

Scoliosis is a curvature of the spine in the coronal plane. It is best visualized by observing the child from behind when the spinous processes of the vertebral bodies are not in a straight line but are curved in an 'S' shape. It can be due to congenital abnormalities of the vertebrae or be secondary to neurological conditions, but most commonly occurs as idiopathic scoliosis which affects up to 1% of all children. The curvature develops gradually for no known reason causing rotation of the ribs and a hump to the chest wall best seen when the child tries to touch his toes while standing with legs straight. A leather, plastic or rarely plaster jacket, can slow or halt the progress of the scoliosis (Fig. 26.5).

Surgery is often required with rods being inserted alongside the whole thoraco-lumbar spine to prevent movement. Scoliosis is frequently found in children with physical handicap, especially spastic quadriplegia, where it is due to poor positioning of the child. If this is not avoided by careful attention to positioning and with physiotherapy, a 'windswept' deformity results which makes dressing and cleaning the child very difficult. In addition, the hips can dislocate resulting in considerable pain. Scoliosis also occurs with progressive muscle weakness, such as Duchenne muscular dystrophy, because the muscles are not strong enough to keep the spine straight against gravity.

KYPHOSIS

A kyphosis is a curvature of the spine in the saggital plane best seen with the child standing, and looking from the side. It is usually due to a congenital abnormality of one or more vertebrae but it can be due to a crush fracture.

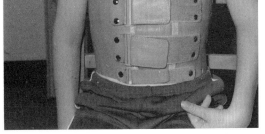

Fig. 26.5 A child with idiopathic scoliosis wearing a scoliosis jacket.

TORTICOLLIS

Pain in the neck due to bone, joint or muscle disease can cause a torticollis or a 'wry' neck where muscle spasm causes limitation of movement. At rest the neck is twisted. This can occur in a child with an upper respiratory tract infection and tender cervical glands. It can also be due to a brain tumour in the posterior cranial fossa. Joint disease as a feature of chronic arthritis causes torticollis because of pain. In Down's syndrome a torticollis or pain in the neck can be due to atlanto-axial dislocation; X-rays of the cervical spine are required urgently. Treatment is to stabilize the neck initially in a cervical collar but if necessary with an arthrodesis.

Trauma to the neck can cause muscle spasm, atlanto-axial dislocation or even a crush fracture of the vertebrae. Diagnosis of a child with torticollis therefore requires careful evaluation of the whole child.

Traumatic disorders

OSGOOD–SCHLATTER DISEASE

Osgood–Schlatter disease is common during adolescence. In this condition, pain occurs below the knee on exercise due to tenderness at the site of the insertion of the patella tendon into the tibial tuberosity. It is usually a sports injury due to vigorous exercise which has to be curtailed if the pain is to resolve. Regular gentle exercise can continue.

PULLED ELBOW

A sudden pull on the arm of an infant or young child, whether given gently to swing the child or jerked to pull the child away from danger, occasionally results in a dislocation of the head of the radius from its fibrous annular ring. The child immediately complains of pain and refuses to use the arm. If the elbow is pronated and then fully supinated, the dislocation is put back in place and the child is immediately relieved of pain.

Genetic disorders

OSTEOGENESIS IMPERFECTA

Osteogenesis imperfecta, or brittle bone disease, is a heterogeneous group of disorders of collagen affecting 1:10 000 children. The defect affects the protein matrix of the bone into which bone minerals are deposited and results in poorly ossified bones which fracture abnormally easily. The joints are often hyperextensible and the sclerae can be abnormally blue. The teeth are affected similarly, a condition called dentigenosis imperfecta. Deafness frequently occurs with increasing age.

The child usually presents with fractures, unless diagnosed asymptomatically because of an affected relative.

Type 1

The majority of cases are of this type which is relatively mild and dominantly inherited. Fractures are most frequent during childhood.

Type 2

This is the lethal variety and can be subdivided further into broad-boned and thin-boned types. Severe fractures during birth usually result in death. Most cases are sporadic but rarely, recessive inheritance occurs. Other types are rare. When treating fractures it is important to keep the child as mobile as possible to prevent further osteoporosis resulting from bed rest. Exercise is important, but the most severe cases can only exercise gently for fear of spontaneous fractures.

OSTEOPETROSIS

This rare genetically inherited disease is sometimes called Albers–Schonberg disease or marble bone disease because on X-rays the bones look highly dense. Despite this the bones fracture easily and have delayed healing. Obliteration of the marrow cavity results in anaemia and hepatosplenomegaly. Cranial nerve palsies result from compression as the nerve passes through bony foramina with resulting deafness and blindness. Hydrocephalus also occurs. Treatment is symptomatic.

CLEIDO-CRANIAL DYSOSTOSIS

This disorder predominantly affects the membranous bones. The clavicles are partially or totally absent resulting in an ability to advance the shoulders towards the sternum. Some children also have delayed ossification of the skull and many have short stature. The disorder is usually asymptomatic and can be familial.

ACHONDROPLASIA

This condition is the most common cause of true adult dwarfism; the adult height usually being 130 cm, and rarely exceeding 140 cm. It is dominantly

Table 26.3 Criteria for the diagnosis of Marfan's syndrome.

Major criteria	Minor criteria
Mitral incompetence with floppy valve	Arachnodactyly
	High arched palate
Aortic incompetence	Funnel chest
Dilated aortic root	Asthenic build
Dissecting aortic aneurysm	Joint laxity (especially ankles)
	Flat feet
Dislocation of the lens	Scoliosis
Trembling iris	Spontaneous pneumothorax
	Floppy mitral valve without incompetence
	Severe myopia (>4 dioptres)

inherited but many cases are new mutations; advanced paternal age is an aetiological factor. The disorder is caused by an abnormality in cartilage production at the epiphyseal growth plate resulting in poor growth especially of the long bones. The head often appears large in contrast, but hydrocephalus can also be present. Mental development is normal. X-rays show a small sciatic notch, a broad flat roof to the acetabulum and short long bones widened at the growth plate. Growth hormone production is normal and treatment is symptomatic.

EHLERS–DANLOS SYNDROME

This is a rare autosomal dominant disorder affecting connective tissue. The joints are hyperextensible as is the skin which is easily traumatized and heals poorly.

MARFAN'S SYNDROME

This is an autosomal dominant condition with a very variable clinical phenotype. No single clinical feature is always present and neither is a specific test available. The two major disadvantages of having Marfan's syndrome are the risk of dissecting aneurysm of the aorta and the risk of dislocation of the lens. Some abnormalities are thought to be more common than others and a system of major and minor criteria help to decide who may be at risk of aortic dissection or rupture (Table 26.3). People with one major and two minor criteria, or five minor criteria and a family history, or seven minor criteria without a family history should have echocardiography of the aortic root. The aortic root size is increased in adults at risk of aortic rupture who require regular repeat echocardiography every 3 months. Beta blockers are thought to reduce the risk of aortic rupture whereas surgery is required if significant aortic incompetence or progressive aortic dilatation occur.

27

SKIN DISORDERS

Skin: structure and function

The skin is derived from two of the primitive germ layers, the ectoderm and the mesoderm. The ectoderm develops into the epidermis and its appendages. The mesoderm becomes the dermis, which lies beneath the epidermis, and makes up the bulk of the skin. The epidermis is a multi-layered structure which renews itself continuously by cell division in its deepest layer – the basal layer. The cells of the basal layer are anchored to the basement membrane which lies between the epidermis and dermis. Cells produced by mitosis in the basal layer ascend through the prickle cell layer. When they reach the granular layer they begin to produce keratin, and they lose their nuclei. The cells on the surface of the skin, forming the horny layer (stratum corneum), are flattened keratin husks which are gradually abraded by day-to-day wear-and-tear from the environment. The cells of the epidermis are held together by inter-cellular bridges (desmosomes).

The pigment-producing cells of the skin, melanocytes, are found amongst the cells of the basal layer. Melanocytes produce melanin which is transferred to adjacent prickle cells via the melanocytes' dendritic processes. The main function of melanin is to protect the cell nucleus from ultraviolet radiation. Another dendritic cell found in the epidermis is the Langerhans' cell. Langerhans' cells are probably modified macrophages, and they play an essential role in antigen recognition and the transference of this information to dermal lymphocytes.

A number of structures arising from the epidermis constitute the epidermal appendages –

hair, sebaceous glands, apocrine and eccrine sweat glands.

The dermis is a layer of connective tissue composed of collagen, elastin, and a mucopolysaccharide ground substance. All these components are produced by dermal fibroblasts. The dermis and epidermis interdigitate via upward projections from the dermis (dermal papillae), and downward extensions from the epidermis (rete ridges). The dermis is richly supplied with nerves, blood vessels and lymphatics.

The skin performs a variety of essential functions. It is a major sensory organ responsible for the perception of heat, cold, pain and touch. The epidermis provides a barrier against external physical and chemical injury, and against water loss from within. Melanin in the skin provides protection against harmful ultraviolet radiation. The skin is essential for body temperature control, by regulation of skin blood flow and eccrine sweat gland activity. It is also responsible for vitamin D synthesis from dehydrocholesterol by the action of ultraviolet light.

HISTORY TAKING IN DERMATOLOGY

An adequate history is as important in dermatology as it is in any other medical or surgical speciality. The questions asked should elucidate:
1 The duration of the skin lesions.
2 Which part of the body was first affected.
3 Whether the lesions itch.
4 If the lesions blister.
5 Whether the lesions come and go or are continuous.

6 If anything appears to make the lesions better or worse.

7 Whether the child has been taking any medicines for another medical problem.

8 What topical medications have been used, including any purchased over-the-counter from the local chemist.

9 Whether anyone else in the family has a similar problem. Is there a family history of psoriasis or eczema?

If atopic eczema is suspected, parents should be asked whether other family members suffer from asthma or hay fever. When scalp ringworm or insect bites are the presenting problems it is important to ask about family pets. A general medical history is also useful as skin lesions may be related to a systemic problem.

EXAMINATION

It is important to examine skin lesions in good light, preferably daylight. It is also essential, for the majority of dermatoses, to examine the whole skin surface, otherwise important diagnostic clues may be missed. Always examine the nappy area in babies. Look inside the mouth; buccal mucosal lesions are associated with some dermatoses. Also examine the hair and nails.

The features of a dermatosis which are important in establishing a diagnosis are listed in Table 27.1.

SPECIAL INVESTIGATIONS

Wood's light

Wood's light is long-wavelength ultraviolet light, and is useful for demonstrating subtle hypopigmented lesions, e.g. ash-leaf macules in tuberous sclerosis, and fluorescence of certain scalp ringworm fungi.

Skin scrapings for mycology

If ringworm is suspected, skin scrapings or plucked hairs are mounted in 10% potassium hydroxide and examined under the microscope for fungal

Table 27.1 Important diagnostic characteristics of skin lesions.

Distribution of lesions
Localized or generalized
Symmetrical or asymmetrical
Do they have a specific pattern of distribution?
    Atopic eczema in limb flexures
    Pityriasis rosea following lines of skin cleavage
    Psoriasis on scalp, elbows and knees
Presence on sites of trauma
    Epidermolysis bullosa
    Koebner phenomenon in psoriasis and lichen planus

Configuration
Annular
    Granuloma annulare
    Erythema annulare
Linear
    Linear lichen planus
    Lichen striatus

Morphology
Note size, shape and colour of lesions

hyphae. Scrapings are also sent to the mycology laboratory for culture on special media.

Skin biopsy

This is a useful procedure for confirmation of a diagnosis, or clarification of the diagnosis when this is uncertain. Skin biopsy is also helpful in categorizing immunologically mediated blistering diseases by immunofluorescence, and in correct classification of cases of epidermolysis bullosa by electron-microscopy. A small piece of skin is removed by excision or punch biopsy, under local anaesthetic. Specimens for routine histology are fixed in formalin, and those for immunofluorescence 'snap frozen' in liquid nitrogen. Special fixatives are required for specimens to be examined by electron-microscopy.

Psoriasis and other papulosquamous

PSORIASIS

Psoriasis is a condition whose precise pathogenesis is unknown. It is a common disorder, affecting approximately 1.5% of the population of Western Europe. Genetic factors are important in its aetiology, and environmental factors may precipitate its onset. Affected individuals often have a family history of the condition, but its exact mode of inheritance is unclear. Psoriasis often has its onset in later childhood and adolescence, but it is rare in infancy and early childhood.

Clinical features

Plaque psoriasis. The commonest type of psoriasis is the chronic plaque variety, in which well-demarcated, raised, erythematous scaly plaques are scattered over the body (Plate 14). Typical sites for these plaques are the scalp, knees, elbows and sacral area. The scale on the surface of the plaques has a characteristic silvery appearance.

Psoriasis may occur at sites of trauma to the skin, such as operation wounds; a reaction known as the Koebner phenomenon.

Guttate psoriasis. This type of psoriasis is not uncommon in children and young adults, and is often precipitated by streptococcal tonsillitis. A profuse eruption of small psoriatic lesions is scattered over the trunk and limbs (Plate 15). These guttate lesions usually resolve gradually over a period of 6–8 weeks, but the subsequent course of events is variable. There may be recurrent episodes of guttate lesions, or persistent psoriatic plaques may develop.

Psoriasis of the nails. The nails are frequently affected by psoriasis, and may show pitting of the nail plate and separation of the nail plate from the nail bed (onycholysis).

Pustular psoriasis. Generalized pustular psoriasis is fortunately a very rare event in childhood, as it is a serious condition. The onset is usually abrupt, with the appearance of sheets of pustules on the skin, accompanied by fever and general malaise.

Treatment

The treatment employed is determined by the type of psoriasis being treated, and the sites affected.

Stable plaque psoriasis on the trunk and limbs may be treated with dithranol (Anthranol). Dithranol in Lassar's paste is often employed in hospital treatment centres, but for use at home there are several proprietary preparations containing dithranol in a cream or ointment base (Psoradrate, Dithrocream, Anthranol, Dithrolan), which are easier to use. In the past, dithranol preparations were left on the skin for several hours, but recent evidence suggests they are equally effective after only a short application time. This has led to their use as 'short contact' therapy, in which the preparations are left on the skin for approximately 30 minutes before being washed off. Dithranol preparations are available in a variety of strengths. Treatment is started with a low concentration of dithranol, and depending upon the response, the concentration is gradually increased until the psoriasis clears. Dithranol is an irritant and will burn the skin if not used with care.

Tar preparations are also useful in the treatment of stable plaque psoriasis. Crude tar is effective but messy, and alternatives include tar creams such as Carbo–Dome (coal tar solution 10%) or Alphosyl (coal tar extract 5%, allantoin 2%) which are cosmetically more acceptable and non-staining.

Scalp psoriasis is difficult to treat effectively, but can usually be improved significantly by the regular use of tar shampoos, keratolytics and topical steroid lotions. Compound coconut oil ointment, which contains coal tar, salicylic acid, sulphur and coconut oil, is a useful preparation, although rather messy. It should be massaged into the scalp 2 or 3 nights each week, and washed out in the morning.

Dithranol and tar preparations are not suitable for the treatment of psoriasis affecting the face, axillae and groin, as they are rather irritant on these sites. These areas should be treated with a mild topical steroid such as a hydrocortisone preparation.

Guttate psoriasis is best treated with a proprietary tar cream such as Carbo–Dome or Alphosyl, and a course of ultraviolet light.

There is no effective treatment for psoriatic nail changes.

Pustular psoriasis is an emergency, and requires in-patient management under the care of a dermatologist.

PITYRIASIS ROSEA

This is a condition which is common in adolescents and young adults, and which may occur in a younger age group. Its aetiology is unknown, although a viral cause has been postulated.

Typically the eruption is preceded by a 'herald patch' which resembles an area of mild eczema. Within a few days of the appearance of the herald patch a more extensive eruption, with a tendency to follow the cleavage lines of the skin in an 'inverted Christmas tree' distribution, occurs on the trunk and the proximal parts of the limbs. The lesions are macular and have a characteristic peripheral collarette of scale (Plate 16). The face and the distal parts of the limbs are only rarely affected. The skin lesions may be itchy, but there is no constitutional upset.

The lesions resolve within 4–6 weeks of the onset. Itching may be treated with a mild topical steroid preparation.

PITYRIASIS LICHENOIDES CHRONICA

In this condition recurrent crops of red-brown papular lesions occur on the trunk and limbs. As these papules gradually fade, the surface of each is covered by a single 'mica-like' scale which can be picked off the skin intact. In a florid variant of this condition the papules are more inflammatory and undergo central necrosis, eventually healing to leave small scars.

Pityriasis lichenoides usually improves with ultraviolet light treatment, but its course may be very protracted, sometimes lasting for several years.

LICHEN PLANUS

Although lichen planus is principally a disease of adults, it may be encountered occasionally in children. It is characterized by an eruption of intensely itchy, flat-topped, violaceous papules which may occur anywhere on the body. The surface of the papules often has a reticulate pattern of white lines (Wickham's striae). The buccal mucosa may also be involved with a similar net-like pattern of white lines. Linear groups of lesions may occur,

particularly on the limbs. Occasionally lichen planus affects the nails.

The aetiology of lichen planus is unknown, but identical lesions may occur as a manifestation of graft-versus-host disease, and as a result of drug provocation. Lichen planus usually resolves spontaneously after several months, and can be helped symptomatically by topical steroid therapy.

Ichthyosis

The ichthyoses are a group of hereditary disorders of keratinization in which the skin is dry and scaly. There are several types, with different modes of inheritance summarized in Table 27.2.

ICHTHYOSIS VULGARIS

This is a common, dominantly inherited disorder. It is not present at birth, but usually develops in early childhood. The skin is covered in small scales (Plate 17) which are more prominent on the extensor aspects of the limbs; the limb flexures are usually spared. Many cases are relatively mild.

Treatment. The regular use of emollients such as emulsifying ointment as a soap substitute, proprietary emollient oils in the bath, the regular application of a urea-containing cream such as Calmurid (urea 10%) or Aquadrate (urea 10%) will help to some extent, but in milder cases treatment is often unnecessary.

X-LINKED ICHTHYOSIS

This condition may be present at birth, or first appear in early infancy. As it is an X-linked

Table 27.2 The ichthyoses.

Dominant
Ichthyosis vulgaris
Bullous ichthyosiform erythroderma

Recessive
Non-bullous ichthyosiform erythroderma
Lamellar ichthyosis

X-linked recessive
X-linked ichthyosis

recessive trait it only occurs in boys. It is known to be associated with a deficiency of the enzyme steroid sulphatase. The skin is more severely affected than in ichthyosis vulgaris and the scales tend to be larger and darker.

Treatment. Emollients are the mainstay of treatment, as in ichthyosis vulgaris.

OTHER TYPES

Other ichthyoses are rare. Generalized erythema and scaling are features of non-bullous ichthyosiform erythroderma which is usually present at birth, or during the neonatal period. Lamellar ichthyosis is similar, but there is less erythema, and the skin is covered in thick brown scales. In bullous ichthyosiform erythroderma there is generalized erythema, scaling and blister formation. These rarer, more severe forms of ichthyosis are frequently treated with the vitamin A derivative etretinate (Tigason), often with considerable benefit.

COLLODION BABY

The term collodion baby is applied to a condition in which a newborn is covered in a shiny cellophane-like membrane (Plate 18). There is usually mild ectropion. Affected babies usually shed the membrane within 2–3 weeks of birth. This appearance may be caused by underlying X-linked ichthyosis, lamellar ichthyosis, or ichthyosiform erythroderma, but in some infants when the membrane is shed the underlying skin is perfectly normal (lamellar desquamation of the newborn).

Collodion babies have an extremely high transepidermal water loss. They should be nursed in a high-humidity environment, and should have a high fluid intake, otherwise they rapidly dehydrate. The skin should be treated with emollients.

HARLEQUIN FETUS

In this severe disorder the infant is covered in thick, fissured plaques. There is gross ectropion and eclabium, and small deformed ears. This condition probably represents a severe form of ichthyosiform erythroderma. Affected infants soon die, but there are reports of the survival of some children following treatment with etretinate.

Eczema

Eczema and dermatitis are terms which are synonymous. Eczema is an inflammatory dermatosis characterized clinically by erythema, oedema, papules, vesicles and exudation. In chronic eczema the affected areas of skin become thickened (lichenification) with prominence of the surface markings. Eczema has a number of causes, often classified as exogenous, when an external factor such as a contact allergen is responsible, and endogenous, when the eczema is constitutional in origin. The commonest type of eczema encountered in childhood is atopic eczema.

ATOPIC ECZEMA

Atopy is a term applied to a genetic predisposition to eczema, asthma and hay fever. A family history of atopy is found in the majority of patients with atopic eczema. The pathogenesis of atopic eczema is complex, and in addition to the genetic predisposition there are several factors such as environmental influences and emotional stimuli which may contribute to the problem.

Clinical features. Atopic eczema is not present at birth, but usually appears during the first year of life, frequently between the ages of 2 and 4 months. In infancy the eczema is often generalized, but in older children there is a characteristic involvement of the limb flexures (Plate 19). The typical picture in an older child is of eczema of the face, hands, limb flexures, and trunk. Itching is intense, and the child will often rub or scratch incessantly, producing raw exuding areas, and eventually lichenification. The course of atopic eczema is typically punctuated by episodic exacerbations. The whole skin tends to be extremely dry in individuals with atopic eczema.

Table 27.3 Summary of treatment of atopic eczema.

Emollients
Topical steroids
Medicated bandages
Sedative antihistamines
Ultraviolet light

Treatment. Perhaps the most important aspect of the management of a child with atopic eczema is sympathetic explanation of the nature of the condition to the parents. Table 27.3 summarizes treatment methods for eczema.

Emollients, which are designed to moisturize the skin, are essential in the management of the dry skin in atopic eczema. A combination of emollients may be used at bathtime – for example, emulsifying ointment as a soap substitute, a bath oil (Oilatum emollient; Alpha Keri bath oil; Balneum) in the water, and Boots E45 cream, Oilatum cream or Unguentum after bathing. It is often necessary to try several different emollients before finding one which apparently suits a particular child.

Topical steroid preparations are also invaluable in the treatment of atopics. In infants and young children it is usually possible to provide adequate control of eczema with mild topical steroids such as hydrocortisone preparations. In older children more potent topical steroids may be required, but the aim should always be to use the weakest possible preparation sufficient to control the disease. A topical steroid/antibacterial combination may be useful in children whose eczema frequently becomes secondarily infected. Topical steroids are available in cream, oily cream and ointment bases. Because of the extremely dry skin in atopic eczema, preparations in oily cream and ointment bases tend to be more beneficial.

Medicated bandages such as Ichthopaste or Coltapaste can be extremely ·useful in the management of severe eczema on the limbs. The bandages may be applied over a topical steroid, and changed every 2 or 3 days until the eczema has improved. The use of sedative antihistamines at night may also be helpful. Ultraviolet light treatment will sometimes improve eczema, but unfortunately relapse occurs quite rapidly when the treatment is discontinued.

The influence of diet on atopic eczema is rather contentious. In some children replacement of cows' milk by a soya preparation results in improvement of the skin, but in others it does not appear to help. Many dermatologists reserve dietary manipulation for those children with very severe eczema who are not responding to other treatment methods. Any dietary alteration should be supervised by a dietitian, in order to avoid nutritional deficiencies.

Complications. The commonest complication of atopic eczema is secondary bacterial infection in the form of folliculitis or impetigo. This should be treated with courses of cloxacillin, flucloxacillin or erythromycin, when necessary.

Children suffering from atopic eczema are more prone to viral warts and molluscum contagiosum, and herpes simplex infection may lead to widespread skin lesions (Plate 20) and a severe illness (eczema herpeticum; Kaposi's varicelliform eruption). Children suffering from eczema herpeticum are usually seen by a dermatologist within a few days of the onset of the condition, and a decision about the most appropriate therapy should be based on whether the lesions are still spreading, and whether the child is systemically unwell. If the lesions are static, and the child is systemically well, anti-viral therapy is probably unnecessary. If, however, lesions are spreading and/or the child is unwell, treatment with intravenous acyclovir (Zovirax i.v.) should be commenced. Eczema herpeticum is often a recurrent phenomenon, but subsequent episodes tend to be less severe than the primary eruption.

Prognosis. In many, atopic eczema will resolve in childhood, but in others it persists into adolescence and adult life. In some, the eczema will resolve in childhood, only to reappear later in life. There is no certain way of predicting the course of the eczema in a particular individual. Those whose eczema has cleared still remain more susceptible to the effects of primary irritants on the skin, and should avoid occupations such as hairdressing and engineering, in which the hands are frequently exposed to primary irritants.

OTHER TYPES OF ECZEMA

Pityriasis alba

This is a common mild eczematous process which produces slightly scaly, hypopigmented areas on the face, and occasionally on the trunk. It is more noticeable on a pigmented skin. It resolves later in childhood, and the only treatment required is an emollient, or a weak hydrocortisone preparation.

Discoid eczema

This is characterized by scattered circumscribed patches of eczema on the trunk and limbs. It is uncommon in childhood. Treatment should be with a mild to moderate potency topical steroid.

Allergic contact dermatitis

Allergic contact dermatitis is considered by most authorities to be rare in childhood, but there are some reports which suggest that routine patch testing of children in whom contact dermatitis is suspected may yield a surprisingly high number of relevant positive results. Nickel is the allergen most frequently responsible for contact dermatitis in children, particularly in girls, where the provoking agents are usually cheap metal earrings or the metal studs on jeans. Other causes include rubber chemicals, topical medicaments, colophony in adhesive plasters, and, in the USA, plant dermatitis from contact with poison ivy.

Infantile seborrhoeic dermatitis

This condition occurs in infants under the age of 3 months. It affects the scalp, the retro-auricular areas, the neck flexures, the axillae, groin, and napkin area. The skin in these areas is erythematous and scaly, and although the eruption may be very extensive it does not appear to be itchy, and there is no constitutional upset. Topical therapy with an emollient and hydrocortisone cream will usually produce a rapid improvement, and in many cases the condition resolves in a few weeks. However, some infants apparently suffering from typical infantile seborrhoeic dermatitis may develop a gradual transition to an atopic pattern of dermatitis, and their subsequent course is that of atopic eczema.

Napkin psoriasis is considered by some to be a variant of infantile seborrhoeic dermatitis, in which the involvement of the nappy area has a sharply demarcated edge (Plate 21), and lesions on the trunk have a psoriasiform appearance. The condition usually resolves after a few weeks, and can be treated with emollients and topical hydrocortisone.

Rare causes of eczema-like eruptions affecting the nappy area include zinc deficiency and histiocytic disorders (p. 472).

Napkin dermatitis

This is a term often used to encompass a number of conditions in which a dermatitis occurs on the nappy area including atopic eczema, infantile seborrhoeic dermatitis and napkin psoriasis. The use of this term should, however, be reserved for dermatitis caused by wearing nappies. True napkin dermatitis is a primary irritant dermatitis, and most infants are affected to some extent. In this condition the nappy area is erythematous and slightly scaly, but the skin creases are spared (Plate 22). In severe cases there may be multiple erosions (Jacquet's ulcers). Various factors may be impliated in the aetiology of irritant napkin dermatitis, including infrequent nappy changes, the effect on the skin of proteolytic and lipolytic enzymes in the faeces, the irritant effects of ammonia generated by the action of urea-splitting organisms in the faeces on urea in the urine, and superinfection with *Candida albicans*. Occlusive plastic nappy covers contribute significantly to the problem.

Treatment should include more frequent nappy changes, using disposable nappies if possible, the use of a barrier cream such as zinc and castor oil cream after cleaning the nappy area, and a topical anti-candida/hydrocortisone preparation such as Nystaform-HC (nystatin, chlorhexidine and hydrocortisone), Daktacort (miconazole, hydrocortisone) or Canesten-HC (clotrimazole, hydrocortisone).

Juvenile plantar dermatosis

The first description of this disorder appeared only a few years ago, and its occurrence seemed to coincide with the widespread use of footwear made of synthetic materials, particularly training shoes. Its exact aetiology, however, remains unknown. It has a characteristic clinical appearance (Plate 23). The weight-bearing areas on the soles of the feet have a scaling, glazed appearance, and the development of painful fissures within these areas can make walking uncomfortable and sporting activities impossible. Treatment is difficult, but the condition does benefit from the liberal use of emollients, and the avoidance of socks and shoes made of synthetic materials may help. Topical steroids are of little value in this condition. Although juvenile plantar dermatosis may persist for many years, it almost invariably resolves in adolescence.

Viral infections

WARTS

Warts are extremely common in childhood. They are benign epidermal neoplasms caused by viruses of the human papilloma virus (HPV) group. There are a number of different strains of HPV which produce different clinical types of warts. The wart viruses probably penetrate the skin via small abrasions.

Common warts

These are raised cauliflower-like lesions which occur most frequently on the hands. They may be scattered, grouped, or periungual in distribution. Common warts in children usually resolve spontaneously eventually.

Treatment. Wart paints are preparations containing salicylic acid (e.g. Salactol – salicylic acid 16.7%, lactic acid 16.7% in collodion), glutaraldehyde (e.g. Glutarol – glutaraldehyde 10%) or formaldehyde (e.g. Veracur gel – formaldehyde 1.5%), and will encourage resolution of warts in the majority of cases. A wart paint should be used for at least 3 months before considering alternative treatment. These preparations are not suitable for use on the face.

Cryotherapy with liquid nitrogen may be applied to warts resistant to topical therapy with wart paints. This procedure is painful and should not be inflicted on young children. If the warts of a young child have not responded to wart paints they are best left alone to resolve spontaneously. In older children warts can be frozen using a simple applicator of cotton wool wrapped around the end of an orange stick. Treatment should be repeated at intervals of 3 weeks until the warts have resolved.

Plantar warts

Plantar warts (verrucae) may be solitary, scattered over the soles of the feet, or grouped together producing so-called mosaic warts (Plate 24). They are frequently painful on walking. The typical appearance of a plantar wart is of a small area of thickened skin which when pared away reveals several black dots produced by thrombosed capillaries.

Treatment. Wart paints are the mainstay of treatment for plantar warts. Cryotherapy is not as effective on the feet as it is on hand warts. A combination of wart paint and cryotherapy can be employed in those cases not responding to either modality alone.

Plane warts

These are tiny, flat-topped, flesh-coloured warts which usually occur on the dorsa of the hands and on the face (Plate 25). They are extremely difficult to treat effectively, and attempts at treatment are likely to do more harm than good. They are best left alone, as they will eventually resolve spontaneously.

Genital warts

The presence of vulval and perianal warts in infants and children may be the result of inoculation of virus from the maternal genital tract during delivery, auto-inoculation of a cutaneous strain of HPV, or innocent non-sexual contact with a parent harbouring genital warts. However, the possibility of sexual abuse must be considered in any child with genital warts. The child should be carefully examined for other signs of abuse (p. 524). The types of HPV associated with genital warts in children have been reported in only a few cases, but the advent of DNA hybridization procedures will permit identification of the virus types, and establish their genital or non-genital origin. The availability of this information may then permit a more accurate assessment of whether or not sexual abuse is responsible for the warts in an individual case.

Treatment. The application of podophyllin paint once weekly, under medical supervision, may be used to treat small numbers of genital warts, but this agent is toxic, and should not be used in large quantities on florid lesions. If the warts are very prolific it is preferable to arrange for surgical ablation under a general anaesthetic.

MOLLUSCUM CONTAGIOSUM

The lesions of molluscum contagiosum are caused by a pox virus. They are typically pearly, pink papules, with a central umbilication filled with a horny plug (Plate 26). The lesions may occur anywhere on the body, but are most commonly encountered on the face and trunk. They are frequently grouped, and may be surrounded by a mild eczematous reaction. They may be very extensive in children with atopic eczema.

Treatment. There is no anti-viral agent which has any effect on the virus of molluscum contagiosum. The lesions will, however, eventually resolve spontaneously. In older children they may be treated by cryotherapy, or carefully pricking the centre of each lesion with a cocktail stick dipped in

phenol. Care is required with phenol and its use should be restricted to lesions on the trunk and limbs. Infants and young children will not tolerate either of these methods, and they should not be inflicted upon them. If parents of young children are anxious that something positive be done to deal with the lesions they can be advised to squeeze each one gently between the thumb-nails to express the central plug. This will often speed their resolution.

HERPES SIMPLEX

There are two antigenic types of the herpes simplex virus. Type 1 is responsible for the common 'cold sore' on the lips or face, and type 2 is associated with genital herpes, and may cause neonatal herpes simplex when acquired from the mother's genital tract.

Primary herpes simplex

Initial contact with the herpes simplex virus usually occurs in early childhood, and any lesions which develop are often so mild they are not noticed. Occasionally, however, a severe primary herpetic gingivostomatitis occurs. Primary cutaneous herpes simplex may also occur. Following a primary infection the virus establishes itself in the dorsal root ganglia and may be triggered to produce recurrent lesions by a variety of stimuli.

Recurrent herpes simplex

Recurrent cold sores on the lips are a common problem. Typically, the eruption of a group of small vesicles is preceded by a sensation of itching and discomfort in the affected area. The vesicles subsequently burst, the lesion crusts over, and resolves within 7–10 days. Usually, topical therapy is not necessary, but a little Betadine paint (povidone-iodine) will help to prevent secondary bacterial infection, and it also has weak anti-viral activity. If the recurrent lesions are more extensive, then topical Herpid (idoxuridine 5% in dimethyl sulphoxide), or Zovirax cream (acyclovir) can be used for treatment.

Eczema herpeticum

In children suffering from atopic eczema, primary herpes simplex infection of the skin can produce extensive lesions, and the child may be systemically unwell (see p. 491).

HERPES ZOSTER

Herpes zoster is uncommon in childhood, but when it does occur the clinical features are exactly the same as those seen in adults. A unilateral eruption of vesicles occurs, limited to the distribution of a dermatome. The lesions usually resolve in 10–14 days.

Treatment. Usually no treatment is required, but if fresh vesicles are appearing, a topical anti-viral agent such as idoxuridine or acyclovir may help to limit the extent of the eruption.

Bacterial infection

IMPETIGO

This is a superficial bacterial infection of the skin caused by *Staphylococcus aureus*, or a combination of this organism and haemolytic streptococci.

Clinical features. The head and neck area are most frequently affected, but lesions can occur anywhere on the body. The initial lesion is a small subcorneal pustule, which rapidly increases in size, and soon ruptures to leave a raw, exuding surface. The exudate dries to form a crust, and the stratum corneum peels back at the margins of the lesion to give a typical appearance (Plate 27). In infants the presenting lesions may be bullous, and this has led to the rather inaccurate term 'pemphigus neonatorum'.

Impetigo may occur as a secondary phenomenon in atopic eczema, scabies, and head louse infestation.

Treatment. Except in the most localized cases, impetigo should be treated with a systemic antibiotic such as cloxacillin, flucloxacillin or erythromycin. Many staphylococci are penicillinase producers, and are therefore resistant to penicillin. A useful topical antibacterial agent to use on localized cases or as an adjunct to systemic therapy is Bactroban ointment (mupirocin 2%).

STAPHYLOCOCCAL SCALDED SKIN SYNDROME

This aptly named condition occurs principally in infants and young children as a result of infection with certain staphylococcal phage types which produce an epidermolytic toxin. This epidermolysin causes a split in the epidermis at the level of the granular layer, and the superficial epidermis peels off in sheets. This condition is distinct from toxic epidermal necrolysis produced by drugs (Lyell's syndrome) where the full thickness of the epidermis is necrotic. It is a potentially life-threatening condition, but responds well to systemic therapy with cloxacillin or flucloxacillin.

Fungal infection

DERMATOPHYTE (RINGWORM) INFECTION

The areas of the body affected by ringworm infection in children differ in some respects from those affected in adults. Scalp ringworm is a disease of childhood, and is rare in adults. Ringworm of the groin and fungal disease of the nails are conditions encountered principally in adults, being rare in childhood.

Scalp ringworm (tinea capitis)

The principal fungi responsible for scalp ringworm vary in different parts of the world. In Britain and other European countries most cases of childhood scalp ringworm are the result of *Microsporum canis* infection (usually acquired from cats); in the USA *Trichophyton tonsurans* is responsible for the majority of infections; in the Indian subcontinent the commonest cause is *Trichophyton violaceum*.

The typical clinical picture is of one or more scaly patches of hair loss on an otherwise normal scalp. The hair in the affected areas is broken off just above the surface of the scalp, producing an irregular stubble (Plate 28). Occasionally the scalp is more diffusely involved, with an appearance resembling seborrhoeic dermatitis.

Diagnosis. Microsporum canis fluoresces a brilliant yellow-green under long-wavelength ultraviolet light (Wood's light) (Plate 28). However, many other fungi do not fluoresce under Wood's light, and the diagnosis must be confirmed by microscopic examination of plucked hairs to demonstrate fungal hyphae and spores. Hair from the affected areas should also be sent to the mycology laboratory for culture, to identify the organism.

Treatment. Scalp ringworm should be treated with oral griseofulvin (10 mg/kg body weight in divided doses daily) for a period of 4–6 weeks. Topical anti-fungal agents are not effective.

Kerion

Kerion is a term applied to a severe inflammatory response to scalp ringworm, usually to *Trichophyton verrucosum*, the organism of cattle ringworm, but other fungi may be responsible for kerion formation. The clinical picture suggests pyogenic bacterial infection, with boggy swelling of the scalp, surface pustulation, and hair loss (Plate 30). An affected child may be left with areas of permanent scarring alopecia once the condition has resolved.

Kerion should be treated with griseofulvin, and the additional use of a potent topical steroid may help to lessen the degree of inflammatory response. It may take several months for the scalp to return to normal.

Tinea corporis

In Britain, ringworm of the trunk and limbs in childhood is usually caused by *Microsporum canis*, and is often associated with scalp ringworm. The lesions are typically annular, with an erythematous, scaly edge and central clearing (Plate 31).

The diagnosis can be confirmed by microscopic examination of skin scrapings for fungal hyphae.

Lesions of tinea corporis are usually multiple and are best treated with a course of griseofulvin for 3–4 weeks.

Tinea pedis (athlete's foot)

Fungal infection of the feet is uncommon in childhood. The clinical appearance is of scaling in the web-spaces between the toes, occasionally extending on to the dorsa of the feet. Sometimes the presentation is more acute, with itchy vesicles on the soles of the feet, leading to diagnostic confusion with eczema. Eczema tends, however, to be symmetrical, whereas fungal infection is usually asymmetrical in distribution.

Treatment. A topical imidazole (clotrimazole, miconazole, econazole) is effective.

PITYRIASIS (TINEA) VERSICOLOR

This condition is uncommon in children living in temperate zones, but is encountered not infrequently in children in tropical climates. It is caused by yeast-like organisms (*Pityrosporum* sp.) which are normal skin commensals present in pilosebaceous follicles. It is presumed that an alteration in the micro-environment of these organisms in affected individuals encourages them to multiply and extend on to the surface of the skin.

Clinical features. On a non-pigmented skin the lesions of pityriasis versicolor are light-brown macules with a fine surface scale, which occur predominantly on the trunk. They are usually asymptomatic. On a pigmented skin the typical appearance is of patchy hypopigmentation.

The diagnosis can be confirmed by microscopic examination of skin scrapings in a mixture of 10% potassium hydroxide and Parker Quink ink, when characteristic clumps of round spores and short, stubby hyphae will be seen.

Treatment. A simple and effective treatment is topical selenium sulphide in the form of Selsun shampoo. This can be left on the skin for 5 minutes each day whilst bathing and is effective within 2 or 3 weeks. Topical imidazoles (clotrimazole, miconazole, econazole) are also effective. The condition does, however, tend to recur and treatment may have to be repeated. Hypopigmented areas of skin may take several months to repigment.

CANDIDIASIS

Candidiasis (moniliasis, 'thrush') is a term applied to infections of the skin and mucous membranes by *Candida albicans*. Although *C. albicans* is a normal gut commensal, certain conditions favour its transition to a pathogenic role: broad spectrum antibiotics, diabetes mellitus, immunosuppressive therapy, primary immunodeficiency disorders, and occlusion in moist, warm areas of skin.

Mucosal candidiasis

Mucosal candidiasis is common in infants, in the absence of any of the above-mentioned predisposing factors. The clinical picture is of white, curd-like patches on the mucosa, which when removed leave a slightly eroded surface.

Treatment. Nystatin oral suspension or Daktarin (miconazole) oral gel.

Cutaneous candidiasis

Candida superinfection of napkin eruptions is very common. It is an organism which flourishes in a moist, warm environment and the occlusive effects of the nappy encourage its growth. Candida may often be isolated on culture from irritant napkin dermatitis, infantile seborrhoeic dermatitis and napkin psoriasis, but it would appear to be a secondary phenomenon in these conditions and is probably not relevant in their aetiology.

Treatment. As cutaneous candidiasis is usually encountered against a background inflammatory dermatosis of the napkin area, it is preferable to use a topical anti-candida agent combined with a weak topical steroid – for example Canesten-HC (clotrimazole, hydrocortisone) or Daktacort (miconazole, hydrocortisone).

Chronic mucocutaneous candidiasis

This is a rare condition in which chronic candidiasis of mucosae, nails and skin is associated with an immune deficiency or an endocrinopathy. Long-term treatment with oral ketoconazole (Nizoral) is often of help in this condition.

Infestations

SCABIES

Aetiology. Scabies is caused by the mite *Sarcoptes scabiei*, and is acquired by close physical contact with another individual harbouring the mite. Holding hands is probably a fairly frequent means of spread, and the close physical contact between children and their parents provides an ideal situation for transmission of the parasite. Scabies is not acquired from contact with fomites. It is a common disorder, and children of all ages are frequently affected, even during the neonatal period.

On the skin of the host the female scabies mite burrows in the epidermis, and following fertilization by the male, she begins to lay eggs in the burrow behind her. The major symptom of scabies is itching, which is characteristically worse at night. The itching is thought to be due principally to a hypersensitivity to mite faeces, although there may be some contribution from the burrowing activity of the mites. The hypersensitivity to mite faeces develops some 4–6 weeks after the infection is first acquired, and there is therefore a latent period during which the host is unaware of the presence of the mites. Once itching commences the host scratches at the burrows, destroying the mites and eggs, and thereby keeping the mite population in check. In the usual case of classical scabies there are often less than a dozen adult female mites on the affected individual.

Clinical features. There are two principal components of the skin lesions in scabies; burrows and

Table 27.4 Clinical features of scabies.

Primary lesions
Burrows
Scabies 'rash'

Secondary lesions
Excoriations
Eczematization
Impetigo

the scabies 'rash' (see Table 27.4). The burrows are the tunnels made in the stratum corneum by the female mites. Each burrow (Plate 32) is a few millimetres long, faintly brown in colour, and usually serpiginous. Burrows are typically found, in older children, on the sides of the fingers, in the web-spaces between the fingers, around the wrists, on the penis and scrotum, and on the borders of the feet. In infants, burrows are frequently present on the palms of the hands and soles of the feet, and they may also occur on the face and scalp. In neonates and infants, skin lesions may include vesicles on the hands and feet, crusted nodules and pustules. Penile and scrotal lesions consist of small inflammatory papules, sometimes surmounted by a burrow; they are pathognomonic of scabies.

The 'rash' of scabies is an eruption of tiny inflammatory papules grouped on the axillary folds, around the umbilicus, and on the thighs (Plate 33). These lesions are thought to be produced by an inflammatory response to immature burrowing mites.

In addition to these primary skin lesions there are often secondary changes, including excoriations, eczematization and bacterial infection. In certain parts of the world secondary infection of scabies lesions with nephritogenic streptococci may result in cases of post-streptococcal glomerulonephritis.

Diagnosis. Absolute confirmation of a diagnosis of scabies can only be made by demonstrating the mites or eggs under the microscope (Plate 34). A burrow is gently scraped off the skin with the edge of a blunt scalpel, and the debris placed in a few drops of 10% potassium hydroxide, or mineral oil, on a microscope slide. If typical burrows cannot be found on a child thought to have scabies, then other members of the family should be examined, as they are often also affected and may have more readily identifiable burrows.

Treatment. Explanatory treatment sheets are extremely useful. Whatever topical therapy is used, the whole family, and any other close physical contacts should be treated simultaneously. The topical therapy should be applied from the neck to the toes with a 2″ paint brush. Itching does not resolve immediately following treatment, but will improve gradually over a period of 1 or 2 weeks as the stratum corneum, containing the allergenic mite faeces, is shed. A topical anti-pruritic such as Eurax-hydrocortisone cream (crotamiton 10% and hydrocortisone 0.25%) can be supplied for use on residual itchy areas. It is not necessary to treat clothing and soft furnishings; washing of underclothes, nightclothes and bed linen is all that is required.

Benzyl benzoate emulsion. Two or three applications in a 24-hour period are usually sufficient. On the evening of day 1 apply the emulsion from neck to toes. Allow to dry, then apply a second coat. The following morning apply a third coat, then wash off the benzyl benzoate on the evening of day 2. Treatment is then complete, and this should be stressed, because the repeated use of benzyl benzoate will produce an irritant dermatitis.

Gamma benzene hexachloride (Quellada lotion). One application from the neck to the toes is sufficient. The lotion should be washed off after 24 hours.

Monosulfiram (Tetmosol solution). Before application Tetmosol should be diluted with two to three parts water. The dilute solution should then be applied from neck to toes, and washed off after 24 hours.

Aqueous malathion (Derbac-M liquid). One application from neck to toes – washed off after 24 hours.

Special considerations in the treatment of infants and young children

Benzyl benzoate is an irritant, and when used on infants it should be diluted to half-strength; the treatment regime may be repeated after an interval of a few days.

Gamma benzene hexachloride is a neurotoxin, and there have been reports of transient neurological problems following its use on babies and young children. Infants have a high skin surface area to body volume ratio, and are therefore more likely to absorb significant amounts of this agent, particularly if they also have large areas of eczematized skin. The debate about its use in infants continues, although many dermatologists have employed it in the treatment of scabies in children for years without any problems.

If burrows are present on the head and neck area in babies, these can be treated by twice-daily application of Eurax cream (crotamiton 10%). Secondary infection should be treated with a systemic antibiotic, and severe secondary eczematization can be treated for a few days with topical Eurax hydrocortisone cream, before using definitive therapy.

Pediculosis

HEAD LICE

Head louse infestation is usually acquired as a result of head-to-head contact with another individual harbouring the parasite. Medical entomologists do not consider that fomites such as caps, brushes and combs, are responsible for transmission of the head louse. In the past, head louse infestation was extremely common. The majority of those affected lived in large industrial conurbations, and belonged to the lower social classes. A survey carried out in 1941 revealed that 50% of pre-school children from industrial areas were infested, whereas less than 5% of children from four rural counties were affected. By 1980 the overall incidence of infestation was much lower, but those principally affected had become rural, suburban and middle class children.

The head louse lives on the surface of the scalp, using its piercing mouthparts to feed on the host's blood. The adult female louse lays eggs which are cemented to the hair shaft close to the scalp. The eggs are flesh-coloured and are difficult to see, but once the louse nymph has emerged the empty egg-case (nit) is more easily seen. Most eggs will have hatched before the hair has grown more than a few millimetres, and any that have not are non-viable.

Itching is the main symptom of head louse infestation. Nits tend to be more numerous in the occipital region of the scalp, and above the ears, and these are the areas to search carefully. Occasionally keratin casts may be mistaken for nits, but not if examined under the microscope. Impetigo may occur as a result of inoculating staphylococci during scratching, and head louse infestation should be considered in any child presenting with scalp impetigo.

Treatment. The insecticides malathion and carbaryl are now the mainstay of treatment for head louse infestation in Britain. They have superseded the use of gamma benzene hexachloride, although this is still used extensively in the USA. Malathion and carbaryl are both effective pediculicides and ovicides, and there are several proprietary preparations of these insecticides available (Table 27.5). Malathion is adsorbed on to keratin, a process which takes about 6 hours, and confers a residual protective effect against re-infestation which lasts for approximately 6 weeks. Carbaryl is not adsorbed in this way, and does not confer any residual protective effect.

Insecticidal shampoos expose the insects to relatively low concentrations of insecticide, and carry

Table 27.5 Treatment of head lice.

Proprietary preparations containing malathion
    Prioderm lotion
    Derbac-M liquid
    Suleo-M

Propietary preparations containing carbaryl
    Carylderm lotion
    Suleo-C

the risk of encouraging insecticide resistance in the lice. It is therefore preferable to use only lotion preparations for the definitive treatment of head lice.

Prioderm lotion, Derbac-M liquid and Caryl-derm lotion should be left on the scalp for 12 hours. Suleo-M and Suleo-C are marketed as 'rapid' treatments of head lice, to be left on the scalp for 2 hours. Both malathion and carbaryl are degraded by heat and should be stored in a cool environment. After their use the hair should be allowed to dry naturally, rather than with the aid of a hot-air-hairdryer. Treatment should be repeated after 7–10 days to deal with any louse nymphs emerging from surviving eggs. All family contacts of an affected child should also be treated. The physical removal of nits from the hair with a nit comb is only necessary for cosmetic reasons.

Crab lice

The crab louse, or pubic louse, may occasionally infest children, usually as a result of contact with parents carrying this parasite. The absence of significant body hair in children results in the crab louse colonizing areas of suitable hair density – the eyelashes and scalp margin. Adults and eggs can be seen on the hairs at the margins of the scalp, and the eyelashes may be festooned with eggs.

Treatment. Any of the proprietary malathion or carbaryl insecticides could be used to treat crab lice on the eyelashes, but most of them are alcohol-based and would irritate the eyes. Derbac-M liquid has an aqueous base, and is an effective, non-irritant treatment. It should be smeared across the eyelids and lashes, and in young children this can be more readily accomplished when they are asleep. The treatment should be repeated after an interval of 7–10 days.

Papular urticaria

Papular urticaria, often referred to as 'heat bumps', is the typical reaction to arthropod bites. The lesions of papular urticaria are usually raised, extremely itchy papules or nodules (Plate 35) but

Table 27.6 Some causes of blistering disease in childhood.

Insect bites
Bullous impetigo
Thermal or chemical burns
Erythema multiforme
Mastocytosis
Porphyria
Fixed drug eruption
Epidermolysis bullosa
Bullous ichthyosiform erythroderma
Incontinentia pigmenti
Chronic bullous dermatosis of childhood
Dermatitis herpetiformis
Bullous pemphigoid
Pemphigus vulgaris

may develop into bullae. They may occur as a result of the bites of a number of winged insects outdoors, but in the home the most likely source of the problem is infestation of household pets, particularly with cat or dog fleas. Papular urticaria may be treated with a topical anti-pruritic such as Eurax hydrocortisone cream, or a mild topical steroid cream.

Blistering diseases

There are numerous skin diseases in which blistering may occur. Blisters may arise within the epidermis, at the dermo-epidermal junction, or beneath the epidermis. Table 27.6 lists some causes of blistering in childhood.

INHERITED BLISTERING DISEASES

Epidermolysis bullosa

The term epidermolysis bullosa is applied to a group of diseases in which blisters develop as a result of trauma or friction. The classification of epidermolysis bullosa is based on inheritance pattern, clinical features, and light and electron-microscopy of skin biopsies. Two major groups are recognized; those in which blisters occur at, or above the level of the epidermal basement membrane and heal without scarring, and those in

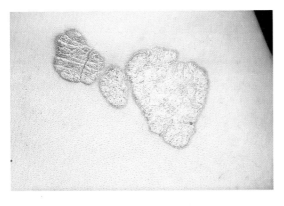

Plate 14 Typical plaques of psoriasis.

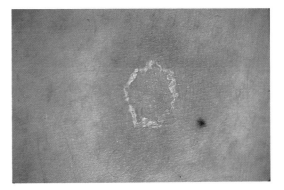

Plate 16 Pink macule with collarette of scale seen in pityriasis rosea.

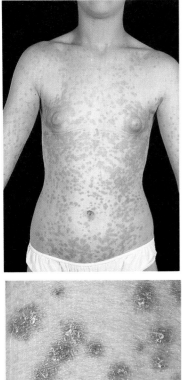

(a)

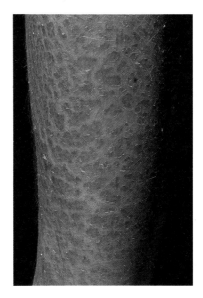

Plate 17 Ichthyosis.

(b)

Plate 15 (a, b) Guttate psoriasis.

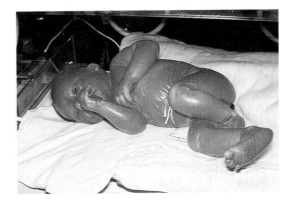

Plate 18 Collodian baby.

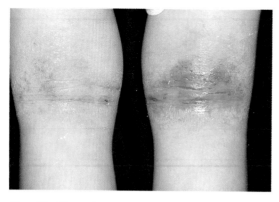

Plate 19 Flexural involvement in atopic eczema.

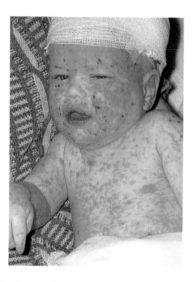

Plate 20 Eczema herpeticum.

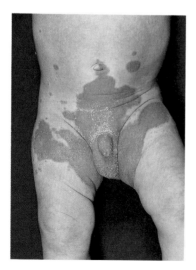

Plate 21 Napkin psoriasis.

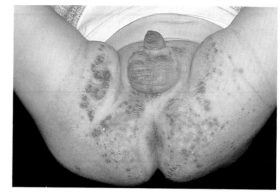

Plate 22 Irritant napkin dermatitis.

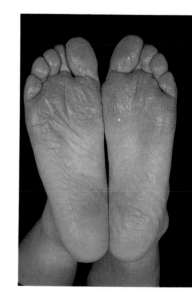

Plate 23 Juvenile plantar dermatosis.

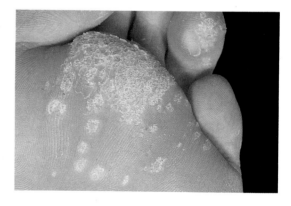

Plate 24 Mosaic plantar warts.

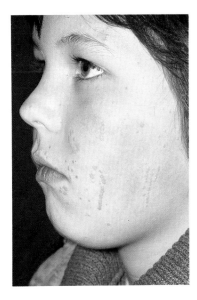

Plate 25 Plane warts.

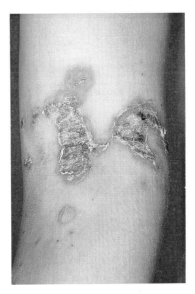

Plate 27 Impetigo.

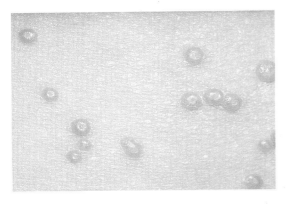

Plate 26 Molluscum contagiosum.

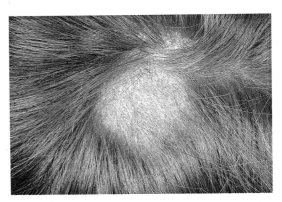

Plate 28 Scalp ringworm.

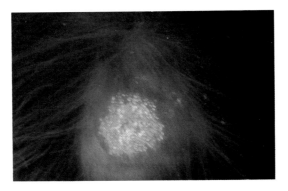

Plate 29 Fluorescence of *M. canis* ringworm under Wood's light.

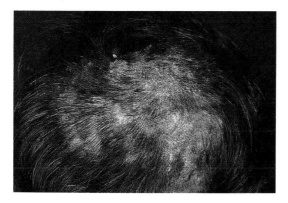

Plate 30 Kerion.

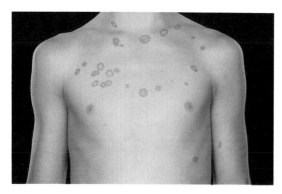

Plate 31 Tinea corporis produced by *M. canis*.

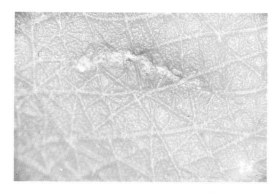

Plate 32 Scabies burrow.

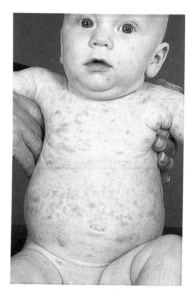

Plate 33 Scabies in an infant.

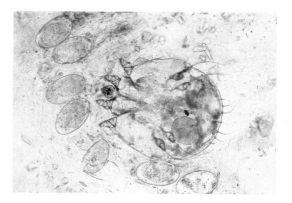

Plate 34 Scabies mite and eggs.

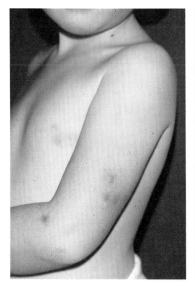 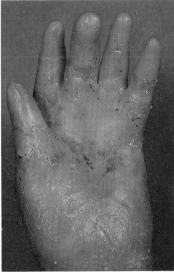 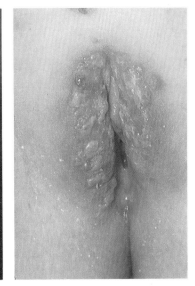

Plate 35 Papular urticaria produced by arthropod bites.

Plate 36 Acquired syndactyly in recessive dystrophic epidermolysis bullosa.

Plate 37 Bullae on the vulva in chronic bullous dermatosis of childhood.

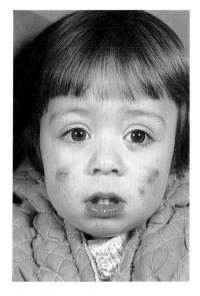 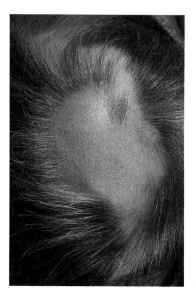

Plate 38 Infantile acne.

Plate 39 Alopecia aereata.

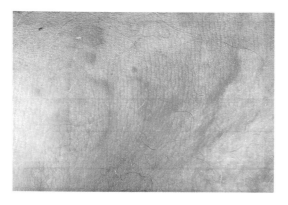

Plate 40   Urticaria.

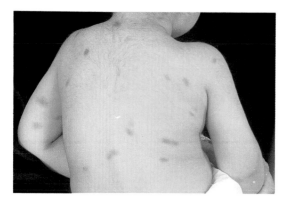

Plate 41   Urticaria pigmentosa.

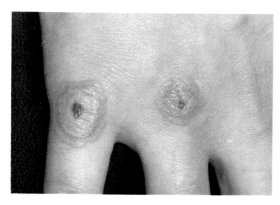

Plate 42   Target lesions in erythema multiforms.

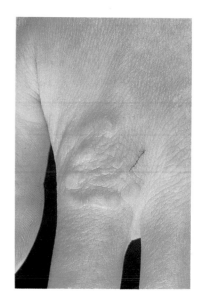

Plate 43   Granuloma annulare.

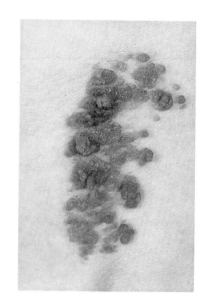

Plate 44   Warty epidermal naevus.

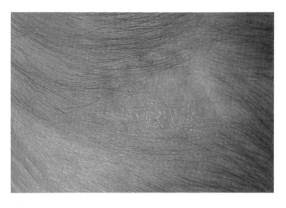

Plate 45 Sebaceous naevus.

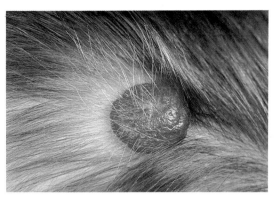

Plate 46 Strawberry naevus.

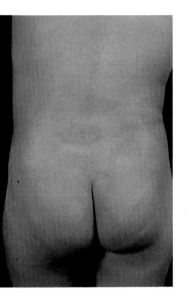

Plate 47 Mongolian spots.

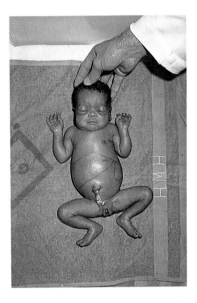

Plate 48 Neonatal syphilis. Note the generalized oedema, scaly skin and hepatosplenomegaly.

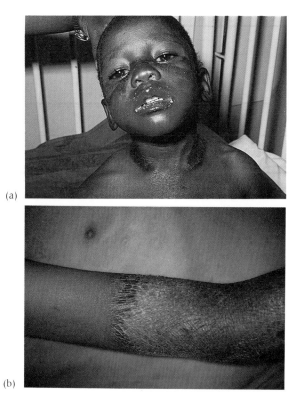

(a)

(b)

Plate 49 Pellagra involving (a) the forearm, and (b) the face. Note the butterfly distribution of the facial rash, Kassel's necklace and the rash on the exposed forearm.

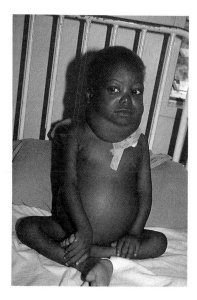

Plate 50 Cervical adenitis due to primary tuberculosis.

which blisters develop within the upper dermis and heal with scarring. The pathogenesis of blister formation in epidermolysis bullosa is not yet fully understood.

In the commonest type, epidermolysis bullosa simplex, which is dominantly inherited, blisters first appear in early infancy on areas subjected to friction. As the child begins to crawl, the hands, feet, elbows and knees are the areas principally involved, but in later childhood usually only the hands and feet are affected. Warmth appears to encourage blister formation, and the condition is considerably worse in summer. The blisters heal without scarring.

The scarring (dystrophic or dermolytic) types of epidermolysis bullosa are divided into dominant and recessive forms, the recessive form being more severe. They are usually present at birth. The slightest trauma provokes blister formation. Severe generalized blistering results in loss of body fluids and susceptibility to secondary bacterial infection. The mucous membranes may be involved in the dominant type, but it is in the recessive form that severe mucosal involvement is seen. This frequently leads to oesophageal stenosis, dysphagia, and consequent failure to thrive. Severe blistering and subsequent scarring on the hands leads to progressive acquired syndactyly of the fingers and a 'mitten' deformity (Plate 36). Death may occur from extensive fluid loss and dehydration, or septicaemia from secondary skin sepsis. Surviving children may be chronically anaemic, malnourished, and show growth retardation. Later in life squamous cell carcinoma may develop in scarred areas, particularly on the legs.

Treatment. In the severe forms of epidermolysis bullosa the major concerns in early childhood are the maintenance of fluid and electrolyte balance, good nutrition, and control of secondary infection. Gentle handling of affected children is absolutely essential. Blistered areas should be kept clean, covered with paraffin gauze, and treated with topical antibacterial agents when necessary.

The nature of the condition should be explained to the parents, and genetic counselling is mandatory. Parents should also be made fully conversant with the routine necessary for day-to-day care of their child.

In later childhood hand problems may require the help of a plastic surgeon, and dental and oesophageal problems will need specialist advice. Although there have been some reports of benefit from treatment with phenytoin and vitamin E, as yet there is no effective oral therapy for epidermolysis bullosa. Prenatal diagnosis by fetoscopy and fetal skin biopsy is now possible. Support groups are of help to many families, and the Dystrophic Epidermolysis Bullosa Research Association (DEBRA) will provide information and advice to parents of affected children.

CHRONIC NON-HEREDITARY BLISTERING DISEASES

The immunologically mediated inflammatory blistering diseases such as dermatitis herpetiformis, bullous pemphigoid, cicatricial pemphigoid and pemphigus vulgaris are all rare in childhood. Each condition has characteristic clinical, histological and immunofluorescence features. Specialized paediatric dermatology texts should be consulted for further details of these conditions.

The commonest of this group of blistering diseases is chronic bullous dermatosis of childhood (CBDC). Its onset is usually before the age of 5 years. Large, tense blisters appear, principally on the lower half of the trunk, genitalia (Plate 37) and thighs, but the head and neck area may also be affected. Histology reveals a subepidermal blister, and direct immunofluorescence shows linear deposition of IgA along the epidermal basement membrane. Treatment with dapsone or sulphapyridine usually controls the condition, but some cases require systemic steroids. The prognosis in the majority of cases is good, with spontaneous remission occurring within 2–3 years.

INCONTINENTIA PIGMENTI (BLOCH–SULZBERGER DISEASE)

This is an X-linked dominant disorder which is usually lethal to males *in utero*. In affected females, skin lesions are present at birth, or appear soon afterwards. Initially these are vesiculo-bullous lesions in linear streaks on the trunk and limbs. There is a marked blood eosinophilia, and the blisters contain many eosinophils. After a few weeks the blisters are replaced by linear warty lesions, and these are followed by streaks and whorls of hyperpigmentation which persist into later childhood or adolescence.

Scarring alopecia, dental and ocular abnormalities, skeletal malformations, and central nervous system disorders are present in a high proportion of patients with incontinentia pigmenti.

Acne vulgaris

Acne is a disorder of the pilosebaceous unit which affects virtually everyone to some extent in adolescence. Its onset is usually around the time of puberty, and its peak severity in the mid- to late-teens.

The development of acne is determined by two principal factors; genetic predisposition and the influence of androgens. Androgens stimulate sebum production by sebaceous glands, and influence keratinization in the pilosebaceous duct. Excess sebum production (seborrhoea) and pilosebaceous duct blockage are two important factors in the pathogenesis of acne. Another essential factor is the presence in the pilosebaceous follicle of the bacterium *Propionibacterium acnes*. This organism produces mediators which are responsible for the inflammatory element of acne.

CLINICAL FEATURES

Acne affects the face, neck, anterior chest and upper back; all areas in which there are pilosebaceous follicles with prominent sebaceous glands. The skin lesions include open comedones (blackheads), in which the pilosebaceous duct is dilated and plugged with keratinous debris and sebum, and closed comedones (whiteheads), in which a narrow blocked duct results in an accumulation of sebum, producing a small cyst, inflammatory papules, pustules, abscesses and scars. Blackheads are simply a cosmetic nuisance, but it is the whiteheads which are the 'time-bombs' of acne. It is around the whiteheads that the inflammatory reaction provoked by mediators from *P. acnes* occurs.

In the severe nodulocystic type of acne, where multiple large abscesses occur, the degree of scarring can be appalling, and even in the milder forms scarring may produce significant cosmetic disability.

TREATMENT

The type of treatment is determined by the severity of the acne. Mild acne is usually controlled by topical therapy alone, whereas those with more severe changes will require a combination of topical and systemic therapy.

Topical therapy

Tretinoin (Retin-A). Available as lotion, gel and cream, this vitamin A derivative influences duct keratinization and helps to 'unplug' the follicles. It is particularly useful in dealing with large numbers of comedones. It is an irritant and should always be tried on a small area of skin before being used more extensively.

Benzoyl peroxide. This is an antibacterial and keratolytic which is available in a number of proprietary preparations, in several concentrations. It is also an irritant, and treatment should be started with lower strength preparations.

Topical antibiotics. At present there are three topical antibiotic preparations marketed for the treatment of acne in Britain: Topicycline (tetracycline hydrochloride), Dalacin T (clindamycin phosphate), and Stiemycin (erythromycin).

Systemic therapy

Antibiotics. Tetracyclines are the mainstay of systemic therapy for acne. Oxytetracycline is usually very effective if taken correctly, and is safe for long-term treatment. An initial dose of 0.5–1 g daily can be reduced when the acne has improved. For maximum benefit oxytetracycline should be taken on an empty stomach, and to ensure this it is best taken as a single dose before breakfast. Alternative tetracycline preparations, which may be of value in individuals who appear unresponsive to oxytetracycline, include Minocin (minocycline hydrochloride), Megaclor (clomocycline sodium), and Vibramycin (doxycycline hydrochloride). Short courses of tetracylines are of little value, and most patients will require prolonged treatment to keep their acne under control.

Tetracyclines should not be given to children under 12 years of age because of the danger of producing staining of the permanent dentition.

Erythromycin or co-trimoxazole may occasionally be useful if tetracyclines prove ineffective.

Isotretinoin. Isotretinoin (Roaccutane) is a vitamin A derivative which is extremely useful in the management of nodulocystic acne and acne unresponsive to systemic antibiotics. Side-effects include cheilitis and erythema and peeling of facial skin. It is a known teratogen.

Diet. There is no scientific evidence that diet has any influence on the severity of acne.

INFANTILE ACNE

Occasionally infants and young children develop facial acne (Plate 38). The majority of those affected under the age of 9 months are boys. In some cases the acne is mild and transient, but in others nodulocystic lesions develop, and the course is protracted. Tetracyclines are contraindicated in this age group, but affected children will often benefit from oral erythromycin, and the lower concentration topical benzoyl peroxide preparations.

Hair abnormalities

There are three types of hair:
1 Lanugo which is present *in utero* and shed by the eighth month of fetal life.
2 Vellus, the fine downy hair present over most of the body except the scalp, eyebrows and eyelashes.

3 Terminal hair, the thick, pigmented hair of the scalp, eyebrows, eyelashes, beard and secondary sexual hair developing at puberty.

Each hair follicle passes through three stages in its growth cycle. *Anagen* – the phase of active growth, which for scalp hair lasts from 3 to 5 years. *Catagen* – a short phase during which the hair follicle atrophies; this is the transition period between growing and resting phases. *Telogen* – the resting stage, which lasts for 3–4 months. At the end of telogen the follicle reactivates, a new hair begins to grow, and the old hair is shed. It is perfectly normal for between 70 and 100 scalp hairs to be shed daily. A normal scalp contains approximately 90% of hairs in anagen and 10% in telogen.

ALOPECIA

This term applies to absence or loss of hair. In assessing a child suffering from alopecia it is useful to consider whether the hair loss is congenital or acquired, diffuse or localized, scarring or non-scarring, whether the affected areas of scalp are scaly or smooth, and whether there are any associated abnormalities of skin and nails. Table 27.7 lists causes of alopecia.

There are numerous genetic disorders in which absence of hair follicles, progressive destruction of hair follicles, or structural abnormalities of the hair shaft lead to varying degress of alopecia. All these conditions are quite rare, and specialized dermatology texts should be consulted for more information about them.

Patchy alopecia

If the hair loss is patchy consider:

Scalp ringworm (see p. 495). Affected areas of scalp are scaly, and the hair in these patches is broken off close to the surface, leaving an irregular stubble.

Alopecia areata. The aetiology of this common condition is unknown, but an auto-immune cause has been suggested. Alopecia areata may be associated

Table 27.7 Commoner causes of alopecia in childhood.

Patchy alopecia
Scalp ringworm
Alopecia areata
Trichotillomania
Traction alopecia

Diffuse alopecia
Telogen effluvium

with other diseases which have an auto-immune basis. There is a family history of alopecia areata in 10–20% of affected individuals. It also occurs quite frequently in patients suffering from Down's syndrome.

The typical clinical picture in alopecia areata is of the sudden onset of patchy hair loss. Sometimes there is only a single patch, but often there are multiple areas. The scalp in these areas is often a light-brown or salmon pink colour, and is not scaly (Plate 39). At the margins of the affected areas it is usually possible to see short, fractured hairs known as 'exclamation mark' hairs. The nails should be examined as they will often show regular lines of small pits.

Occasionally alopecia areata will progress to complete loss of scalp hair (alopecia totalis) or loss of all body hair (alopecia universalis).

Treatment of alopecia areata is not very satisfactory, but fortunately in most cases of mild alopecia areata spontaneous regrowth begins after a few weeks. When there is no evidence of regrowth the affected areas can be treated with intradermal injections of Adcortyl (triamcinolone). Adults will usually tolerate this, but children certainly will not. Scalp hyperaemia encourages hair growth, and numerous methods of inducing an inflammatory response, with accompanying hyperaemia, have been tried. These include ultraviolet light, dithranol, and induced contact dermatitis using a variety of allergens. These methods may stimulate regrowth, but it is often not maintained. In the more extensive cases a wig should be provided.

In some patients lesions continue to develop episodically for many years. In extensive cases the prognosis for regrowth is poor, particularly if the onset is in early childhood.

Trichotillomania. This is a compulsion to pull or twist the hair which results in irregular patchy hair loss in which the broken strands of hair are of varying length. The underlying scalp usually appears normal. In children this condition is usually the result of a habit, although it may indicate underlying emotional stress. Its occurrence in adolescence could be associated with a significant psychological problem requiring psychiatric help (see Chapter 20).

Traction alopecia. Certain hair styles, such as the pony tail, and short plaited styles adopted by black people, exert considerable traction on hair follicles, and may lead to patchy hair loss. The hair on the temples is particularly susceptible to traction alopecia. The hair usually recovers rapidly in children, once the hair style is changed.

Acquired diffuse alopecia

Telogen effluvium is the commonest cause of acquired diffuse alopecia. Any severe physical stress, such as a severe febrile illness, may result in many more hairs entering the telogen phase of their growth cycle. The hair loss in telogen effluvium occurs some 2–3 months after the initiating event, when the telogen hairs are shed. This process does not damage the follicles, and the hair will subsequently regrow completely.

Disorders of pigmentation

Melanin is the pigment responsible for the colour of skin and hair. It is synthesized in melanocytes from the amino acid tyrosine. The enzyme tyrosinase is essential for the first step in the synthetic pathway. Melanin is stored in organelles known as melanosomes which are transferred to the prickle cells of the epidermis via the melanocytes' dendrites.

HYPOPIGMENTATION/DE-PIGMENTATION

Loss of skin and hair pigment may occur as a result of absence of melanocytes or defective production of melanin. These melanocyte abnormalities may be congenital or acquired.

Congenital abnormalities

Albinism. Oculocutaneous albinism is a recessively inherited disorder in which a deficiency of tyrosinase results in failure of melanin synthesis. The skin is very light, the hair is white to yellowish in colour, the pupils are pink and the irides are grey or blue. Because of the absence of melanin in the skin, affected individuals are extremely photosensitive and burn very easily in the sun. The ocular abnormalities are associated with severe photophobia. Loss of the protective effect of melanin leads to early ultraviolet damage to the skin and development of skin neoplasia. Patients with oculocutaneous albinism should avoid exposure to strong sunlight, and should protect the exposed parts of the skin with a high sun protection factor (SPF) sunscreen.

Piebaldism. This is a dominantly inherited disorder in which there is patchy hypopigmentation or depigmentation on an otherwise normal skin. The affected areas are present from birth. A frequent feature of the condition is a white forelock. There are reduced numbers of melanocytes containing abnormal melanosomes in the affected areas of skin.

Miscellaneous. In *Waardenburg's syndrome* a white forelock is associated with heterochromia irides, lateral displacement of the medial canthi, and sensorineural deafness.

Ash-leaf-shaped areas of hypopigmentation on the trunk and limbs are the earliest cutaneous manifestation of *tuberous sclerosis*, and their presence may permit early diagnosis of this condition in a child with seizures (p. 302). The hypopigmented areas are more easily seen under Wood's light.

There is marked dilution of pigment in the skin, eyes and hair of children with untreated *phenylketonuria*.

Acquired abnormalities

Acquired pigment loss in childhood is much more frequently encountered than congenital pigmentary problems, and the commonest causes are vitiligo and post-inflammatory hypopigmentation.

Vitiligo. This common disorder frequently first appears in childhood. Forty to fifty per cent of affected individuals have a positive family history of vitiligo. Its exact aetiology is unknown, but it is thought to be an auto-immune process in which melanocytes are destroyed. There is a significant association between vitiligo and other auto-immune disorders.

The clinical picture is of well-demarcated depigmented areas which are usually symmetrically distributed, and frequently affect the face, the dorsa of the hands and feet, the axillae and groin, and the elbows, knees and shins.

Spontaneous re-pigmentation may occur in patches of vitiligo, but in many cases the pigment loss is permanent. The changes may remain localized to certain areas for years, but in some cases there is gradual extension of the de-pigmented patches until most of the body is affected.

Treatment for this is not very satisfactory. Occasionally the use of a potent topical steroid will stimulate re-pigmentation, but in the majority of cases topical steroids are of no benefit. PUVA therapy (psoralens + UVA) has had limited success in the management of vitiligo, but treatment is very prolonged, and frequently not justifiable.

In most cases management will consist of advice on the use of sunscreens to protect areas of vitiligo on exposed parts of the body, and cosmetic camouflage on the face and hands to make the affected areas less conspicuous.

Post-inflammatory hypopigmentation. This is a common phenomenon in pigmented races, and is also frequently seen on tanned Caucasian skin. Partial pigment loss is particularly common following resolution of eczema, psoriasis, pityriasis lichenoides and pityriasis rosea. As there is no permanent damage to melanocytes, affected areas will eventually re-pigment.

The commonest cause of increased pigmentation of the skin is as a post-inflammatory phenomenon. This is particularly likely to occur in races whose skin is naturally pigmented, and is a frequent accompaniment of eczema and lichen planus.

Urticaria and angioedema

Urticaria (nettle-rash or hives) is characterized by the development of raised, extremely itchy weals scattered over the body (Plate 40). The lesions are transient, lasting only a few hours before fading, but are continually replaced by new crops of weals. Histamine liberated from mast cells is probably the principal mediator responsible for these changes, but other substances such as kinins and prostaglandins appear to play a part. The lesions develop as a result of dilatation and increased permeability of small blood vessels in the skin, allowing fluid to escape into the surrounding tissues. If this process occurs in subcutaneous tissues, marked localized oedema (angioedema) results. Angioedema frequently affects the eyelids and the lips, but occasionally the throat is involved, causing respiratory obstruction.

Urticaria may be acute, lasting for a few days, or chronic, lasting months or years. It is sometimes classified as 'allergic' and 'non-allergic' in aetiology. Allergic urticaria is usually due to a Type I hypersensitivity reaction, whereas in the non-allergic type the release of histamine and other mediators is not associated with immunological factors.

There are several agents known to trigger urticaria, including:

Drugs. Acute urticaria is a manifestation of hypersensitivity to some drugs, particularly penicillins. Other drugs such as salicylates and morphine derivatives are direct histamine liberators.

Foods. Eggs, strawberries, nuts, fish and shellfish may provoke acute urticaria by either allergic or non-allergic mechanisms. Affected individuals frequently have an atopic constitution. Food allergy is rarely responsible for chronic urticaria.

Food additives. Food dyes and preservatives may be responsible for some cases of chronic urticaria.

Contact urticaria. Weals appear at the site of contact with an allergen; for example, lesions on the lips and mouth produced by certain foods.

Physical urticarias. Occasionally, urticaria may be provoked by heat, cold, sunlight, pressure, or contact with water.

Miscellaneous. Infections with bacteria, viruses, Candida, and parasites, may be associated with urticaria.

Establishing the cause of urticaria is often difficult, and in the majority of cases of chronic urticaria the cause is never established. A careful history is the most important part of the assessment, and may suggest a possible cause for an acute urticaria. Extensive investigation is rarely rewarding. In occasional refractory cases provocation tests with food additives are undertaken.

Treatment. If there is no obvious cause which can be eliminated, treatment is based on control of the urticaria with antihistamines. There is a wide choice of antihistamines available, but the author has found Atarax (hydroxyzine hydrochloride) and Triludan (terfenadine) particularly useful. A sedative antihistamine such as Phenergan (promethazine hydrochloride) may be taken at night.

In chronic refractory urticaria it may be worthwhile trying food-dye and preservative-free diets.

In severe acute urticaria a short course of systemic steroids can be helpful, but there is no place for steroids in the management of chronic urticaria.

Urticaria pigmentosa (mastocytosis)

This is a disorder produced by the presence of increased numbers of mast cells in the dermis. Typical childhood urticaria pigmentosa is present at birth, or develops within the first few months of life. The clinical picture is of scattered pigmented macules, papules or plaques which urticate when rubbed (Plate 41). Usually no treatment is required, and in the majority of cases the condition resolves in later childhood.

Erythema multiforme

Erythema multiforme is a reaction pattern in the skin which can be precipitated by a number of different agents, including drugs, herpes simplex and mycoplasma infections. In a severe form of erythema multiforme known as *Stevens–Johnson syndrome*, the mucous membranes are involved. The typical 'iris' or 'target' lesions on the skin have a slightly raised red margin, and a rather cyanotic centre (Plate 42). They develop in crops over a few days on the hands, feet, elbows and knees, and they may become bullous. The skin lesions fade over a period of 2–3 weeks. In Stevens–Johnson syndrome, bullae and erosions develop in the mouth and on the genitalia, and there may be a severe conjunctivitis. There is an accompanying pyrexia and malaise.

Recurrent herpes simplex may trigger repeated episodes of erythema multiforme.

Treatment. In the milder forms no treatment is required, in fact there is evidence that in children systemic steroid therapy may prolong the course of the eruption. The value of systemic steroids in the management of Stevens–Johnson syndrome is debatable, but nevertheless they are usually recommended.

Granuloma annulare

This condition presents with grouped, flat-topped papules, often in an annular configuration (Plate 43). The lesions commonly occur on the dorsa of the hands or feet, but may affect other parts of the body. The aetiology of granuloma annulare is unknown, and although it is often stated that there is an association with diabetes, there is little real evidence for this.

Treatment. The use of a potent topical steroid will often help to clear the lesions, but in small children they are best left alone, as their natural history is for eventual spontaneous regression.

Naevi

The term naevus is a synonym for a cutaneous hamartoma; an abnormal mixture of a tissue's usual components. Some of the commoner naevi are described below.

EPITHELIAL NAEVI

Warty epidermal naevus

This naevus is usually present at birth, and becomes more prominent with age. Most warty epidermal naevi are relatively small linear lesions (Plate 44), but occasionally extensive areas of the body are affected. The smaller lesions can be dealt with by excision.

Sebaceous naevus

This naevus is most commonly seen on the scalp as an orange–yellow area devoid of hair (Plate 45). At birth the lesion is flat, but in later childhood it becomes slightly raised, with a rather warty surface. Dermatologists usually recommend excision of these lesions in adolescence or early adult life because there is a risk of basal cell epithelioma developing within the naevus in later life.

VASCULAR NAEVI

Salmon patches

These pink areas, produced by dilated dermal capillaries, are very common in neonates. They occur on the forehead, eyelids and nape of the neck. Unna's naevus, the lesion on the neck, often referred to as the 'stork bite', persists into adult life, but the facial marks gradually fade in the first year of life.

Port wine stain (naevus flammeus)

Port wine stains are present at birth, and are produced by a congenital malformation of capillaries. They most commonly involve the face, but may be present on any part of the body. They persist into adult life and represent a significant cosmetic problem when they affect the face. Laser therapy may improve some lesions in adults, but this form of treatment is rarely employed in children. Cosmetic camouflage is useful in making facial lesions less conspicuous, and children with port wine stains should be referred to a beautician with experience of cosmetic camouflage techniques.

In the *Sturge–Weber syndrome* a facial port wine stain is associated with an intracranial angioma, epilepsy and mental retardation. Typical 'tramline' calcification associated with the intracranial angioma can be seen on skull X-ray.

Angiomatous naevi

Angiomatous naevi are probably best classified as superficial or deep, although mixed types are not uncommon.

Superficial angiomatous naevus (strawberry naevus). Usually solitary, but occasionally multiple, these vascular lesions are hardly visible at birth, but enlarge rapidly over the first 6–9 months of life (Plate 46). They then gradually involute, and most smaller lesions have regressed completely by school age. It is extremely rare for significant bleeding to occur from these lesions.

Deep angiomatous naevus. Entirely subcutaneous angiomatous naevi are relatively uncommon. They present as soft, bluish subcutaneous swellings. These lesions also gradually regress, but complete resolution is less likely than with the superficial type.

A rare complication of large angiomatous naevi is platelet sequestration within the naevus, and the development of a consumption coagulopathy (*Kasabach–Merritt syndrome*).

In the majority of cases angiomatous naevi should be allowed to regress spontaneously, as the

eventual cosmetic result will be superior to that which can be achieved by surgery or other means. Active intervention is, however, required for lesions which interfere with vision (producing amblyopia in the occluded eye), feeding, or respiration. High-dose systemic steroid therapy may be useful in these circumstances.

PIGMENTED NAEVI

Café-au-lait patches

These are light brown, uniformly pigmented macules of varying size and shape. It is common to encounter children with a few café-au-lait patches, but numerous lesions may be associated with neurofibromatosis, tuberous sclerosis and Albright's syndrome.

Mongolian spots

These slate-blue areas of discolouration on the lower back and buttocks are common in infants of dark-skinned races (Plate 47). The colour is produced by melanocytes lying deep in the dermis. Mongolian spots have usually disappeared by the age of 5 or 6 years.

Melanocytic naevi (moles)

Moles are uncommon in infancy, but occur with increasing frequency in childhood and adolescence. In childhood the majority of moles are flat, and dark brown in colour. They are produced by melanocyte proliferation at the dermo-epidermal junction. In later childhood and adolescence moles tend to become more prominent as melanocytes migrate into the dermis where they form nests.

Congenital melanocytic naevi

Some melanocytic naevi are present at birth, and these tend to be larger than those which develop later. They are dark brown in colour, have a mammillated surface, and a tendency to grow coarse, dark hair. Occasionally, very large lesions cover extensive areas of skin, and carry a significant risk of the development of malignant melanoma within them.

Sutton's halo naevus

In this harmless condition one or more moles become surrounded by a halo of de-pigmentation. The mole gradually disappears, and the affected area subsequently re-pigments.

Further reading

Verbov J, Morley N. *Colour Atlas of Paediatric Dermatology.* MTP Press Ltd, Lancaster 1983.

Harper J. *Handbook of Paediatric Dermatology.* Butterworths, London 1985.

Verbov J. (Ed.) *Modern Topics in Paediatric Dermatology.* William Heinemann Medical Books Ltd, London 1979.

Hurwitz S. *Clinical Paediatric Dermatology.* WB Saunders Company, Philadelphia 1981.

28

SUDDEN INFANT DEATH, ACCIDENTAL INJURY AND CHILD ABUSE

Whereas the incidence of disease in children is steadily decreasing, the number of accidents is steadily rising. Injury and poisoning account for 10% of all deaths in children aged 15 years and less and is the commonest cause of death in children over 1 year of age. Non-fatal injury due to accidents accounts for a much higher number of children who require admission to hospital each year, a significant proportion of which leave the child disabled. It is estimated that 10% of the child population of Britain attend hospital because of an accident at some time.

Children are highly vulnerable to injury due to a number of factors including their dependence on adults, inexperience of their potentially dangerous environment, their enquiring nature and their small size. Accidents in the home account for considerably more deaths in children than accidents outside the home, suggesting that many of these may be preventable.

Approximately 300 children a year die as a direct result of injury deliberately inflicted by an adult (the so-called 'non-accidental injury') but the number suffering abuse not severe enough to kill them is vastly greater than this. Accidents, poisonings and child abuse will be discussed separately in this chapter.

Sudden infant death syndrome

Sudden infant death syndrome (SIDS) is the commonest cause of post-neonatal deaths – those occurring between 1 month and 1 year of age.

SIDS is also known as cot or crib death'. Its inclusion in this chapter does not indicate it has anything to do with child abuse, but its sudden and unexpected nature requires the paediatrician and pathologist to consider a larger number of possible causes.

The definition of SIDS is the sudden and unexpected death of an infant or young child in whom post-mortem examination reveals no adequate explanation for the death. The incidence of SIDS in most developed countries is 1–2 : 1000 babies and in UK approaches 1 : 500 babies. This represents almost 1400 totally unexpected and unexplained deaths per year in the UK. The peak age for SIDS to occur is at 3 months and is very rare after 1 year.

RISK FACTORS

A number of risk factors have been recognized which will predict a higher risk of SIDS. These are summarized in Table 28.1.

Maternal factors

Young age of the mother, and short intervals between pregnancies are well recognized risk factors. Young mothers are also likely to be unmarried and unsupported, living in inferior housing and may themselves be subject to physical abuse by their partners. Maternal smoking during pregnancy is another risk factor; those who smoke more than 20 cigarettes a day have a four-fold increased risk of their baby dying unexpectedly at home. These

Table 28.1   Risk factors for 'SIDS' identifiable at birth.

Maternal factors
Young age
Short interval between pregnancies (<1 year)
Smoking

Infant factors
Male
Prematurity
Low birth weight
Multiple birth

Nurture
Low socioeconomic class
Formula feeding
Birth in winter months

risk factors are similar to those recognized for 'non-accidental injury'.

Infant factors

Male sex increases the risk of SIDS. Premature delivery and low birth weight also predispose to this condition. Those severely premature infants who have required mechanical ventilation and particularly those who develop chronic lung disease (p. 93) have a significantly increased chance of SIDS.

Nurture

Feeding practices are important. SIDS is more likely to occur in bottle-fed infants and the risk amongst babies who are breast fed appears to fall in proportion to the duration of time that they receive breast milk. SIDS is commoner in the winter months and this may be associated with a greater risk of respiratory tract infection.

AETIOLOGY

At autopsy the pathologist is able to define the nature of the death more accurately. Four groups can be recognized on the basis of post-mortem information:

1 An obvious cause for death in which case the term SIDS is not appropriate.

2 A definite abnormality at autopsy (such as a ventricular septal defect) that was unlikely to cause, but possibly contributed to the death.

3 Minor abnormalities such as mild inflammatory changes in the upper or lower respiratory tract which could not be considered, on their own, to be the direct cause of death.

4 No abnormality discovered at all.

The term SIDS does not imply one single cause of death, but rather a number of different and quite separate causes, all probably producing death in a different manner. Table 28.2 lists the possible causes of SIDS, and many of these are discussed in detail elsewhere in this book.

It has been suggested that overheated babies are more at risk of SIDS. It has been shown that nursing some babies at too high an environmental temperature causes the respiratory pattern to become unstable with more periods of short apnoea. Many mothers wrap their babies up when mildly unwell and this should be discouraged. Babies require to be nursed in a room with a constant temperature of 18°C (65°F) and dressed in a thin vest and an all-in-one baby outfit (or equivalent) and require no more than one or two thin blankets. If a baby has a fever then the blankets should be removed rather than the number of bed clothes increased.

It has been suggested that some cases of SIDS are due to smothering, asphyxia or deliberate infanticide. It is not possible to know how often this occurs but it is probably in the order of 1–2% of cases. All parents whose baby dies will be devas-

Table 28.2   Some causes of apparent 'SIDS'.

Unstable respiratory activity
  Sleep apnoea
  Ondine's curse
Cardiac arrhythmia
Infection
Immune-deficiency disorder
Overheating
Allergic hypersensitivity
Gastro-oesophageal reflux
Surfactant deficiency
Inborn error of biochemical function
Suffocation/asphyxia

tated by the event and any suggestion of foul play is entirely unwarranted on the first meeting. If there is any suspicion, this should be investigated by the appropriate authorities and a decision made whether to pursue this at a later stage.

The parents need special help in order to relieve them as much as possible of their inevitable feelings of guilt. A full clinical history should be taken as for any other patient. In another room the doctor will make a complete clinical examination and take appropriate bacterial and viral specimens, including cerebrospinal fluid. This is important for research and is also therapeutic for the parents, being very different from just referring them to the coroner's officer. Arrangements should be made for them to be seen the next day by the same doctor, ideally with a social worker experienced in this field who will provide ongoing care.

CLINICAL FEATURES

In about one-half of cases of SIDS, a history of the child being unwell immediately prior to death will be obtained. This is usually minor, such as snuffles, occasional vomits or cough. In some cases the parents may have underestimated the severity of the child's symptoms. If there has been a previous history of SIDS, then the child should be admitted to hospital even if the symptoms appear only minor. There is an increased risk of a twin also dying if his twin pair has sustained SIDS; this is particularly likely in identical (monozygotic) twins.

Sometimes the baby may be found in a collapsed state in his cot. This is sometimes referred to as 'near miss' SIDS. Resuscitation may be possible and the child should be evaluated carefully for possible causes of the collapse. If severe, home monitoring is advised (see later). Rarely a baby can be resuscitated and the heart beat returns but the child's brain has been irreversibly damaged and eventually ventilatory support must be withdrawn.

COUNSELLING

It is essential that all parents whose baby has died with a diagnosis of SIDS be seen 6–8 weeks after the death by an experienced paediatrician. The parents are bewildered by the loss of their baby and confused as to why it occurred. They will have strong feelings of guilt concerning the death and fears that it might happen to subsequent babies.

The paediatrician should inform the parents of the findings at autopsy. These are often negative and the possible causes of SIDS should be discussed. Parents are often helped by being put into contact with a parents' support group run by parents who themselves have had a baby die of SIDS. It is often helpful to meet with them again some months later to ensure that they have come to terms with their baby's death.

PREVENTION

The prevention of SIDS can be considered at the community level and at the individual level when considering the new sibling of a SIDS baby.

As mentioned above, some women can be identified at delivery to be at high risk of their baby dying of SIDS. It has been shown that close supervision of those families by health visitors reduces the risk of death in the first year of life. Daily weighing to detect those babies who show early evidence of failing to thrive may identify those who are most at risk of SIDS.

Newborn siblings of SIDS babies have an increased risk of this condition compared to other babies. The risk is four- to five-fold greater than for the general population. The GP, health visitor and paediatrician need to be particularly sensitive to the parents' fear that their next baby may also die and need to give appropriate advice. Most paediatricians believe that giving an apnoea monitor allays parents' anxieties and may also protect the baby. There is, however, no convincing evidence that apnoea monitors save lives.

Apnoea monitors. These are usually the sort that are stuck to the baby's anterior abdominal skin and click with each respiration. They are programmed to sound an alarm if there is apparent apnoea lasting more than 20 seconds. They have the advantage of being relatively cheap (about £250), but do require some care with application. They detect cessation of respiratory movements and will ring during periods of central apnoea but will not detect obstructive apnoea. In this condition, the baby's airway becomes obstructed due to a variety of causes and the infant will make vigorous respiratory efforts to try and overcome the obstruction. The monitor will detect these breathing movements and not ring, despite the baby moving no air in or out of his chest and possibly being severely compromised. The monitor will of course ring when the baby eventually stops struggling.

Nevertheless, most parents feel reassured by having a home monitor and use it for 6–12 months. Paediatric departments should have a supply of monitors available to lend to parents. It is essential to show parents what to do if the apnoea alarm goes off. Basic resuscitation skills are necessary if home apnoea monitoring is to be effective. The indications for home apnoea monitoring are listed in Table 28.3.

Accidental injury

In Britain, on an average day, two children die due to accidents or fire. The numbers who are injured or permanently disabled are not known, but certainly constitute a large group. Accidents and their prevention can be divided into those occurring at home and those that happen outside the home.

Accidents in the home

More accidents occurs in the home than on the roads, and relatively few occur in school. Accidental poisoning is considered separately below. Death by fire or smoke inhalation is the commonest cause of mortality from accidents in the

Table 28.3 Indications for home apnoea monitoring.

Sibling of a SIDS infant
'Near-miss' episode of SIDS
Premature infants with continued apnoea
Conditions associated with hypoventilation

home and the management of burns is considered below.

The greatest risk lies in the under-5-years age group; boys being more susceptible after the age of 1 year than girls. Overcrowding increases the risk of accidents. The lack of outside play facilities with modern housing, especially flats, is a further reason for the increased number of accidents in the home. They also occur more often when the home routine is altered, such as when moving house, during decorating or when there has been a death in the home. Staying in other people's houses increases the dangers because the usual safety precautions for children may be lacking. Elderly relatives often leave dangerous medicines lying around; some are routinely kept under the bed by old people. These and many other situations are associated with increased parental tension so that supervision of the children is less efficient.

Lacerations are the commonest type of injury and may occur as a result of playing with knives or falling through glass doors. Head injuries from falls are also common in the home and occur particularly in toddlers who fall down stairs. The occurrence of one accident in a family is the signal for redoubled efforts in preventive education for the family. Parents who have made one mistake are more likely to make others. The causes in the home are parental carelessness and ignorance, combined with a lack of instruction and supervision of the children. Marital unhappiness is an important factor. Most accidents in the home can be prevented by forethought. When an accident does occur, the GP or health visitor should go round the house and look, together with the parents, for danger points. Particular attention should be paid to:

Fires. All open fires must be protected by a guard, this being fixed to the wall. Electric fires should also be fixed to the wall. In England it is illegal for an electric fire to be sold unless equipped with a guard. Unfortunately, however, these guards are often removed in the home. No matches should be left lying about. Gas taps should be left in a position in which they cannot be turned on by children. Drip-feed portable oil burners are particularly liable to cause fires.

Clothes. Long loose-fitting clothing is always a danger; therefore, pyjamas should be worn in preference to nightdresses. All children's clothing should be made of flame-resistant fabrics.

Electric points. Three-point plugs should be supplied and, when not in use, should be protected by an unused or dummy plug. Trailing flexes must be avoided.

Saucepans. No handles should be left protruding over the edge of the cooker where they can be grabbed by a toddler. Preferably, the use of a saucepan with a long handle should be avoided; if used, the handle should be turned inwards. The only exception is if the cooker is fitted with a special rack into which the handles fit so that they cannot be moved from below.

Teapots. These should not be left on the table where they can be reached by a toddler.

Tablecloths. These should be turned in, rather than left hanging over the edge where they can be pulled down, together with any hot fluids placed on the table.

Feeding bottles. These should never be left propped up against the pillow for the baby to suck, since he is liable to vomit and inhale the vomitus.

Stairs. Stair rods must be carefully secured since, if loose, they can cause falls down stairs. A gate should be fixed at the top and bottom of the staircase if there are toddlers in the house. Quite young children can be taught how to go down the stairs backwards, this being safer than a gate.

Upstairs windows. These should always have guards. These guards should be placed so that the child's head cannot get stuck between the bars. They should be vertical so that they cannot be used as a climbing frame. An alternative safety method is to insert a screw so that only limited opening of the window is possible.

Pillows. Babies should not have pillows, owing to the possibility of suffocation. However, the risk of asphyxia from this cause is much less than previously believed; the majority of babies found dead in cots and thought to have died from suffocation fall into the group of sudden infant death syndrome (p. 510).

Plastic bags. These should not be brought into the homes of young children since they may draw them over their heads and then suffocate.

Fireworks. These should never be carried in trouser pockets since they are liable to explode when the child goes near a bonfire, causing appalling burns of the genitalia.

Baths. Bath water for babies must not be too hot. The temperature should be tested by the mother's elbow before the baby is put in. Since the bottom of a bath retains heat, cold water must be put in first. If hot water is used first the bath may burn the child even though the temperature of the water is correct.

Accidents outside the home

Road traffic accidents are common in developed countries. The child may be involved as a pedestrian, cyclist or occupant of a car. An unrestrained young child in the back seat of a car may sustain major injury in collisions at velocities of no more than 25 m.p.h.

PLAYGROUND ACCIDENTS

The most likely causes of injury in the playground are falls from climbing frames or slides. These are particularly likely to produce serious injury if the height of the fall exceeds 2.5 m, and playground equipment should not exceed this height. A fall on to a hard concrete surface is more likely to be damaging than one on to cinders, turf or bark chippings. Limb fractures and head injuries are the most common serious injury sustained in the playground.

VEHICLE ACCIDENTS

Cyclists are particularly vulnerable to serious injury or death. Children should only be allowed to cycle on the open road if they have passsed a cycling proficiency test. Protective head gear is particularly important in preventing serious head injury.

All infants and children should be restrained when in the back seat of cars. An adult holding a child on his or her lap cannot protect him in the event of a collision. In Britain, it is illegal for a child below the age of 12 years to sit in the front seat of a car.

DROWNING AND NEAR-DROWNING

This is one of the commonest causes of death or serious injury in children living in hot climates where open water for swimming is readily available. Even in temperate northern climates, drowning accidents are becoming more common.

Immersion in water causes three distinct problems; asphyxia, water intoxication and hypothermia. Immediate resuscitation is necessary and the hypothermia may be important in this context as complete recovery is well recognized following prolonged cardiac arrest. In these cases, hypothermia may protect the brain from major asphyxial damage. Fresh water may be more damaging than the sea as water intoxication is more likely to occur.

Head injuries

These are extremely common and half are due to road traffic accidents. In infancy the commonest cause is non-accidental injury (p. 521).

It is important to take a careful history of the injury. A description of the blow to the head, together with the duration of unconsciousness is best taken from a witness. If the child is old enough and well enough to communicate, the period of amnesia prior to the accident is an important prognostic feature. If the child is unconscious, the airway must be secured by either tracheal intubation or passing an oral airway. Prior to this the patient must be laid semi-prone to avoid aspiration of vomitus.

The level of consciousness should be determined. If the child is conscious and the blow to the head has been severe, or if the child had been knocked out, he should be admitted to hospital and hourly observation of pulse, respiratory rate, and state of consciousness undertaken. The pupils should regularly be examined for size and their reaction to light. This is traditionally undertaken for 24 hours after the head injury, but if the child is normal 6 hours after the incident, he is most unlikely to show later evidence of cerebral compromise. A pupil which is progressively dilating and losing its light reaction indicates imparied function of the third nerve from expanding intracranial pressure on the same side. As the pressure increases, both sides become similarly affected. Bilaterally fixed dilated pupils are of grave prognostic significance. The examination of the child then determines the presence of focal neurological signs and whether there are injuries to other parts of the body. Deterioration is shown by fixed dilated pupils, slowing of the pulse, increase in the pulse pressure, increase or decrease in the respiratory rate (especially Cheyne–Stokes respiration) and the development of paresis.

The child should be examined carefully on admission to the Accident and Emergency department for injury to the rest of the body. Particular attention should be paid to CSF draining from the ear or nose, subconjunctival haemorrhage without a clearly defined edge and bilateral periorbital oedema.

Admission to hospital is necessary if the child has been unconscious, if there is regular vomiting or if any of the above physical signs are present. An uncomplicated linear skull fracture does not necessarily require hospital admission.

Management. Major head injury may be treatable or non-treatable. The two major treatable conditions are subdural and extradural haemorrhage (see later). A CT scan should be performed on all children who are either unconscious or semiconscious. Generalized cerebral oedema may be present and this is best treated with elective mechanical hyperventilation.

Irreversible cerebral injury may have occurred as a result of the original injury or may develop whilst the child is in hospital. Brain stem death can be diagnosed in children over 2 months of age (p. 245) and organ transplantation discussed with the parents.

EXTRADURAL HAEMATOMA

This is due to bleeding from the middle cerebral artery, usually in association with a linear fracture overlying the vessel. There is sometimes a lucid interval before the development of coma, but this is less common than in adults. Dilatation of the pupil and an extensor plantar response on the side of the lesion are common but not invariable. These signs may be followed by the development of contra-lateral hemiparesis, but children tend to pass directly from the stage of unequal pupils into a state of decerebrate rigidity.

Diagnosis is confirmed by CT scan and treatment is by drainage of the clot through a craniotomy.

SUBDURAL HAEMORRHAGE

This occurs most commonly in infants and is often bilateral. It may be associated with birth trauma, but this is uncommon these days. Non-accidental injury is the commonest cause of this condition today. Subdural haemorrhage is due either to tearing of the dura from distortion of the head shape as occurs during rapid delivery, or rupture of bridging veins associated with a shaking injury. Subdural clots expand due to an osmotic effect and may gradually enlarge causing symptoms to be progressive.

Bleeding may be insidious and the child shows gradually increasing irritability and signs of raised intracranial pressure. Vomiting and convulsions are common. The anterior fontanelle may be tense. Retinal and subhyaloid haemorrhage are important and common diagnostic findings. Papilloedema occurs less commonly.

Diagnosis is made by ultrasound or CT scan.

Management involves evacuation of the collection by repeated subdural taps. Not more than 20 ml should be removed at any one time because of the effects of sudden volume or pressure changes possibly inducing further bleeding.

Burns and scalds

Scalding is particularly common in infants and young children. Deliberate scalding of the child by a parent is a relatively common form of non-accidental injury and this should always be considered in scalded children. Burns and scalds are a particularly distressing form of injury as scarring, disfigurement and psychological trauma may continue to affect the child for the rest of his life.

On admission to the Accident and Emergency department the child should be carefully assessed. An adequate airway is essential and if the child has inhaled hot gases then airway obstruction may rapidly occur. Adequate analgesia is also important.

The severity of the burn can be graded by the percentage of the body involved. If less than 50% of the surface is burnt the child should survive; children can survive burns of up to 75%. A more useful grading is between partial and full thickness burns involving the epidermis and dermis, respectively. If a pinprick can be felt it is probably a partial thickness burn and the skin will regenerate. Full thickness burns require grafting. Infection can convert partial thickness into full thickness.

Management. An intravenous infusion should be set up for burns involving 10% or more of the surface area. Particular attention must be paid to acid–base control. Fluid replacement with plasma or other colloid solution is given immediately and the volumes depend on the size of the burn and the weight of the child. Major burns must be treated in specialized burns centres with close supervision by paediatricians and plastic surgeons.

Poisoning

The risk of poisoning from drugs and household chemicals is very great. The most common drugs are aspirin and paracetamol. Iron tablets used to be a common cause of poisoning but this has been reduced by education, while the drive to stop doctors from prescribing barbiturates has largely eliminated this cause. The commonest household chemicals are paraffin, turpentine, disinfectants and cleaning agents. Approximately 1:5 of all medical admissions of children to hospital are for poisoning. The sex incidence is equal. Two per cent of all 2 year olds are admitted to hospital with poisoning. In England and Wales, about 140 children die from this cause every year.

Although there are many aspects of prevention, basically it is a matter of making these substances inaccessible to the children by ensuring that they are always in locked cupboards. However, the major cause of accidental poisoning is disturbed family relationships. The hazard must, of course, be reduced in all homes but the remarkable fact is that children from undisturbed families have few accidents even when other risk factors are high. The risk of ingestion of poisons is intimately associated with parental psychopathology and disturbed family relationships.

Parental ignorance accounts for part of the problem, there being many who have no idea of the dangers to children of household paraffin or iron tablets. Not only should these substances be in locked cupboards but they should be clearly marked 'keep away from children' to remind mothers of the risks. Parents should never take pills in front of their children as this increases the chance that the child will later try them for himself. Strip packing and blister packing of individual tablets as well as the use of child-proof containers have helped to reduce the risk of accidental poisoning.

Drugs should not be made attractive so that children mistake them for sweets. Parents should not refer to them as 'sweets' when they are prescribed, as this may lead the child to help himself on some future occasion. Ideally, all dangerous drugs should be dispensed in separate cellophane strips, but this increases their expense. The introduction of child-resistant containers has been important in reducing the risk of accidental poisoning.

In cases of accidental poisoning, it is essential that the doctor treating the child should know what poison he is treating and whether there is a specific management for the agent. National Poison Reference Centres have been set up which will give detailed advice over the telephone as to the management of any ingested agent and these should be consulted whenever necessary.

GENERAL MANAGEMENT OF POISONING

The management of a child who has swallowed a poison is always an emergency. There are three basic principles:

Removal of the poison

The child should be made to vomit by giving ipecacuanha syrup. There are three important exceptions to this rule. First, the child who is either semi-conscious or unconscious may aspirate if vomiting is induced. Secondly, the child who has ingested caustic or corrosive poison may exacerbate the oesophageal injury by vomiting, and thirdly, paraffin, kerosene or petrol may be aspirated during vomiting which may cause lipoid pneumonia.

Activated charcoal (Medicoal), an absorbent, can reduce the absorption of many drugs including aspirin, paracetamol, barbiturates and tricyclic antidepressants. It in no way replaces emesis or gastric lavage but may be a useful adjunct. It must not be given until the ipecacuanha has been effective.

Whenever possible, blood levels of the ingested poison should be measured in order to assess the severity of poisoning and the efficacy of treatment. The significance of the level relates to the time of ingestion. Forced alkaline diuresis increases the rate at which certain drugs are eliminated from the body. This is mainly of use in salicylate and phenobarbitone poisoning. It is not of value with other barbiturates because these are more highly protein-bound and are more widely distributed in the body, resulting in a lower plasma concentration.

Administration of an antidote

An antidote is a drug given to minimize the severity of the poison. There are specific antagonist antidotes such as naloxane in opiate overdosage and non-specific antidotes such as acetylcysteine for paracetamol poisoning. There are in fact very few specific antidotes but a Poison Reference Centre will give the most up-to-date advice concerning management.

Supportive therapy

Respiratory and/or cardiovascular failure are important and common complications of many forms of poisoning. It is important to assess carefully and regularly the child's conscious level and spontaneous respiratory activity. Mechanical ventilation may become necessary. Blood pressure and cardiac activity must also be carefully assessed and plasma given if hypotension occurs. Some drugs such as the tricyclics may cause cardiac arrhythmias and this should be anticipated in such cases (see p. 519).

SALICYLATE POISONING

Owing to its easy availability in many homes, aspirin is the most common drug to be ingested accidentally by children. The physical and laboratory findings show a considerable similarity to those found in cases of diabetic coma. The first change is a respiratory alkalosis resulting from the direct stimulant action of the salicylate on the respiratory centre. This only lasts 6–8 hours, and is followed by a metabolic acidosis which is due to interference with carbohydrate metabolism, renal dysfunction and the acidity of the salicylate. Ketosis results from the increased rate of fat catabolism and the disturbance of carbohydrate metabolism, the latter also causing hyperglycaemia and glycosuria. Hypernatraemia and hypokalaemia develop in severe cases. Salicylates also cause hypoprothrombinaemia, leading to bleeding.

The earliest clinical feature is over-breathing, this being associated with vomiting and diarrhoea. Sweating occurs at first but stops once dehydration develops. The child becomes pale and collapsed, haemorrhages may occur, finally there is loss of consciousness followed by death.

Diagnosis. The similarity of the clinical and biochemical features to diabetic coma is striking. Differentiation requires an accurate history, either of salicylate administration or previous polyuria and thirst suggesting the onset of diabetes. Serum level of salicylate should be measured.

Treatment. Salicylates are retained in the stomach for a long time, vomiting should therefore be induced immediately, even if it is some hours since the salicylate was taken. The vomit should be tested with ferric chloride for the presence of a salicylate.

Sodium bicarbonate should be given intravenously in acidotic patients since this promotes the renal excretion of salicylate. Full biochemical control is necessary, additional potassium being required once dehydration has been corrected. Vitamin K should be given to counteract hypoprothrombinaemia.

If the child is unconscious, additional methods to remove the salicylate should be used, such as renal dialysis. If this is not available, an exchange transfusion or peritoneal dialysis should be performed.

PARACETAMOL POISONING

This analgesic is found in many households and accidental poisoning occurs commonly. Rarely is enough taken to cause serious problems but liver failure is the major risk if more than 150 mg/kg is ingested. The liver function tests become abnormal after 12–24 hours and the most sensitive investigation is the prothrombin time. If this is prolonged then significant hepatic damage is likely to occur. Clinically apparent liver failure develops some time after the second day. Successful treatment depends on early recognition and institution of adequate treatment. Vomiting should be induced in all cases. In patients at risk of liver damage, oral methionine or *N*-acetyl-cysteine reduces the severity of liver necrosis. The decision to use these agents depends on the serum level of para-cetamol 4 hours after ingestion.

BARBITURATE POISONING

Fortunately children do not usually obtain a fatal dose. In mild cases there is drowsiness only. In more severe cases the patient is in a light coma from which he can be aroused by vigorous manual stimulation; nystagmus and dysarthria occur and respirations are shallow. In the most severe cases the child is in deep coma associated with shock; respirations and reflexes are depressed.

Treatment. In mild cases the child's level of consciousness should be carefully monitored but no specific treatment is usually necessary. In severe cases, symptomatic treatment and the maintenance of respiratory function is the basis of management, and blood or plasma is given for shock. Mechanical ventilation may be necessary for respiratory depression. If available, dialysis should be used to increase the elimination of the drug. Failing this, exchange transfusion or peritoneal dialysis should be performed. All severe cases should receive prophylactic antibiotic therapy and a close watch should be kept on the urinary output. If acute renal failure develops, indicated by oliguria, treatment should be given as discussed on p. 265.

IRON POISONING

The source is almost always iron tablets which are freely given out to expectant mothers, often with no warning of their potential danger to children. Many of the tablets are highly coloured and look like sweets.

The immediate effect of the iron is its corrosive action on the gastric musosa which may be sufficient to perforate the stomach. Vomiting is followed very rapidly by profound shock and coma. The child may then appear to improve for a few hours before symptoms from cerebral and hepatic damage appear. These are indicated by renewed restlessness, collapse, convulsions and coma. Jaundice may appear and there is biochemical evidence of a metabolic acidosis. If the child survives, pyloric stenosis may develop from scarring.

If death occurs in the acute phase, oedema and ulceration of the stomach are found, associated with a characteristic brown staining of the mucous membrane. The liver is always affected, a striking periportal necrosis occurring from the direct toxic action of the metal.

Treatment. Emesis should be induced as soon as possible. Following this, 50 ml sodium dihydrogen phosphate or sodium bicarbonate are introduced into the stomach by mouth or tube. A serum iron level above 90 µmol/l indicates serious poisoning.

Desferrioxamine (Desferal), a specific iron-chelating agent, is then given intravenously, intramuscularly or by mouth.

The iron tablets are radio-opaque so that a plain film of the abdomen will show whether they have all been removed by the washout.

TRICYCLIC ANTIDEPRESSANT POISONING

These drugs may be ingested by children in one of two forms. Amitryptyline (Trypitzol) is widely prescribed for depression, particularly in adult women, and imipramine (Tofranil) is used in the treatment of enuresis. Overdoses of these drugs cause atropine-like effects, cerebral irritability, cardiac arrhythmias and respiratory depression.

Management. Vomiting should be induced and activated charcoal may be helpful. The child should be carefully observed for neurological complications and these may require supportive treatment. Cardiac arrhythmias are the most serious complication and the child should be carefully monitored in hospital.

INGESTION OF HOUSEHOLD PRODUCTS

This accounts for about half of all accidental poisoning cases in children. Advice should be obtained from a Poison's Reference Centre about each case.

Bleaches

Ingestion is usually minor due to the unpleasant taste of the substance. Bleaches usually contain sodium hypochlorite which is mildly corrosive. Milk should be given and vomiting should not be induced.

Batteries

Small button batteries are now common in many households and may easily be swallowed by young children. The alkali batteries are highly corrosive and very dangerous. They may lodge in the oesophagus but more commonly are retained in the stomach. They are radio-opaque and their position can be verified by X-ray. They should be removed endoscopically if they have not been passed within 8 hours.

Weed-killers

Paraquat is the most dangerous commercially available herbicide. It causes liver, kidney and respiratory damage and may be fatal. Treatment involves induced vomiting and the oral administration of activated charcoal. Measurement of plasma paraquat levels may help to indicate the prognosis.

Paraffin (kerosene) poisoning

The accidental ingestion of household paraffin is particularly liable to occur since it is so often stored in old fruit juice bottles. Moreover, many parents are unaware of its danger; much more information regarding this is required. In some developing countries there is the additional problem that kerosene is used as a 'medicine' for various ailments.

The kerosene causes acute gastric symptoms but the greatest danger is from its inhalation which occurs during vomiting, causing a lipoid pneumonia. For this reason the stomach should not be washed out, nor vomiting induced, since the risk of lipoid pneumonia is thereby increased.

CHRONIC LEAD POISONING

In childhood the commonest cause of lead poisoning is the ingestion of flakes of paint containing lead. Lead is no longer permitted in commercially available paints but may be present in paint applied many years ago. Outbreaks of lead poisoning have occurred from the burning of old car batteries, with subsequent accidental ingestion of the ash which contains a high content of lead, rather than the inhalation of fumes.

The earliest symptoms are irritability, pallor, colic, vomiting and constipation, often associated with pica. These symptoms may continue for some weeks before their seriousness is realized and the dramatic development of lead encephalopathy may be the occasion when the doctor is first called. This complication, resulting from acute cerebral oedema, is particularly liable to occur in young children. Severe vomiting is followed by convulsions, coma and death. Peripheral nerve palsies and a lead line on the gums are uncommon in children.

Laboratory studies show a moderate anaemia and there may be punctate basophilia. Glycosuria may occur and red cells are sometimes present in the urine; amino-aciduria also occurs. These features result from renal tubular damage. There may be an excess of coproporphyrins in the urine. Lead is deposited in the growing ends of bone where it may be seen as a dense line on X-ray. Radio-opaque material may be visible within the intestine.

The most valuable test is the blood lead level; a reading of over 40 µg/dl is very suggestive of lead poisoning. Punctate basophilia and an excess of urinary coproporphyrins may both be negative so that a blood lead level is essential in all suspicious cases. There is also an increased urinary and faecal excretion of lead.

Florid cases of lead poisoning are now becoming uncommon with the reduction in the use of lead paint. Interest is now centred on lead in petrol and lead pollution in the atmosphere and in water. It is thought that elevated lead levels may contribute to mental handicap, hyperactivity and other forms of neuropsychological dysfunction. Symptom-free children living near a lead-emitting smelter and with a blood lead level above 40 µg/dl were found to have a lower age-adjusted performance IQ and a slower performance in a finger–wrist tapping test compared with similar children whose level was below 40 µg/dl. There may be an association between hyperactivity and raised blood lead levels. Lead levels above 24.5 µg/dl are probably potentially dangerous.

Treatment. The use of the chelating agent calcium disodium edanthamil (EDTA), given intramuscularly is highly effective. Unfortunately, its action in lead encephalopathy is often delayed for up to 48 hours and cerebral symptoms may be exacerbated during this time. Dexamethasone and mannitol may be needed for up to 24 hours before the administration of EDTA in order to reduce raised intracranial pressure.

Penicillamine is a drug which increases the excretion of lead and is an important additional form of therapy.

Prognosis. Apart from the immediate risk of death from lead encephalopathy (probably 25% of such cases die) there is a risk of mental handicap if the child survives. It is hoped that the use of EDTA and penicillamine will reduce the incidence of this complication. Other sequelae are convulsions, blindness and speech defect.

GLUE SNIFFING (SOLVENT ABUSE)

This has become a major problem in the UK over the last 15 years. It is particularly common in young underprivileged males, 13–15 years of age, living in inner city slums, and should be regarded as a manifestation of delinquent behaviour. Toluene is the main solvent in glue and produces a period of euphoria for up to 30 minutes after inhalation. The glue is usually squeezed into a rag or poured into a plastic bag and the fumes deeply inhaled. Other solvents abused include benzene (petrol) and dry cleaning fluid. The main danger from glue sniffing is trauma related to falls following intoxication or to suffocation from the plastic bag. Rarely solvent encephalopathy has been reported with convulsions, ataxia and coma.

Treatment is difficult. The dangers of suffocation must be stressed to the children. Family therapy may be a successful approach in breaking the child

of the habit. Unfortunately the families of these children are usually severely disrupted, absence of fathers being common, and are unreliable in giving adequate support. There is little evidence that glue sniffing progresses to drug addiction and most children eventually break the habit spontaneously. Shopkeepers should be discouraged from selling glue to children unaccompanied by a responsible adult.

Child abuse

Physical battering, although the most dramatic and best-known form of child abuse, is only one end of the spectrum of the disorder. At the other end lie those children who are passively battered by being emotionally starved of affection. The problem has reached enormous prominence in the last decade because it is so widespread and may have such tragic results for the child concerned and for the whole family. Child abuse has existed for generations but the increasing frequency with which it is now recognized is probably due to an actual increase, as well as to a greater awareness of the problem.

In addition to physical abuse, child sexual abuse has recently become a 'headline' issue and is an important and controversial condition. That child sexual abuse exists is unquestioned amongst those caring for children, it is rather its frequency and precise diagnostic criteria that are most controversial at the present time.

Physical abuse

Physical abuse may be described as either 'non-accidental injury' or the 'battered baby syndrome'. Frequently the nature of physical injuries is not clear or there is an incomplete explanation. The paediatrician's first responsibility is to the child and physical abuse must always be considered in such cases. In recent years a new form of physical abuse has been recognized which takes the form of a parent simulating illness in the child; a condition referred to as *Munchausen's syndrome by proxy* (see p. 528).

The injury to the child, whether physical or

emotional, is almost always caused by the parents. At least 90% of those who batter their children do so because they were insufficiently mothered as children. 'Mothering' has nothing to do with mothercraft, which is the technical aspect of baby care, such as bathing, changing and feeding. Mothering is the ability to give her baby loving attention 24 hours every day without feeling resentful or expecting something in return. It includes fathers, though with a different emphasis, and is included in 'parenting'. The ability to 'mother' is acquired from normal mothering experiences as a very young child; it failure leads to the 'cycle of deprivation', whereby harsh childhood experiences are repeated in the next generation. These deprived parents are not mentally ill. A very small proportion of battering parents are psychopathic and there are some who communicate by 'bashing', either verbally or physically, everyone they meet.

Mothers are more liable to abuse babies whereas fathers are more likely to harm older children. The normal response of a mother to her crying baby is to comfort him by cuddling. Every mother feels exasperated by her baby's cries at times; the normal reaction when these cries become intolerable is to leave the baby crying for a time and go to another room to make herself a cup of tea or to have a smoke. The pathological response of the unmothered mother is to feel that she must make her baby stop crying. This may cause her to shake or smack him and at worst to kill her baby.

Such a mother does not hate her baby in the usually accepted sense of the word but the baby's demanding cries evoke responses which relate to her own childhood experiences. They make her feel inadequate as though her baby's cries are accusing her of not being able to make him happy. To her the baby represents herself as a baby and reminds her of her own unhappy childhood, whereas she expected the baby to supply her with the warmth of feeling which she had never received as a child. Parents who were strictly disciplined as children expect their children to conform and to behave properly. Fear of 'spoiling' the child is often strong.

Child abuse affects parents from every social

Table 28.4 Important risk factors in families where physical abuse of children is most likely.

Parental factors
Unsupported mother
Young mother
History of being abused as a child
Personality disorder (recurrent difficulties in making and
    maintaining intimate social relationships)
Mental illness
Violence between mother and other adults in the family

Child factors
Prematurity
Adverse temperament

class and of all levels of intellect. The only reason for the apparently larger numbers from the poorer social classes is their inability to be able to get away from their babies because of overcrowding and financial hardship. In the old days, grandmothers were more often available; it is the loss of this support together with the increasing anxieties of modern life which, in part, account for the increase in the problem. Mothers who batter are very frightened of being left alone with their babies. They are exquisitely sensitive to loss of support from the environment and they cannot stand criticism because it makes them feel rejected.

The causes of physical abuse of the child can be divided into a number of categories. It can be conveniently classified as being due to either parental or child factors (Table 28.4), but in practice is usually a combination of the two.

Bonding between a mother and her new baby is not automatic. It is particularly liable to fail if the two are separated for any length of time, for example, if the baby is in a special care unit. The same happens with animals separated from their young. This explains the higher incidence of battering in low birth weight babies and in those delivered by Caesarean section. It emphasizes the need for such mothers to be allowed to handle their babies even if the baby is in an incubator. Routine removal of babies delivered by Caesarean section or by forceps to nurseries 'for observation' should be discouraged.

Mothers should be warned that 'instant love' for the newborn baby is often a myth. It takes many mothers time to fall in love with their babies just as it does with future husbands. Mothers who find they do not immediately love their babies often suffer guilt feelings because they have never been told that this is a common experience.

DIAGNOSIS

The reaction of the infant or toddler to repeated physical abuse may be one of 'frozen watchfulness' — he moves very little and just stares out of his unsmiling face. To survive he may undergo role reversal, whereby he mothers his mother, patting her knee and trying to make her happy. With his strict father he becomes excessively obedient in order to avoid his father's punishments. Some children who lack mothering become precocious in order to mother themselves or become the over-active demanding child whose needs cannot be met by his parents.

Parents who batter do not hide their children from doctors but they do not give an accurate history. It is the discrepancies in the history which lead to the diagnosis; for example the baby of 2 weeks who is stated to have bruised his cheek by banging it on the side of the cot, or the spiral fracture of the humerus which is described as being due to a fall when this type of fracture can only result from the arm being twisted. Often a denial of the actual cause is based on a wish that it had never happened; sometimes true amnesia occurs. A second vital point in the history is that there is commonly a delay of a day or more between the time of injury and the visit to the doctor. The possibility of child abuse should be particularly considered in children brought in during the night. The mother's aggitation is often out of proportion to the signs in the child and strange parental behaviour may lead them to leaving the child before the admission procedure has been completed.

When the child is examined, he is likely to be found bruised or to show other signs on the skin. Sometimes the injury fits a cigarette burn or

where a sharp stone ring has been bored into the skin. The shape of an adult human bite may be apparent. The frenulum of the upper lip in a baby may be torn or the lips or gum margins bruised because the bottle or fist has been rammed into his mouth to stop him crying. The child's height and weight should be carefully plotted on the appropriate centile charts to detect failure to thrive. The fundi should be carefully examined to detect retinal or subhyaloid haemorrhages resulting from shaking the baby. If the child shows any abnormal neurological signs, subdural haemorrhage (p. 516) should be excluded with a CT scan.

In coming to a diagnosis the doctor should not try to be a detective. There is no need to attempt to discover which parent caused the injury because the other parent is usually also aware of the situation. Sometimes the injury has been caused by another child in this disturbed family. What is helpful is to learn what the mother feels about her baby's crying; does it worry her and does her baby make her feel angry?

A mother's reply as to why she chose to bottle feed can be very informative but the question must be most sensitively asked to avoid seeming critical. One mother replied that she did not want her baby to come to rely on her; a vital indication of her own childhood experiences and their effect on her feelings towards her own baby.

Doctors find the diagnosis of physical abuse difficult to make because it is so unpleasant and difficult to imagine that any parent could do such things to a child. Moreover, this difficulty may be increased by not knowing what to do once the diagnosis has been made.

INVESTIGATIONS

X-ray changes have been overemphasized so that their absence has led to a failure to make the diagnosis. The changes which may be found and which require the whole skeleton to be X-rayed are evidence of new or old fractures, epiphyseal fractures or displacements and periosteal new bone formation. Metaphyseal flakes result from pulling on a limb and epiphyseal stippling from a crushing injury. Films should be repeated after 2 weeks since recent injury may not show until callus or periosteal new bone formation occurs.

In children where bruising is the main feature of possible physical abuse, coagulopathy must be excluded by appropriate haematological investigations (p. 433).

All visible injuries should be photographed by a medical photographer and these may subsequently be necessary to present in a courtroom as evidence.

MANAGEMENT

The suspicion of physical abuse of a child should always be considered in any injured child. Suspicion may be aroused in teachers, social workers, health visitors, GPs, community paediatricians, accident and emergency staff, or hospital paediatric staff. It is most important that if suspicion is aroused, the professionals are equipped with clear procedures worked out by a multi-disciplinary Area Review Committee (now known in Britain as Area Child Protection Committees). One role of this group is to set up 'At risk registers' to ensure that information can rapidly be obtained as to whether any professional agency has had serious concern about an individual child previously.

Whenever child abuse is suspected, the child should be examined by a doctor experienced in this area. In the majority of cases this does not need to be a hospital paediatrician and is often more appropriately a community paediatrician. Careful written documentation of all the injuries must be made. Whether a child requires admission to hospital depends on two factors; the severity of the injury, and the risk of further injury. Although the hospital is often referred to as a 'place of safety' this is only relative. The risk of the child (particularly a baby) developing gastro-enteritis or respiratory infection in hospital is relatively high and this should be considered before admitting a well child. Short-term foster care may be a better alternative.

A multi-disciplinary team should meet at the earliest opportunity to consider the case; this is

often referred to as a 'case conference'. This team should include the local Social Services or in some areas the National Society for the Prevention of Cruelty to Children (NSPCC), a paediatrician (community or hospital), and where appropriate the police, probation services and a representative from the education authority. It is most important that as much *accurate* information as possible is available at this conference. The conference should make a decision as to the further management of the child and the family and whether the needs of the child should be protected by legal constraint (see p. 21). The parents must be kept aware of what is happening and although it is often inappropriate that they should be present at a case conference they should know when it will take place and be told immediately of its decisions. A 'key worker' should be nominated by the conference to communicate and work with the family.

The psychological management of the child and the family is discussed in Chapter 20. It is important to recognize that only one child in a family may be battered but that, whatever the situation, the whole family is in need of help. This will require the mobilization of many services, especially the Social Services. Successful treatment not only requires an end to abuse of the child at risk, but also the prevention of recurrence in future children. Removal from the family of a child at risk, without adequate ongoing therapy, results in the rapid replacement of the lost child by a new baby who is at grave risk of the same fate.

Sexual abuse

Child sexual abuse (CSA) is not new, but in recent years it has provoked much discussion. When considering the problem of CSA a broader definition should be considered. This includes all situations where children are used by adults to obtain any form of sexual gratification such as fondling children's genitals, involvement in pornography as well as any form of sexual interference (vaginal, anal or oral) or any form of masturbation. Discussions of CSA are often painful, distressing and sometimes revolting and for these reasons some individuals have actually denied that it occurs. This is a great mistake and exposes children to further exploitation. Only by discussing this problem openly can society hope to protect children from it adequately.

The prevalence of CSA is unknown but it is becoming considerably more common. This is probably due to the fact that it is being increasingly recognized but it is also possible that its actual frequency is increasing. The vast majority of cases of CSA occur in the family context. Fathers or adult males living in the home are the usual culprits, but occasionally mothers or older females may interfere with small boys.

It is often helpful to view the severity of CSA on a continuum. At one pole it is the result of a major breakdown in family relationships where the daughter has moved into the mother's role. At the other extreme, a disturbed individual may have moved into the household as a stepparent, sometimes with the specific intention of violating the children. The vast majority of abusers are men and the majority of victims are girls, although homosexual abuse of boys is also common.

Sexual abuse should always be considered when children are seen because of physical abuse; up to 15% of children with non-accidental injury are also sexually abused. Sexual abuse may present in a number of ways:

Disclosure by the child. This should always be taken seriously when he or she discloses that sexual abuse may have occurred. The doctor should listen carefully to the child and the onus is on the paediatrician to pursue the allegations actively. It is most unlikely that children will fabricate stories of CSA *ab ignitio*, but leading questions should be avoided as it is easy to make a child agree with any suggestions put by an authorative figure.

Behavioural abnormalities. Table 28.5 lists the features that should alert the paediatrician to the possibility of CSA. None of these behavioural abnormalities prove abuse but should make the doctor suspicious of sexual abuse.

Table 28.5 Behavioural features which should make the doctor suspicious of the possibility of CSA.

Sexually provocative behaviour to adults
Sexually explicit descriptions
Preoccupation with sexual fantasies and behaviour
Specific fear towards a mature male living in the family
Unexplained changes in behaviour
Fearful of men
Running away from home with no obvious reason

Physical abnormalities. Certain physical abnormalities should alert the paediatrician to the possibility of CSA. These include vulvovaginitis with soreness and discharge, recurrent dysuria without evidence of infection, unexplained vaginal bleeding, genital laceration or injury, dilated vagina and other genital abnormalities (see below), sexually transmitted diseases, or pregnancy in young adolescent girls where the father is apparently unknown.

CLINICAL FEATURES

All children in whom CSA is suspected should be carefully examined by an experienced paediatrician. This should be performed in the same way as in a child presenting with any problem. General examination of the child should precede examination of the genitalia and anus. If there is strong evidence of CSA then the child should be referred to a doctor with special expertise in this area. The number of examinations the child undergoes must be kept to a minimum, and if it is felt necessary for a police surgeon also to see the child the examination should be delayed until the paediatrician and police surgeon can perform a joint examination. The child should only be examined in a children's department and never in a police station. Clinical photography to record any possible evidence should be done at the time of this examination.

There are no pathognomic signs of CSA, but there are some physical signs which strongly suggest this diagnosis. These include bruises, burns or bite marks particularly around the genitalia. The labia should be inspected for redness or bruising or signs of chronic friction in cases of long-standing abuse. The vulva and hymen should also be carefully examined for evidence of trauma. The hymenal opening in pre-pubertal girls should normally be less than 7 mm in diameter.

The anus should also be carefully examined. In cases of acute abuse, there may be local inflammation and bruising, tears of the anal mucosa or dilated veins in either a ring or arc around the anus. The reflex anal dilatation (RAD) test has been widely publicized and should be performed on all children where CSA is considered.

The reflex anal dilatation test. The child should be laid in the left lateral position with the knees tucked up to the chest. The buttocks are gently parted by the examiner and the anus observed. In a positive RAD test, the external sphincter relaxes within 30 seconds so that the interior of the anal canal and lower rectum can be seen and this dilatation should remain for at least 2–3 seconds. A positive test suggests incompetence of the internal sphincter and this may be due to penetration and stretching. It may also be due to constipation, particularly in small children.

As mentioned above, there is no pathognomic test for CSA and the diagnosis is made by consideration of many factors. It is equally important to be aware of the converse which is that CSA may have occurred with *no* physical signs. In older children (over 5 years) a disclosure interview may be helpful. This is undertaken by specially trained people and involves the use of anatomically correct dolls. The way the child plays with the dolls is very important in understanding what has happened to the child. This interview should be recorded on videotape.

MANAGEMENT

Once the diagnosis is confirmed or strongly suspected a multi-disciplinary case conference should be convened as described on p. 524. A decision should be made on the need for legal proceedings and/or notification of the Child Protection ('At risk') Register. Many children who have suffered sexual abuse are emotionally traumatized by the experience which may have been going on for several years. Referral to a child psychiatrist is essential and this is discussed in Chapter 20.

Failure to thrive

Failure to thrive is not a diagnosis, but a symptom and one which must be carefully investigated and treated. There are critical periods of growth and development and if a child's growth is restricted for too long, complete catch-up is not possible. Although the causes of failure to thrive are numerous, a very important and often neglected cause is a form of child abuse where 'nurturing' is withheld.

Nurturing refers to the process of rearing. It includes attention to physical needs such as adequate nutrition but also caring for the general development of the child with the giving of love, comfort and security. Poor nurturing may be associated with failure to thrive and unless considered, is easily neglected when investigating other, more physical causes. No child can thrive unless mothered. This passive battering is by far the commonest cause of 'failure to thrive' in young children, accounting for at least 20% of such cases.

DIAGNOSIS

The diagnosis of failure to thrive is made by accurate measurements of the child's growth including weight, length and head circumference. These are then related to appropriate centile charts as discussed on p. 39. The diagnosis is made if there has been falling off in these measurements (particularly weight) over a period of time or if there is a discrepancy in weight when compared with head circumference.

Table 28.6 lists the major causes of failure to thrive. All the organic causes are discussed elsewhere in this book.

Non-organic failure to thrive is a major feature of child abuse. Physical or sexual abuse may be associated with this condition. Sudden failure to thrive may precede physical abuse and is often a warning sign of the acute onset of serious family disruption. Non-organic failure to thrive is a diagnosis of exclusion. A careful history must be

Table 28.6 Major causes of failure to thrive.

Impaired intake
Faulty breast-feeding technique
Malnutrition
Child abuse
Emotional deprivation

Impaired absorption
Carbohydrate
   Disaccharidase deficiency (p. 200)
   Galactosaemia (p. 370)
   Fructosaemia (p. 371)
Fat malabsorption causing steatorrhoea
   Cystic fibrosis (p. 199)
   Coeliac disease (p. 196)
   Parasites
   Pancreatic insufficiency
   Jaundice (p. 207)
Protein malabsorption
   Any cause of chronic diarrhoea (p. 195)
   Cow's milk intolerance (p. 198)

Chronic disease
Nervous system
   Cerebral palsy (p. 320)
   Neuro-degenerative disorders (p. 305)
   Severe mental retardation
Cardiovascular disease
   Cyanotic heart disease (p. 219)
   Cardiac failure (p. 222)
Respiratory disease
   Severe chronic asthma (p. 183)
   Bronchiectasis (p. 181)
Gastrointestinal disease
Renal disease
   Chronic renal failure (p. 266)
Long-standing liver disease (cirrhosis) (p. 211)
Haematological disorders
   Sickle cell disease (p. 431)
   Thalassaemia (p. 430)

Chronic infection
Tuberculosis (p. 555)
Malaria (p. 572)
AIDS

Chromosomal disorders
Down's syndrome, etc. (p. 119)

Drugs
Long-term steroids

taken including detailed enquiry into dietary factors, assessment of how the family works and whether there is evidence of strife in the household. Unemployment, low intelligence, trouble with the police and maternal depression are important factors to ascertain. The mother may be very inexperienced and it is important to watch how she feeds her baby.

The child should be examined carefully both for evidence of organic disease and also for signs of physical or sexual abuse. Bruises and scratches should be carefully recorded. A careful developmental assessment should also be performed as many children with neglect also have developmental delay.

INVESTIGATIONS

Routine investigations should include urinalysis, full blood count, serum electrolytes, and liver, urine and bone function tests as well as examination of the stool for malabsorption or infection. If cystic fibrosis or coeliac disease is suspected specific investigations should also be performed.

If non-organic failure to thrive is seriously considered, then the child should be admitted to hospital for investigation. With adequate diet, children should put on up to 70 g/day whilst in hospital, but some children who have had long-standing non-organic failure to thrive may take a week or more before they start to thrive. The child's mood should also be noted. Initially, the child is often withdrawn and sullen but later starts to blossom and become interested in his environment. The period of hospitalization should also be used to befriend the mother and observe her handling of the child.

MANAGEMENT

The management of the family is important in treating the child who has not been nurtured properly. Intervention by a sensitive social worker and sometimes a psychologist or child psychiatrist may be very helpful. In some areas a programme to teach the mother mothering skills has proven to be very helpful. Often an older 'grandmother'-type figure can befriend the mother and offer counselling and practical advice.

Unfortunately, the long-term outlook for the child may not be very good as permanent growth or developmental impairment may have occurred. The child's IQ may be permanently lowered.

Munchausen's syndrome by proxy

This condition refers to a parent fabricating features of an illness in their child and represents a serious form of child abuse. It usually occurs in children below the age of 6 years, and most commonly in children of around 3 years of age. The children usually present with symptoms often originating in more than one system and which may have been investigated by a variety of doctors, on a number of occasions, for more than 1 year. The realization that the illness is fabricated by the parents (almost always the mother) takes some time.

PRESENTING FEATURES

Presenting symptoms or signs vary and usually affect a number of systems. Bleeding is the most common sign and usually occurs in the urine, vomitus or stool. The blood is subsequently found to be the mother's which has surreptitiously been mixed with the child's urine or vomit. The next most common presentation is with neurological features including drowsiness (due to the administration of sedative drugs) or seizures (either induced by carotid sinus pressure or invented). Rashes induced by painting the skin with a variety of agents and fever induced by tampering with the thermometer are both other relatively common symptoms deliberately fabricated by the mother.

A feature of this condition is that the mothers often have some rudimentary medical knowledge (up to half have been nurses or have started nurse training). Some of the mothers have had a history of producing factitious symptoms or signs in themselves (Munchausen's syndrome).

This condition should be suspected in any child where the persistent symptoms or signs cannot be explained, or where the relatively severe clinical features do not correlate with general health of the child who appears bright and healthy. Munchausen's syndrome by proxy is considerably less rare than some of the very obscure diagnoses considered in children with mothers who fabricate disease.

MANAGEMENT

Once the diagnosis is strongly suspected, contact between the mother and child should be restricted to discover whether the symptoms and signs disappear with her absence. In some circumstances a 'place of safety' order may be necessary in order to do this. When the diagnosis is clear, the mother (assuming she is responsible for the fabricated symptoms) should be confronted with the facts. This should not be done in a punitive manner, but rather with the intent of offering her understanding and help. Legal proceedings and psychiatric referral may be necessary, but once the mother has been confronted with the knowledge that she has been found out, the symptoms abate and the relationship may improve. Careful long-term surveillance is of course essential.

29

PAEDIATRICS IN
DEVELOPING COUNTRIES

By the year 2000, there will be 2.5 billion children aged 14 years or less alive in the world, of whom 80% will be living in developing countries and at risk from the infectious, parasitic and nutritional disorders described in this chapter. Although many of these conditions are now rare in Western countries, they do still occur: air travel and immigration facilitate the spread of infectious diseases, while in pockets of poverty and deprivation, nutritional deficiencies exist, and may be increasing.

Child health provision

There are three major factors which make child health provision difficult.

1 Geographical factors. In many countries, 70–80% of the population live in rural areas, and where there has been urbanization this has often been unplanned, giving rise to shanty towns, which create their own problems.

2 Numbers of children. In many countries, 50% of the population are below the age of 14 years, thus falling into the paediatric age range. Children are without a political voice and although one would expect that they would receive an appropriate proportion of the health budget, this is rarely so.

3 Population increase. High birth rates, with falling infant mortality, have led in some countries to a potential to double the total population within 17–25 years. Increased numbers of infants surviving to childhood may reduce the amount per head

which can be spent on health and the amount of food available.

High birth rates are stimulated by many factors, including cultural and religious beliefs, lack of security in old age, and by the desire to replace children lost because of the high infant mortality rate. One way in which the paediatrician can contribute to the problem of excessive fertility is by working to reduce the infant mortality rate. Once the population perceives that most children born alive will survive, spontaneous family spacing and limitation will follow, after a 'lag' period of about a generation. It is very difficult to reverse the equation, urging people to limit their families in number as a means to improve health and survival of their children.

Priorities

Many developing countries suffer from a lack of data relating to the causes of morbidity and mortality in childhood on which to base health priorities. The paediatrician therefore needs to organize the collection of useful information at several levels. The cause of death and reason for admission to hospital are usually easily collected, and will highlight the importance of conditions such as diarrhoeal disease, common to most developing countries, also drawing attention to the problems which may be of a local nature, such as tetanus, malaria or sickle cell disease.

Data collected from clinics may reinforce the priorities derived from hospital data, but may also uncover conditions, such as bilharzia, which rarely

Causes of death	Reasons for admission	Reasons for clinic attendance
Malnutrition	Pneumonia	Acute gastro-enteritis
Tetanus	Malnutrition	Respiratory tract infections
Measles	Measles	Skin conditions
Acute gastro-enteritis	Pharyngitis	Measles
Pneumonia	Acute gastro-enteritis	Malaria
Meningitis	Tetanus	Bilharzia

Table 29.1 The commonest causes of death in Zimbabwe (1974). The commonest reasons for admission to hospital and clinic attendances are also shown.

need hospital admission, but are none the less significant causes of morbidity (Table 29.1).

Once the disease patterns are known, priorities can be set at different levels. In hospital, for instance, simple, rational guidelines for the management of the common conditions can be laid down. At the community level, the priorities may turn out to be measles immunization, maternal tetanus immunization or treatment of vitamin A deficiency.

Local child care practices

All societies have evolved traditional ways of caring for children. These can have positive or negative effects on child health, or may be harmless. The paediatrician must examine these practices and decide which should be reinforced (e.g. prolonged breast feeding, attending herbalists for psychosomatic problems), which should be discouraged (e.g. cupping, burning and scarification) and which may be ignored.

Many countries now encourage herbalists and witch doctors to participate in child care by teaching them to recognize conditions which they can treat and those best referred to clinic or hospital.

The doctor's role

The doctor's role in a developing country, be he paediatrician or a general doctor with a major paediatric interest, differs from his role in, for example, Europe or the USA. He is much less likely to be seeing mothers and children in a one-to-one relationship, and more likely to be heading a team where much of the doctor's traditional responsibility for diagnosis and treatment has to be

delegated. The doctor will be more involved with the education and management of his team, of hospital and clinic staff, and with the collection of data aimed at improving the delivery of the service. He is likely to have close links with key people in the community, who themselves can influence child health positively through the spread of ideas and practical knowledge, for example, school teachers, traditional leaders, hydrologists and agriculturalists. This is not an easy task, but unless a doctor is prepared to withdraw somewhat from the overwhelming clinical load and find areas where problems can be tackled at their roots, the service provided may turn out to be inappropriate and under-used, and in the long term have little effect on the community it is designed to serve.

Delegation

The number of doctors per head of the population varies from approximately 1:1000 in Britain to 1:25 000 in some of the less economically developed countries. This latter figure may be made worse by an uneven distribution of doctors between rural and urban areas. Much of the traditional doctor's work will have to be delegated to other workers, implying that these workers' skills need to be expanded. One of the doctor's functions is to ensure that they receive appropriate training and support in their expanded roles, and to issue protocols and guidelines for the management of the more common conditions and emergencies they will meet in their daily practice. It is also important that their responsibilities are well defined, that they receive guidance in what they can and cannot be expected to handle, and appropriate instruction on when to refer for second opinions. The importance of keeping up morale among health workers, especially if they are working in comparative isolation cannot be overstressed. This can be done in a number of ways including through personal contact with the doctor, time off for further education, and by encouraging innovations.

Delivery of service

Health care is provided in all countries at three levels:

1 Home or village.
2 Regional.
3 National.

The state of development of each level will depend on past history and present political climate of the country and on factors such as per-capita spending on health and the number of trained health workers. In many countries past neglect of the provision of care, at home and village level, is being corrected rapidly through involvement of the people themselves in community planning and decision making. If there is to be lasting improvement in child health it has to be based on services provided at a local level being readily accessible and accepted by the population. It is also at this level that the introduction of relatively cheap and simple preventive and curative measures such as oral rehydration, can have such a profound influence on morbidity and mortality. Similarly, it is at this level that the contribution of other disciplines is so important.

Integration of service

It is usually accepted that the health of the mother is inextricably bound up with that of her dependent infants and children. The provision of a fragmented service, with ante-natal clinics, immunization clinics and clinics to treat minor illness on different days or at different times, may discourage attendance. Maternal and child health clinics, which integrate the care of the mothers and children under 5 years old, have been developed to answer this criticism.

Managing a ward

The importance of prevention and early treatment of childhood illnesses in the out-patient setting has been stressed, but many children will need to be admitted to hospital for initial therapy. Most hospital wards in developing countries are overcrowded, and there is a danger in seeing the solution as providing more beds, rather than positively managing the existing facilities to maximum effect. Overcrowding leads to cross-infection, with increased length of stay and hence further overcrowding. Many children admitted are malnourished and are therefore in danger from infectious illnesses. Overcrowding also leads to a dilution of medical and nursing care, further lengthening hospital stay.

Positive steps need to be taken against overcrowding by managing children if possible as out-patients, or as day cases. Many clinics treat acute gastro-enteritis on an out-patient basis, mothers attending for 6–12 hours per day. They treat their children under supervision and return home at night. Many children with measles can be handled in the same way.

Mothers should be admitted with their children. This not only cuts down cross-infection, as the mother is the only one who handles the child, but also gives an opportunity to assess the mother's ability to handle her sick child when he goes home, and to begin preventive health education.

Length of stay in a hospital ward should be kept to the minimum necessary to ensure that the child is recovering. The consolidation of treatment can hen be continued from out-patient or local clinics. Communication with these clinics and providing them with the knowledge and medication needed, will be vital.

Measles vaccination of all children over 5 months old should be given within 24 hours of admission, to cut down measles cross-infections (see p. 535).

Preventive versus curative

What a population wants may differ from what it really needs. Most mothers, if asked about what they would like provided will opt for a service which offers to cure their ill children. The concept of prevention, acting when the child is well to forestall some possible future illness, may be alien. Many health-care advisors believe that preventive and curative services should be provided in tandem; the initial attraction will be the offer to cure, but as confidence in the service builds up, the message of prevention will begin to take hold.

NEONATAL SERVICES

The provision of an appropriate service for the newborn, within the economic constraints, will tax the organizing ability and ingenuity of all paediatricians working in developing countries. Although it is said that the overall state of a country's development is reflected in its perinatal statistics, the perinatal period is in fact a time when comparatively simple and cheap innovations, such as the cervicograph and prompt resuscitation at birth can result in dramatic improvements in mortality and morbidity.

Zimbabwean figures collected 10 years ago showed that the booked perinatal mortality rate in a large city was 35:1000. The unbooked rate was five times greater. The definition of 'booked' was that a women had attended an ante-natal clinic on a single occasion. This highlights the importance of discovering those women whose babies are at risk. Some of the maternal conditions which are likely to produce problems in their newborn are shown in Table 29.2.

Table 29.2 Maternal risk factors predisposing to neonatal problems.

Young or old age of mother
Grand multiparity
Pelvic deformity
Maternal infection
   Malaria
   Anaemia
   Bilharzia
   Tuberculosis
Maternal malnutrition
Prolonged labour
Late presentation in labour

Definition of priorities

Each country has differing problems, so local causes for perinatal morbidity and mortality should be recorded. In developing countries, most of the problems will arise from the high incidence of prematurity and small-for-gestational-age babies and their associated complications (see Fig. 29.1). Local variations will be found in the incidence of infections such as tetanus, syphilis, gonorrhoea and AIDS.

Provision of service

Some of the day-to-day management of babies, normally undertaken by a doctor, will need to be delegated to nursing staff. An active teaching programme for the staff therefore needs to be established and written protocols for the management of common neonatal problems formulated. Regular liason meetings between the obstetric and paediatric staff should be held to review the statistics and decide on joint policies. Facilities for investigation, monitoring and treatment will vary widely between units, but the most important provisions for the neonate are warmth, food and an infection-free environment. The following protocols are given as examples of the level of care which should be available at most hospitals and clinics. A more detailed discussion of the management and treatment of neonatal problems is given in Chapter 7.

Management

The normal newborn. This should include facilities for:
- prompt resuscitation at birth;
- cord care to prevent tetanus;
- vitamin K, 1 mg intramuscularly or orally;
- early start to breast feeding;
- routine examination for congenital abnormalities;
- BCG before discharge;

Most of the day-to-day care of the baby should be given by the mother both to reduce cross-infection and release staff for nursing more sick infants. Teaching sessions for mothers, covering topics such as infant feeding, cord care and immunization, should be given.

Pre-term babies. Particular attention should be paid to:
• prompt resuscitation and oxygenation at birth;
• prevention of heat loss and the maintenance of body temperature;
• vitamin K, 0.5 mg intramuscularly or orally;
• early feeding with mother's own milk, by tube if necessary.

Most mothers can learn to express their milk and are able to feed their babies under supervision. A feeding schedule needs to be worked out, starting at about 60 ml/kg/day on the first day of life rising to approximately 200–220 ml/kg/day by the seventh to tenth day. The rate of increase will depend on toleration of the previous days feeds as shown by a lack of vomiting and abdominal distension.
• Daily weighing and examination for signs of jaundice and infection.
• Pre-discharge BCG immunization.
• Vitamin and iron supplements on discharge for those of less than 36 weeks gestation.

Most of the day-to-day care of the baby can be given by the mother. Discharge from the unit should not depend on weight alone, but on whether the baby can suck and maintain his body temperature, and on the mother's ability to handle a small baby.

Respiratory distress syndrome (RDS). The importance of prompt resuscitation, oxygenation and warmth has already been stressed, and is particularly so in preventing the development of RDS. If RDS does develop in the pre-term, management will depend on the facilities available. The most important provisions are:
• maintain hydration, by naso-gastric or intravenous fluids;
• maintain blood sugar level between 2 and 5 mmol/l;
• maintain the body temperature as close to normal as possible;

• provide oxygen by head box. This may be life saving, but there are dangers of over-oxygenation (p. 112);
• give antibiotics if there is a history of premature rupture of membranes;
• Group B beta haemolytic *Streptococcus* infections may mimic RDS so many units prescribe penicillin prophylactically until the diagnosis becomes clearer;
• in the absence of ventilators, there is little else that can be done if the baby's condition deteriorates. Positive end-expiratory pressure through nasal prongs or a face mask may help the moderately severe cases, particularly if applied early.

Ventilation of newborns with RDS is beyond the resources of many countries. If ventilators are available, they should in the first instance be reserved for babies with a reasonable chance of survival, and not used as a last resort.

Jaundice. Rational management of jaundice depends to a large extent on quick and accurate measurement of serum bilirubin (p. 106). Much can be done by simple methods to minimize the rate of rise of bilirubin:
• feeding early, particularly in pre-term babies;
• maintain hydration with extra glucose water if needed;
• phototherapy. Raising the intensity of lighting in the unit by painting the walls white and nursing babies naked in reflected sunlight will help

Babies whose jaundice appears within 24 hours of birth and those who become severely jaundiced later will need to be referred to a centre for further investigation and management.

Neonatal syphilis. Syphilis should be suspected in any newborn with pneumonia, anaemia, jaundice, hepatomegaly, a dry scaly skin or oedema (Plate 48). Later manifestations include bloody nasal discharge, weeping lesions around the mouth and anus, tender long bones and haematuria. A firm diagnosis can be made rapidly from the X-ray changes in the long bones and confirmed by a WR or TPI test. Treatment should be with intramuscular penicillin daily for 10 days, or a single injection of long-acting penicillin if follow-up is likely to be

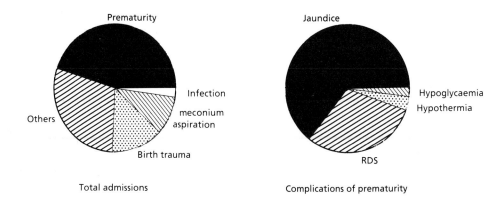

Fig. 29.1 Breakdown of the commoner reasons for admissions to a neonatal unit in Zimbabwe (1977).

difficult. In advanced cases, penicillin makes little difference to the liver or renal pathology, which will progress.

Tetanus (see also p. 354). Neonatal tetanus can be prevented if mothers are fully immunized. Accidental contamination of the moist umbilicus, or treatment with inappropriate powders containing cow dung or charcoal are the usual source of infection. Typically, presentation is with failure to suck between the fifth and fourteenth days of life, followed by rapid progression to stiffness and then convulsions. Early presentation indicates poor prognosis. In severe cases, profuse sweating and tachycardia are manifestations of sympathetic over-activity. Death usually results from a combination of hypoxia and exhaustion. Treatment without ventilation is difficult, but with assiduous attention to the details of nursing care, mortality can be reduced to about 50%.

Anti-tetanic serum (ATS) and penicillin should be given, followed by naso-gastric feeds with expressed breast milk. Frequent suction of secretions is needed, but this often precipitates spasms. Oxygen will be needed during hypoxic spells. Basic sedation with phenobarbitone and chlorpromazine or diazepam, with additional paraldehyde as needed, should be given.

The baby should be nursed in a quite room, and sudden stimuli such as light, vibration or sound should be avoided. Although spasms may cease after 1–2 weeks, stiffness which interferes with

feeding may persist for several weeks. On recovery a full course of tetanus toxoid should be given. Neither intrathecal ATS nor systemic steroids have been shown to affect outcome.

IMMUNIZATIONS APPROPRIATE TO DEVELOPING COUNTRIES

The different epidemiology of infectious diseases in developed countries may make the traditional immunization schedules used in more developed countries inappropriate. In addition, as the epidemiology of individual infectious diseases change with time, immunization policies may need to be adapted to suit the changed circumstances. One must also question the traditional contraindications to immunizations. In countries where measles has an overall mortality of 2–5% it would seem appropriate to immunize even in the presence of mild upper respiratory tract infections and malnutrition, rather than risk measles during an epidemic. Similar arguments can be made for other immunization procedures. Table 29.3 summarizes a recommended immunization regime for developing countries.

Diphtheria, pertussis, tetanus (DPT)

During epidemics of pertussis it is justifiable to give the first DPT injection at birth or within the first month of life. Pertussis in infants under 6 months of age is particularly severe and often

Table 29.3 Suggested immunization regime for developing countries.

Time	Immunization
Birth or first clinic visit	BCG
0–2 months	DPT + OPV
2–4 months	DPT + OPV
4–9 months	DPT + OPV (+ measles, see below)
12–14 months	Measles or MMR (see below)
4–5 years	DT + OPV
11–13 years	DT + OPV, Heaf test and BCG

D: diphtheria; P: pertussis; T: tetanus; OPV: oral polio vaccine.

atypical. Immunization in the neonatal period has been shown to modify the clinical picture.

Oral polio vaccine

In most developing countries polio is common and often under-reported. It tends to be seen in younger age groups than in Britain or the USA, occurring from the time when passive protection from maternal antibodies has ceased. Apart from immunosuppression, and known immunological abnormalities, there are no contraindications to live oral polio vaccine.

BCG

The ideal time to give BCG is at birth, or at the first clinic visit. Although not as effective in preventing tuberculosis as measles vaccine is in preventing measles, protection rates of 60–80% are reported and in particular, miliary tuberculosis and tubercular meningitis are very rare in immunized children. BCG also gives some protection against leprosy. BCG leaves a small scar which means those immunized can be readily identified at a later date. Most authorities therefore recommend using the left deltoid area for immunization, now that smallpox vaccine is no longer necessary.

Heaf or Mantoux testing before giving BCG at birth is obviously not required, but when BCG is given after the age of 3 months, it is probably wise to do so, particularly if tuberculosis is common in the community. If BCG is given to a child with active tuberculosis, the response to the BCG will be similar to that after a Mantoux test with an area of induration, reddening and possibly blistering. This is the so-called accelerated reaction, which can be painful, may take weeks to heal, and may leave an unsightly scar. Contraindications to BCG include active tuberculosis, severe malnutrition, other severe illness and immunosuppression (see also p. 355).

Measles

Measles immunization is a safe and very effective procedure, giving life-long protection in 98% of those immunized. The vaccine is live and it is important that there is no break in the 'cold chain' from manufacturer, through transport to the clinic, to the actual administration of the vaccine. Determining the optimal time at which to vaccinate is difficult and policies vary from country to country.

Maternal antibodies against measles cross the placenta and protect the newborn from the disease, but will also inactivate measles vaccine. The rate at which maternal antibodies disappear varies from child to child. Virtually 100% of children will still have antibodies at the age of 5 months, whereas by 14 months, no child will possess antibodies. If, however, immunization is delayed to 14 months, as recommended in Britain and the USA, many children in developing countries will already have suffered from measles, commonly at the time when they were being weaned from the breast on to an often inadequate diet. Immunization at 9 months will lead to a failure rate of between 10 and 15% because of persisting maternal antibodies, while immunization at 6 months will give a failure rate of around 50–60%.

The following recommendations can be made:

Measles endemic

In rural areas or towns the spread of measles can be slow.
1 Few cases below the age of 12 months: immunize at 12–14 months.

2 Significant numbers of cases below 12 months: immunize at 6–9 months and repeat at 12–14 months.

Once the measles incidence has been reduced, and the age of catching the disease has increased, as it should following this plan, continue with a single dose at 12–14 months.

Measles epidemic

1 In severe epidemics, large scale campaigns aiming to immunize all children over 6 months of age, should halt the epidemic (e.g. in refugee camps).

2 Once the epidemic has waned, continue vaccination at 9 months, with repeat dose at 12–14 months, for all those vaccinated at under the age of 12 months.

3 If the above measures are very successful and reporting shows very few cases below the age of 1 year, it may be possible to return to a single dose at 12–14 months.

None of these recommendations is ideal, but all should result in at least 90–95% of children receiving protection. The only contraindication to two doses is the added cost.

Measles vaccine can be used to protect children recently exposed to measles, provided that they are immunized within 48–72 hours of exposure. In this situation, antibodies to the vaccine are produced within 6–7 days which interfere with the replication of the wild measles virus, effectively preventing the disease. Immunization beyond 72 hours will not be effective, but as the effects of measles itself and the effects of the vaccine do not summate no harm will be done. The child will simply suffer from measles as he would have done without the vaccine.

Admission to a hospital ward, or a visit to a clinic, is often the time of contact with measles. In this situation vaccine should be used to prevent measles, despite the presence of severe malnutrition or other major illnesses. The alternative use of gamma globulin is extremely expensive.

The author's experience of open paediatric wards in Africa showed that provided every child over 5 months of age, regardless of admission diagnosis, was immunized within 48 hours of admission, measles cross-infection did not occur. There was no evidence that the vaccine reactions were more dangerous, or more frequent, in children with kwashiorkor, in whom a death rate of 20% from wild measles would have been expected if cross-infection had been allowed to occur.

At the moment we do not know if the antibody levels produced after immunizing malnourished or ill children are as high, or last as long, as after immunizing well children. It would seem wise therefore to re-immunize such children when they are fully recovered.

Other vaccinations

Some large cities routinely immunize all 11–13-year-old girls with rubella vaccine. Care must be taken during publicity campaigns to make sure that the immunization is not misinterpreted as a forced method of family planning. Few developing countries give priority to rubella vaccine, but when the cost of MMR (measles, mumps, rubella vaccine) comes down, there would be a good incentive to use this new vaccine instead of measles vaccine at 12–14 months, or as recommended locally.

Meningococcal vaccine, against types A and C meningococcus, has been used during epidemics in sub-Saharan Africa. Unfortunately protection is short-lived and no country includes this vaccine routinely in its schedule.

Where populations are thinly scattered and access to static clinics difficult, immunization rates will only approach the effective 90–95% range if the vaccines are taken to children by travelling clinics. Considerable thought needs to be given to storage and transport of the live vaccines and to advance publicity to ensure an effective programme. Where roads are only open for a few months each year, it should be possible to construct an immunization schedule appropriate to the circumstances by giving several vaccines at once; something which would not normally be done in developed countries.

INFANT FEEDING

Breast feeding

The advantages of breast feeding and the grave consequences of bottle feeding in the developing countries are well recognized. All health workers need to promote breast feeding through every available channel, starting at school and continuing through adult education projects and antenatal clinics. Almost every women is able to breast feed given the necessary support. Infant contraindications to breast feeding are galactosaemia, congenital lactose intolerance and phenylketonuria − all of which are extremely rare. Neither malnutrition nor disease in the mother are absolute contraindications, providing they are under treatment. Even severely malnourished women provide some milk of normal composition. Women with tuberculosis can breast feed provided they are receiving treatment and the baby receiving prophylactic isoniazid (INAH). Conditions in the baby which make sucking difficult, such as cleft palate, can be managed by maternal expression of milk and by feeding with a cup and spoon.

Introduction of solids

The majority of babies in developing countries can be fed for 5−6 months from the breast alone. Provided there is evidence of satisfactory growth, no additional foods are necessary. At some point, which varies from baby to baby, weight gain will tail off. Physiologically the limiting factor here is the provision of energy; growth ceases and protein is converted to energy to sustain life, a very wasteful use of breast milk protein. A source of energy needs to be introduced at this stage, the exact food varying from culture to culture, but usually consisting of a porridge made from the local staple, rice, maize, cassava or plantain. Once the extra energy needs are satisfied, growth will resume and the breast milk protein can be used efficiently. An additional source of protein is not physiologically needed at this point provided breast feeding continues.

Some time during the second 6 months of life, additional protein will become necessary as the baby's protein needs outstrip the production of milk. There are sound economic reasons for this protein to be provided from vegetable sources. No one vegetable contains all the amino acids in amounts or ratios which will allow optimum growth, but by mixing several sources of vegetable protein in one meal, a balanced amino acid composition can be built up. Providing breast feeding continues, no other source of expensive 'first class' protein is necessary until breast feeding ceases during the second year of life.

Bulk factor

Adults have lower needs for energy than infants and young children and their daily needs can be supplied almost entirely from a dietary staple such as maize. In infants, however, the volume of staple needed to provide the necessary energy may be too much to be consumed and this is referred to as the 'bulk factor'. Certain staples need, therefore, to be fortified by the addition of an alternative source of concentrated energy such as sugar or vegetable oil. This has the advantage of making the staple more palatable.

A summary of infant feeding recommendations is given in Table 29.4. Paediatricians and nutritionists in each country need to obtain data on the nutritional content of their foodstuffs and construct children's diets to suit the local circumstances, while bearing in mind availability, palatability, cost, cooking and storage. Recommendations regarding the introduction of local iron- and vitamin-containing foods must also be made.

From the age of 6 months, when the maternal antibody protection is waning, until the age of 2 years, infants are susceptible to a variety of diseases, including gastro-enteritis. Adequate nutrition during this time helps to lessen the severity of these illnesses and is particularly important in preventing the vicious cycle of infection begetting malnutrition, and malnutrition increasing the severity and duration of illness. The importance of good nutrition during the critical weaning period cannot be overstressed.

Birth to 5–6 months	Breast feed exclusively
5–6 months	Introduce additional energy source (local 'porridge') Continue breast feeding
6 months and over	'Porridge' Vegetable mixes (two or three together), continue to breast feed Fruit juices and green vegetables for additional vitamins C and A.
1 year and over	Vegetable mixes, staples Local diet (consider bulk factor) Introduce available local animal protein in small amounts Breast feed into the second year if possible

Table 29.4 Summary of a feeding regime suitable for developing countries. Exposure to sunshine is important for production of vitamin D.

Malnutrition

Protein–energy malnutrition

The World Health Organization (WHO) definitions of the types of protein–energy malnutrition (PEM) are shown in Figure 29.2.

Marasmus. A child is defined as suffering from marasmus if his weight is below 60% of the expected weight (fiftieth centile) for his age.

Kwashiorkor. This is defined as weight between 60 and 80% of that expected for age, together with the presence of oedema. Eighty per cent of expected weight for age corresponds roughly to the third centile.

No definition can cover every situation, but the WHO classification is useful in that it allows international comparison of data, and experience in management of malnutrition. The contribution made by kwashiorkor to the total number of malnourished children varies from country to country, and within countries there may be seasonal variations. There may also be differences in the peak age incidence and in the details of clinical descriptions. Cultural, nutritional and environmental factors account for most of the variation, rather than an inherent racial difference. Length of breast feeding, customs surrounding weaning, differences in the protein and amino acid content of the local dietary staples, and the incidence of gastro-enteritis and measles are all important variables. Nutritional marasmus appears most common

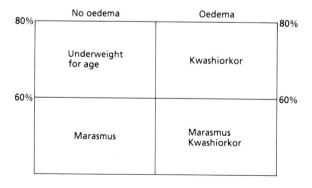

Fig. 29.2 WHO definitions of protein–energy malnutrition.

in societies where the period of breast feeding is short, or where bottle feeding is widespread.

Aetiology

When protein and energy intakes fall below requirements, linear growth ceases and weight remains static or drops. A state of malnutrition develops. The words malnutrition and malnourished imply that a child is receiving either an imbalanced or inadequate diet and that the correction of the dietary abnormality will cure the condition. This is only half the story and does not stress the importance of infection in the aetiology of clinical malnutrition. The ways in which infection may influence the state of nutrition are listed in Table 29.5.

Gastro-enteritis is particularly common in developing countries and has a very important influence on nutritional state, working through each of the mechanisms shown in Table 29.5. During acute viral or bacterial enteritis, the epithelial cells lining the gut are damaged, but in well-nourished children repair and replacement occur within 48–72 hours leading to spontaneous recovery. In the child with little nutritional reserve, the repair process is slower and frequently associated with chronic diarrhoea. There may be associated histological changes in the gut mucosa, including stunting of the villi and decrease in mucosal disaccharidases

Table 29.5 The influence of infection on the child's state of nutrition.

Fever	Increased temperature raises basal metabolic rate and energy requirements
Anorexia	Decreases intake in the face of increased needs.
Diarrhoea	
Acute	Causes loss of ingested energy, protein, K^+ and Na^+
Chronic	Causes secondary gut changes leading to malabsorption
Vomiting	Decreases nutrient intake
Tissue damage	Increases need of protein and energy

and peptidases. A vicious circle develops in which the gut is damaged and nutrient absorption impaired, but until nutrient absorption can be improved, no healing of the gut can take place. It is this interaction which accounts for the close association between recurrent and chronic diarrhoea and malnutrition.

A second example illustrating the profound effect of infection on nutritional state is measles, again working through the same five mechanisms. Epidemics of kwashiorkor often follow epidemics of measles, with a lag period of 2–3 months. In some areas of Africa 30–50% of children presenting with oedematous malnutrition have suffered from measles during the previous few months. In contrast to the clinical picture in well-nourished children, measles in malnourished children is frequently associated with bloody diarrhoea, followed by more prolonged diarrhoea lasting weeks or months. Significant protein loss from the gut has been documented, as well as structural alterations to the jejunal mucosa.

These two examples of how infection can influence nutrition emphasize that the approach to improving nutritional status in developing countries should not just concentrate on providing an increased supply of more nutritious food. Prevention of infection through improved water supplies and hygiene and through immunization, has an equally important role. One could also postulate that many children in poorer areas of the world are receiving a diet which would allow optimal growth, were it not for the influence of repeated infections.

KWASHIORKOR

Oedematous malnutrition has been recognized for centuries but it was Cecily Williams who first drew attention to the condition we now call kwashiorkor in Ghanain children who had recently been weaned from the breast. Subsequently it was described in many parts of the world and various aetiologies postulated. Because the skin changes were similar to those of pellagra, first thoughts were that the cause was a vitamin or multiple vitamin deficiency. Later workers developed the theory that kwashiorkor was a syndrome associated with lack of protein, but normal energy intake. This theory appeared to explain most of the clinical and biochemical findings, but it proved very difficult to reproduce a syndrome similar to kwashiorkor in laboratory animals by reducing protein intake and feeding normal or excessive amounts of energy. It was also found in India that the diets of children who subsequently developed kwashiorkor, as opposed to marasmus, were identical. This prompted a search for other aetiological factors.

The classification of malnutrition in childhood into the strict categories of either kwashiorkor or marasmus has on the one hand helped define progress and management of the conditions, but on the other hand tended to obscure the fact that there are many children who fall between the two definitions. The continuum of malnutrition in childhood can be represented in Figure 29.3.

The question to be asked is why should some children follow the path to kwashiorkor and others to marasmus? In addition, why do some with marasmus then go on to the clinical syndrome of kwashiorkor when their diets appear similar? Marasmus can be viewed as an adaption to reduced protein and energy intake. Biochemical and haematological tests are usually within normal limits and growth and energy expenditure

have been cut in response to dietary stress. Kwashiorkor, however, can be seen as a failure of adaptation, with abnormalities in a wide range of biochemical and haematological tests. These include low serum and body potassium, low serum sodium with an excess of body sodium, low haemoglobin, contracted intravascular volume, and high renin and cortisol levels. In addition there are low serum proteins (by definition) and abnormalities of carbohydrate metabolism.

Recent work on kwashiorkor and marasmus has centred on finding a precipitating cause for the 'maladaptation' in kwashiorkor. As already discussed, an attack of gastro-enteritis or measles often precedes the development of frank kwashiorkor in a child with marasmus, or one who is underweight for age. This has focused attention on the sudden loss of body potassium, through diarrhoea, as the mechanism.

The relationship between the various forms of childhood malnutrition can therefore be re-drawn as shown in Figure 29.4.

In addition to aiding our understanding of the aetiology of kwashiorkor, this hypothesis has important implications for treatment (potassium supplementation) and for prevention. The hypothesis also removes undernutrition, particularly protein deficiency, from the central point it has occupied in the aetiology of kwashiorkor, and sets it alongside infection as an important but not exclusive aetiological factor. Recent reports suggest a role for aflatoxin, found in poorly stored foods, in the aetiology of kwashiorkor but not marasmus.

Clinical features

The typical picture of kwashiorkor is unmistakeable. The child is usually between 10 months and 3 years old, intensely miserable and with symmetrical oedema of the arms and legs. The face is rounded, partly from oedema and partly from the preservation of the cheek fat pads. There is muscle wasting beneath the oedema. Motor development has often regressed and clinically the child may be hypotonic. The skin may be paler than expected, with areas of scaly hyperpigmentation over the extensor surfaces. Where desquamation has occurred,

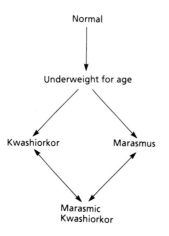

Fig. 29.3 Inter-relationships between kwashiorkor and marasmus.

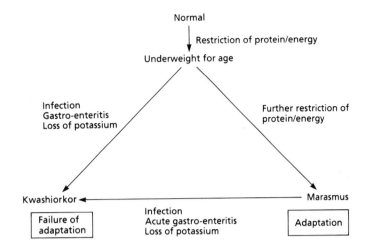

Fig. 29.4 Relationship between adaptation and failure of adaptation in states of protein–energy malnutrition.

the areas exposed are red and weeping, and show little sign of healing at the edges. Desquamation is particularly marked in the napkin area and in the axillae. The hair is usually lighter and more sparse than expected from the racial background, particularly if kwashiorkor has developed slowly. In cases of rapid onset, particularly following recent infection, the absence of skin and hair changes can be misleading and the diagnosis may not be suspected.

Misery and apathy are profound, often accompanied by a continuous, weak cry. The child will be inconsolable. There is little spontaneous activity and the child will be unable to feed himself even if presented with appetizing food. The hands and feet are cold and frequently the core temperature is below normal. The mucous membranes are pale, but severe pallor would suggest a complicating anaemia or heart failure.

Systemic examination reveals no abnormality of the heart and lungs unless there is an associated disease. The abdomen is protuberant due to a combination of muscle laxity and liver enlargement, which in the majority of cases is palpable 2–5 cm below the costal margin, firm and smooth. The spleen in not enlarged unless there is coexistent bacterial or protozoal infection. Ascites is very rare in uncomplicated kwashiorkor. Careful examination should be made for sites of infection, including the ears, mouth and throat.

Laboratory investigations will depend on facilities available. Table 29.6 gives a guide to those most commonly helpful in management.

Management

Kwashiorkor may be managed either in or out of hospital.

Out-patients. Mild and moderate kwashiorkor can be managed successfully outside hospital, provided that the appetite is fair and that there are no adverse clinical signs (see Table 29.7). Mothers can be instructed on the local foods to give, backed up with protein and energy supplements for the first week or so if needed. Multi-vitamin syrup and potassium supplements should be given. Oral iron therapy, if indicated, is started in the second week. Clinical infection should be treated with an oral antibiotic, but antibiotic prophylaxis should be avoided. Response to treatment is shown by a return of appetite and smile and loss of oedema, which should occur by the end of the first week. Children who fail to respond, or who deteriorate, should be examined carefully, and re-investigated for missed infection.

In-patient. Kwashiorkor and marasmic-kwashiorkor are the result of weeks or months of slow deterioration and attempting to correct some of

Investigation	Usual result in kwashiorkor	Comments
Haemoglobin*	7–10 g/dl	Lower levels suggest malaria, hookworm, iron-deficiency anaemia, sickle cell disease
Blood film*	Normochromic Normocytic	Microcytes – iron deficient Macrocytes – folate deficient Detection of malaria parasites or sickle cells
Urine*	Normal	Exclude infection, including bilharzia
Stool microscopy*	Giardia, hookworm, ascaris *S. mansoni* common in some areas	RBCs and WBCs also found in shigella and salmonella infections
Stool culture	Pathogens often found	
Blood glucose*	Low normal (2–3 mmol/l)	Symptomatic hypoglycaemia has poor prognosis
Mantoux/Heaf*	Negative	Often negative in presence of active TB
Chest X-ray	Normal	Helpful in diagnosis of occult TB or pneumonia
Blood culture		Often reveals occult Gram-negative infection

Table 29.6 Investigations undertaken in children presenting with kwashiorkor.

* These tests should be routine as they are cheap and can be performed with simple methods.

Table 29.7 Adverse clinical signs in kwashiorkor which suggest the need for admission to hospital.

Profound anorexia
Drowsiness, fits, coma
Shortness of breath (pneumonia and/or cardiac failure)
Severe anaemia
Diarrhoea with dehydration
Hypothermia or unexplained fever
Widespread weeping skin lesions

the clinical and biochemical abnormalities rapidly can be dangerous. Hyponatraemia will correct itself slowly, provided the child is given fluids containing sodium and potassium supplements. Rapid infusion of sodium chloride intravenously may result in worsening of oedema and the precipitation of heart failure. Enthusiastic correction of anaemia by blood transfusion is similarly dangerous to an already weak heart. Inappropriate use of diuretics to treat oedema will result in further depletion of intravascular volume with ensuing shock and death.

The first 24 hours in hospital should be spent stabilizing the clinical condition. Particular attention should be paid to preventing heat loss and maintaining the core (rectal) temperature in the normal range. Naso-gastric or intravenous fluids containing sodium and potassium, with extra glucose, in a volume of 100–120 ml/kg/day should be given. Half-strength Darrow's solution, made up to 7–10% dextrose is widely used. The blood glucose should be checked and extra glucose given intravenously if necessary. Baseline laboratory investigation should be undertaken and treatment of infection started if clinically indicated. Oral potassium supplements (6 mmol/kg/day) should be started, along with a multi-vitamin preparation and folic acid. In some areas, routine magnesium supplements are given.

During the second day, a fluid diet based on dried skimmed milk as the source of protein, with glucose or sucrose and a vegetable oil as the source of energy, is fed by naso-gastric tube. The exact recipe will vary from country to country, but the aim should be to build up to an intake of 3–4 g protein/kg/day and 150 cal/kg/day by the end of the first week of treatment. Solids in the form of porridge, vegetable mixes, bananas, etc. should be introduced as the appetite returns.

At the point where the appetite is returning and oedema disappearing most children can be discharged, either home with regular supervision, or to a nutritional rehabilitation unit, for the consolidation phase of treatment. This phase involves supervising the mother in the cooking and feeding of locally available protein- and energy-rich food. In this way she sees that it is the food, not medicine, that is curing her child. Unfortunately, management of severe cases of kwashiorkor will involve intravenous therapy and antibiotics, thus detracting from this message.

If improvement does not occur as expected towards the end of the first week of treatment, a vigorous search for infection, particularly tuberculosis and intestinal parasites, should be undertaken.

COMPLICATIONS

Infection

There is considerable circumstantial and experimental evidence that malnutrition (particularly kwashiorkor) has a profound influence on immunological status (Table 29.8). The evidence points to suppression of cell-mediated immunity (CMI) rather than to any gross interference in the production of immunoglobulins.

Immunoglobulins in both kwashiorkor and marasmus are within the normal range, or raised, suggesting response to earlier infections. Depression of CMI is reflected in the severity of such infections as measles, with giant cell pneumonia, and prolonged giant cell excretion from the nasal mucosa, similar to the situation in leukaemia or artificial immunosuppression. The child with kwashiorkor responds to infection in many ways like the newborn; often with a lack of fever, no rise in white cells and an inability to localize infection, which leads to early bacteraemia and septicaemia. The types of infecting organisms are also similar, with disseminated herpes simplex, candida and Gram-negative bacteria being particularly common.

Infection and kwashiorkor are so frequently associated that there is a temptation to use antibiotics prophylactically, but the range of organisms and antibiotic sensitivities are so great that very broad spectrum, expensive antibiotics would be needed.

A suggested approach is as follows:

1 Mild to moderate kwashiorkor with no

Table 29.8 Immunological status in kwashiorkor.

T-cell function	B-cell function
Thymic atrophy with decrease in cortical lymphocytes Decreased tonsillar size Decreased total lymphocyte count	Splenic histology normal IgG, IgM, IgA normal or raised
False negative Mantoux test False negative candida skin test Decreased lymphocyte transformation to phytohaemagglutinin	Normal response to antigens (TAB, tetanus toxoid)

hypothermia, and no obvious signs of septicaemia. Investigate, but no antibiotic unless clinical evidence of infection, e.g. otitis media.

2 The ill child with signs of pneumonia, skin sepsis or severe enteritis. Investigate and start treatment with, for example intramuscular penicillin and gentamicin or oral ampicillin, chloramphenicol or Septrin.

3 The severely ill child. Investigate and treat with intravenous antibiotics (e.g. ampicillin and gentamicin or penicillin and chloramphenicol).

Subsequent treatment may need to be modified in light of laboratory results. If this simple guide is followed, the more expensive antibiotics can be reserved for those most in need.

Hypothermia

A low core (rectal) temperature is common in children with kwashiorkor, particularly during the first night or two after admission. This may be due to removal from contact with the mother's warm body, or inappropriate exposure and cooling by bathing the child. It is frequently associated with hypoglycaemia, when the progress is poor. Treatment is aimed at preventing further heat loss by wrapping and nursing in a warm environment which includes using the mother as a source of warmth. Active warming with hot water bottles or radiant heat cradles may cause skin burns and shock through cutaneous vasodilation.

Anaemia

A moderate degree of anaemia is usual in kwashiorkor, with haemoglobin levels between 8 and 10 g/dl. The anaemia has been shown to be due to lack of protein needed to manufacture globin and not primarily due to iron or folate deficiency. During recovery, there is at first a drop in haemoglobin concentration associated with expanding blood volume. Following this the level begins to rise as haemoglobin synthesis recommences. It is during this recovery phase that iron stores may be used up and iron supplements become necessary. In some areas, folic acid may also be lacking and supplements are needed.

Severe anaemia at diagnosis should raise the question of pre-existing conditions such as sickle cell disease, malaria, hookworm or iron deficiency. If a blood transfusion is needed, as it may be if the haemoglobin is below 5–6 g/dl, then a small transfusion of packed cells, sufficient to raise the haemoglobin to 8–9 g/dl should be given slowly, together with a diuretic. Larger transfusions may easily tip the child into heart failure.

Hypoglycaemia

Asymptomatic hypoglycaemia is common and usually responds to oral feeding. If possible the blood sugar should be checked a few times a day until the child is out of danger. A very low blood sugar is often found associated with hypothermia, coma and fits, but unfortunately raising the blood sugar may not improve the neurological state in these very ill children.

Diarrhoea

Almost all children with kwashiorkor have an associated diarrhoea. Jejunal histology shows changes similar to those found in moderate to severe coeliac disease, but without lymphocytic infiltration. There may be specific pathogens such as giardia, amoeba and salmonella, or a non-specific overgrowth of normal gut flora in the ileum and jejunum. Functionally, there may be decreased disaccharidase and peptidase levels. The introduction of feeding may precipitate a temporary worsening of diarrhoea in many children with kwashiorkor. If this does not lead to serious dehydration, feeding should continue, in the hope that improved gut function will follow an improvement in the nutritional state. However, if the diarrhoea is severe and watery and contains reducing substances, a lactose-free feeding schedule may be needed. In rare cases, other disaccharides or even monosaccharides may need to be eliminated from the diet.

Lactose intolerance is common in many tropical countries and a case has been made for starting treatment in all children with a lactose-free diet, but as milk is cheap and a good source of protein, it is probably best to reserve the more expensive lactose-free diets for children selected on the criteria mentioned. Although the structural changes in the gut take many months to improve, functional improvement occurs within the first week or two.

Tuberculosis

Tuberculosis may accompany malnutrition and may be one reason for failure to respond to re-feeding. The Heaf or Mantoux test is often negative in severely malnourished children in the presence of active tuberculosis. A chest X-ray and gastric washings should be taken if tuberculosis is suspected. On occasions it may be necessary to start treatment on suspicion and to review the diagnosis after a month or two. If the nutritional state has improved, then the Heaf or Mantoux test should reflect the child's true sensitivity to tuberculin (see also p. 556).

Changes in conscious level

Some children with kwashiorkor are admitted drowsy, fitting or unconscious. Often the blood sugar is unrecordable, but correction with intravenous glucose may not help. The prognosis in these cases is very poor. Severe septicaemia, liver failure, poisoning, encephalitis or severe electrolyte imbalance accounts for some cases but it does not appear that there is a specific encephalopathy associated with kwashiorkor.

NUTRITIONAL MARASMUS

The definition and aetiology of nutritional marasmus has already been discussed. Clinically, children with marasmus are thin and wizened, with lack of subcutaneous fat and reduced muscle bulk. There is no oedema, by definition, nor do they show the skin and hair changes seen with kwashiorkor. Spontaneous movement is lacking and most children have a wide-eyed unsmiling appearance. In contrast to kwashiorkor there are no characteristic biochemical or haematological changes. Clinical and bacteriological examination should be undertaken, as in kwashiorkor, to exclude infection.

Management. The treatment of nutritional marasmus is more straightforward than that of kwashiorkor, as the appetite is frequently preserved, and complications rarer. Tube feeding with a fluid diet is rarely needed, and many children can be managed by out-patient supervision. Numbers of children, despite having a good appetite, and being free of infection will fail to gain weight unless particular attention is paid to their caloric needs. In calculating calorie requirements, the child's expected weight rather than actual weight should be used. Calorie requirements per day may work out at over 200 kcal/kg of actual weight. During the first week of treatment it may be impossible to achieve this level of intake. Three main meals a day, together with energy-rich snacks are needed, but in some children, further calorie supplementation will be required in the form of vegetable oil or medium-chain triglycerides. Once weight gain begins, recovery is usually rapid, although catch-up will continue for many months, or years.

Malnutrition, brain growth and development

The literature on this subject, both clinical and experimental is large and controversial but there does seem to be broad agreement in the following areas.
1 Human brain growth is maximal at 22−24 weeks gestational age, and continues until about 18 months. Periods of severe and prolonged malnutrition reduce the number of neuronal cells, the effect being more marked the closer the stress is to the period of maximum cell division. If the stress of malnutrition is removed and re-feeding started, a certain amount of catch-up growth is possible. Adequate nutrition after a period of intra-uterine malnutrition allows catch-up, whereas a combination of intra-uterine malnutrition with marasmus in the first year of life is very likely to lead to permanent restriction in brain growth. On the other hand, in kwashiorkor, no consistent abnormalities have been reported as the main stress of malnutrition comes after the age of 12−18 months when brain growth has largely ceased.

2 IQ and developmental testing broadly reflect the histological and anatomical findings. Children most severely impaired are those who have undergone a period of intra-uterine plus early extra-uterine malnutrition. Children suffering from kwashiorkor are less affected than those with marasmus, as would be expected. Most long-term studies stress that improvement after correction of malnutrition will continue for many years.

Many workers believe that periods of malnutrition, independent of other environmental factors, do adversely affect IQ, but not to the extent of producing mental retardation in a child who would otherwise have been normal. Although, in the individual child loss of potential IQ may not be great, in terms of the community, the accumulated loss may be very significant.

Cancrum oris (Noma)

Cancrum oris is a condition often associated geographically with protein–energy malnutrition. Particularly destructive ulceration with widespread loss of tissue round the mouth occurs, usually after an infection such as measles or herpes (or both together). No individual bacterium has been consistently associated with the lesions. Similar lesions to those of cancrum oris may involve the nose or ears, occasionally with complete loss of

both structures. Lesions of the mouth often involve the upper or lower jaw, with loss of teeth and eventually sequestration (Fig. 29.5).

Management. There is no specific treatment. An antibiotic should be prescribed and attention given to cleaning the mouth and removal of loose teeth, bone or skin. Formal debridement should be delayed until the child's general condition has improved. Anaemia should be treated. The first sign of healing is the appearance of healthy skin and granulation tissue at the edge of the lesion. Eventually dead skin and bone will slough leaving a defect which will need major plastic surgery over many months.

Prevention. Dental hygiene, measles vaccination and improved nutritional state all play a part in prevention of cancrum oris. Early treatment of herpes simplex mouth infections, with attention to oral hygiene, fluid intake and nutrition are also important.

Vitamin deficiency states

VITAMIN A DEFICIENCY

Vitamin A is a fat-soluble vitamin found in cheese, eggs, liver and fish oils, with precursors in carrots

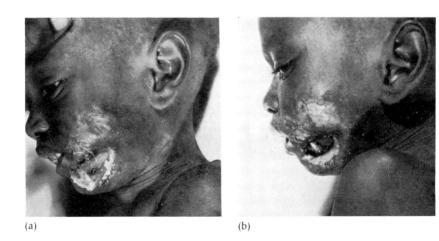

(a)   (b)

Fig. 29.5 Cancrum oris. (a) The child presented with a visible sequestrum of the mandible. (b) The sequestrum was removed without difficulty, revealing a large skin defect.

and green vegetables. It is not surprising, therefore, that vitamin A deficiency is frequently associated with protein–energy malnutrition. Vitamin A is necessary for the integrity of epithelial surfaces and early signs of vitamin A deficiency include a dry scaly skin and follicular hyperkeratosis. Keratinization of the epithelium of the eye causes xerophthalmia. The conjunctiva becomes dry with Bitot's spots appearing on the scleral conjunctiva. The cornea may become soft, hazy and ulcerated. An attack of measles may accelerate the corneal changes, leading to opacification, rapid perforation and permanent blindness. Vitamin A deficiency may also increase the severity of measles and pneumonia in malnourished children through synergistic action on the lung epithelium. Daily requirements of vitamin A are 2000 U. In clinical deficiency, particularly in children with malnutrition and measles, 20 000–50 000 U should be given by intramuscular injection immediately, followed by daily supplementation orally.

VITAMIN B GROUP DEFICIENCIES

Vitamin B_1 (thiamine)

Lack of vitamin B_1 (thiamine) results in beri-beri. Thiamine-containing foods include meat, liver, fish, eggs, milk products, green vegetables and fruit.

Beri-beri (thiamine deficiency). Clinical features include anorexia, listlessness, vomiting and oedema. Cardiac failure follows enlargement of the heart and neurological features include paraesthesia and peripheral neuritis. Beri-beri should be included in the differential diagnosis of heart failure in children in developing countries, particularly in areas where the staple food is rice. Daily requirements are 0.4–1.0 mg, while in acute cases 10–20 mg can be given either intramuscularly or intravenously.

Vitamin B_2 (riboflavin)

Riboflavin is present in the foods listed above containing vitamin B_1. Lack of riboflavin mainly affects the mucous membrane of the mouth, leading to angular ceilitis and a magenta-coloured tongue with flattened papillae. Daily requirements are 0.2–2.0 mg. Doses of 3–10 mg are required for treatment of the deficiency state.

Pellagra (nicotinic acid deficiency). The vitamin is present in meat, liver, milk and whole wheat and maize. Lack of nicotinic acid causes pellagra. This is particularly common in areas where maize is the staple, particularly if the maize has been refined into flour after removal of the germ. A photosensitive dermatitis develops, with skin lesions in the necklace area, over the face and on the forearms (Plate 49). The tongue becomes red and smooth. Vomiting and diarrhoea occur, and later apathy, sleeplessness and delirium. Gastrointestinal infections and typhoid may precipitate the onset of acute neurological symptoms in subclinical nicotinic acid deficiency. Daily requirements of nicotinic acid are 5–15 mg. Deficiency states are treated with 50–300 mg of vitamin B_2 daily by mouth, or in a combined intravenous preparation.

VITAMIN C

Vitamin C is contained in fruit juices and fresh green vegetables; its lack causes scurvy. Breast milk has a high content of vitamin C so that scurvy is extremely uncommon in breast-fed infants. On the other hand, even fresh cow's milk has only one-quarter the amount of vitamin C in breast milk, presumably because the calf is less able to synthesize the vitamin. The amount in bottled cow's milk is very low. Modern formula milks are supplemented with vitamin C and other vitamins.

Scurvy

Deficiency of ascorbic acid causes increased capillary permeability with consequent haemorrhage. Bone formation ceases, but calcification of cartilage continues so that a dense line of calcification appears at the growing ends of long bones. Delayed healing occurs since ascorbic acid is necessary for the repair of tissues.

Scurvy may occur at any age but is seen mainly

in infants of 7–12 months of age. The limbs become acutely painful and tender from the haemorrhages under the tight periosteum, this being the chief feature of the disease. The child is irritable and very apprehensive when approached, from fear of pain on handling. He lies quite still (pseudo-paralysis) since the slightest movement of the bed causes pain. The limbs adopt the characteristic 'frog position' with the thighs abducted and the knees slightly flexed. Subperiosteal haemorrhages may be large enough to be palpable or even visible as swellings in the limb. The costochondral junctions become prominent, forming a 'rosary' from subluxation of the sternum at these joints. The rosary in scurvy differs from that in rickets. In scurvy it is angular and sharp because it is due to epiphyseal separation of the upper ribs with backward displacement of the costosternal plate. In rickets it is dome-shaped and semicircular because it is due to expansion of the rib ends.

Haemorrhages may be present in the skin or orbit and haematuria or melaena may occur. The gums become spongy and swollen, though bleeding occurs only if the teeth have erupted. Anaemia results from the loss of blood but possibly also from a specific effect of lack of vitamin C on the bone marrow. The anaemia may be megaloblastic and, although this is sometimes corrected by vitamin C, folic acid also may be required.

X-rays of the long bones show generalized osteoporosis. There is a characteristic dense line of calcification at the epiphysis, with a thin subepiphyseal line of rarefaction; this represents a break in the continuity of bone and may be the site of epiphyseal separation. The dense line of calcification is sometimes continued beyond the edge of the shaft to form a spur (Fig. 29.6). When healing occurs the subperiosteal haemorrhage calcifies, causing a very striking picture as it may involve the whole length of the shaft. Absorption of this calcified mass eventually occurs, leaving no deformity.

Red cells are almost always found on microscopic examination of the urine so that normal urine is strong evidence against the diagnosis. Further confirmation of the diagnosis is provided by a saturation test in which a known quantity of

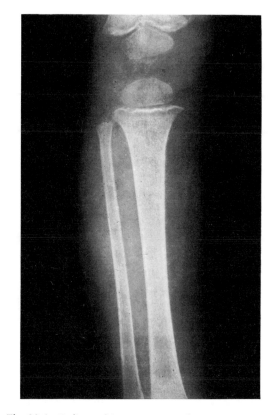

Fig. 29.6 Radiographic appearances of scurvy. There is a characteristic dense line of calcification at the upper end of the tibia, extending medially to form a short spur. A thin subepiphyseal line of rarefaction lies just below this.

ascorbic acid is given. The amount of ascorbic acid excreted in the urine is then determined; this is less in scurvy than in a normal individual because of the amount taken up by the body.

Prophylaxis. Infants require 30–50 mg of ascorbic acid per day. If mothers are well fed, breast milk contains sufficient for the baby's needs, and formula milks are now fortified with vitamin C. However, it is probably wise to give an alternative source, in the form of fruit juice, to all children from about 3 months, and to those fed on modified cow's milk, from birth.

Treatment. Between 100 and 500 mg ascorbic acid daily or an equivalent amount from fruit juice concentrates should be given. Nursing must be extremely gentle, the child should not be taken out of the cot and a cradle should be provided to keep the weight of the bed clothes off the legs. Wrapping the limbs with cotton wool reduces some of the pain and analgesics may be required at first. Pain is dramatically relieved within 1–2 days of starting ascorbic acid.

VITAMIN D

There are two sources of vitamin D in man; from foods such as fish, eggs and liver, and from the synthesis within the body through the action of sunlight on 7 dehydrocholesterol in the skin. In many parts of the world, the diet is deficient in vitamin D, so children rely heavily on sunlight for its manufacture. The absorbed or synthesized vitamin D is initially in an inactive form, in which it may be stored in fat or muscle, or transported to the liver, where it is hydroxylated to 25 hydroxy-vitamin D. A further hydroxylation step occurs in the kidneys, under the influence of parathyroid hormone, before the active dihydroxyvitamin D is produced. Vitamin D increases absorption of calcium and phosphorus from the gut, aids calcium reabsorption from the renal tubules, and in synergism with parathyroid hormone, liberates calcium from bone.

Rickets

Lack of vitamin D causes a fall in blood phosphorus. In the early stages the calcium level does not fall since, although its absorption is affected, increased parathyroid activity maintains the normal serum level. This is achieved at the expense of the bones from which calcium is withdrawn, with consequent osteoporosis. If this mechanism breaks down, the serum calcium level falls and tetany may result.

A knowledge of normal bone growth is necessary if the mechanism of vitamin D deficiency on bone development is to be understood. At the growing end of the bone there are four zones. In the first are resting cartilage cells. In the second these have arranged themselves in orderly columns. The third is the zone of preparatory calcification in which the cartilage cells have become swollen and degenerate; here the matrix is impregnated with calcium salts. In the fourth zone the spaces left by the degenerated cartilage cells are invaded by capillaries accompanied by osteoblasts which deposit a layer of osteoid on the calcified cartilaginous trabeculae. This osteoid is converted into bone by the deposition of calcium and phosphorus, the calcified cartilage being reabsorbed. As a result of these processes the zone of preparatory calcification lies between the layers of cartilage and osteoid, being seen as a straight line on the X-ray.

In rickets the cartilage cells fail both to arrange themselves in columns and also to undergo normal degeneration. Consequently, the invasion of capillaries occurs in an irregular manner. The matrix is not impregnated with calcium and the osteoid, which remains uncalcified, is deposited irregularly. The result is a wide irregular zone of non-calcified cartilage and osteoid which has none of the rigidity of normal bone. Under normal circumstances bone is also formed under the periosteum, but in rickets a shell of osteoid is formed which surrounds the whole length of the shaft.

Rickets may also be due to renal disease; the so-called 'renal rickets' and this is discussed in Chapter 22.

Geographical and social factors. Although in temperate climates rickets is classically associated with undernutrition and lack of sunshine, it is nevertheless common in the tropics and subtropics. Its distribution is remarkably patchy, even in areas with long hours of sunshine. In Zimbabwe and Zambia it is much less common than in South Africa and Ethiopia, although in all four places there is plenty of sunshine. In the former two countries, many children spend their early months in the fields, strapped to their mother's back, with their heads exposed to sunlight. Even an hour or two of exposure per day in this way appears to protect against rickets. In Ethiopia, despite similar feeding practices, rickets is common and often severely deforming. Mothers often shun sunshine during the latter part of their pregnancy, wear clothing which covers most of the body and head, and avoid exposing their children to sunlight during the first year of life. Although breast fed, these infants receive little vitamin D from their mothers and are unable to manufacture their own. In Soweto, Johannesberg, a combination of bottle feeding, and industrial and home-fire air pollution may be responsible. In Saudi Arabia, where there is probably more sunshine than anywhere else in the world, rickets appears to be on the increase. A recent social change from cooking on open fires out of doors, to cooking on stoves in a kitchen may have reduced mothers' exposure to sunlight, and hence reduced vitamin D in their milk.

Clinical features. Rickets is a disorder of growing bones and therefore the bones affected in any patient are those which are growing fastest at the time of deficiency. Children who are not growing, such as those with kwashiorkor, marasmus and coeliac disease will not exhibit clinical rickets. They may, however, do so when treatment allows growth to restart, if vitamin D is not given.

Rickets mainly occurs between 6 months and 2 years of age. If it occurs in the first year, the skull is principally involved as it is growing the fastest. The excess of osteoid and the non-calcified cartilage is heaped-up, forming bosses over the frontal bones. Craniotabes indicates an abnormal softening of the skull bones which can often be indented; it is a common feature of rickets but it is also found in normal babies, particularly those born pre-term. There is also delay in the closure of the anterior fontanelle.

The long bones are particularly affected from the second year onwards when they grow the fastest. Widening of the epiphyses at the wrists and ankles is visible and palpable (Fig. 29.7). The wrist deformity is increased by pressure from crawling on the soft radius and ulna. Similarly, walking causes bowing of the long bones of the legs and a green stick fracture may occur.

Prominence of the costochondral junctions results in the 'rickety rosary' and a wide Harrison's sulcus may develop with flaring of the costal margins. The sternum may be depressed or excessively prominent (pigeon chest). The spine may be deformed by kyphosis or scoliosis and deformities of the pelvis also result. Eruption of the teeth is delayed and dental caries is likely.

In addition to bone deformities, children with rickets are fretful, hypotonic, pot-bellied and have a tendency to head-sweating. Sitting up and walking may be delayed; a child who develops rickets when he has already started to walk may go off his legs because they are painful. Nasal catarrh and iron-deficiency anaemia are common and the child is subject to attacks of bronchitis.

Diagnosis. Confirmation of rickets is obtained from X-rays, the changes being seen best at the wrist. The lower ends of the radius and ulna are widened, cupped and indistinct. The appearance has been aptly likened to a frothing champagne glass (Fig. 29.8). The distance between the epiphyses and the calcified portion of the shaft is greater than normal and when healing takes place, irregular calcification occurs in this area. There is

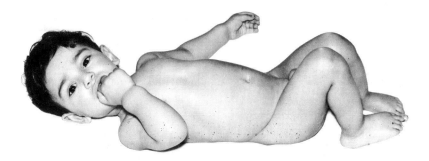

Fig. 29.7   Rickets. Appearances in an 18-month-old child showing widening of the wrists and ankles.

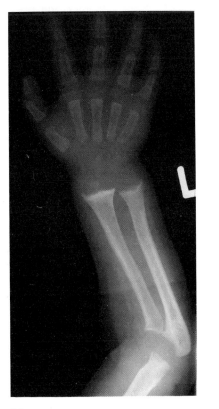

(a)

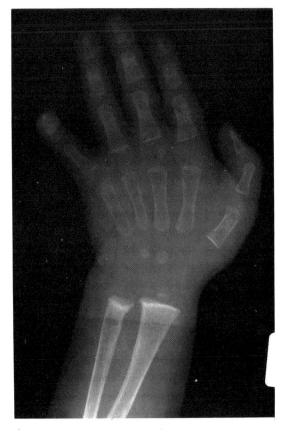

(b)

Fig. 29.8 Radiographic appearances of rickets. (a) X-ray of the forearm and wrist showing the typical changes of rickets in a growing child. The lower ends of the radius and ulna are widened, cupped and indistinct. (b) Minor changes of rickets in a marasmic child in whom growth had ceased. There is a line of increased density across the lower end of both the radius and ulna, with mild cupping of the ulna.

generalized osteoporosis and the bone age is delayed. A periosteal reaction suggests concomitant scurvy since this does not occur in pure rickets.

The serum calcium is usually normal but the phosphorus is decreased and there is a considerable rise in the alkaline phosphatase. An increased urinary output of amino acids occurs.

Prophylaxis. Infants require 400 IU vitamin D daily. In well-nourished populations where rickets is now rare, vitamin D supplementation is probably not needed for either breast- or bottle-fed term infants. Formula milk contains approximately 400

IU per litre, but extra vitamin D supplementation should be given to pre-term babies, children with malnutrition and to special groups known to be susceptible, such as children of Asian or Caribbean origin living in Britain.

Where rickets is common, vitamin supplementation should be given to pregnant and lactating women, and to both breast- and bottle-fed babies. In addition, exposure to sunlight, by both women and children should be encouraged.

Treatment. Approximately 10 000 IU of vitamin D daily is sufficient for cure, along with a pint of milk a day to cover calcium requirements. Weight bearing should be postponed until there is clinical evidence of healing. Vitamin D-resistant rickets is discussed on p. 000.

Acute gastro-enteritis

Acute gastro-enteritis (AGE) in infants between 6 months and 2 years of age is, after upper respiratory tract infections, the commonest cause for seeking medical attention in developing countries. Despite many recent advances in understanding and treating the condition, it remains the largest single killer in this age group. Furthermore, repeated attacks of AGE lead to chronic diarrhoea and malnutrition, and delayed death, in an additional group of children.

McNeish has produced a conceptual model of the inter-relationship between the various factors involved (Fig. 29.9). AGE can enter the model through either malnutrition or chronic diarrhoea.

AETIOLOGY

The majority of children with AGE in all areas of the world are suffering from viral infection, most commonly rotavirus. In developing countries the contribution from epidemics of salmonella and

shigella infection, giardia, campylobacter and amoeba, varies both with time and place. From the point of view of community control of diarrhoeal disease, knowledge of the aetiology is important, but has little bearing on the initial treatment.

TREATMENT

The key alterations in management over the past 10–20 years involve the widespread introduction of oral rehydration therapy (ORT), a shift to early re-introduction of feeds, and the abandoning of routine antibiotics and anti-diarrhoeal agents.

Oral rehydration

Even during the early stages of AGE, water, sodium, potassium and chloride are still absorbed from the bowel. Absorption is aided by the presence of glucose or a disaccharide, with optimal absorption from solutions containing between 5 and 10% sugar. Several solutions are available, usually packed in powder form to be made up with clean water before use. The standard WHO rehydration fluid contains 90 mmol/l of sodium and 110 mmol/l of glucose. The amount of sodium

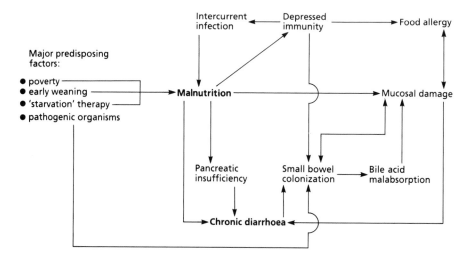

Fig. 29.9 The relationship between diarrhoea and malnutrition. (With permission of Walker-Smith JA and McNeish AS (Eds) and *Diarrhoea and Malnutrition in Childhood.* Butterworths 1986, p.5.)

s more than recommended for use in developed countries. Once rehydration is complete the WHO oral rehydration solution (ORS) should be diluted 2 parts to 1 with water for maintenence. In breast-ed infants, the re-introduction of breast milk will supply the necessary diluting fluid. This approach minimizes the danger of hypernatraemia, while preserving a single solution for use in the field.

In addition to aiding absorption of water and electrolytes, glucose provides energy which is needed particularly by the malnourished. Attempts to provide more energy are hampered by the osmotic effect of glucose in concentrations greater than 10%. Trials with sucrose, which has half the osmotic effect of glucose, have been successful despite the theoretical disadvantage of reduced disaccharidase levels in the intestinal mucosa both in malnutrition and during AGE. Initial trials with large-chain sugar molecules (e.g. rice water) to provide extra energy have shown as good results as with glucose or sucrose.

ORS has not eliminated the need for intravenous fluid replacement which will still be necessary in severely shocked and dehydrated children. The importance of ORS is that if it is started early, preferably at home, most children will not progress to the stage of needing intravenous therapy.

Re-feeding

AGE in breast-fed infants should be treated with an ORS and continuation of breast feeding. This provides additional hypotonic fluid, energy and a non-allergic source of protein.

In bottle-fed infants, ORS alone for 24 hours is followed by either a quick (2-day) or slow (4-day) regrade on to full-strength milk. The less severely ill can usually follow a quick regrade. If diarrhoea recurs during the regrade, lactose or cow's milk intolerance may be the cause. Management may be difficult and expensive, and entails a lactose-free, low-allergenic milk (e.g. Pregestimil) or soya-based preparation. A cheap alternative which can be made up as needed, uses eggs as the source of protein, with glucose and oil to provide calories. One must beware of the danger of further calorie deprivation associated with repeated regradings in the malnourished child. It is probably better to push on with the regrade despite a temporary increase in stool volume and frequency, unless the diarrhoea becomes life threatening.

The toddler with diarrhoea is treated with ORS for 24 hours, followed by the rapid re-introduction of a nutritious diet over 2–3 days.

During admission, or in the out-patient clinic, the mother should be taught the elements of home ORT, hygiene and nutrition in an attempt to prevent or alleviate further attacks of AGE. During the follow-up period, emphasis should be placed on improving the nutritional state.

Antibiotics and anti-diarrhoeals

In the well-nourished child, AGE caused by viruses, salmonellae, shigellae, cholera and *E. coli* responds to ORT, and antibiotics have not been shown to influence the outcome. The routine use of non-absorbable antibiotics such as neomycin, and sulphas should be abandoned. The situation is less straightforward in the malnourished, particularly if severely ill on admission, and when septicaemia cannot be ruled out. In these cases an absorbable or parenteral broad spectrum antibiotic may help. In severe shigellosis, particularly in the form associated with DIC, furazolidone and nalidixic acid have been found to be effective.

After investigation, specific treatment will be needed for giardia and amoeba. Other parasites found during stool examination such as bilharzia, hookworm and trichuris, while not causes of AGE are best treated when the child has recovered and the nutritional state is improving.

So-called anti-diarrhoeals, such as kaolin and pectin have no general or physiological effect, lull the provider into a false sense of security, and are best abandoned.

Measles in developing countries

Until the beginning of this century, measles was a severe and often fatal disease in Europe and the USA. Mortality and morbidity have dropped steadily since 1900, to the present death rate of about 1:10 000 attacks in Britain. Almost half the deaths are now in immunosuppressed children. Measles as it relates to developed countries is discussed in Chapter 21. Figures for overall mortality in developing countries are difficult to obtain, but in some epidemics 5–10% of children will die during the acute attack, and an unknown number will die during the subsequent months from complications directly or indirectly attributable to measles.

Most paediatricians relate the severity of measles to underlying malnutrition, coincidental conditions such as anaemia, malaria and tuberculosis, to inappropriate treatment at home, or to late hospital or clinic attendance. Recent reports from the Gambia, citing a particularly high mortality during epidemics, have suggested that the explanation lies in the larger number of virus particles inhaled where measles is epidemic, as opposed to endemic.

In many countries, measles occurs in epidemics every 2 years with the peak incidence between 15 and 36 months, coinciding with peaks for marasmus and kwashiorkor. Unimmunized or partially immunized populations, living close together in cities or refugee camps are particularly liable to explosive epidemics. To prevent epidemics in such populations, a very high level of immunization, of 95% or more, is required. The timing of vaccination is discussed on p. 535.

CLINICAL FEATURES

The early course of measles, from the prodrome through to the development of Koplik spots and the appearance of the rash, does not differ greatly from country to country. However, at the time when one would normally expect a fall in temperature, and the start of recovery, about 2–3 days after the rash has appeared, children in developing countries often deteriorate with evidence of pneumonia, diarrhoea and high fever.

TREATMENT

The basic treatment of measles includes rehydration, attention to temperature control and nutrition, and a search for secondary bacterial infection. Eye and mouth care are particularly important. In many countries where there is coincidental vitamin A deficiency, intramuscular or oral vitamin A is given routinely. Unless there is evidence of bacterial infection, prophylactic antibiotics are best avoided. There is evidence that the routine administration of penicillin predisposes to staphylococcal pneumonia. Early treatment concentrating on fluid and nutrition therapy, starting as soon as the diagnosis is apparent, will prevent the need for hospital admission.

COMPLICATIONS

Ocular

Bacterial conjunctivitis, superimposed on the viral conjunctivitis, often associated with vitamin A deficiency, produces corneal ulcers and in some cases perforation of the globe. This can occur very rapidly and measles is a significant cause of blindness in many countries. Urgent treatment with systemic and local antibiotics, and intramuscular vitamin A should be given.

Stomatitis and mouth ulcers

Dehydration and bacterial invasion working together with the mucosal damage produced by measles may lead to severe gingivitis and necrotic ulcers of the lips and cheeks. These lesions are indistinguishable from cancrum oris, and herpes simplex virus (coexisting or reactivated) may be a further synergistic factor. Treatment consists of rehydration, antibiotics, attention to anaemia and the nutritional state, and mild antiseptic mouth washes.

Pneumonia

By the third or fourth day after the rash has appeared, the pneumonia in many cases will be due to bacterial superinfection, although, in some, measles giant cell pneumonia may develop. Common bacterial pathogens are the staphylococcus and klebsiella pneumoniae, which may lead to abscess and bullous formation, complicated by pneumothorax and empyema. Broad spectrum antibiotic cover will be needed until the aetiology is known.

Diarrhoea

Many children experience a complicating diarrhoea, either coinciding with the appearance of the rash or during the week following. The diarrhoea may resemble that of shigella dysentry, with blood and mucus. The rectosigmoid mucosa is affected by measles in a similar way to the skin and significant loss of protein and fluid occurs into the gut. There is no specific treatment and diarrhoea improves as the state of hydration and nutrition improves.

Disseminated intravascular coagulation

DIC has been reported with measles, associated with shock lung and peripheral symmetrical gangrene.

Skin sepsis

In malnourished children, large areas of the skin may desquamate after measles allowing the entry of bacteria, particularly staphylococci. This causes enlarged, suppurating lymph nodes, abscesses, and on occasions, large areas of skin and subcutaneous tissue loss, particularly in the groin and axillae.

Tuberculosis

If a child is going through a primary TB infection at the time he suffers measles, there may be a rapid deterioration and dissemination of the tuberculosis bacteria. Diagnosis may be difficult as the Heaf or Mantoux tests are often negative for several months after measles. Anti-tuberculous treatment may have to be started on suspicion and continued until the diagnosis becomes clearer.

Central nervous system

There is no evidence that CNS complications are more common or severe in developing countries.

Fever is the commonest cause of convulsions, but some children will suffer from measles encephalitis and very rarely subacute sclerosing panencephalopathy (p. 283).

Effects on nutritional state

Measles has a profound effect on the state of nutrition. Figures from several African states south of the Sahara show epidemics of kwashiorkor occurring 2–3 months after epidemics of measles. In some areas 30–50% of children admitted with kwashiorkor have a history of recent measles. Measles exerts its effect through the five mechanisms discussed on p. 554.

Influence on cell-mediated immunity (CMI)

An attack of measles depresses CMI for some weeks or months. The tuberculin skin test may be falsely negative, and the bacteria may disseminate rapidly. In some children measles virus infection persists, as shown by prolonged excretion of giant cells, and a giant cell pneumonia, which is often fatal.

There is probably no other infectious disease in which the differences in mortality and morbidity between developed and developing countries is so great. Measles vaccination must have very high priority in all countries, but is particularly cost effective and life saving in the tropics and subtropics.

Tuberculosis

Tuberculosis (TB) is a world-wide disease, now comparatively rare in Europe and North America, but unfortunately still common in developing countries where overcrowded cities and poor general health help to sustain its steady passage through the population. In Britain now there are two main sources of childhood infection; the elderly and recent immigrants.

The elderly population lived through the last major epidemic of TB in the UK, which started with the Second World War and ended with the introduction of anti-tuberculous therapy in the early 1950s. For years this generation has carried live TB bacilli inside calcified lesions in their lungs. With declining immunity, from old age, carcinomatosis or leukaemia enable the bacilli to break out and cause cavitating disease, which may not be diagnosed before death. These old people may infect their children or grandchildren. The second source in the UK is recent immigrants from countries where TB is still common.

NATURAL HISTORY

Two factors determine the response of an individual to infection with tuberculosis; resistance and the size of the infecting dose of bacilli. Resistance is of two types: natural which is present at birth and may be dependent on race, family and individual variations; and acquired which depends on immunity from a previous infection. Response also depends on the number of TB bacilli taken into the body; the greater the number, the more likely infection is to take place.

SCREENING FOR TUBERCULOSIS

The likely response of an individual to infection with tuberculosis can be determined by his reaction to the tuberculin test. Six weeks after first infection the patient develops a positive tuberculin test. This is a specific reaction to the intradermal injection of tuberculin protein, indicating a state of allergy but not immunity. A positive test shows that the individual has at some time been infected with tubercle bacilli, unless he has previously received BCG vaccination, which has the same effect. It gives no indication when the infection

occurred, except that it must have been at least 6 weeks previously: it might have been 60 years or more before. This can be determined only by knowing when the test was previously negative, and therefore, when conversion to positive could have taken place. Nor does the tuberculin test give any indication whether the patient is now suffering from active tuberculosis. An individual with a positive test might by reason of natural and acquired resistance, be immune to the disease, another might be dying from it owing to lack of immunity. The test cannot differentiate between human and bovine infection. A list of conditions in which there may be a reduced or absent reaction to tuberculin is given in Table 29.9.

It is probable that in most individuals with a positive test, living tubercle bacilli are present in the body. Surveys planned to determine the tuberculosis attack rate in those whose tuberculin state was previously known, have shown that the highest morbidity is now in those already positive whereas until recently the reverse was the case. This emphasizes the error of regarding the tuberculin positive state from a natural infection as a form of protection and underlines the need to follow all such children through adolescence when their risk of adult tuberculosis is greatest.

Tuberculin test

Two tuberculin tests are widely used, the Mantoux test available in three dilutions, and the Heaf test.

Mantoux test. For routine Mantoux testing 0.1 ml of 1:1000 dilution of old tuberculin is injected intradermally into the flexor surface of the left forearm (equivalent to 10 units). The test is read

Severe overwhelming TB infection
Infection with TB within past 6–8 weeks
Other severe illness
Recent measles or measles vaccination
Recent pertussis
Leukaemia, or other disease affecting immunological status
Severe malnutrition

Table 29.9 Causes of a negative tuberculin test in the presence of active TB.

at 72 hours, a positive result being a palpable area of induration greater than 6 mm across. In children with erythema nodosum, a 1:10 000 solution is used (1 unit) as the response to 1:1000 solution may include ulceration. Non-specific reactions may occur when 1:100 strength solution is used, indicating previous contact with non-pathogenic mycobacteria.

Heaf test. The Heaf test uses a special gun, the six needles of which simultaneously pierce the skin to the correct depth. It has the advantage of ease, accuracy and absence of pain. The method was designed for use in Africa, the result being much more easy to read on black skin than the single Mantoux mark. The solution used is tuberculin PPD (purified protein derivative) containing 100 000 units per ml. The test is not a quantitative one but is considered to be equivalent to the 1:1000 Mantoux test. It is most important that the correct solution is used, this being more viscous than that used for a Mantoux test. A small drop of this solution is placed on the skin using a sterile platinum loop. The end plate of the Heaf gun must be held at right angles to the skin, being pressed firmly on the centre of the film of tuberculin solution. The removable head containing the needles is sterilized by autoclave, or flaming in methylated spirit. The result is read in 72 hours but can be delayed up to 7 days. A positive result is indicated by the development of palpable induration at the site of at least four of the puncture points.

It is important to check the sharpness of the six needle points at frequent intervals, as false negative results will occur from lack of skin penetration.

PATHOGENESIS

When infection with TB bacilli occurs, there are broadly two possible reactions: a primary focus is produced which heals spontaneously leaving the patient sensitized, or the primary focus cannot be contained and progression of the disease occurs. Progressive primary TB tends to occur in infants and young children, and is clinically manifest in TB pneumonia, miliary TB and TB of the lymph nodes.

Older children and adults, in whom initial infection was overcome, remain sensitized. Further contact with TB bacilli, or a breakdown in the original primary infection leads to the more 'adult' manifestation of TB, where there is an additional sensitivity reaction to the invading organisms. These manifestations include phlyctenular conjunctivitis, erythema nodosum, pleural effusions, cavitation and fibrosis. This is summarized in Figure 29.10.

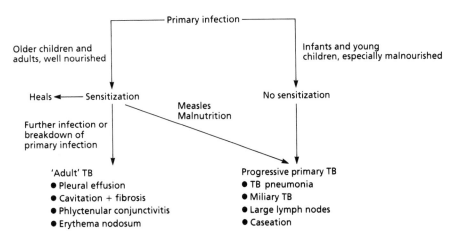

Fig. 29.10 Diagram to show the possible outcomes in a child with primary tuberculosis.

Primary infection

Effects in the non-immune

Primary infection results in a lesion with two components which together are known as the 'primary complex'; these components bear the same relationship to each other wherever the site of the lesion. One is the parenchymal component or tubercle, whose site is dependent on the route of infection. The other component is glandular, resulting from lymphatic spread to the glands draining the parenchymal lesion. There are two types of infection, human and bovine. Human infection is now by far the most important, usually occurring by droplet spread from a patient with open pulmonary tuberculosis. Bovine tuberculosis reaches the body by the ingestion of infected milk. Bovine disease is now uncommon in Britain as tuberculosis amongst cattle has been largely eradicated. As the major route of infection is droplet inhalation, the most common site for the primary complex is the lung. Ingestion of the bacilli causes a primary lesion in the intestine; direct contact often associated with local trauma causes a lesion on the skin, or less commonly, in the mouth.

The primary focus in the lung (the Ghon focus) usually lies immediately under the pleura, most often in the right upper lobe. The glandular element involves the mediastinal nodes. In the abdomen, the parenchymal lesion is in the intestine, the mesenteric glands being involved. The tonsils are sometimes the primary site, the tonsillar glands then comprising the second component of the primary complex. Involvement of the skin or mouth causes a similar enlargement of the appropriate regional glands.

Both components of the primary complex may heal or extend and undergo caseation, but extension and caseation are far more likely to occur in the glandular component than in the parenchymal. Involvement of the glands accounts for the majority of the clinical features of the primary complex, their effect varying greatly according to the site. Enlarged cervical glands cause no trouble from pressure, but similar enlargement in the mediastinum results in serious bronchial damage.

Healing takes place by fibrosis and calcification is common later. Calcification in the neck causes little disturbance but in the chest may cause bronchial stenosis. Even though healing has proceeded to calcification, living tubercle bacilli may remain in the lesion for many years. Extension may occur from either of the components, taking place by local spread or via the bronchi, blood or lymphatics.

If direct or bronchial spread of the primary infection occurs, it usually does so within a few months of the original infection. Lymphatic spread to the group of glands draining the primary gland usually appears within a year, but may be delayed as long as 7 years. Blood-stream spread results from the erosion of a blood vessel and, if it occurs, usually does so soon after the onset of the primary infection, often before this has been detected. This liability continues with diminishing frequency for about 2 years, being very rare after that time. Haematogenous spread, causing miliary tuberculosis or meningitis, occurs earlier than spread to bone or kidneys which often takes place during the second year after the primary infection. Part of this longer interval may be due to the fact that bone and kidney lesions take longer to manifest themselves. Needle biopsy of the liver has shown evidence of hepatic spread in a significant proportion of cases of primary tuberculosis, although there are no symptoms referable to the liver in these cases. There is no enlargement of the regional glands from a haematogenous deposit.

The age at first infection is important in deciding the subsequent clinical pattern. Active tuberculosis is far more likely to follow infection in infancy than in older children, the type of lesion also being affected by the age at which first infection occurs. The younger the child, the larger the lymph gland component and the more often does the disease become disseminated. The older the child, the more often does a pleural effusion occur. Pleural effusions may result from blood stream spread or from direct involvement of the pleura and usually occur about 6 months after the primary infection. In older children and adolescents the risk that the adult type of the disease will supervene is much greater than in younger children.

Infection after previous sensitization

The entry of tubercle bacilli into a patient who has already developed some immunity as the result of a primary infection is much more violent, but remains local; it is known as the adult type of the disease. The local reaction is one of acute inflammation and may be sufficiently intense to proceed to caseation and necrosis with consequent cavity formation. Cavitation is common with this type of reaction as distinct from a primary complex in which cavitation is rarely seen. Alternatively, depending on the degree of resistance and the size of the infecting dose, it may resolve completely with or without fibrosis. Unlike the primary lesion, which may occur anywhere in the lungs, this lesion is most often posterior, either in the subapical region of the upper lobe or, less commonly, in a similar position in the lower lobe. There is no enlargement of the regional lymph glands and haematogenous spread is rare.

It is still uncertain whether this secondary form of tuberculosis is the result of spread from the primary complex or re-infection from outside. The balance of evidence, including the constant site of the lesion, favours a bronchogenic spread from breakdown of the primary lesion.

PRIMARY TUBERCULOSIS

Before describing the clinical features of primary tuberculosis it is necessary to consider erythema nodosum and phlyctenular conjunctivitis. These are hypersensitivity states which represent an allergic reaction to infection with the tubercle bacilli or the haemolytic *Streptococcus*. Their recognition is therefore of paramount importance since they may be the only indication of primary tuberculosis. Both conditions are very rare in the first 2 years of life. They differ in that erythema nodosum is seen only in the early phase of the primary complex and, if of tubercular origin, occurs once only, whereas phlyctenular conjunctivitis may occur during all stages of activity of the primary complex and has a tendency to relapse. When erythema nodosum is of streptococcal origin, repeated attacks may occur.

Table 29.10 Causes of erythema nodosum.

Tuberculosis
Streptococcal infection
Crohn's disease
Ulcerative colitis
Histoplasmosis
Systemic lupus erythematosus
Leprosy
Yersinia infections
Sulphonamide therapy

Erythema nodosum

Tender mauve nodules appear on the front of the shins and occasionally on the extensor aspects of the forearms. They have a similar appearance to that produced by a positive Mantoux test. The lesions always disappear in about 2 weeks, going through the colour changes of a fading bruise. Unfortunately, parents mistake erythema nodosum for bruises and fail to alert the doctor.

Unusually there is sufficient pain to warrant local therapy but if this is required calamine lotion is soothing. No other treatment is necessary, though a full investigation for tuberculosis is indicated. If the significance of this exceedingly important condition is missed, it may be months before the effects of the primary infection become detectable again; in the interval much harm may have been done.

The frequency of a tuberculous origin of erythema nodosum is declining in England but it is still the commonest cause in young children. Table 29.10 lists causes of erythema nodosum.

Phlyctenular conjunctivitis

A phlyctenule is a minute vesicle or ulcerated nodule found on the cornea or conjunctiva. It is best seen by examining the eye obliquely, when a granular surface can be observed. The lesion occurs most often at the corneoscleral junction, its site being clearly marked by a triangular leash of the blood vessels, the apex of which lies at the site of the phlyctenule.

Lacrimation and photophobia occur if corneal

ulceration has taken place. But in many cases the condition is mild and its serious relationship to tuberculosis is not appreciated. Cortisone eye drops relieve the local symptoms, but if corneal ulceration has occurred healing leaves an opacity.

Intrathoracic primary tuberculosis

Most often an uncomplicated primary infection passes unnoticed, having either produced no symptoms or only a period of vague ill health which may have been regarded as 'influenza'. It cannot be emphasized too strongly that night sweats, haemoptysis and a severe illness, as seen in adults with tuberculosis, are not features of primary infection and that loss of appetite and tiredness are the main presenting symptoms. Pain in the limb muscles sometimes occurs, which may be ascribed to 'growing pains'; occasionally pain may be felt in the joints.

Cough is not a prominent feature unless there is

pressure on a bronchus by enlarged hilar glands, when it is likely to be 'brassy'. Physical signs in the chest may not be obvious and it is surprising how large a shadow on the X-ray can be without clinical signs, emphasizing the need for radiography in all suspected cases. It is often this discrepancy between the clinical signs and X-ray changes which first points to a diagnosis of TB.

The most common complication of the primary complex is the segmental lesion which occurs more often in younger patients. This lesion is due to aspiration tuberculosis pneumonia, with or without caseation, resulting from perforation of a caseous lymph gland through the bronchial wall. The X-ray shadow is composed of the enlarged glands and the pulmonary lesion. It is seldom possible to determine their respective limits (Fig. 29.11). Caseous lymph glands often contain large numbers of tubercle bacilli and it is understandable that simple collapse, rarely if ever, occurs. Consequently, clearing of the opacity results from

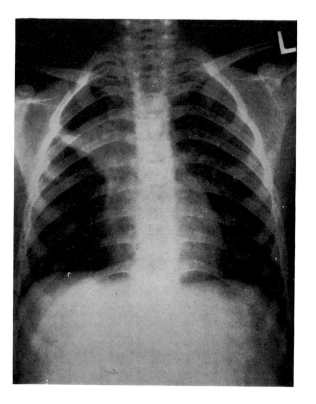

Fig. 29.11 Chest radiograph showing primary tuberculosis. The segmental opacity in the right upper zone comprises enlarged hilar glands together with consolidation and collapse in the upper lobe.

the resolution of the tuberculous exudate and not from simple re-aeration of a collapsed lobe. The term 'epituberculosis' was used in the past to describe these shadows, but should now be discarded in view of the more detailed pathology available. The primary complex occurs more often on the right, and a right-sided lesion is more liable to extend than one of the left. Cavitation of a primary lung lesion is rare in comparison with that in adult-type tuberculosis.

Obstructive emphysema is a serious complication which is not rare but is easily missed. Partial obstruction of the bronchus by an eroding gland permits more air to enter the lung than can come out; the lobe becoming over-distended. Wheezing may occur with diminished movement and air entry on the affected side. An inspiratory film may show no difference between the two sides but, on expiration the diseased lung, remaining aerated, appears clearer than the normal side. Later, the gland entirely blocks the lumen, causing complete collapse of the lung with ensuing tuberculous pneumonia and bronchiectasis. In children under 1 year old, a clinical picture resembling bronchiolitis is sometimes seen, which is due to the reaction to inhaled bacilli from an ulcerating mediastinal lymph node. Bilateral hilar gland enlargement, with partial bronchial obstruction, mimics asthma in the older child.

Rupture of the primary focus into the pleural sac may result in a pleural effusion. This is more common in well-nourished children with good sensitization. The pleural fluid is straw-coloured, and contains lymphocytes and a high level of protein. The bacilli may not be seen in the centrifuged deposit, and culture should be undertaken. Rarely the effusion progresses to a TB empyema. It is probably best to remove most of the pleural fluid at the diagnostic tap. Once treatment has started further removal is usually unnecessary. If despite several taps, fluid continues to accumulate, a short course of oral steroids may help.

Tuberculous pericarditis and pericardial effusion are rare and should be considered in any child with TB who deteriorates unexpectedly, particularly one showing shock, enlarging liver and dyspnoea.

Abdominal primary TB

The source of infection is most commonly from the lung lesion, either by swallowing the bacilli or from haematogenous spread. Those patients with no evidence of pulmonary TB may have contracted bovine TB from the ingestion of infected milk. A small proportion of patients develop TB peritonitis, with severe wasting, abdominal distention and signs of partial or intermittent intestinal obstruction.

Cervical adenitis

The primary source of this infection is most often in the tonsil but may be in the adenoids, middle ear or teeth. The tonsils may look diseased but are just as likely to look entirely normal. The evidence points to human infection being more common than bovine infection.

The glands cause no pain and no systemic illness and are therefore often disregarded until the condition is far advanced (Plate 50). So long as the infection in the gland is purely tuberculous, the gland remains discrete and mobile, not being fixed from periadenitis. Caseation is common, as shown by the incidence of radiological calcification, but not all those glands which caseate develop clinical abscesses. The development of an abscess appears to be determined by size and is more likely to occur once the diameter of the gland is greater than 2 cm.

A mixture of tuberculous and streptococcal infections in the gland is common. The tuberculous infection progresses steadily, but the streptococcal infection waxes and wanes. A mixed infection causes periadenitis and once this has occurred the skin is likely to break down. The first evidence of this is the gland becoming tethered to the overlying skin. The skin initially becomes pink and then mauve and thinned, followed by a discharge of caseous material. Finally an indolent discharging ulcer remains.

Generalized lymphadenitis is rare in Britain but is seen quite frequently in older children in Africa. In such cases the enlargement of the axillary lymph nodes is usually greater than any other groups.

Chronic otitis media may be caused by tuberculosis and should be suspected if neck glands are enlarged on the same side as a discharging ear.

Tuberculous meningitis (TBM)

The symptoms and signs at the onset of TBM can be divided broadly into three groups.

General. The child is non-specifically unwell. He may be miserable or irritable, or wanting to be left alone. Older children may complain of headache. Fever and vomiting are often present.

Meningeal. In older children, a stiff neck with positive Kernig's sign will be present. There may be difficulty kissing the knees. As with other forms of meningitis, these signs are unreliable in infants.

Brain and cranial nerve involvement. Sixth nerve or palsy of the other ocular nerves may occur. Drowsiness increases and leads to coma.

Most children, untreated, take 10–14 days to pass from the non-specific onset to coma with signs of brain involvement. If morbidity and mortality from TBM are to improve, treatment must be started as soon as possible. Those children presenting with coma and cranial nerve palsies rarely recover fully.

Clinical examination of the child may not help differentiate TBM from other forms of meningitis. Close examination of the fundi sometimes reveals choroidal tubercles. Chest X-ray often helps by showing miliary mottling or other evidence of TB but the chest X-ray may initially be normal with bacteriologically proven TBM.

Investigations. Lumbar puncture findings are usually characteristic with turbidity and a cell count of 200–400/mm³, which are mainly lymphocytes. The protein is raised, in late cases to very high levels (1–2 g/l). CSF glucose will be below 2.8 mmol/l in the majority of cases. In very early TBM more polymorphs than lymphocytes may be seen and the glucose may not have fallen to a diagnostically low level. The CSF changes can therefore mimic those of a partially treated bacterial meningitis, or early viral meningitis (p. 281). A careful search for acid-fast bacilli in centrifuged CSF will often resolve the dilemma. On occasion, treatment for both bacterial and tuberculous meningitis must be started until the diagnosis becomes clear.

MILIARY TUBERCULOSIS

The disease is so named because the parenchymal lesions disseminated throughout the body resemble millet seeds. The patient is often described as presenting with dyspnoea and cyanosis, but more usually these children are picked up on chest X-ray for the investigation of vague ill-health. A careful ophthalmoscopic examination may reveal choroidal tubercles before they are seen on chest X-ray due to the magnification provided by the ophthalmoscope.

SKIN OR MUCOUS MEMBRANE LESIONS

The primary focus occurs in a visible situation more often than is appreciated. The majority of such lesions occur on the skin, but they may be found in the eye or mouth. In the latter case they may be seen either on the buccal mucous membrane or, more often, on the gum. There is often a history of trauma causing a break in the continuity of the epithelium which allows the entrance of the tubercle bacilli. In all cases there is enlargement of the regional glands. The appearance of the lesions is variable but all are indolent and indurated, ulceration being common. In some cases 'apple jelly' nodules are seen at the edge of the lesion. The possibility of a tuberculous skin infection must be considered in any child whose skin wound has healed and then breaks down, and where painless enlargement of the regional lymph glands also exists.

BONE AND JOINT TUBERCULOSIS

The most common sites in children are the spine (Pott's disease) and hip. Tuberculous dactylitis is a rare manifestation. Trauma is an aetiological factor, influencing the localization of the disease. Synovial lesions usually present earlier than bone lesions and their course is more rapid so that they may simulate acute suppurative arthritis or rheumatic fever.

SPINAL TUBERCULOSIS

The disease most often affects the lower back and thoracic spine, causing limitation of movement and local pain, although this may sometimes be referred to the abdomen. Muscle spasm causes the affected area of the spine to be held rigid. Paraplegia occurs in a considerable proportion of the patients and may be the presenting feature. It is due to pressure from tuberculous granulations and caseous material rather than to the collapse of the vertebrae. A psoas abscess, which is 'cold' may develop, and if this presents externally it appears immediately above the inguinal ligament; less often a lumbar abscess develops. These abscesses may be the first manifestation of the disease. X-rays may show one or more vertebrae to be involved; these will be decalcified and have often collapsed, causing considerable deformity.

TUBERCULOSIS OF THE HIP

These patients are usually under 5 years of age and present with a limp or pain in the hip, though this is sometimes referred to the knee. Examination reveals wasting of the hip muscles and limitation of joint movement. The X-ray shows rarefaction of the bone around the joint.

RENAL TUBERCULOSIS

This is much less common in children than adults, rarely occurring under the age of 10 years. It results from haematogenous spread, usually from a pulmonary lesion and often produces no clinical features. The fact that the kidney is involved may be discovered only on routine urinary examination in a child with tuberculosis, or at autopsy. The possibility must always be considered in cases of sterile pyuria.

METASTATIC ABSCESSES

These abscesses are haematogenous in origin, forming in the subcutaneous tissues. They are usually painless and slowly involve the overlying skin to produce one or more discharging sinuses from which indolent ulcers develop. Healing eventually takes place, with an area of puckered, tethered skin remaining.

CONGENITAL TUBERCULOSIS

Congenital TB is rare, and the mother is usually clinically very ill. Spread to the baby via the placenta leads to miliary TB with enlargement of the liver and spleen. Inhalation of infected amniotic fluid leads to TB pneumonia, with an X-ray picture not unlike meconium aspiration, with additional hilar gland enlargement. The Mantoux test may be negative. Diagnosis rests on suspicion and can be confirmed by examination of gastric washings.

Diagnosis of tuberculosis in children

History

A recent history of a respiratory tract infection or measles is often obtained. Viral infections may lower resistance and damage lung tissue, allowing TB bacilli to gain a foothold. Measles, in particular, is often followed by a rapid extension and dissemination of a primary focus, through its effect on nutritional status and through depression of cell-mediated immunity.

A history of TB in a contact of the patient is strong evidence in favour of the diagnosis. In all cases a wide search for possible contacts should be made, which primarily involves the close family, but may need to be extended to school teachers, doctors and family friends. Two recent epidemics in Britain among schoolchildren were traced to open TB in their teachers. Similarly, doctors with TB are liable to pass the disease to their patients, particularly if they are working with the newborn.

Identification of TB bacilli

The only direct proof that a child is suffering from TB is to find the bacilli. Children swallow their sputum so examination of gastric washings, from an empty stomach, on three consecutive mornings, is an alternative method of obtaining bacteriological confirmation. CSF, pleural and pericardial fluid can be examined after concentration by centrifuging. Pus from discharging glands or otitis media can be examined directly for acid-fast bacilli. If renal TB is suspected, a 24–hour collection of urine should be spun down and examined.

Culture and sensitivity testing

Culture methods are now more rapid than in the past and animal inoculation is no longer necessary. Sensitivity testing of TB bacilli is difficult and time-consuming, and can be performed in only a few centres in each country. Nevertheless, it is important to know the national pattern of drug resistance in order to define a policy of treatment.

Tuberculin test

A positive tuberculin test is helpful in diagnosing TB, but a negative test may be falsely negative for reasons given in Table 29.9. In children with malnutrition, and after measles, it is justifiable to use Mantoux 1:100 solution in the expectation that a negative response will be obtained from solutions of greater dilution.

Radiography

Wherever the site of suspected tuberculosis, the chest should be X-rayed since the majority of non-pulmonary lesions have resulted from pulmonary tuberculosis. Miliary tuberculosis can be diagnosed on sight by its typical 'snow storm' appearance but none of the other pulmonary shadows is diagnostic.

Biopsy

This may involve the removal of an enlarged regional gland or portion of skin. In bone and joint tuberculosis a biopsy of the synovial membrane is taken, or occasionally, a portion of bone.

PREVENTION

Contact tracing. As already stated, TB in children indicates an adult reservoir of bacilli. TB very rarely spreads from child to child. The child's contacts should be traced, starting with the immediate family, then widening the net to include lodgers, neighbours and school teachers if indicated.

Mass radiography. Mass radiography is cost effective where there is still a significant amount of adult TB in a population. As it is voluntary, it may not reach the population at risk. Those people who are health conscious and less liable to be suffering from TB are those most likely to come forward for X-ray. Routine X-ray for certain groups at particular risk of spreading TB to children, such as teachers, nurses and doctors is undertaken in some countries.

Sputum examination. Sputum examination in the field, by trained microscopists, has been used in parts of Africa. Adults known to have chronic cough are asked to provide a sputum sample, which is stained and examined under a special microscope using the sun's illumination.

Mass screening of children. Screening of schoolchildren using the Heaf test is a simple and cheap procedure. Those who are Heaf negative can receive BCG. Those with positive reactions, in the absence of a BCG scar, should be examined and sent for a chest X-ray.

Pasteurization of milk. In many developed countries milk is pasteurized, largely preventing the spread of bovine TB. In developing countries where raw cow's milk forms part of the diet of young children, this potential mode of spread of TB should be remembered.

Prophylactic treatment

The treatment of active TB is considered below. In many countries, children, particularly those under 5–8 years old, who have a positive tuberculin test, or who are known to have recently converted from tuberculin negative to positive, but have no evidence of active TB, are treated prophylactically. This group is known to be at risk of developing active TB during the 2 years after conversion. Six to 12 months of isoniazid (INAH) alone is the standard regime.

BCG vaccination (see also p. 355). When the tuberculosis rate in a country is high, as in most tropical countries, all newborn babies should be vaccinated. If the tuberculosis rate is low, vaccination is given in later childhood to those whose tuberculin test is negative. BCG given to a child who is already tuberculin positive will produce an accelerated response. Late BCG vaccination avoids its higher complication rate in infancy and maintains the tuberculin test as an epidemiological tool. The recommended age for this vaccination is between the tenth and fourteenth birthdays, thus ensuring protection before the higher risk period of adolescence. BCG should also be given to those at special risk, such as diabetics, hospital workers and contacts who are found to be tuberculin negative. In view of the high incidence of TB among immigrants it is recommended that their children should receive BCG at birth. When vaccination is undertaken during infancy no preliminary tuberculin testing is required.

A freeze-dried vaccine is now available which maintains its activity for a year, if kept in a refrigerator, and obviates the problem of the short life of the liquid preparations. The vaccine is injected intradermally in a dose of 0.05 ml. After 3–6 weeks a small red papule appears, which in most cases, breaks down to a shallow ulcer after 4 weeks. Healing is slow and may take as long as a year, leaving a small puckered scar. Occasionally, painless axillary adenitis develops which may break down to form an abscess. They are best left alone and should not be incised as they are liable to leave a discharging sinus. Aspiration should be undertaken only if they are very large. If an indolent ulcer develops, para-aminosalicylic acid ointment will hasten the healing.

An isoniazid-resistant BCG is of great value in countries where breast feeding is essential for the survival of newborn infants. By this means the baby of a mother with open tuberculosis can be protected with INAH and INAH-resistant BCG and breast feeding permitted. The INAH should be given to the baby from birth and he should be vaccinated as soon as possible with INAH-resistant BCG. The mother should receive full anti-tuberculous treatment, the baby being isolated from her for the first 48 hours to allow the protective blood level of INAH to be reached. Thereafter, feeding at the breast is permitted and INAH continued until Mantoux conversion has occurred. Where INAH-resistant BCG is still not available the baby should be given INAH by mouth until the mother's TB has healed and the baby maintained on the breast. The baby should then be vaccinated with ordinary BCG.

It must be emphasized that BCG vaccination cannot produce complete immunity to tuberculosis any more than a subclinical infection can. It is only one weapon in the fight against tuberculosis and should only be used in combination with all the other measures.

Treatment of tuberculosis

GENERAL MANAGEMENT

Bed rest has not been shown to help recovery from TB in children, who should be allowed out of bed if they feel well enough. Many children can be treated as out-patients, provided compliance with treatment is assured. A good diet and vitamin supplements should be prescribed, and regular weighing undertaken to gauge recovery. After completion of treatment, children should be followed-up through puberty which is the time when relapse is most likely to occur. Isolation of children with TB is unnecessary, as they rarely have cavitating disease.

SPECIFIC THERAPY

The emergence of drug-resistant strains of TB bacilli is encouraged by use of drugs singly, intermittently, or by giving inappropriately short courses. Each country needs, therefore, to have a defined policy towards treating the disease, and a way of enforcing the policy. In some areas TB officers with responsibility for case finding, prevention and supervision of treatment are appointed. They may have the power to remove the licence to prescribe anti-TB medication from those doctors who refuse to follow the national treatment guidelines. In countries where TB is now rare, it is all the more important that treatment should be supervised by those doctors who still see TB, usually chest physicians or specialists in infectious diseases.

As treatment schedules vary so much from country to country, depending on local policy, resistance patterns and money available for treatment, only a very broad guide to specific therapy will be given. Table 29.11 summarizes an approach to the use of anti-tuberculous therapy. The following drugs are available.

Rifampicin. This has largely replaced streptomycin as a first-line drug. It has the great advantage of being given orally, but is more expensive than streptomycin; however, if one considers the cost of syringes and needles for the administration of streptomycin, and the shorter course of rifampicin needed, the cost difference is less apparent. Dose 10–20 mg/kg/day; maximum dose 600 mg/day.

Streptomycin. Streptomycin may be still used in the first 6–8 weeks. Dose 20 mg/kg once daily intramuscularly. It is given intrathecally daily, or on alternate days in a dose of 1 mg/kg (maximum 50 mg) for tuberculous meningitis.

Isoniazid (INAH). Isoniazid forms part of every therapeutic regime against TB. It is cheap, relatively non-toxic, and crosses the blood–brain barrier. Dose 5–10 mg/kg/day; the higher dose being used in TB meningitis. Formulations for giving INAH intravenously and intrathecally are available for very ill children with TB meningitis.

Ethambutol. Ethambutol is a useful adjunct to treatment with rifampicin and INAH, but as optic neuritis is a complication it should be restricted to children whose age permits the detection of deteriorating eyesight. Dose 15–30 mg/kg/day.

Table 29.11 Summary of treatment for tuberculosis.

Manifestation	Treatment
Primary TB TB neck glands Child not ill	Rifampicin + INAH continue for 6 months
Miliary TB without meningitis Severe TB of any type Ill child	Rifampicin + INAH + ethambutol for 12 months ? stop rifampicin after 6 months

TB meningitis	Rifampicin + INAH + ethambutol
	    + pyrazinamide
	    ± intrathecal streptomycin
	Stop streptomycin and
	    pyrazinamide when CSF
	    normal
	Treat for 12 months

Child <8 years, with positive
    tuberculin test, but no
    evidence of active TB
	INAH for 6–12 months

Ethionamide. This is a useful drug when used in combination. Dose 10–15 mg/kg/day.

Para-aminosalicylic acid (PAS). Although the use of PAS is declining in developed countries, it is nevertheless a useful and cheap drug when used in combination with INAH for consolidation therapy.

Pyrazinamide. Pyrazinamide attacks TB bacteria within macrophages and is useful in short course regimens, and in TB meningitis. Dose 40 mg/kg/day.

As a general rule, anti-TB drugs are never given alone. Rifampicin and INAH together form the basis of initial treatment for most forms of TB in children. For uncomplicated respiratory TB both drugs should be given for 6 months. In miliary TB, organ TB and extensive pulmonary TB, ethambutol and pyrazinamide might be added for the first few months, after which treatment with rifampicin and INAH, or INAH and ethambutol, would continue for a total of 9–12 months.

In TB meningitis, initial treatment with rifampicin, INAH, ethambutol and pyrazinamide is usually given, and in some cases intrathecal streptomycin added. Once the CSF has returned to normal, consolidation with rifampicin and INAH continues for a total of 12 months. If the CSF protein is high, prednisolone intrathecally with streptomycin may help reduce the danger of spinal block and hydrocephalus.

Steroid therapy. Steroid therapy may be useful in the following situations:

1 Severely ill children, where the general anti-inflammatory effect of steroids may buy time until anti-TB therapy starts to exert its effect.

2 Children with enlarged hilar nodes, which are causing bronchial obstruction, particularly if bilateral.

3 Children with TB meningitis and high CSF proteins (see above).

4 In the occasional case of recurrent pleural effusion.

Leprosy

This chronic disease is widespread in Asia and India. It particularly affects children, since they are more easily infected than adults. The disease is due to *Mycobacterium leprae* (Hansen's bacillus) which is difficult to study because it cannot be cultured on microbiological medium and has only recently been successfully grown in animals.

Prolonged and intimate contact is necessary for the transfer of infection so that congenital leprosy does not occur. The incubation period is usually 2–4 years. It used to be thought that the infection was transmitted by direct person-to-person skin contact, but studies have shown that insignificant numbers of the bacilli are shed from the intact skin of lepromatous patients, whereas large numbers are shed from the nose which is therefore the main source of infection.

Unfortuately there is no skin test comparable to the tuberculin test to indicate susceptibility to previous infection. The lepromin test indicates potential resistance to the antigen. This is prepared from macerated tissue containing large numbers of bacilli. The test is negative in lepromatous leprosy and positive in the tuberculoid type.

CLINICAL MANIFESTATIONS

The earliest variety is called indeterminate leprosy. Thereafter, the type of disease is determined by the body's resistance and therefore its reaction to the bacilli. If resistance is low there is free multiplication of the organisms with widespread dissemination causing lepromatous leprosy. If resistance is high there is intense cellular activity with minimal spread of bacteria resulting in tuberculoid leprosy. Cases of borderline leprosy exist between these two extremes. Figure 29.12 summarizes these types.

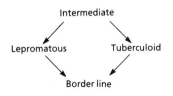

Fig. 29.12 The clinical manifestations of leprosy.

Intermediate leprosy

These early signs occur anywhere on the skin. The lesions are slightly hypopigmented macules which sometimes correspond to an area where paraesthesiae is felt. There is no impairment of sensation.

Lepromatous leprosy

The early skin lesions are ill-defined, smooth, hypopigmented macules mainly over the trunk. Skin snips show these to be teeming with bacilli. Infiltration is the feature of this type and it is this which leads to the production of nodules, especially on the face and ear lobes (Fig. 29.13), eventually creating the 'leonine facies'. There is generalized involvement of nerves but this is minimal in the early stages, in contrast to the tuberculoid type, so that anaesthesia is slight. Later there is increasing nerve involvement with enlargement and hardening of the nerves which can be felt under the skin, together with loss of function. Destruction of the autonomic pathways leads to loss of sweating. The mucosa of the nose, throat and eyes is frequently involved.

The bacilli pass rapidly to the lymph nodes and then by the blood stream to the eyes and testes, and to the liver, spleen and bone marrow.

Tuberculoid leprosy

The term 'tuberculoid' refers to the histological tubercles which are present in most lesions. Skin and nerves only are involved. The skin lesions are clearly demarcated, hypopigmented, anaesthetic areas with a raised border and saucer-like centre (Fig. 29.14). The surface is often rough. The skin is negative for bacilli.

Borderline leprosy

This is an unstable form of the disease with skin lesions of both the main types present at the same time. The lepromin test may be positive or negative and may later reverse. Skin snips are always positive.

REACTIONS IN LEPROSY

Two types of reaction occur in untreated leprosy, or after treatment has started.

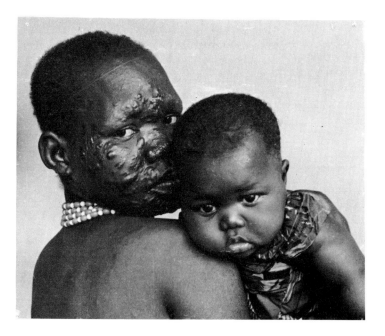

Fig. 29.13 Lepromatous leprosy. Numerous nodules present on the mother's face. The right ear is also involved. The baby looks clinically unaffected, but the mother's milk contained large numbers of leprosy bacilli.

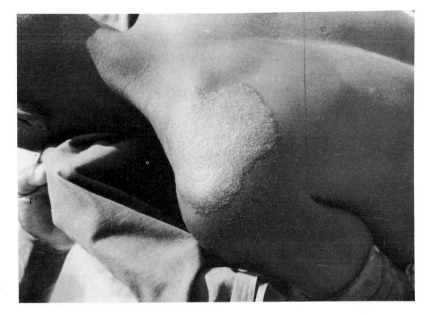

Fig. 29.14 Tuberculoid leprosy. Clearly demarcated hypopigmented lesion with raised border. The surface is rough and dry. No sweating occurred in the affected area which was also anaesthetic. This was the only skin lesion present.

Type 1 lepra reaction

This occurs in pauci-bacillary or tuberculoid leprosy where the reaction is manifested by cellular hyperactivity. There is swelling and pain in skin and nerve lesions, and rapid loss of function.

Type 2 lepra reaction

This occurs in multi-bacillary leprosy (lepromatous or borderline) and is caused by the body's reaction to degenerating bacilli. Clinical manifestations include erythema nodosum leprosum, iritis, dactylitis and orchitis.

TREATMENT

Some protection against leprosy is given by BCG. Table 29.12 summarizes the treatment of leprosy. Triple therapy is recommended for patients with leprosy who have multi-bacillary disease to reduce the possibility of drug resistance.

Mild Type 1 reaction can be treated with aspirin or chloroquine, and if more severe by prednisolone at a high dose initially, reducing rapidly and tailing off over months. The Type 2 reaction responds to thalidomide, prednisolone or to increasing the dose of clofazimine to once daily.

Streptococcal disease

In most developing countries streptococcal disease is more common than in Britain or the USA and often its manifestations can be more severe. Overcrowded living conditions allow the easy spread of the haemolytic *Streptococcus* by droplet, and with sparse primary care facilities, a child with a streptococcal sore throat is much less likely to receive an adequate course of penicillin. Reduced host immunity from malnutrition and other coincidental disease may also contribute to the differing clinical pattern. Overcrowding and lack of water for washing encourages the rapid spread of scabies with subsequent inoculation of haemolytic streptococci into the skin, followed by acute glomerulonephritis.

ACUTE RHEUMATIC FEVER

This is also discussed in Chapter 26. Classically associated with overcrowding, damp and temperate climates, acute rheumatic fever is never-

	Drug	Dose	Frequency
Pauci-bacillary (tuberculoid or borderline)	Rifampicin + dapsone	20 mg/kg 2 mg/kg/day	2 days a month daily Treat for 1 year
Multi-bacillary (lepromatous or borderline)	Rifampicin	20 mg/kg	2 days a month or daily for 1 month
	Clofazimine	5–10 mg/week	Three divided doses, alternate days
	Dapsone	2 mg/kg/day	Daily Treat for 2 years

Table 29.12 Drug management of leprosy.

theless common in warm, dry climates. In contrast to the clinical picture seen 30–40 years ago in Britain, rheumatic fever is often severe, and established valvular disease is seen at a younger age. On a dark skin the accompanying rashes are easily missed, and subcutaneous nodules are rare. The first attack is often subclinical, or in the parents' eyes the illness is not severe enough to warrant seeking medical help. Children are therefore often seen in a second attack with advanced valve damage.

The diagnosis of rheumatic fever is based on the clinical and laboratory criteria discussed on p. 477. The differential diagnosis includes sickle cell disease (with limb pains from avascular necrosis of bone, and a cardiac murmur from anaemia), rheumatoid arthritis, which appears to be rare in children in the tropics, and leukaemia. Treatment is discussed on p. 477. Prophylactic penicillin is best given by monthly injections of a long-acting preparation and should continue at least through puberty.

RHEUMATIC CHOREA

By the time of presentation, both ESR and ASO titre are characteristically normal. Swallowing may be impossible during attacks, necessitating nasogastric tube feeds, with additional calories to compensate for the continuous movement during waking hours.

ACUTE GLOMERULONEPHRITIS

Studies of extensive epidemics of acute glomerulonephritis in the tropics have shown a clinical picture and complication rate similar to that found in more developed areas (see Chapter 15). This is true whether the precipitating streptococcal infection has been in the throat, or on the skin following inoculation by scratching scabetic lesions. Treatment is described on p. 260. During epidemics many children can be managed on an out-patient basis, with daily attendance for clinical examination and measurement of blood pressure. Those with hypertension, fits, heart failure and anuria should be admitted to hospital.

SCARLET FEVER

Alone among the manifestations of streptococcal disease, scarlet fever does not appear to be either more serious or more common in the tropics. However, it may be underdiagnosed as the rash is not easily visible on a pigmented skin. The diagnosis may be made in retrospect from observing desquamation of the palms and soles (p. 362).

PREVENTION OF STREPTOCOCCAL DISEASE

During the past 90 years both the incidence and severity of all forms of streptococcal disease have fallen steadily in Britain. The virulence of the streptococci is not known to have changed, and a considerable part of the improvement occurred before the discovery of penicillin. The major contribution to the improved picture seems to have come from better childhood nutrition and less overcrowded homes. If this is so, as socioeconomic conditions improve in developing countries, so should the incidence and severity of streptococcal disease decline. Programmes to prevent streptococcal infection and its aftermath should include guidelines for the treatment of sore throat and tonsillitis and should emphasize the importance of scabies in relation to streptococcal disease.

Anaemia in children (see also p. 423)

In developing countries, chronic anaemia in children is common, and although rarely the direct cause of death, undermines general health and the response to infection and is therefore an important contributing cause to ill health and mortality. Anaemia can be considered under the broad headings in Table 29.13.

Iron-deficiency anaemia from lack of dietary iron is probably the single most common anaemia throughout the world. In developing countries with a high incidence of prematurity, prolonged breast feeding without the introduction of iron-rich foods, and widespread parasitic infestations of the gut, anaemia is particularly common. The history will often be sufficient to make a clinical diagnosis, confirmed by examination of the peripheral blood film which shows a microcytic, hypochromic anaemia. If further investigations, such as serum iron and haemoglobin electrophoresis are not available, it would be reasonable to treat with oral iron and observe the result after 1–2 months. Stools and urine should be inspected for parasites and treatment given if necessary. Failure to respond to iron therapy would suggest thalassaemia (p. 430), undetected blood loss or chronic infection.

The two main causes of haemolytic anaemia in the developing world are malaria (p. 572) and sickle cell disease (p. 431). Malaria is thought to contribute to about a million childhood deaths a

Table 29.13 Common causes of anaemia seen in developing countries.

Mechanism	Common causes	History	Blood film
Nutritional	Iron deficiency	Prolonged breast feeding with lack of iron-containing foods Prematurity	Hypochromic/microcytic
	Protein–energy malnutrition		Normochromic/normocytic Occasionally macrocytic
	Folic acid	Chronic diarrhoea or haemolytic anaemia	Macrocytic
Blood loss	Hookworm *Schistosoma mansoni*	Macroscopic or microscopic blood in stool Ova in stool	Hypochromic/microcytic
Haemolytic	Malaria	Geographical area, fever, splenomegaly	Parasites in thick/thin film
	Sickle cell disease	Geographical area, crises (p. 432), bone pain	Sickle cells

year in Africa alone. In areas where it is common, the diagnosis is usually straightforward from the history, clinical findings and positive blood films. Appropriate treatment (p. 431) results in a rapid rise in haemoglobin level. If this does not occur then other causes of anaemia should be investigated.

Parasitic diseases

MALARIA

This disease is distributed throughout the tropics, but its incidence is less in dry places and at high altitudes. Four types of parasite are known to affect man: (1) *Plasmodium malaria*, the cause of quartan malaria, (2) and (3) *P. vivax* and *P. ovale* which cause benign tertian malaria, and (4) *P. falciparum* which causes malignant malaria, the type responsible for the more serious complications, including cerebral malaria.

In the first stage of the life cycle in human beings the parasites develop in the liver. They then pass out into red blood cells, for the asexual cycle, destroying them in the process. The length of the asexual cycle determines the interval between bouts of fever in the classic form of the disease. However, infection by two different types of parasite, or by the same parasite from mosquito bites at different times may upset the typical periodicity of the fever.

After a time, certain of the parasites of the asexual cycle become sexually differentiated, developing into male and female gametocytes. When a patient is bitten by a mosquito these gametocytes complete their development, and migrate to the mosquito salivary glands ready to infect humans again.

Clinical features

The classical disease with recurring bouts of high fever is seen only in the non-immune child. For the child living in an endemic area the illness is quite different depending on age and degree of immunity. The newborn baby has a degree of passive immunity from his mother lasting several months. Early infections are therefore modified and may be asymptomatic, despite the presence of parasitaemia.

As maternal protection wanes symptoms of fever, anorexia and diarrhoea develop, but gradually the child's own immunity builds up, leading to a state where he lives in symbiosis with the parasite. During this time there may be an increased mortality from pneumonia, diarrhoeal diseases and other infections, and the contribution of malaria to these deaths is underestimated. Clinically, as the child grows his spleen becomes progressively smaller until in areas holendemic for *P. falciparum*, it becomes impalpable. There is usually a moderate to severe compensated anaemia.

It is very important to remember that in developing countries multiple pathology is common. Thus in children from malarious areas, with a fever, the presence of parasites in the blood does not necessarily mean that the fever is caused by malaria. It is important to search for other causes, such as pneumonia or meningitis.

In the partially immune, or non-immune child, malaria is a more severe illness, particularly if caused by *P. falciparum*. A well-recognized situation is the town-dwelling child who visits grandparents in a rural area and who subsequently develops cerebral malaria. The symptoms of malaria may mimic many other illnesses and include fevers and rigors, muscle pains, cough, drowsiness, convulsions and coma. Profuse diarrhoea and abdominal distension (algid malaria) may be mistaken for enteric infection, and suggests that a search for parasites should be made in all children with diarrhoea from a malarial area.

In cerebral malaria, the capillaries of the brain become blocked by masses of parasites of *P. falciparum* which may lead to multiple areas of brain ischaemia or infarction. The death rate is high and survival may be associated with permanent brain damage. Some children do survive to make a remarkable recovery over the course of 2–3 months.

Treatment and prophylaxis

There are many general measures which can be taken against malaria, including residual insecticide spraying of houses, draining stagnant water to prevent mosquito breeding, and sleeping under nets. In endemic areas, where malaria contributes significantly to infant and child mortality and morbidity, regular drug prophylaxis improves growth and health. The haemoglobin level also remains higher than in untreated children. Prophylaxis may, however, interfere with the development of immunity, so once started, it should not be stopped. In areas where malaria control is poor, it may be better to provide treatment for acute attacks, hoping to control morbidity, without interfering with the development of immunity.

In severe malaria, including cerebral malaria, intravenous quinine may be used in a dose of 10 mg/kg, repeated in 12 hours. Once there is improvement, treatment can continue orally with 10–15 mg/kg 8-hourly. Intravenous chloroquine is best avoided in children.

Drug prophylaxis for malaria is becoming more difficult with the emergence of resistant strains. Local advice should always be sought. In areas where resistance is not a problem, proguanil daily, pyrimethamine weekly or chloroquine weekly are useful. Where chloroquine resistance exists, combinations of pyrimethamine and dapsone (Maloprim) or pyrimethamine and sulfadoxine (Fansidar) are useful.

HOOKWORM (*ANCYLOSTOMA DUODENALE* AND *NECATOR AMERICANUS*)

In some areas this is the cause of serious chronic ill-health and anaemia. Man is the host. Eggs are passed in the faeces, and develop into larvae in damp soil. They enter the body by penetration of the skin of the feet, pass into the blood stream and migrate through the lungs, to be swallowed and eventually reach the small intestine. Here they attach themselves to the mucosa and feed by sucking blood. Occasionally the larvae do not enter blood vessels, but migrate through the skin causing lava migrans.

A few worms cause negligible blood loss, but heavy infestation causes a severe chronic iron-deficiency anaemia with eventual death from heart failure. The diagnosis is confirmed by finding blood and ova in the stools.

Methods of prevention include controlled disposal of faeces, and the wearing of shoes. Mebendazole or thiabendazole are effective as specific treatments (see Ascaris, below). In severe anaemia with heart failure, specific treatment should be delayed until the general condition can be improved by blood transfusion. Post-treatment iron should be given for 2–3 months to replenish body stores.

ASCARIS

Ascaris lumbricoides inhabits the small intestine, and looks like a white earthworm, but is pointed at both ends. Ova are passed in the stools, and where insanitary conditions exist the ova may contaminate food or earth, and may be ingested by children. The ova hatch in the small intestine from where the larvae are carried by the blood stream to the lungs. Here they pass up the trachea to be swallowed and develop into adult worms in the intestine. During passage through the lungs, there may be asthma-like symptoms, with dry cough, wheeze and mild fever. An X-ray may show diffuse infiltration associated with a high peripheral blood eosinophil count (Loeffler's syndrome).

The presence of a few worms in the intestine gives rise to no symptoms. Larger loads may be associated with abdominal pain, and in some children, signs of intestinal obstruction. A mass of worms may be felt abdominally and confirmed by the typical X-ray appearance of tram-line lucencies.

The treatment is piperazine 100 mg/kg, maximum 4 g in a single dose or thiabendazole 25 mg/kg/day for 2 days.

TOXOCARIASIS

This disorder is caused by the migration of toxocara larvae from the roundworms which commonly infest dogs and cats. It occurs in both temperate and tropical climates. Toxocara eggs are ingested and hatch in the intestine, releasing larvae which penetrate the gut wall. The severity of the illness relates to the number of larvae, the host reaction and the organs invaded by the larvae. These rarely mature into the adult worm but cause granulomata to form round them. Some patients develop fever, hepatosplenomegaly and eosinophilia. Pulmonary involvement can cause Loeffler's syndrome. Visual disturbance results from a single granuloma on, or under, the retina or in the ciliary body. Epilepsy can result from a granuloma in the brain. Diagnosis is made by a positive serological test, usually the toxocara fluorescent antibody test.

Management. Diethylcarbamazine 9 mg/kg daily in divided doses for 3 weeks or thiabendazole 25 mg/kg twice a day for 7–28 days.

TRICHURIS TRICHURIA (WHIPWORM)

This parasite is about 5 cm long and is widely distributed in warm, moist climates. The anterior portion of the worm is elongated into a thin whip-like filament with which it bores into the superficial mucosa of the caecum, lower ileum or ascending colon. The thicker posterior portion of the worm projects into the lumen of the bowel. The eggs are passed in the stools where they can easily be recognized microscopically. If deposited on moist soil the eggs hatch into larvae in 2 weeks. If ripe eggs are swallowed they hatch out in the duodenum and then become attached to the mucous membrane of the caecum or nearby bowel.

Infestation is frequently so mild that there are no symptoms. Heavy infestation causes abdominal pain, anaemia, bloody diarrhoea, prolapsed rectum, and growth stunting in children. An unexplained association is finger clubbing.

Management. Mebendazole 100 mg daily for 3–4 days for children over 2 years.

STRONGYLOIDES STERCORALIS

In America this parasite is known as the threadworm. The parasite is only just visible to the naked eye as a delicate thread. It lives in the depths of the mucous membrane anywhere in the intestine,

but mainly in the duodenum. The eggs hatch out in the intestine to form larvae which undergo further development in warm soil. These larvae penetrate the skin, travelling through the lungs in the same way as the hookworm and may produce the same clinical effects. Chronic infestation causes epigastric pain and diarrhoea leading to emaciation.

Strongyloides is unusual in that it can multiply in the body, thus keeping infection active for decades. In the immunosuppressed patient severe illness may result from the worm migrating through the intestinal wall into the peritoneal cavity.

Management. Mebendazole 25 mg/kg every 12 hours for 3 days.

TAPEWORM

Infestation results from eating undercooked pork (*T. solium*) or beef (*T. saginata*). Symptoms are rare and the diagnosis is usually made when segments of the worms are passed in the faeces. Man is also liable to infestation by the cysticercus stage of *T. solium* after ingestion of the eggs. Cysticerci may lodge in the brain, causing convulsions, a syndrome mimicking cerebral tumour or, in massive infection, progressive dementia. CT scan and muscle X-ray are helpful in diagnosis.

Management. In cases of *T. solium* and *T. saginata* intestinal infection, niclosamide (500 mg) is given in a child up to 2 years and in older children (2–6 years) a dose of 1 g is used.

Cerebral cysticercosis is treated with praziquantel (50 mg/kg/day) in divided doses for 15 days. Cerebral signs may become worse, so treatment should be undertaken in hospital. Dexamethasone cover is often used.

TRICHINIASIS

Trichinella spiralis is one of the smallest roundworms parasitic in man and it is acquired through eating inadequately cooked pork. The adult worms are 1–4 mm long and burrow into the mucosa of the small intestine. The larvae are not expelled with the faeces like other intestinal helminths, but pass into the blood stream and settle in the skeletal muscle fibres where they form fibrotic nodules.

Fever is usual and gastrointestinal symptoms may be marked during the acute stage, although they have been minimal in some outbreaks. There is stiffness and weakness of muscles and often there are signs that the CNS or the peripheral nerves have been affected. Two characteristic features are oedema of the eyelids and splinter haemorrhages under the nails. Eosinophilia is almost invariable.

Management. Steroids will reduce symptoms and a course of mebendazole may be effective if the larvae have not been too well encysted.

SCHISTOSOMIASIS (BILHARZIA)

Schistosoma mansoni and *S. japonicum* affect mainly the intestines and abdominal viscera, while *S. haematobium* affects the bladder and ureters. Man is the primary host, with adult worms laying eggs which are passed in either stools or urine. In water, the eggs hatch into larvae (miracidia) which invade species of water snail, where they undergo maturation into larvae (cercariae). These escape from the snail and enter humans through the skin, so close contact with water, such as washing or swimming is necessary for this part of the life cycle. Bilharzia cannot be caught by drinking contaminated water. Once under the skin, the cercariae make their way via the blood stream and the lungs to the liver where they mature. After sexual maturation, moving through the portal blood stream, the female schistosomes deposit their ova in viscera; *S. mansoni* and *S. japonicum* in the large bowel wall, *S. haematobium* in the bladder wall and ureters.

Clinical manifestations depend on the size of the infecting load of cercariae, and on previous exposure. In non-immune subjects, a heavy infestation with *S. mansoni* or *S. japonicum* may result in Katayama syndrome, in which there is a high fever, headache, allergic skin rashes and eosinophilia. In subjects repeatedly exposed to small infecting loads, there may be few symptoms until terminal haematuria (*S. haematobium*) or dysentery-like symptoms (*S. mansoni, S. japonicum*) develop. Repeated exposure to large numbers of any of these parasites may lead to death in early teenage from cor pulmonale, due to pulmonary fibrosis around the eggs and to a lesser extent around the parasites within the lungs. Heavy and repeated infestation by *S. mansoni* and *S. japonicum* may lead to hepatic fibrosis and portal symptoms by a similar mechanism. In long-standing *S. haematobium* infestation, calcification of the bladder and ureters is often found, and chronic renal failure may supervene.

Infection by schistosomes tends to occur early in life, when the passage of eggs will be maximal. As the child grows older and gains immunity fewer eggs will be passed and in adults an active search for eggs by bladder or rectal mucosal biopsy may have to be made. In many areas of Africa double infection with *S. mansoni* and *S. haematobium* is common, and particularly near rivers or lakes, virtually 100% of children will be affected, undermining their general health.

Control of bilharzial spread involves preventing contamination of rivers and lakes with excreta, killing the secondary host (snails), advice against wading or swimming in contaminated water and treatment of individual cases.

Management. Praziquantel is effective in all forms of schistosomiasis. It is given as a single dose of 40 mg/kg. Oxamiquin is only effective in *S. mansoni* (15–30 mg/kg daily for 1–3 days). Metrifonate only affects *S. haematobium* and is given in three doses of 7.5 mg/kg, 2 weeks apart.

Further reading

Morley D. *Paediatric Priorities in the Developing World.* Butterworths London 1973.

Coóvadia HM, Loening WEK. (Eds) *Paediatrics and Child Health.* Oxford University Press, Oxford 1984.

Walker-Smith JA, McNeish AS. (Eds) *Diarrhoea and Malnutrition in Childhood.* Butterworths London 1986.

Ross JD, Horne NW. *Modern Drug Treatment in Tuberculosis,* 6th Edn. The Chest and Stroke Association Edinburgh 1983.

INDEX

Principal references are given in **bold**
Table references are given in *italic*

abdomen
  examination, 11–12
  newborn examination, 58–9
abdominal distension, 193
  causes, *193*
abdominal pain, 204–6
  acute appendicitis, 205–6
  Meckel's diverticulum, 206
  in neuroblastoma, 458
  peptic ulceration, 204–5
  psychosomatic, 347
abetalipoproteinaemia, 372
ABO incompatibility, *106, 107*, 432
abortion, spontaneous, chromosome
    abnormalities and, 119
abscess
  breast, 68
  cerebral, 284
  lung, 178
  orbital, 158
  peritonsillar, 161
acanthocytes, in abetalipoproteinaemia,
  372
accident and emergency department,
  20–1, 515
accidental injury, **513–21**
  birth trauma, 111–12
  burns and scalds, 516
  drowning/near-drowning, *240*, 515
  head injury, *170, 240*, 515–16
  playground accidents, 514
  poisoning, 516–21
  vehicle accidents, 514, 515
achondroplasia, *128*, 484–5
acid-base balance, 276–8
acidosis, 275
  metabolic, 76, 275, **276–7**
  respiratory, 170, 276
acne vulgaris, 502–3
  infantile, 503, *Plate 38*
acquired immune deficiency syndrome
    (AIDS), 361, 369, *527*
acrocyanosis, 56
active tone, 5
adaptation to birth, 53

addiction, drug abuse, 349–50
Addison's disease, 416–17
additives (food)
  hyperactivity and, 294
  urticaria due to, 506
adenocarcinoma, vaginal, 444
adenoids, hypertrophy of, 30, 158–9
adenoma
  islet cell, 407
  pituitary, 417
adipose tissue growth, 38
adoption agencies, 21
adrenal disorders, **413–18**
  congenital hyperplasia, *131*, 278,
    413–15
adrenal failure, post-meningitis, 283
adrenal tumours, 417
adreno-genital syndrome, 413
adult polycystic kidney disease, 256
aerophagy, 74, 193
aflatoxin, 540
agammaglobulinaemia, *131*, 440
agnosia, 332
AIDS, 361, 369, *527*
Alagille's syndrome, 209
Albers–Schoenberg disease, 484
albinism, 317, 505
  ocular, 317
Albright's syndrome, 421
  café-au-lait patches in, 508
alcohol, fetal alcohol syndrome, *391*
alcohol abuse, 349–50
  mental retardation and, *329*
alkalosis, 275
  metabolic, 275, 277–8
  respiratory, 276
allergic disorders
  allergic contact dermatitis, 492
  alveolitis, 187
  aspergillosis, 186–7
  in asthma, 183, 184
  atopic eczema, 490–2
  egg allergy, 199, 506
  history taking, 4
  in hyperactivity, 294
  in Sydenham's chorea, 293
  to animal hair/fur, 183
  urticarial, 506
  see also cow's milk protein intolerance

allergic rhinitis, 157
alopecia, 503–4
  areata, 503–4, *Plate 39*
alpha fetoprotein
  in liver tumour diagnosis, 471
  neural tube defects and, 143–4
alpha-1-antitrypsin deficiency, *107, 131,*
  443
  neonatal hepatitis due to, 189, 208–9
  respiratory disorders due to, *169*, 189
Alport's syndrome, *128*
Alzheimer's disease, 120
  Down's syndrome and, 120
ambiguous genitalia, 418–20
amblyopia, due to persistent squint, 314
amino acid metabolism disorders, 376–8
  Hartnup disease, 377
  homocystinuria, 377, 391
  maple syrup disease, 377
  organic acidaemias, 378
  phenylketonuria, 74, 329, **376–7**, 505
  tyrosinaemia, *107*, 377–8, *443*
  urea cycle disorders, 378
amino acid requirements, of infants, 64
aminoacidaemias, *104*
aminoaciduria, 247
aminophylline, in asthma management,
  185
ammonia dermatitis, 35
  meatal ulcer and, 31
amnesia, following head injury, 515
amoebiasis, 211
amphetamine abuse, 350
anaemia, **423–33**
  aplastic, **428–30**, 452
  B-12 deficiency, 428
  in cancer patient, 446–7
  classification, *425*
  in developing countries, 571–2
  folate deficiency, 427–8, *571*
  glucose-6-phosphate dehydrogenase
    deficiency, *106, 107, 131*, 433
  haemolytic, **430–3**
  hyperactivity and, 294
  investigation of, *426*
  iron-deficiency, 426–7, 571
  in malnutrition, 544
  neonatal, 105–6, 432
  physiological, 105

pica and, 30, 425
in scurvy, 548
sideroblastic, 427
in systemic onset arthritis, 476
see also sickle cell disease; thalassaemia
anal atresia, 142
in Down's syndrome, *119*
anal fissure, 30, 203
neonatal, *203*
analgesia, in cancer management, 447–8
'anaphylactoid purpura', 261
anencephaly, 144
angioedema, 506
animal hair/fur allergy, 183
ankylosing spondylitis, juvenile onset,
476
anorexia nervosa, 341, **348**
delayed puberty in, 397
antenatal diagnosis
in congenital nephrotic syndrome, 264
in Duchenne muscular dystrophy, 135
antibiotic therapy
in acne, 502–3
in acute gastroenteritis in developing
countries, 553
in critically ill child, 242
in cystic fibrosis, 188
in meningitis, 281
in newborn, 96
in pneumonia, *178*
in urinary tract infection, 258–9, *259*
antibody, classification, 352
anticonvulsant therapy, 290
in epilepsy treatment, 290
in newborn, 103
antidepressants
poisoning due to, 519
use in children, 343
antidiarrhoeals, 553
antigen agglutination tests, 351
antispasmodics, for evening colic, 75
antiviral agents, in pneumonia, 180
aorta, coarctation of, *122*, 232
aortic stenosis, 232–3
heart sounds in, 9
pulse assessment in, 8
sudden death due to, 226, 232
Apert's syndrome, *137*
apex beat, 8
Apgar score, 55–6, *56*
aplastic anaemias, **428–30**
classification, *429*
Diamond–Blackfan, 429–30
Fanconi's, *391*, 429, *443*
versus acute lymphoblastic leukaemia,
452
apnoea, neonatal, 97–100
'apnoea of prematurity', 97–8
causes, *97*
intrapartum asphyxia, 54, *111*
obstructive, 98–100
apnoea monitors, 512–13
appendicitis
acute, 205–6
threadworm infestation and, 33
aqueduct stenosis, 295
Area Child Protection Committee, 524
Arnold–Chiari malformation, 146
arrhythmias *see* cardiac arrhythmias
arthritis, **474–6**

pauciarticular, 475
polyarticular disease, 476
psoriatic, 476
reactive arthropathy, 476
Reiter's disease, 476
in rubella infection, 356–7
septic, 479, 480–1
spondiloarthritis, 476
systemic, 476
terminology problems, 475
torticollis due to, 483
arthrogryposis multiplex, 150–1
in trisomy-18, 122
ascaris, 573
Asperger's syndrome, 345
aspergillosis, 186–7
asphyxia
crying and, 29
in drowning/near-drowning, 515
due to suffocation from pillow, 514
handicap risks following, *103*
intrapartum, 54, *111*
perinatal, 100–1
in sudden infant death syndrome, 511
aspirin
Reye's syndrome and, 211
in rheumatic fever treatment, 477
aspirin poisoning *see* salicylate poisoning
asthma, 165–9, **183–7**
aspergillosis and, 186
atopic eczema and, 490
chest pain in, 225
failure to thrive due to, *527*
respiratory failure due to, *170*
astigmatism, 316
astrocytomas, 464
At-Risk Register, 524, 526
ataxia, **292–3**
in abetalipoproteinaemia, 372
acute cerebellar, 292–3
in cerebral palsy, 323–4
Friedreich's, 293
in Hartnup disease, 377
in medulloblastoma, 463
in metachromatic leukodystrophy, 374
in neuroblastoma, 458
in solvent abuse, 521
ataxia-telangiectasia, 293, *301*
immunodeficiency and, 440
tumour predisposition in, *443*
athetosis, 293
in cerebral palsy, 323
athlete's foot, 496
atopic eczema, 490–2, *Plate 19*
molluscum contagiosum and, 494
atopy *see* allergic disorders
atrial flutter/fibrillation, 226–7
atrial septal defect, 228–9
in Down's syndrome, *119*
heart sounds in, 9
recurrence risk for siblings, *133*
attachment behaviour, abnormal, 334–5
attention deficit disorder, 341
amphetamines in, 343
audiometry, 309–10
autism, 335, 341–2, **345–6**
cataracts and, 25
crying and, 29
educational therapies, 344
in fragile X syndrome, 127

autopsy
following fatal illness, 245
following sudden infant death
syndrome, 512
autosomal dominant disorders, 127–9
autosomal recessive disorders, 129–31
Axline, Virginia, 344

B-12 deficiency, 428
Bacillus Calmette-Guérin *see* BCG
vaccination
bacterial endocarditis, prevention, 239
bacterial infections, **362–6**
diagnosis, 351, *352*
in immunosuppressed child, 446–7
of liver, 211
of skin, 495
see also under specific infection
bacterial meningitis, 280–2, 366
bag-and-mask resuscitation, 55
balance, disorders of, 307–8
ataxia, 292–3
balanoposthitis, 31
banding, 118
barbiturate abuse, 350
barbiturate poisoning, 519
Barlow's test, 60
Bartter's syndrome, 278
bath temperature, 514
Batten's disease, 374
battered baby syndrome *see* non-
accidental injury
battery ingestion, 520
BCG vaccination, 189, 355–6, 565
in developing countries, 535, 565
immunization schedule, 353
Becker-type muscular dystrophy, 298
Beckwith–Wiedeman syndrome, *104*, *137*
Beckwith's syndrome, *443*
beclomethasone, in asthma management,
186
bed-wetting, 26–7
behaviour therapy, 344
behavioural disorders, **334–50**
assessment, 335–42
classification, 338–42
diagnosis, 338–42
encopresis, 27–8, 201, **348–9**
high intelligence and, 332
in mentally handicapped, 330, 340
minor, **23–9**
negativistic phase and, 23, 25, 28, 201,
303
positive reinforcement and, 27
in sexually abused child, *525*
speech problems and, 303
'star chart' and, 27, 201, 349
in temporal lobe epilepsy, 288
treatment, 343–5
see also emotional disorders
Bell's palsy, 300
benign focal epilepsy of childhood, 288
benign intracranial hypertension, 297
benign paroxysmal vertigo, 307–8
benzodiazepine abuse, 350
benzodiazepines, as anticonvulsants, 290
bereavement, reactions, 346
Berger's disease, 261
beri-beri, 547

bicarbonate, normal plasma levels, 276
bilharzia (schistosomiasis), 530, 575
biliary atresia
  extrahepatic, 209
  neonatal jaundice and, *107*, 108
biopsy
  in cancer diagnosis, 451
  renal, 250
  skin, 487
birth, adaptation of fetus, 53
birth asphyxia, 100–1
  cerebral palsy due to, *321*, 324
birth injury, 111–12
  subdural haemorrhage, 516
birth weight, 52, 77
  see also low birth weight
blackheads, 502
bladder extrophy, 255–6
bleach ingestion, 520
bleeding disorders, **433–9**
  acquired, 438–9
  inherited, 436–8
  investigations, *434*
  in newborn, 110–11
blindness, 315–17, 319
  causes, *315*
  in cerebral palsy, 322
  cortical, 317, 322
  in osteopetrosis, 485
blistering skin diseases, 500–2
Bloch-Sulzberger disease, 501–2
blood cultures, 351
blood groups, ABO incompatibility, *106*,
  107, 432
blood pressure
  measurement technique, 10
  normal values, 269, *271*
  raised *see* hypertension
blood transfusion, neonatal exchange
  transfusion, 110
Bloom's syndrome, tumour predisposition
  in, *443*
body water, composition at different ages,
  273
boils, 36
bonding of mother–child, 522–3
bone
  skeletal growth, 38, 474
  tuberculosis of, 562–3
bone disorders, **474–85**
  see also under specific disorder
bone marrow transplantation
  in acute lymphoblastic leukaemia, 455
  in acute myeloid leukaemia, 456
  in aplastic anaemia, 429
  in severe immunodeficiency, 440
bone scans, role in cancer diagnosis, 450,
  460
bone tumours, **466–70**
  osteosarcoma, 466–9
  see also Ewing's sarcoma
Bornholm disease, 174
bottom shuffling, 42, 325
  in cerebral palsy, 325
botulism, 365
bow legs, 33
bowing of the tibia, 34
brachial plexus injury, due to birth
  trauma, 112
brachiofemoral delay, 226

brachycephaly, 148
brain disorders, disability due to, 319–33
brain growth, 37
brain stem death, 245, 295, 516
brain stem glioma, 465
brain tumours, 445, **462–5**
  torticollis due to, 483
branchial cleft cysts, 163
breast abscess, 68
breast engorgement
  in mother, 67–8
  in newborn, 58
breast feeding, **64–70**
  complement formula feeds, 67
  contraindications, 68–9, 200
  in developing countries, 537
  guide to use of common drugs, *69*
  infection risks and, 32
  neonatal rickets and, 114
  non-nutritive sucking, 67
  as protection against gastroenteritis,
    193
  respiratory infections and, 189
  SIDS risks and, 511
  technique, 67
  weaning, 72–3
breast milk, 63–7
  anti-infective properties, 68
  bank, 69–70
  compared to cow's and formula milk,
    63, 70
  drugs in, *69*, 69
  expression of, for sick infant, 84
  human immunodeficiency virus (HIV)
    in, 70, 361
  pasteurization, 69–70
  variations in, 65–6
breast milk jaundice, 107
breath-holding attacks, 31–2
  versus convulsions, 289
breath sounds
  bronchial, 10–11
  crepitations, 11
  rhonchi, 11
  vesicular, 10–11
British Ability Scales, 327
brittle bone disease, 484
bronchial abnormalities, 172–3
bronchiectasis, 181–2
  failure to thrive due to, *527*
  predisposing factors, *181*
  wheeze due to, *169*
bronchiolitis, 179–80
bronchitis, 180–1
bronchogenic cysts, 173, 189
bronchopulmonary dysplasia, *86*, 94
brucellosis, 364
Bruton's disease, *131*, 440
  tumour predisposition in, *443*
Budd-Chiari syndrome, 212–13
budesonide, in asthma management, 186
bullous dermatosis of childhood, chronic,
  501, *Plate 37*
bullous icthyosiform erythroderma, 490
bullous pemphigoid, 501
buphthalmos (glaucoma), 316–17
Burkitt's lymphoma, **458**
  genetic factors, 442
  viral factors, 444
burns, 516

shock due to, *240*
buzzer alarm, in enuresis treatment, 27

Caesarean section
  mother–child bonding following, 522
  role in premature infant delivery, 80
café-au-lait patches, 508
calcium metabolism disorders *see*
  hypocalcaemia; hypercalcaemia
cancer, **442–73**
  aetiology, 442–4
  bone tumours, 466–70
  brain tumours, **462–5**, 483
  genetic factors, 442–4
  germ cell tumours, 471–2
  liver tumours, 471
  management, 444–5
  out-patient care, 448
  presentation, 448
  see also under specific tumour
cancrum oris, 546
candida infection, 497
  nappy rash due to, 35–6
  of throat, 161
car accidents, 514, 515
carbamazepine, as anticonvulsant, 290
carbohydrate intolerance, 74, 200
  abdominal distension due to, *193*
carbohydrate metabolism disorders,
  370–2
  fructosaemia, *107, 208*, 371, *527*
carbohydrate requirements, of infants, 64
cardiac arrhythmias, **226–7**
  collapse due to, 222
  faints and, 32
  shock due to, *240*
  sudden infant death syndrome and, *511*
  versus convulsions, 289
cardiac catheterization, 219
cardiac failure
  causes, 222
  failure to thrive due to, *527*
  neonatal respiratory distress and, *86*
  in Pompe's disease, 372
  in rheumatic fever, 476
  wheeze due to, *169*
cardiac murmurs *see* murmurs
cardiac pain, 225
cardiomyopathy, 238
cardiorespiratory arrest
  causes, *240*
  management, 241–2, *242*
cardiovascular disorders, **214–39**
  acquired, 237–9
  congenital, 227–37
  investigative techniques, 216–19
  pulse abnormalities, 226
  see also cardiac arrhythmias
cardiovascular system
  examination, 8–10
  newborn examination, 58
care order, 21
case conference, in child abuse, 524, 526
cataract, 315–16
  autism and, 25
  causes, *316*
  congenital, 57
  in galactosaemia, 370, 371
catarrhal otitis media, 155

'catch up growth', 37
  following malnutrition, 545–6
catheterization, cardiac, 219
cellulitis, *versus* osteomyelitis, 482
central venous catheters, in cancer
    patient, 447
cephalhaematoma, 57, 106, *111*, 112
cerebellar astrocytoma, 465
cerebellar ataxia, 292–3
cerebral abscess, following meningitis,
    284
cerebral gigantism, 392
cerebral palsy, **320–7**
  causes, *321*
  classification *321*
  due to kernicterus, 109, 293, 321
  dysphagia and, 191
  early diagnosis, 324–5
  failure to thrive due to, *527*
  following meningitis, 283, *321*
  microcephaly and, 147
  pertussis vaccination and, 354
cerebrospinal fluid, culture, 351
cervical adenitis, in tuberculosis, 561–2,
    Plate 50
Charcot–Marie–Tooth disease, 300
chemotherapy, 444–5
  complications, 446–7
cherry-red spot
  in metachromatic leukodystrophy, 374
  in Niemann–Pick disease, 373
  in Tay–Sachs disease, 373
chest expansion, assessment, 10
chest pain, in cardiovascular disorders,
    225
chest wall deformities, 171–2
chickenpox (varicella), **358–9**
  in cancer patient, 448, 454
  cerebellar ataxia and, 292
  chickenpox pneumonitis, 179
  vaccine, 356
chilblains, 36
  child abuse, 345, **521–8**
  failure to thrive, 526–8
  Munchausen syndrome by proxy, 248,
    521, **528**
  police involvement, 21–2
  psychological management, 345
  somatic pains and, 347
  see also non-accidental injury; sexual
    abuse
child development unit, 320
  in cerebral palsy evaluation, 325–6
child guidance service, 21
child health provision, in developing
    countries, **529–36**
Child Protection (At-Risk) Register, 524,
    526
chlamydial infection
  diagnostic test, 351
  neonatal pneumonitis, 89, *94*
chloramphenicol, use in newborn, 96
chloridorrhoea, 200
choanal atresia, 156
choledochal cyst, neonatal jaundice and,
    107
chorea, 293
  athetoid cerebral palsy, 323
  rheumatic, 570
  in rheumatic fever, 476

versus habit spasm, 28
chorioretinitis, in congenital
    toxoplasmosis, 369
christmas disease, *110, 111, 131*, 437
chromosome disorders, **119–27**, 137
  karyotype-XXX, 392
  in malignant disease, 442–3
  mental retardation due to, *329*
  see also under specific disorder
chromosome(s)
  normal karyotype, 117–18
  Philadelphia, 454, 455
  structure/function, 117
chronic granulocytic leukaemia 455
  oncogenes and, 443
chronic lung disease, neonatal, 93–5
chronic lymphocytic leukaemia, 455
chronic pulmonary insufficiency of
    prematurity, *86, 94*, 95
chronic pyelonephritis, 257
chronic renal failure, 266–8
cicatricial pemphigoid, 501
circumcision, in paraphimosis treatment,
    30
cirrhosis, 211–12
  abdominal distension due to, *193*
  failure to thrive due to, *527*
cleft lip/palate, 57, 138–9
  breast feeding and, 68
  otitis media and, 154
  recurrence risk for siblings, *133*
  in trisomy-13, *122*
cleido-cranial dysostosis, 484
clinical examination, *4–14*
  in child abuse, 523–4
  in dermatology, 487
  neonatal hearing assessment, 308
  neonatal visual assessment, 312
  of nervous system, 279
  of newborn, 56–62
  in sexual abuse, 525–6
clonazepan, in newborn, 103
clonus, 322
Clostridia botulinum poisoning, 365
clotting factor deficiency, 111
club foot (talipes), 149–50
clubbing, 5
  in bronchiectasis, 181
  due to whipworm, 574
clumsy child, 331–2
cluster headaches, 291–2
coagulation disorders, **433–9**
  acute idiopathic thrombocytopenic
    purpura, 438
  haemophilia A, 436–7
  haemophilia B (christmas disease), *110,
    111, 131*, 437
  von Willebrand's disease, *128*, 437–8
  see also disseminated intravascular
    coagulation
coarctation of aorta, 232
  in trisomy-18, *122*
cocaine abuse, 350
coeliac disease, 196–8, *Plate 3*
  abdominal distension due to, *193*
  diabetes and, 402
  failure to thrive due to, *527*
  folate deficiency in, 428
  short stature and, 391
cold sores, 494

colic, 74–5
  crying and, *29*
colitis, cow's milk, 199
collodion baby, 490, *Plate 18*
coloboma, ocular, 317
colostrum, 66–7
  protein content, 64
  secretion in third trimester, 65
colour vision defects, *131*, 314
coma, 294–5
  following barbiturate poisoning, 519
comedones (blackheads), 502
common cold (coryza), 32, 157
community child health care, 18
community services for children, 18–19
complement, 352
  levels in glomerulonephritis, 260, 261
computerized tomography (CT)
  in cancer diagnosis, 450
  in kidney disorders, 250
  in nervous system disorders, 279
concomitant squint, 314
conduct disorders, 338–40
congenital abnormalities, **136–51**
  see also under specific abnormality
congenital adrenal hyperplasia, 413–15
  biochemical abnormalities, *415*
congenital adrenal hypoplasia, 415–16
congenital diaphragmatic hernia, 90–1
congenital dislocation of hips, 34, 59–60,
    150
congenital heart disease, **227–37**
  aetiology, *215*
  recurrence risk for siblings, *133*
  see also under specific disease
congenital infections, 367–9
  cytomegalovirus, 367
  HIV infection, 367–8
  rubella, 367
  syphilis, 369
  toxoplasmosis, 369
congenital lobar emphysema, 173
congenital microvillous atrophy, 200
congenital myasthenia, 299
congenital myopathy, 301
congenital nephrotic syndrome, 264
congenital tuberculosis, 563
conjunctivitis
  in chlamydia pneumonia, 89
  in Kawasaki's disease, 479
  in tuberculosis, 559–60
consciousness, in head injuries, 515
constipation, 28, **200–2**
  abdominal distension due to, *193*
  in acute appendicitis, 206
  anal fissure and, 30
  encopresis and, 348, 349
  enuresis due to, 27
  in Hirschsprung's disease, 201
  in infancy; 75
  reflex anal dilatation test and, 526
convulsions, **284–90**
  definition, 284
  differential diagnosis, 289
  due to cardiac arrhythmias, 226
  febrile, 285–6
  following tapeworm infestation, 574
  hypoglycaemic, 104
  management, 290
  neonatal, 100–3, 105

convulsions *contd*
  in solvent abuse, 521
  in spastic hemiplegia, 322
  teething and, 29
  in trisomy-13, 123
  see also epilepsy; seizures
Cooley's anaemia, 430
Coombs' test, 108
cor pulmonale, 94
  in cystic fibrosis, 187
  due to adenoidal hypertrophy, 158
  due to schistosomiasis, 575
cortical blindness, 317
  in cerebral palsy, 322
coryza, 32, 157
cot death *see* sudden infant death
      syndrome
cough, 166–8
  causes, *167*
  psychogenic, 168
counselling
  genetic *see* genetic counselling
  of mother of non-thriving child, 527
  of parents of SIDS baby, 512
Court Report (1976), 16–17
cover test, 313
cow's milk colitis, 199
  rectal bleeding due to, *203*
cow's milk protein intolerance, 74,
      198–9, *Plate 4*
  abdominal distension due to, *193*
  failure to thrive due to, *527*
  pulmonary haemosiderosis and, 189
  versus gastroenteritis, 195
coxsackie virus infection, neonatal
      hepatitis syndrome due to, *208*
crab lice, 500
cracked nipples, 67
cradle cap (seborrhoeic dermatitis), 36
cranial nerve palsy, due to brain tumour,
      463
cranio-pharyngioma, 465
cranio-synostosis, 147–8, 474
craniotabes, 57
'cretinism', 411
Creutzfeldt–Jacob disease, due to growth
      hormone therapy, 389
cri du chat syndrome, crying and, *29*
crib death *see* sudden infant death
      syndrome
Crigler–Najjar syndrome, *107*
critically ill child, **240–5**
Crohn's disease, 202
  versus anorexia, 348
croup, 159–60
Crouzon's syndrome, *137*
crying, 28–9
  at night, 26
  in meningitis, 280
  normal, 28–9, 51
  organic causes, *29*
cryotherapy, in wart treatment, 493
CSF (cerebrospinal fluid), culture, 351
CT scans *see* computerized tomography
curd, 64, 70
curly toes, 35
Cushing's response, 296
Cushing's syndrome, 278, 386, 417
cyanosis
  cardiac *versus* respiratory, 217, 220

lesions associated with, 234–7
  neonatal causes, *220*
  as sign of cardiovascular disease,
      219–22
cyanotic heart disease, 217, 220, *233*
cystic adenomatous malformation, 174
cystic fibrosis, *131*, **187–9**, 199
  abdominal distension due to, *193*
  chronic diarrhoea in, 199
  failure to thrive due to, *527*
  fat intolerance in, 74, 187, 199
  haemoptysis due to, *167*
  neonatal jaundice and, *107*
  pancreatic lipase deficiency in, 74, 199
  portal hypertension in, 212
  rectal prolapse in, 187, 204
  respiratory failure due to, *170*
  wheeze due to, *169*
cystic hygroma, 163–4
  differential diagnosis, *450*
cystic peri-ventricular leukomalacia,
      cerebral palsy due to, 324
cystinosis, 268, 379–80
cystinuria, 380
  renal stones and, 268
cysts (congenital)
  bronchogenic, 173, 189
  of gastrointestinal tract, 189
  of lung, 189
  of pericardium, 189
cytomegalovirus infection, 360
  in cancer patient, 446
  cerebral palsy due to, *321*
  congenital, 367
  prenatal, 77, 78, *106*
cytotoxic agents, malignancy risks of, 444

'dancing eyes' syndrome, in
      neuroblastoma, 458
Dandy–Walker malformation, 295
day case procedures, 20
de Toni–Febre–Fanconi syndrome, 380
deafness, **308–11**
  in cerebral palsy, 323
  following meningitis, 283
  in genetic bone disorders, 484
  in Hunter's syndrome, 375
  management of deaf child, 310–11
  sensorineural, 109
  speech delay and, 42, 303
  see also hearing impairment
death
  brain stem death, 245, 295, 516
  causes in children 1–14 years, *16*
  of critically ill child, 244, 245
  from asthma, 186
  mortality rates, *15*, 15–17, *16*, *17*
  neonatal, 21
  sudden infant death syndrome, 15,
      510–13, 365
  terminal care, 448
DEBRA (Dystrophic Epidermolysis
      Bullosa Research Association), 501
dehydration, 274–6
  clinical assessment, *194*, *274*
  management, 194–5, 275–6
Dejerine–Sottas disease, 300
delayed development, 42, 340, 390, 527
delayed visual maturation, 317
delinquency, 340

dementia
  in Batten's disease, 374
  following tapeworm infestation, 574
dental maturation, *41*, 41
dentigenesis imperfecta, 484
depressive illness, 346
dermatitis
  ammonia, 35
  herpetiformis, 501
  napkin, 492–3, *Plate 22*
  seborrhoeic, 35, 36
  see also eczema
dermatomyositis, 477–8, *Plates 10–11*
dermatophyte infection, 495–6
desferrioxamine, 431
detachment, 335
development
  assessment, 43–50
  normal, **37–51**
developmental anomalies, 147–8
  craniosynostosis, 147–8
  microcephaly, 147
  plagiocephaly, 148
developmental delay, 42, 340, 390
  in child abuse, 527
developmental dysphasia, 304
developmental impairment, following
      cancer treatment, 445–6
developmental milestones, *42*
developmental psychopathology, 334–5
developmental quotient (DQ), 41, 328
dexamethasone, in bronchopulmonary
      dysplasia management, 94
di George syndrome, 420
diabetes insipidus, 408–9
  enuresis due to, *27*
  in Langerhans' cell histiocytosis, 473
  nephrogenetic, 269
diabetes mellitus, **397–405**
  diabetic coma *versus* salicylate
      poisoning, 518
  enuresis due to, *27*
  in infancy, 405
  infants of diabetic mothers, 86, 104
  in Klinefelter's syndrome, 126
  recurrent boils and, 36
  versus hypernatraemic dehydration,
      275
diabetic ketoacidosis (DKA), 398, **403–4**
dialysis
  in acute renal failure, 265
  in chronic renal failure, 266–7
Diamond–Blackfan anaemia, 429–30
diaphragmatic abnormalities, 189
  see also diaphragmatic hernia
diaphragmatic hernia (congenital), *86*,
      90–1, *93*
  prenatal surgery for, 165
  pulmonary abnormalities, 165, 173
diarrhoea, **193–200**
  acute, 193–5
  in cancer patient, 447
  chronic, 195–200, *527*
  in infancy, 75
  in malnutrition, 544–5
  in measles, 555
  in salmonella infections, 364
  toddler's, 30, 196
  see also gastroenteritis
diastematomyelia, enuresis due to, *27*

DIC *see* disseminated intravascular coagulation
diet
in coeliac disease, 197
in diabetes, 400
of infants in developing countries, 537, *538*
role in acne, 503
role in constipation, 201
role in eczema, 491
role in hyperactivity, 294
role in urticaria, 506
specialized diets in infancy, 73–4
see also feeding problems
diethylenetriaminepentacetic (DTPA) scan, 249
dimercaptosuccinic acid (DMSA) scan, 249
diphtheria, **362–3**
heart block in, 227
immunization, *353*, 354
immunization in developing countries, 535
stridor due to, *159*
disability, *definition*, 319
disaccharide deficiency, failure to thrive due to, *527*
discoid eczema, 492
dislocated hips (congenital), 34, 59–60, 150
in cerebral palsy, 325
disseminated intravascular coagulation, *106*, 110, **438–9**
in acute myeloid leukaemia, 455
in measles, 375, 555
distraction test of hearing, 308–9
district handicap team (DHT), 320
district nurses, 18
DMSA scan, 249
Down's syndrome, **119–21**
alopecia areata in, 504
atrial septal defect in, 229
chromosome abnormalities in, *121*
common abnormalities in, *119*
educational needs, 330–1
failure to thrive due to, *527*
intrauterine growth retardation, 78
maternal age-specific risk, *121*
otitis media in, 154
short stature in, *391*
torticollis in, 483
doxapram, in obstructive apnoea management, 100
DQ (developmental quotient), 41
drowning/near-drowning, *240*, 515
drug abuse, 349–50
drug allergy, urticaria due to, 506
dry cleaning fluid, solvent abuse of, 521
D^{T}PA scan, 249
Dubin–Johnson syndrome, neonatal jaundice and, *107*
Dubowitz method, 80–4
Duchenne muscular dystrophy, 298
cardiomyopathy in, 238
clinical features, *131*
genetic counselling, 134–5
genetics of, 117, 134–5
scoliosis in, 483
ductus arteriosus, function of, 53
ductus arteriosus, patent, *88, 94*, 114

prostaglandin therapy and, 221
duodenal atresia, 142
in Down's syndrome, *119*
dwarfism, *128*, 484–5
dysarthria, 304
dyschondrosteosis, 388
dysentry, *versus* ulcerative colitis, 203
dyslexia, 304, 332–3
dysmotile cilia syndrome, 181, **182–3**
dysphagia, 191
dysphasia, 304
dyspnoea, 168–9
dyspraxia
clumsiness due to, 332
verbal, 304
dystrophia myotonia congenita, 301
Dystrophic Epidermolysis Bullosa Research Association, 501
dystrophin, 117
dysuria, 31
due to bladder tumour, 465
due to sexual abuse, 525

ear, examination, 13–14, 152–4
ear disorders, **152–6, 307–11**
balance disorders, 307–8
earache, 156
glue ear, 153, 155, 158
mastoiditis, 155
otitis externa, 154
otitis media *see* otitis media
see also deafness; hearing impairment
earache, 156
Ebstein's anomaly, 226–7
ecchymoses, 434
ECG, 216
features of cardiac abnormalities, *216*
low potassium effects, 275
normal values, *216*
echolalia, in autism, 345
ectopia vesica, enuresis due to, 27
ectopic ureter, enuresis due to, 27
ectropion, in collodion baby, 490
eczema, **490–3**
allergic contact dermatitis, 492
atopic, 490–2, *Plate 19*
cradle cap and, 36
discoid, 492
herpeticum, 359, 491, 495, *Plates 8 and 20*
history taking, 487
hypopigmentation following, 505
infantile seborrhoeic dermatitis, 492, *Plate 21*
juvenile plantar dermatosis, 493, *Plate 23*
molluscum contagiosum and, 494
napkin dermatitis, 492–3, *Plate 22*
in phenylketonuria, 376
pityriasis alba, 492
versus athlete's foot, 496
education
of deaf child, 311
educational subnormality, 328, 331
of handicapped child, 320
history taking, 3
in hospital, 20
of mentally handicapped, 330–1
role of education department, 21

school absenteeism due to respiratory problems, 165
school behaviour *versus* home behaviour, 336
school difficulties in depressive illness, 346
school medical services, 18–19
school refusal/truancy, 335, 346–7
'special educational needs', 320
special educational therapies, 344
Edwards' syndrome *see* trisomy-18
EEG
in epilepsy diagnosis, 284
hypsarrhythmia, 287
egg allergy, 199, 506
Ehlers–Danlos syndrome, 434, 485
Eisenmenger complex, 221, **228**
elbow, pulled, 484
electrocardiogram, 216
features of cardiac abnormalities, *216*
low potassium effects, 275
normal values, *216*
electroencephalogram (EEG)
in epilepsy diagnosis, 284
hypsarrhythmia, 287
electrolyte problems, **273–8**
electrolyte requirements, normal, 273–4
Ellis–van Creveld syndrome, heart disease in, *215*
emergency management of critically ill child, 241–5
emollients, in eczema management, 491
emotional deprivation
developmental delay and, 42, 390
failure to thrive due to, *527*
mental retardation due to, *329*
role in child abuse, 522
emotional disorders, **334–50**
in diabetic families, 404–5
due to dysphasia/dyslexia, 304
hyperactivity and, 294
in mentally handicaped, 331, 341–2
periodic syndrome, 292
precocious puberty and, 396
trichotillomania in, 504
see also behavioural disorders
empyema, 175
encephalitis, 283–4
deafness and, 310
measles, 357
respiratory failure due to, *170*
encephalocele, 144
encephalopathy
causes, *294*
lead, 520
measles, 555
post-asphyxial, *100*
solvent, 521
encopresis, 27–8, 201, **348–9**
endocardial fibroelastosis, 237
endocrine disorders, **382–442**
see also under specific disorder
energy requirement, of infants, 63
engorgement of breast
in mother, 67–8
in newborn, 58
enteric fever, 365
enuresis, 26–7, 349
age for treatment, 334
causes, 27

enuresis *contd*
  management, 27, 349
  threadworm infestation and, 33
environmental factors
  in cancer aetiology, 444
  in leukaemia aetiology, 451
eosinophilic granuloma, *versus*
    osteosarcoma, 467
ependymomas, 464
ephedrine, in coryza treatment, 32
epidemic myalgia (Bornholm disease),
    174
epidermolysis bullosa, 500–1, *Plate 36*
  skin biopsy in, 487
epididymitis, 31
  versus testicular torsion, 394
epididymo-orchitis, following mumps,
    358
epiglottitis
  acute, 160
  respiratory failure due to, *170*
epilepsia partialis continua, 288
epilepsy, **284–90**
  benign focal, 288
  in cerebral palsy, 321
  in mentally handicapped, 331
  pertussis vaccination and, 354
  status epilepticus, 286
  in systemic lupus erythematosus, *478*
  temporal lobe, 288–9
  treatment, 290
  versus breath-holding attacks, 32, 289
  versus faints, 32, 33, 289
epispadias, 59
  bladder extrophy and, 256
  enuresis due to, *27*
epistaxis, 157
  causes, *156*
Epstein–Barr virus, 360, 444
Epstein's pearls, 57
Erb's palsy, *111*, 112
erythema infectiosum, 357–8, *Plate 7*
erythema marginatum, in rheumatic
    fever, 476
erythema multiforme, 507, *Plate 42*
erythema, nodosum, 559
  causes, *559*
  Mantoux test in, 557
erythema pernio, 36
erythropoietin, management of renal
    failure, 266
ethmoiditis, acute, 158
Eustachian tube dysfunction, 154
evening colic, 74–5
Ewing's sarcoma, 469–70
  differential diagnosis, *450*
  pleural effusion due to, *175*
  versus osteosarcoma, 467
examination *see* clinical examination
exanthem subitum, 358
exomphalos, 143
  in trisomy-13, *122*
exons, 117
extradural haematoma, 516
extrahepatic biliary atresia, 209
extrinsic allergic alveolitis, 187
eye disorders, **311–18**
  in albinism, 317, 505
  coloboma, 317
  colour blindness, *131*, 314

in congenital rubella, 367
in congenital toxoplasmosis, 369
cortical blindness, 317, 322
delayed visual maturation, 317
in erythema multiforme, 507
in facial nerve palsy, 112
glaucoma, 316–17
Leber's amaurosis, 317
in Marfan's syndrome, 485
in measles, 554
in neonatal chlamydial infection, 89
in pauciarticular arthritis, 475
refractive errors, 316
see also blindness; cataract; nystagmus;
    retinoblastoma; squint
eye examination, 5
  in newborn, 57
eye movements, assessment, 5
eyelashes, crab lice on, 500

facial nerve palsy, 300
  assessment, 5
  due to birth trauma, *111*, 112, 300
faints, 32
  due to cardiac arrhythmias, 226
  hyperventilation and, 170
  versus convulsions, 289
Fallot's tetralogy, 235–6
  cyanosis in, 221
  in Down's syndrome, *119*
familial dysautonomia, *131*
familial hypercholesterolaemia, *128*
familial short stature, 388
family interviews, 338–42
family therapy, 344
Fanconi's anaemia, 429
  short stature and, *391*
  tumour predisposition in, *443*
Fanconi's syndrome (tubular rickets), 379
fat child, 392
  see also obesity
fat intolerance, 74
fat requirements, of infants, 63
favism, 433
fears and tantrums, 334
febrile convulsions, 285–6
  treatment, 290
feeding
  of critically ill child, 243
  of infants, **63–76**
  of infants in developing countries, 537
  see also diet
feeding problems
  in cerebral palsy, 324
  food fads, 24
  food refusal, 23–4
  in infancy, 74–5
  obesity development, 38
femoral anteversion, 33–4
femoral retroversion, 34
ferritin, 426
fetal alcohol syndrome, short stature and,
    391
fever, crying and, *29*
fever of unknown origin, 369
  investigations, *368*
  in Munchausen syndrome by proxy,
    528
  systemic arthritis following, 476

'fifth day fits', *100*, 102, *102*,
fifth disease, **357–8**, *Plate 7*
fine motor development, 49–50
fingers
  extra, 35
  fused, 35
fire hazards, 513
fireguards, 513
fireworks, 514
first aid, management of critically ill child,
    241
fish allergy, 506
fits *see* convulsions; seizures
flat foot, 34
floppy infant, causes, *300*
flu vaccine, 356
fluid and electrolyte problems, **273–8**
fluid requirements
  of infants, 63
  normal, 273–4
fluoride, in breast milk, 64
focal seizures, 288
folate deficiency, 427–8, *571*
folliculitis, 36
Fontan procedure, 235
fontanelle examination, 5, 56
food additives
  hyperactivity and, 294
  urticaria due to, 506
food allergies, 199, 506
  see also cow's milk protein intolerance
food fads, 24
food poisoning, 365
food refusal, 23–4
forced alkaline diuresis, in poisoning
    management, 517
foreign body
  in ear, 166
  inhaled, *170*
formula feeds, 70–3
  specialized diets, 73
fragile X syndrome, 126–7
  autism and, 345
Freud, Anna, 337
Freud, Sigmund, 343–4
Friedreich's ataxia, 293
fructosaemia, 371
  failure to thrive due to, 527
  neonatal, *107*, *208*
fructosuria, 371
fungal infections
  Candida, 35–6, 161
  histoplasmosis, 366–7
  of skin, 495–7
funnel chest, 172
funny turns, cardiac causes, 225–6
furunculosis, 36

galactosaemia, 74, *104*, **370–1**
  failure to thrive due to, *527*
  neonatal hepatitis syndrome due to, *208*
  rickets due to, 379
  tumour predisposition in, *443*
gamma benzene hexachloride, 498–9
ganglioneuroblastoma, differential
    diagnosis, *450*
ganglioneuroma, 418, 460
  differential diagnosis, *450*
gangliosidoses, 373

'gargoylism', 375
gastro-oesophageal reflux, 24, 98, 192
    sudden infant death syndrome and, *511*
gastroenteritis, 194
    in developing countries, **552–3**
    infective, 193–5
    lactose intolerance following, 74
    in newborn, 65
    Salmonella, 364
gastrointestinal disorders, **191–213**
    abdominal distension, 193
    abdominal pain, 204–6
    dysphagia, 191
    hepatic disease, 206–13
    inflammatory bowel disease, 202–3
    minor, **29–30**
    rectal bleeding, 203–4
    see also constipation; diarrhoea;
        vomiting
gastrointestinal malformations, **137–43**
    anal atresia, 142
    duodenal atresia, 142
    exomphalos, 143
    gastroschisis, 143
    inguinal hernia, 143
    intestinal obstruction, 140–2
    malrotation, 142
    Meckel's diverticulum, 142–3
    oesophageal atresia, 139–40
    small bowel atresia, 142
    tracheo-oesophageal fistula, 139–40
    see also cleft lip/palate
gastroschisis, 143
Gaucher's disease, 373
    neonatal hepatitis syndrome due to, *208*
gender, in child with ambiguous genitalia,
        418–20
genetic counselling, **134–5**
    in Down's syndrome, 120
    in fragile X syndrome, 127
    in multifactorial disorders, 133
    in Tay–Sachs disease, 373
    in thalassaemia, 430, 431
genetic disorders, **116–35**
    see also under specific disorder
genetic finger-printing, 116
genetics, 116–18
    autosomal dominant inheritance,
        127–9
    autosomal recessive inheritance, 129–
        30
    chromosome structure/function, 117
    gene structure, 116–17
    normal karyotype, 117–18
genital herpes, 494
genital warts, 494
genitalia
    ambiguous, 414, **418–20**
    examination, 13
    examination in sexual abuse, 525–6
    newborn examination, 59
genitourinary system disorders, minor,
        30–1
genitourinary tract malformations, 148–9
    hypospadias, 59, 148–9
    renal agenesis, 148
genu valgum, 33
germ cell tumours, 471–2
    ovarian tumours, 472
    sacrococcygeal teratoma, 472

testicular teratoma, 471–2
german measles *see* rubella
germinal matrix haemorrhage, 101
gestation
    assessment, 80–4
    Dubowitz assessment method, 80–4
giardiasis, 199
'gifted' child, 332
gigantism, 391
    cerebral (Soto's syndrome), 392
Gilles de la Tourette syndrome, 341, 343
glandular fever, 360
glaucoma (buphthalmos), 316–17
    in retinoblastoma, 470
glomerular filtration rate, 248
glomerulonephritis
    following scabies infestation, 498
    post-streptococcal, 260, 569, 570
glucocorticoid deficiency, 407
glucose-6-phosphate dehydrogenase
        deficiency, *106, 107, 131*, 433
glucose-galactose malabsorption, 200
glue ear, 153, 155
    due to adenoidal hypertrophy, 158
glue sniffing (solvent abuse), 349, 521
glycogen storage disease, *104*, 371–2
glycosuria, renal tubular defects and,
        247
goitre, *163*, 412
gonads, disorders of, **392–7**
goniotomy, 317
gonococcus, vulvovaginitis and, 31
Goodpastures syndrome, 189
Gowers' sign, 297, 298
grand mal convulsions, 285, 290
    treatment, 290
granulocyte abnormalities, **439–40**
    in cancer patient, 446–7
granuloma annulare, 507, *Plate 43*
granulomatous disease, chronic, 439–40
grasp reflex, 43, 49
    persistence in cerebral palsy, 325
Grave's disease, 412–13
    maternal, 412
'grey baby syndrome', 96
Griffiths Developmental Scale, 327
gross motor development, 47–9
growth and development, **37–51**
    at puberty, 395
    of bones, 474
    endocrine growth disorders, 386–92
    growth assessment, 382–6
    of lungs, 165
    non-organic failure to thrive, 526–8
    radiation-related defects, 445–6
    of SGA infants, 78–9
    the tall child, 391–2
growth hormone deficiency, 388–90
growth hormone replacement therapy,
        following cancer treatment, 445
Guillain-Barré syndrome, 299–300
Guthrie test, 376–7

habit spasm (tic), 28, 293, 341, 343
haemachromatosis, tumour predisposition
        in, *443*
haemangioma
    differential diagnosis, *450*
    liver, 471

haematological disorders, **423–41**
    see also under specific disorder
haematuria, 247
    acute nephritic syndrome and, 260
    causes, *247*
    due to bladder tumour, 465
    in Henoch–Schönlein purpura, 262
    in scurvy, 548
    in Wilm's tumour, *247*, 461
haemochromatosis, 427
haemodialysis, in chronic renal failure,
        267
haemoglobin
    fetal, 53, 423
    normal levels in childhood, *425*
haemolysis
    chronic, 433
    drug-induced, 433
    neonatal, *105*, 106–10
haemolytic anaemias, **430–3**
    glucose-6-phosphate dehydrogenase
        deficiency, 433
    haemolytic disease of newborn, 432
    hereditary spherocytosis, 432–3
    see also sickle cell disease; thalassaemia
haemolytic disease of newborn, 432
haemolytic uraemic syndrome, 265–6
haemophilia, *110, 111, 131*, 436–7
haemophilia A, 436–7
haemophilia B (Christmas disease), *110,
        111, 131*, 437
HIV infection and, 361
Haemophilus influenzae
    acute osteomyelitis following, 482
    septic arthritis following, 480
    vaccine, 356
haemoptysis, causes, *167*
haemorrhage
    neonatal anaemia and, 105–6
    neonatal intracranial, 101–2
    shock due to, *240*
    subdural, 516
haemorrhagic disease of the newborn, 64,
        110–11
haemosiderosis, 427
    haemoptysis due to, *167*
haemostatis, normal, 433–4
hair abnormalities, 503–4
    alopecia, 503–4
Hand–Schuller–Christian disease, 472
handicapped child, **319–33**
    definition, 319
    management, 319–20
harlequin colour change, 56
harlequin fetus, 490
Harrison's sulci 172, *Plate 1*
    asthma and, 184
    in rickets, 550
Hartnup disease, 377
Hashimoto's chronic lymphocytic
        thyroiditis, 412
hay fever, 157
    atopic eczema and, 490
head banging, in mentally handicapped,
        330
head circumference, assessment, 39–40
head injury, **515–16**
    cardiorespiratory arrest due to, *240*
    from falls in the home, 513
    respiratory failure due to, *170*

head lice, 499–500
head tilt, squint and, 315
head-rolling/head-banging, 25
headache, **291–2**
  cluster headaches, 291–2
  due to brain tumours, 463
  intracranial hypertension and, 292, 296
  migraine, 291
  psychosomatic, 347
  short stature and, 386
  tension headaches, 292
Heaf test, 355, 356, **557**, 564
  after measles infection, 555
  in developing countries, 535
  in malnourished children, 545
health visitors, 18
  hearing testing by, 308–9
  liaison, 20
hearing, anatomical pathways, 308
hearing aid, 311
hearing assessment, 308–10
  in newborn, 62
hearing impairment
  in cerebral palsy, 321
  due to congenital cytomegalovirus infection, 367
  due to congenital rubella, 367
  in glue ear, 155
  see also deafness
heart block, 227
heart disease *see* cardiovascular disorders
heart murmurs *see* murmurs
heat bumps, 500
heat rash, 36
height
  changes at puberty, 395
  measurement, 39, 382–5
  parental, 387, 388, 391
Henderson–Hasselbach equation, 276
Henoch–Schönlein purpura, 206, 261–2, 434
hepatic disease, **206–13**
  in paracetamol poisoning, 518
  see also jaundice
hepatitis
  chronic, 210–11
  hepatitis A, 209–10
  hepatitis B, 210
  neonatal, 208–9
  neonatal hepatitis syndrome, *208*
  neonatal, *versus* conjugated hyperbilirubinaemia, 108
  vaccine, 356
hepatoblastoma, 471
hepatocarcinoma, 471
hepatomegaly
  assessment, 11
  in fructosaemia, 371
herbalists, role in developing countries, 530
hereditary haemorrhagic telangiectasia, 434
hereditary spherocytosis, *106, 107*, 432–3
hernia, *31*
  strangulated, *29*
heroin abuse, 350
herpes simplex
  infections in cancer patient, 446
  skin disorders, 494–5

herpes zoster, 358–9, 495
  infections in cancer patients, 446
heterozygote, *definition*, 118
hiatus hernia, gastro-oesophageal reflux and, 192
hip
  congenital dislocation of, 34, 59–60, 150
  dislocated in cerebral palsy, 325
  examination, 13
  irritable, 479
  irritable hip *versus* neuroblastoma, 458
  newborn examination, 59–60
  painful, **479–83**
  tuberculosis of, 563
Hirschsprung's disease, 201–2
  abdominal distension due to, *193*
  constipation in, 75
  necrotizing enterocolitis in, 114
histiocytic disorders, 472–3
  dermatitis due to, 492
histiocytosis-X, 472
histoplasmosis, 366–7
history taking, 1–4
  in dermatology, 486–7
  in emotional disorders, 335–40
  in suspected child abuse, 523
  talking to children, 336–8
HIV infection, 361–2
  BCG vaccination and, 356, 361
  in breast milk, 70, 361
  congenital, 367–8
  polio vaccination and, 355, 361
  role in inducing malignancy, 444
hives, 506
hoarseness, 162
Hodgkin's disease, **455–7**
  differential diagnosis, *450*
  second tumours in, 446
Holt–Oram syndrome, *128*
  heart disease in, *215*
home apnoea monitors, 512–13
homocystinuria, 377, 391
homozygote, *definition*, 118
hookworm, **573**
  anaemia due to, *571*, 573
horseshoe kidney, 254
hospital services for children, 19–21
human immunodeficiency virus *see* HIV infection
Hunter's syndrome, 375
Huntington's chorea, *128*, 293
Hurler's disease, pseudo, 373
Hurler's syndrome, 375
hyaline membrane disease, 86–8
hyaluronidase, in paraphimosis treatment, 30
hydatid disease, 211
hydranencephaly, 147, 295–6
hydrocephalus, 102, 146–7, 295
  external, 296
  following meningitis, 282
  intracranial hypertension management, 296–7
  in osteopetrosis, 484
hydrogen breath test, 200
hydronephrosis, abdominal distension due to, *193*
hydrops, erythema infectiosum and, 358
hymenal skin tags, 59

hyperactivity, 294, 332, 339–40
  blood lead levels and, 520
  in clumsy child, 332
hyperacusis, in Tay–Sachs disease, 373
hyperaldosteronism, 278
hyperammonaemia, transient, 378
hyperbilirubinaemia, 107–10
  conjugated, 108
hyperbilirubinaemia, unconjugated, 106
hypercalcaemia, 380–1, 421–2
  cardiorespiratory arrest due to, *240*
hypercapnia, 170
hypercholesterolaemia, in nephrotic syndrome, 262
hyperglycaemia
  in salicylate poisoning, 518
  in von Gierke's disease, 372
hyperinsulinism, *104*
hyperkalaemia, cardiorespiratory arrest due to, *240*
hyperlipoproteinaemia, 372–3
hypermetropia, 316
hypernatraemic dehydration, 274–5
  management, 275–6
hyperoxia test, 217
hyperparathyroidism, 380, **421–2**
  in glomerular rickets, 379
hypertension, **260–72**
  causes in childhood, *271*
  epistaxis due to, *156*
  in neuroblastoma, 458
  portal, 212
  in Wilm's tumour, 461
  see also intracranial hypertension
hyperthyroidism, 412–13
hypertrophic obstructive cardiomyopathy, 226
hyperventilation, 169–70
hypoadrenalism, 415–16
hypoalbuminaemia
  in nephrotic syndrome, 262
  shock due to, *240*
hypocalcaemia, 420–1
  following high phosphorus intake, 64
  handicap risks following, *103*
  neonatal fits and, *100*, 102
hypogammaglobulinaemia, transient, of infancy, 440
hypoglycaemia, **405–7**
  asymptomatic, 105
  causes, *405*
  ketotic, 407
  in malnutrition, 544
  neonatal, *100, 103*, 370
  recognition in diabetes management, 402, 403
  symptoms, *402*, 405–6
hypokalaemia, 275
  cardiorespiratory arrest due to, *240*
hypomagnesaemia, neonatal fits and, 102
hyponatraemic dehydration, 274
  management, 276
hypoparathyroidism, **420–1**
  pseudo, *391*
hypophosphataemia, rickets due to, 379
hypophosphatasia, 380–1
hypopigmentation disorders, 504–5
hypopituitarism, neonatal hepatitis syndrome due to, *208*

hypoplastic left heart syndrome, 223, **231–2**
 pulse assessment in, 8
hypospadias, 59, 148–9
hypotension, pulse assessment in, 8
hypothermia
 in drowning/near-drowning, 515
 in malnutrition, 544
hypothyroidism, **410–12**
 causes, *409*
 diabetes and, 402
 neonatal hepatitis syndrome due to, *208*
 neonatal jaundice and, *107*
hypotonia, in cerebral palsy, 324
hypoxaemia, in respiratory failure, 170
hypsarrhythmia, 287
hysteria
 faints and, 32
 hysterical conversion states, 342

icthyosis, 489–90
 icthyosis vulgaris, 489, *Plate 17*
 inheritance, *489*
 X-linked, 489–90
ICU, neonatal, 84
idiopathic fibrosing alveolitis, 187
idiopathic thrombocytopenia, maternal, 110
imipramine, in enuresis treatment, 27
immotile cilia syndrome, 181, **182–3**
immune response 351–2
immunity
 active, 353
 adaptive, 352
 natural, 351–2
 passive, 353
immunization, 189, 190, **351–6**
 in developing countries, **534–6**
 history taking, 3–4
 schedules, *353*
immunocompromised hosts, pneumonia in, 179
immunoglobulin therapy, in cancer patient, 448
immunoglobulins, classification, 352
impairment, *definition*, 319
impetigo 495, *Plate 27*
 following head lice infestation, 499
in-toeing, 33–4
inborn errors of metabolism, **370–81**
 crying and, *29*
 sudden infant death syndrome and, *511*
 see also under specific disorder
incomitant squint, 314
incontinentia pigmenti, *131, 301*, 501–2
infant feeding, **63–76**
infant mortality rate
 definition, 16
 in developing countries, 529, 532
 social class and, *17*
infanticide, deliberate, 511
infantile spasms, 286–7
 causes, *287*
infections
 diagnosis, 351–2
 effects on nutrition, 539
 in kwashiorkor, 543–4
 minor, **32–3**
 neonatal *see below*

of nervous system, **280–4**
pleural diseases, 174–6
of throat, 160–2
see also infectious diseases *and under specific infection*
infections, neonatal, 84, **95–7**
 apnoea and, 97
 convulsions and, 102
 pneumonia, 88–9
infectious diseases, 351–2, **356–69**
 hazards for cancer patient, 448, 454
infectious mononucleosis, 360
infective endocarditis, 238–9
infertility, irradiation and, 446
infestations, 33
inflammatory bowel disease, 202–3
 Crohn's disease, 202, 348
 ulcerative colitis, 203
influenza, 360–1
 septic arthritis following, 480
 vaccine, 356
inguinal hernia, 143
inheritance of disease, 118–19
 genetic disorders, **116–35**
injury *see* accidental injury; non-accidental injury
insect bites, history taking, 487
inspissated bile syndrome, neonatal jaundice and, *107*
insulin therapy
 in diabetes management, 398–402
 in diabetic ketoacidosis management, 403
insulinoma, 407
intelligence
 behavioural disturbances and, 332
 'gifted child', 332
intelligence quotient (IQ), 41, 327
 in irradiated leukaemic child, 445–6, 453
 in mentally handicapped, 327–8
 psychometric tests, 327
intensive care
 of critically ill child, 243–4
 neonatal units, 84
 withdrawal, 243–5
interferon, 352
intertrigo, 36
intestinal lymphangiectasia, 200
intestinal obstruction
 due to ascaris, 573
 neonatal, 140–2
intracranial haemorrhage, neonatal, 101–2
intracranial hypertension, **296–7**
 benign, 297
 cardiorespiratory arrest due to, *240*
 crying and, *29*
 due to brain tumours, 463
 headache and, 292, 296
 in hydrocephalus, 146–7
 sunsetting sign, *Plate 5*
intrauterine growth retardation, 77–84
 causes, 77
 hypoglycaemia due to, *405*
 mental retardation due to, 328
 short stature and, 389
intravenous urogram (IVU), 248
intraventricular haemorrhage, neonatal, 101–2

introns, 117
intubation, of newborn, 55
intussusception, 204
 crying and, *29*
 rectal bleeding due to, *203*
inverted nipples, 67
involuntary movement disorders, 293–4
IQ tests, 41, 327
iridocyclitis, in pauciarticular arthritis, 475
iron deficiency
 anaemia, 426–7
 in premature infant, 105
iron poisoning, 519
iron requirements, of infants 64
iron toxicity, 427
 in thalassaemia, 431
irritable hip, 458, **479**
Ishihara charts, 314
islet cell adenoma, 407
isoimmune thrombocytopenia, 110
itching
 in eczema, 490
 in head lice infestation, 499
 in scabies, 497

Jacquet's ulcers, 492
jaundice, **206–11**
 failure to thrive due to, *527*
 following iron poisoning, 519
 in galactosaemia, 370
 neonatal *see below*
jaundice, neonatal, 106–10, 208–9
 breast feeding and, 69
 causes, *107*
 in developing countries, 533
 in glucose-6-phosphate dehydrogenase deficiency, 433
 in haemolytic disease of newborn, 432
 in hereditary spherocytosis, 432
 prolonged, 208–9
 total parenteral nutrition and, 76
joints
 congenital abnormalities, 149–50
 disorders of, **474–85**
 tuberculosis of, 562–3
Joubert's syndrome, hyperventilation in, 170
juvenile chronic arthritis (JCA), 474–6
 terminology problems, 475
juvenile hypothyroidism, 412
juvenile plantar dermatosis, 493, *Plate 23*
juvenile thyrotoxicosis, 413–14

Kallmann's syndrome, 397
Kaposi's varicelliform eruption, 359, *Plate 8*
Kartagener's syndrome, 182
karyotype
 abnormalities in tumour cells, 443
 in child with ambiguous genitalia, 418–19
 normal, 117–18
 XXX-karyotype, 392
Kasabach–Merritt syndrome, 508
Katamaya syndrome, 575
Kawasaki's disease **478–9**, *Plate 13*
 chest pain in, 225

Kawasaki's disease *contd*
  sudden death in, 226
Kayser–Fleischer ring, 212
kerion, 496, *Plate 30*
kernicterus, 106, 108–9
  cerebral palsy due to, 321, 323
Kernig's sign, 280
kerosene poisoning, 520
kidney
  development/function, 246
  examination, 12
  horseshoe, 254
  polycystic disease, 256
  see also renal
kidney transplantation, 266, 267–8
Klinefelter's syndrome, 126, 392
  delayed puberty in, 396
Klumpke's palsy, *111*, 112
knock knees, 33
Koebner phenomenon, 488
koilonychia, 427
Koplik's spots, 357, 554
Kostmann's disease, 439
Krabbe's disease, 374
kwashiorkor, **539–45**
  aetiology, 539
  definition, 538
  following measles epidemics, 555
  investigations, *542*
kyphosis, 483
  in rickets, 550

lacerations, 513
lactalbumin, 64
lactation, physiology of, 65
lactoferrin, in breast milk, 68
lactose deficiency
  following gastroenteritis, 195
  in necrotizing enterocolitis, 115
lactose intolerance, 74, 200
  in tropical countries, 544–5
lamellar icthyosis, 490
Langerhans' cell histiocytosis, 472–3
language development, 44, 47, 335
  disorders, 335, 345–5
  Reynell Developmental Language Scale,
    327
language disorders, **302–5**
lanugo, 81
laryngeal disease, cough characteristics,
  168
laryngeal disorders, 159–60
  congenital obstruction, 159
  laryngotracheobronchitis, 159–60
  papillomata, 162
laryngitis
  acute, 162
  chronic, 162
  following measles, 357
laryngomalacia, 159
Laurence–Moon–Biedl syndrome, *137*
LBW *see* low birth weight
lead poisoning, 520–1
  mental retardation due to, *329*
  pica and, 30
learning disability, 332
Leber's amaurosis, 317
leishmaniasis, 211
length, measurement in infant, 385
lepromin test, 567

leprosy, **567–9**
  BCG vaccination and, 535
  management, *570*
leptospirosis, 365
Lesch–Nyhan syndrome, *131*
let-down reflex, 65
Letterer–Siwe disease, 472
leucine sensitivity hypoglycaemia, *405*,
  407
leucodystrophies, 306
leukaemia, **451–5**
  acute lymphoblastic, 442, 452–5
  brain irradiation and IQ impairment,
    445–6, 453
  classification, *452*
  in Down's syndrome, *119*
  epistaxis due to, *156*
  late diagnosis, 449
  neonatal, *110*
  nuclear installations and leukaemic
    clusters, 444, 451
  pleural effusion due to, *175*
  second tumours in, 446
  versus rheumatic fever, 570
leukodystrophies, 306, 374
  Krabbe's disease, 374
lice, 499–500
lichen planus, 489
lipid metabolism disorders, 372–3
  abetalipoproteinaemia, 372
  hyperlipoproteinaemias, 372–3
  lipoprotein deficiencies, 372
liver disease, chronic, 210–13
liver failure, following paracetamol
  poisoning, 518
liver transplantation, 208, 212
liver tumours, 471
Loeffler's syndrome, 573
long sightedness, 316
loperamide, for toddler's diarrhoea, 30
low birth weight (LBW)
  definition, 52, 77
  formula feeds, 72
lumbar puncture, technique, 279
lung
  anatomy and function, 165–6
  congenital abnormalities, 173–4
  development, 165
  tumours, 189
lung disease, **187–9**
  alpha-antitrypsin deficiency, *169*, 189
  neonatal, 93–5
  preventative aspects, 189–90
  pulmonary haemosiderosis, 189
  SIDS risk and, 511
  see also cystic fibrosis
lung volumes, standard, 166, *167*
Lyell's syndrome, 495
lymph nodes, examination, 13
lymphadenopathy, 13, 32–3, 164, 455
  generalized, 440–1
  in Hodgkin's disease, 456
  in malignant histiocytosis, 473
  in non-Hodgkin's lymphoma, 457
lymphoid tissue growth, 37–8
lymphomas, *163*, 444, **455–8**
  Burkitt's, 442, 444, **458**
  differential diagnosis, *450*
  Hodgkin's, 446, 450, **455–7**
  of neck, 164

non-Hodgkin's, *450*, 457–8
  pleural effusion due to, *175*
  versus osteosarcoma, 467
lysozyme, 352

Mcleod's syndrome, 180
macrocephaly
  definition, 295
  due to brain tumour, 463
  without hydrocephalus, 296
magnetic resonance imaging (MRI)
  in kidney disorders, 250
  of nervous system, 279
  role in cancer diagnosis 450
Maladie de Roger, 230
malaria, 571–2, **572–3**
  failure to thrive due to, *527*
  nephrotic syndrome and, 262
malignant disease *see* cancer; tumours
malignant histiocytosis, 473
malnutrition
  anaemia due to, *571*
  in developing countries, **538–46**
  failure to thrive due to, *527*
  following measles epidemics, 555
  maternal, during pregnancy, 77–8
  mental retardation due to, 328
malrotation (of bowel), 142
mania, 341
manic depressive psychosis, 341
Mantoux test, **556–7**, 564
  after measles infection, 555
  in developing countries, 535
  in malnourished children, 545
maple syrup disease, 377
marasmus, **545–6**
  aetiology, 539–40
  definition, 538
marble bone disease, 484
Marfan's syndrome, *128*, 485
  funnel chest in, 172
  height problems in, 391
  versus homocystinuria, 377
Maroteaux–Lamy syndrome, 376
mastocytosis, 506–7
mastoiditis, 155
masturbation, 24–5
  in mentally handicapped, 330
  vulvovaginitis and, 31
measles 357, *Plate 6*
  in cancer patient, 448, 454
  complications, 554–5
  in developing countries, 535–6, **553–5**
  encephalitis, 283
  epidemics, 536, 554
  immunization, 190, *353*, 355
  immunization, in developing countries,
    535–6
  subacute sclerosing panencephalitis,
    283–4
  tuberculosis and, 563
meatal stenosis, 31
meatal ulcer, 31
mechanical ventilation, in respiratory
  distress syndrome, 87–8
Meckel's diverticulum, 142–3, *203*, 206
meconium aspiration syndrome, *86*, 89–
  90, 93
meconium ileus, incystic fibrosis, 187, 199

medulloblastoma, 463, **464–5**
megacustis-megaureter syndrome, 254
megalencephaly, 295, 296
melanin, function of, 486, 504
melanocytic naevi, 508–9
menarche, normal 395
meningismus, 280
meningitis, **280–3, 366**
  bacterial, 280–2, 366
  cerebral palsy due to, 321
  crying and, *29*, 280
  deafness and, 283, 310
  laboratory findings, *352*
  in leptospirosis, 365
  neonatal, 95, 102, *103*, **282**
  pneumococcal, 179, *281*
  respiratory failure due to, *170*
  tuberculous, 280, *281*, 562
  viral, 282–3
meningocele, 144
meningococcal disease, 366
meningococcal septicaemia, emergency
  management, 242
meningococcal vaccines, 356
  in developing countries, 536
meningoencephalitis, 280, 283
mental retardation, **327–31**, 340
  causes, *329*
  cerebral palsy and, 321
  developmental delay and, 42
  in Down's syndrome, 120
  due to kernicterus, 109
  failure to thrive due to, *527*
  following meningitis, 283
  in fragile X syndrome, 127
  in galactosaemia, 370, 371
  in Klinefelter's syndrome, 126
  in lead poisoning, 520
  speech delay and, 304
  in trisomy-13, 123
mercury toxicity, cerebral palsy due to,
  321
Merrill Palmer psychometric test, 327
mesangial IgA nephropathy, 261
mesenteric adenitis
  tonsillitis and, 161
  versus acute appendicitis, 206
metabolic acidosis, 275, **276–7**
  total parenteral nutrition and, 76
metabolic alkalosis, 275, 277–8
metabolic disorders, **370–81**
  see also under specific disorder
metachromatic leukodystrophy, 374
metatarsus varus, 34
methyl xanthines, in obstructive apnoea
  management, 98, 100
microcephaly, 147
  in trisomy-13, *122*
micrognathia, 57
microscopy, of urine, 247–8
micturating cystourethrogram, 248–9
  in UTI investigation, 259
micturating renogram, indirect, 249
micturition, painful, 31
migraine, 291
milestones in development, *42*
milia, 36
miliaria rubra, 36
milk allergy *see* cow's milk protein
  intolerance

milk aspiration, *86*, 90
mineral requirements, of infants, 64
minimal brain dysfunction, 331
minimal valve disorders, 237
MMR vaccination, 355
  in developing countries, 536
  schedule, *353*
Mobius syndrome, 300
mole (pigmented naevus), 36, **508–9**
molluscum contagiosum, 494, *Plate 26*
Mongolian spots, 508, *Plate 47*
Moro reflex, 43
  persistence in cerebral palsy, 325
morphoea, 478
Morquio's syndrome, 375–6
mortality rates, **15–17**, 52
  in developing countries, 529, 532
mouth, newborn examination, 57
mouth breathing, 30
  due to adenoidal hypertrophy, 158
mouth ulcers, in measles, 554
MRI *see* magnetic resonance imaging
muco-cutaneous lymph node syndrome,
  479
mucolipidoses, *305*
mucopolysaccharidoses, 306, 374–6
  Hunter's syndrome, 375
  Hurler's syndrome, 375
  Maroteaux-Lamy syndrome, 376
  Morquio's syndrome, 375–6
  Sanfilippo syndrome, 375
mucositis, in cancer patient, 447
mucus vomiting, in neonates, 74
mumps, *163*, **358**
  cause of earache, *156*
  deafness and, 310
  vaccination, *353*, 355
Munchausen syndrome by proxy, 521,
  528
  fictitious haematuria in, 248, 528
murmurs (cardiac), 9–10, **223–5**
  intracranial bruits, 224
  in rheumatic fever, 476
  Still's murmur, 224
  venous hum, 10, 224
muscular dystrophy, 298–9
  congenital, 301
Mustard operation, 234
myasthenia gravis, 299
myelomeningocele, 144
myocarditis, 238
  cardiorespiratory arrest due to, *240*
myoclonic seizures, 287–8
myopia, 316
  in Marfan's syndrome, *485*
myotonic dystrophy, 128
myringotomy, in otitis media
  management, 154

naevi, 36, **507–9**
NAI *see* non-accidental injury
nail-biting, 25
nails, psoriasis of, 488
napkin dermatitis 492–3, *Plate 22*
  candida superinfection, 497
napkin psoriasis, *Plate 21*
nappy rash, 35–6
  candida superinfection, 497
  napkin dermatitis, 492–3, *Plate 22*

narcotics, intrauterine growth retardation
  due to, 77
nasojejunal feeding route, in premature
  infants, 72
natal teeth, 29
National Association for the Welfare of
  Children in Hospital, 22
National Society for the Prevention of
  Cruelty to Children, 22, 524
NAWCH, 22
neck swelling, 162–4
  causes, *163*
necrotizing enterocolitis, 75, 114–15
  nasojejunal tubes and, 72
negativistic behaviour
  food refusal, 23
  sleep refusal, 25
  speech refusal, 303
  stool holding, 28, 201
neonatal convulsions, 100–2
neonatal hepatitis, 208–9
  versus conjugated hyperbilirubinaemia,
  108
neonatal herpes simplex, 494
neonatal meningitis, 95, 102, *103*, 280,
  282
neonatal mortality rate, *definition*, 16
neonatal myasthenia, transient, 299
neonatal rickets, 114
neonatal seizures, treatment, *290*
neonatal syphilis, in developing countries,
  533–4, *Plate 48*
neonatal thyrotoxicosis, 413
neonates
  normal newborn infant, **52–62**
  problems in developing countries,
  532–4
  special care of sick, **77–115**
  wards for, 21
nephritic syndrome, acute, 260–1
  in systemic lupus erythematosis, *478*
nephroblastoma *see* Wilm's tumour
nephrocalcinosis, 268, 380
nephropathy, mesangial IgA, 261
nephrotic syndrome, 262–4
  abdominal distension due to, *193*
  congenital, 264
  pleural effusion due to, *175*
  secondary causes, 264
nervous system
  examination, 5–6 279
  infections, 280–4
  newborn examination, 60, 62
  normal development, 41–3
nervous system, disorders of, **279–306**
  congenital malformations, 143–7,
  295–6
  degenerative disorders, 305–6
  floppy infant, 300–1
  handicapped child, **319–33**
  infections, 280–4
  involuntary movements, 293–4
  minor neurological deficits, 331–3
  speech/language disorders, 302–5,
  332–3
  weak child, 297–300
  see also convulsions; headache; seizures
nesidioblastosis, *104*, 104, 105, 407
nettle-rash, 506
neural crest tumours, 418

neural tube defects, 143–4
   recurrence risk for siblings, 133
neuroblastoma, *163*, 418, **458–61**
   abdominal distension due to, *193*
   cure rates, 450, 460, 461
   differential diagnosis, *450*
   stage IVS, 461
   versus osteosarcoma, 467
neurocutaneous disorders, 301–2
   ataxia-telangiectasia, 293, *301*, 440, *443*
   incontinentia pigmenti, *131*, *301*, 501–2
   neurofibromatosis, *128*, *301*, 302, *443*, 508
   Sturge–Weber syndrome, *301*, 302, 508
   see also tuberous sclerosis
neurodegenerative disorders, **305–6**
   leukodystrophies, 306, 374
   mucolipidoses, *305*
   mucopolysaccharidoses, 306, 374–6
   neuronal storage diseases, 306
neuroectodermal tumours, 464
neurofibroma, differential diagnosis, *450*
neurofibromatosis, *128*, 302
   café-au-lait patches in, 508
   tumour predisposition in, *443*
neurological disorders, minor, **31–2**
neurological system
   examination, 5–6, 279
   newborn examination, 60, 62
neuromuscular disorders, 297–301
   the floppy infant, 300–1
neuronal storage diseases, 306
neutropenia, 439
   in cancer, 446–7
neutrophil function, defective, 439
newborn
   examination of, 58–62
   special care of sick, **77–115**
   see also neonates
nickel allergy, 492
nicotinic acid deficiency, 547, *Plate 49*
Niemann–Pick disease, 373–4
   neonatal hepatitis syndrome due to, *208*
night terrors, 26
nightmares, 26
nipples
   cracked, 67
   inverted, 67
nitrogen washout test, 217
nits, 499, 500
noma (cancrum oris), 546
non-accidental injury, **521–8**
   deaths following, 510
   head injury, 515, 516
   police involvement, 21–2
   scalding, 516
   subdural haemorrhage, 516
   see also child abuse; sexual abuse
non-Hodgkin's lymphoma, 457–8
   differential diagnosis, *450*
non-paralytic squint, 314
Noonan's syndrome, 125, *128*
   heart disease in, *215*
nose, disorder of, 156–9
   acute ethmoiditis, 158
   adenoidal hypertrophy, 158–9
   choanal atresia, 156
   epistaxis, *156*, 157
   rhinitis, 157
   sinusitis, 158

NSPCC, 22
nut allergy, 506
nystagmus, 317
   in cerebral palsy, 324
   in medulloblastoma, 463
   in neuroblastoma, 458

obesity
   hypertension and, 270
   knock knees and, 33
   stature and, 391, 392
obstetric care
   importance in premature infant survival, 79–80
   see also pregnancy
obstruction
   bowel, 29
   urinary, 27
obstructive apnoea, 98–100
occipito-frontal head circumference, 39–40
occupational therapy, in cerebral palsy management, 327
ocular albinism, 317
ocular disorders *see* eye disorders
ocular examination, 5
   in newborn, 57
ocular movements, assessment, 5
oculocutaneous albinism, 505
oesophageal atresia, 139–40
   in trisomy-18, *122*
oesophageal disorders, 191
oncogenes, 119, 443–4
Ondine's curse, sudden infant death syndrome and, *511*
onycholysis, 488
opiate addiction, withdrawal from maternal, 29
opiate analgesia in labour, neonatal effects, 55–6
opisthotonus, due to kernicterus, 109
optic atrophy, in Batten's disease, 374
optic glioma, 465
oral hydration solution (ORS), 195
oral rehydration, in developing countries, 552–3
orbital abscess, 158
orbital tumours, 465
orchidopexy, 394
orchitis, *31*
   following mumps, 358
   versus testicular torsion, 394
organ donation, brain stem death and, 244
organic acidaemias, 378
orthopaedic abnormalities
   congenital, 149–50
   minor, **33–5**, 59
orthopaedic intervention, in cerebral palsy, 327
Ortolani's test, 59–60
Osgood–Schlatter disease, 484
osmolality, urinary, 246–7
ossification centres, 38
osteogenesis imperfecta, *128*, 484
osteomyelitis
   acute, 481–3
   neonatal, 96
   versus osteosarcoma, 467

osteopetrosis, 484
osteoporosis, in scurvy, 548
osteosarcoma, 466–9
otitis externa, 154
otitis media, 153, 154–5, 310
   crying and, 29
   due to adenoidal hypertrophy, 158
   following measles, 357
   serous, 155
   in tuberculosis, 562
ovarian disorders, 394–5, 472
ovarian tumours, 395, 472
over-riding of toes, 35
oxygen dissociation curve, fetal blood, 53
oxytocin, 'after pains' and, 65

pain
   abdominal, **204–6**, 347, 458
   cardiac, 225
   chest, in cardiovascular disorders, 225
   hip, **479–83**
   on micturiton, 31
   psychosomatic, 347
   somatic, 347–8
paint, chronic lead poisoning and, 520
pallid syncope, 289
palpitations, 225
pancreatic lipase deficiency, 74
pancreatitis, 204
pancuronium, in pneumothorax management, 89
papilloedema
   in diabetic ketoacidosis, 404
   in intracranial hypertension, 292
papular urticaria, 500, *Plate 35*
paracetamol poisoning, 517, 518–19
parachute reflex, 6
   in cerebral palsy, 325
paraffin poisoning, 520
paraldehyde, in newborn, 103
paralytic squint, 314
paraphimosis, 30
paraplegia, in spinal tuberculosis, 563
paraquat poisoning, 520
parasitic infections
   in developing countries, **572–5**
   gastroenteritis, 194
   of liver, 211
   threadworm, 33
parasternal heave, 8
parathyroid gland disorders, 420–2
parenteral nutrition
   in cancer patient, 447
   in critically ill child, 243
   in infancy, 75–6
parents
   of abused child, 522–3
   autopsy consent from, 245
   of critically ill child, 243
   follow-up needs after child's death, 245
   of ill newborn infant, 84
   interview techniques in emotional disorders, 338
   in Munchausen syndrome by proxy, 528
   reaction to mental handicap diagnosis, 330
   role in emotional/behavioural disorders, 334–50

passive tone, 5
Patau's syndrome *see* trisomy-13
patent ductus arteriosus, *88, 94,* 114,
230–1
  in Down's syndrome, *119*
  recurrence risk for siblings, *133*
  in trisomy-18, *122*
pauciarticular arthritis, 475
Paul Bunnell tests 360
peak flow meter, 166
peas and carrots diarrhoea, 30, 196
pectus carinatum, 172
pectus excavatum, 172
pediculosis, 499–500
pellagra, 547, *Plate 49*
pelviureteric junction obstruction, 252
pemphigus neonatorum, 495
pemphigus vlugaris, 501
penis, newborn examination, 59
peptic ulcer, 204–5
percussion, chest, 10–11
pericarditis, 237–8
perinatal mortality rate, in developing
  countries, 532
perinatal mortality rates
  definition, 16, 52
  as health service index, 15
  social class and, *17*
periodic syndrome, headaches and, 292
peritonitis, shock due to, *240*
periventricular haemorrhage, 101
periventricular leukomalacia, 102–3
peroneal muscular atrophy, *128*, 300
persistent fetal circulation, *86*, 93
persistent pulmonary hypertension, 93
Perthe's disease, 479–80
  versus irritable hip, 479
pertussis, 180, **363–4**
  cough treatment, 168
  vaccination, *353*, 354
  wheeze due to, *169*
pes planus, 34
petit mal convulsions, 287
  treatment, 290
petrol abuse, 521
Peutz–Jegher syndrome, *128*, 203–4
  tumour predisposition in, *443*
pH
  plasma, 276
  urine, 246–7
phaeochromocytoma, 418
  differential diagnosis, *450*
pharyngitis, acute, 161
phenobarbitone
  as anticonvulsant, 290
  in newborn, 103
phenylketonuria, 74, **376–7**
  de-pigmentation in, 505
  undiagnosed maternal, 329
phenytoin, in newborn, 103
Philadelphia chromosome, 454, 455
phimosis, 30
phlyctenular conjunctivitis, in
  tuberculosis, 559–60
photosensitivity, in Hartnup disease, 377
phototherapy, 110
  in developing countries, 533
phrenic nerve injury, 189
phrenic nerve palsy, 189
physiotherapy

in cerebral palsy management, 326–7
in cystic fibrosis, 188
pica, 30
  in anaemia, 30, 425
  in lead poisoning, 520
piebaldism, 505
Pierre Robin syndrome, *137*, 138
pigeon chest, 172
pigeon toes, 33–4
pigmentation disorders, 504–6
pigmented naevus, 36, 508–9
pillows, risk of asphyxia, 514
pityriasis alba, 492
pityriasis lichenoides, hypopigmentation
  following, 505
pityriasis lichenoides chronica, 489
pityriasis rosea 489, *Plate 16*
  hypopigmentation following, 505
pityriasis (tinea) versicolor, 496–7
Place of Safety Order, 21
plagiocephaly, 148
plane warts, 493, *Plate 25*
plant dermatitis, 492
plantar dermatosis, juvenile, 493, *Plate 23*
plantar warts, 493, *Plate 24*
platelet disorders, 434–6
  classification, *436*
play therapist, 20
playground accidents, 514
pleural diseases, 174–6
pleural effusion, 174–5
  causes, *175*
  respiratory failure due to, *170*
pleurisy, 174
  in systemic lupus erythematosus, *478*
pleurodynia, 174
pneumococcal meningitis, 179
pneumococcal vaccine, 356
pneumomediastinum, 89
pneumonia, **176–9**
  in cancer patient, 448
  following measles, 357
  haemoptysis due to, *167*
  lipoid pneumonia following paraffin
    poisoning, 520
  in measles, 554–5
  neonatal, *86*, 88–9, 95
  pleural effusion due to, *175*
  versus acute appendicitis, 206
pneumopericardium, 89
pneumoperitoneum, 89
pneumothorax, 175–6
  neonatal, *86, 88,* 89
poisoning, **516–21**
  barbiturate, 519
  glue sniffing (solvent abuse), 349, 521
  household product ingestion, 519–20
  iron, 519
  lead, 520–1
  management principles, 517–18
  paracetamol, 518–19
  salicylate, 518
  tricyclic antidepressant, 519
polio vaccination, *353*, 355
  in developing countries, 535
polyarticular disease, 476
polycystic kidney disease
  abdominal distension due to, *193*
  infantile, 256
polycythaemia

necrotizing enterocolitis and, 114
neonatal jaundice and, *107*
polydactyly, 35
polydipsia, 407–9
  short stature and, 386
polygenic defects, 118–19
polyhydramnios, 79
  in chloridorrhoea, 200
polyposis coli, *128*
polyuria, 407–9
  enuresis due to, *27*
  shock due to, *240*
Pompe's disease, 372
port wine stain, 508
Portage scheme, 330–1
portal hypertension, 212
possitting, 24, 75, 191
post-infectious encephalitis, 283
post-neonatal mortality rate, *definition*, 16
posterior urethral valves, 255, 265
potassium, in kwashiorkor, 540
potassium disorders, *240*, 275
Potter's syndrome, *93*, 250, 256
Pott's disease, 562–3
Prader–Willi syndrome, *300*, 392
  delayed puberty in, 397
  short stature and, *391*
prednisolone
  in asthma management, 186
  in nephrotic syndrome management,
    263
pregnancy
  gestation assessment, 52, 80–4
  hypertension during, 78
  maternal malnutrition, 77–8
  placental haemorrhage, 105
  premature labour, 79, 80
  rubella infection, 356, 367
  toxaemia of, 78
  varicella infection, 359
  see also intrauterine growth retardation
premature infant/prematurity, **79–85**
  anaemia and, 105
  apnoea and, 97–8
  cerebral palsy and, 321
  chest wall deformities in, 171
  chronic pulmonary insufficiency of, 95
  definition, 52
  in developing countries, 533
  factors associated with, 79
  fat and carbohydrate malabsorption, 71
  feeding, 71–2
  fluid requirements, 273–4
  general care principles, 84–5
  growth assessment, 39
  immunization schedules, 354
  iron supplements, 64
  SIDS risks and, 511
prenatal diagnosis
  in congenital nephrotic syndrome, 264
  in Duchenne muscular dystrophy, 135
prenatal infections
  cerebral palsy due to, *321*
  mental retardation due to, *329*
prenatal surgery, for diaphragmatic
  hernia, 165
prickly heat, 36
primary health care, 18
primitive reflexes, 6, 43
  persistence in cerebral palsy, 324–5

probation officers, 21–2
prostaglandin therapy, in cardiac disease, 221, 223, 231
protein intolerance, 74
protein losing enteropathy, abdominal distension due to, *193*
protein requirements, of infants, 64
protein-energy malnutrition, in developing countries, **538–46**
proteinuria, 247
protozoal infestations
  giardiasis, 199
  see also toxoplasmosis
prune belly syndrome
  chronic renal failure in, 266
  enuresis due to, 27
  urinary tract abnormalities, 254
pruritis, liver disease and, 208
pseudohypoparathyroidism, *131*
Pseudomonas infection, in cystic fibrosis, 188
psoriasis, 487–9
  guttate, 488, *Plate 15*
  hypopigmentation following, 505
  napkin, *Plate 21*
  plaque, 488, *Plate 14*
  psoriatic arthritis, 476
psychiatric disorder
  definition, 341
  see also behavioural disorders; emotional disorders
psycho-social support, in cancer, 447
psychodynamic therapy, 343–4
psychogenic cough, 168
psychometric tests, 327
psychotherapy, 343–5
  for anorexia nervosa, 348
  in mentally handicapped management, 331
puberty
  ambiguous genitalia and, 420
  delayed, 389, 396–7
  delayed in Crohn's disease, 202
  delayed in Turner's syndrome, 125
  disorders of, 395–7
  normal, 41, 395
  precocious, 395–6
pubic lice, 500
pulmonary abnormalities, 173–4
  arterio-venous malformations, 174
  atresia, 236–7
  haemosiderosis, 189
  neonatal hypoplasia, *86*, 91–3
  stenosis, 9, 233–4
pulmonary interstitial emphysema, 89
pulse
  abnormalities, 226
  assessment of, 8
  collapsing or waterhammer, 8
pyloric stenosis, 192–3
  following iron poisoning, 519
  recurrence risk for siblings, 133
pyridoxine deficiency, *100*

quinsy, 161

RAD (reflex anal dilatation) test, 526
radiography
  in cancer diagnosis, 450

chest, 216–7
  in child abuse, 523–4
  in heart disease, 216–17
  in urinary tract disorders, 248–50
radiotherapy, 445
  late effects, 445
  radiation-induced tumours, 444
ranula, 57
Raynaud's phenomenon, in scleroderma, 478
RDS *see* respiratory distress syndrome
rectal bleeding, 203–4
  anal fissure and, 30
  causes in neonate, *203*
rectal examination, 12
rectal polyp, 203
rectal prolapse, in cystic fibrosis, 187, 204
red reflex, 57, 312–13
  in retinoblastoma, 313, 470
reflex anal dilatation test, 526
reflex anoxic seizures, 289
reflex apnoea, 98
reflex epilepsy, 285
reflexes
  assessment, 6, 62
  assessment in newborn, 43, 62
  asymmetrical tonic neck, 43
  in cerebral palsy, 324–5
  development of, 43
  Moro, 43
  palmar grasp, 43, 49
  parachute, 6,
  primitive, 6, 43
  tendon jerk, 6
reflux nephropathy, 257
refractive errors, 316
Refsum's disease, 300
regurgitation, in infancy, 24, 75, 191
rehydration therapy, 275–6
Reiter's disease, 476
renal agenesis, 148
  unilateral, 251
renal biopsy, 250
renal dialysis *see* dialysis
renal disease *see under* urinary tract disorders
renal dysplasia, 251–2
renal failure, **264–8**
  acute, 264–5
  chronic, 266–8
  following barbiturate poisoning, 519
  following schistosomiasis, 575
  haemolytic uraemic syndrome, 265–6
  management, 265
renal function tests, 246–50
renal hypoplasia, 251–2
renal osteodystrophy, 379
renal rickets, 378–9
  in tyrosinaemia, 377
renal stones, 268
renal transplantation, 266, 267–8
renal tuberculosis, 563
renal tubular acidosis, 268–9
  in fructosaemia, 371
  urinary pH in, 246
renal tubular disorders, 268–9
respiratory acidosis, 170, 276
respiratory alkalosis, 276
respiratory disorders, **165–90**
  neonatal, **85–95**

respiratory distress syndrome (RDS), *86*, 86–8
  in developing countries, 533
respiratory failure, 170–1
  causes, *170*
respiratory infections
  recurrent, 32
  of throat, 160–2
  see also pneumonia
respiratory syncytial viral infection, 179, 180
respiratory system, examination, 10–11
respiratory tract, congenital abnormalities
  bronchial, 172–3
  laryngeal, 159–60
  pulmonary, 173–4
  tracheal, 172
resuscitation, emergency procedures, 240–5
resuscitation, of newborn, 55–6
  pneumothorax following, 89
reticuloendothelial system, examination, 13
retinal degeneration, in abetalipoproteinaemia, 372
retinal haemorrhage
  following child abuse, 523
  following head injury, 516
retinitis pigmentosa, Leber's amaurosis and, 317
retinoblastoma, **470**
  genetics, 127
  inheritance, 442–3
  loss of red reflex, 313, 470
retinopathy of prematurity (ROP), *88*, **112–13**
  loss of red reflex, 313
retrolental fibroplasia *see* retinopathy of prematurity
Reye's syndrome, 211
  aspirin and, 359
Reynell Developmental Language Scale, 327
rhabdomyosarcoma, *163*, 465–6
  differential diagnosis, *449*
rhesus incompatibility, *107*, 107–8, 432
  neonatal hypoglycaemia and, *104*
rheumatic fever, 238, **476–7**
  in developing countries, 569–70
  following scarlet fever, 362
  heart block in, 227, 476
rheumatoid arthritis
  pleural effusion due to, *175*
  terminology problems, 475
  versus rheumatic fever, 570
rhinitis, 157
  allergic, 157
  common cold (coryza), 32, 157
rhinoviral infections, 32
Ribavirin, 180
riboflavin deficiency, in developing countries, 547
rickets, **378–9**, **549–52**
  bow legs and, 33
  chest wall deformities and, 171
  craniotabes and, 57
  glomerular, 379
  in hyperparathyroidism, 422
  neonatal, *94*, 114

of prematurity, 72
renal, 378–9
tubular, 379
in tyrosinaemia, 377
vitamin D-resistant, *131*
weaning and, 72
rifampicin, prophylaxis in meningococcal
meningitis, 281
right ventricular hypertrophy, parasternal
heave in, 8
right-to-left shunting, 235–6
Riley-Day syndrome, 300
ringworm 495–6, *Plates 28–9*
alopecia due to, 503
history taking, 487
investigations, 487
road traffic accidents, 514, 515
RDP (retinopathy of prematurity), *88,*
112–12, *313*
roseola infantum, 358
rotavirus, gastroenteritis due to, 194, 552
Rotor syndrome, *107, 208*
RTA (road traffic accidents), 514, 515
rubella, **356–7**
congenital, 367
intrauterine growth retardation due to,
77
vaccination, *353,* 355
vaccination, in developing countries,
536

sacral agenesis, enuresis due to, *27*
sacrococcygeal teratoma, 472
safety in the home, 513–14
salbutamol, in asthma management, 185
salicylate poisoning, 518
salicylate toxicity
Reye's syndrome and, 211
in rheumatic fever treatment, 477
salicylates, hyperactivity due to, 294
salmon patches, 507
salmonella infections, 364
Sanfilippo syndrome, 375
sarcoma
differential diagnosis, *450*
soft tissue, 446, **465–6**
scabies 497–9, *Plates 32–4*
impetigo and, 495
streptococcal infection following, 570
scalded skin syndrome, 495
scalding, 516
scalp ringworm 495–6, *Plate 28*
alopecia due to, 503
scaphocephaly, 147
scarlet fever 362, *Plate 9*
post-streptococcal, 570
Scheie's syndrome, 375
Schick test, 354
Schistosoma mansoni (hookworm), *571*
schistosomiasis, 575
nephrotic syndrome and, 262
schizophrenia, 342
schools/schooling *see under* education
Schwann cell tumour, differential
diagnosis, *450*
'scissoring', in spastic quadriplegia, 324
scleroderma, 478
scoliosis, *172,* **483**
in cerebral palsy, 325, 327

in Klinefelter's syndrome, 126
respiratory failure due to, *170*
in rickets, 550
screening
child health clinics, 18
for congenital cataract, 312
for cystic fibrosis, 188
for growth disorders, 383–5
for hearing impairment, 308
for hypothyroidism, 410–11
visual assessment, 312
scrotum
causes of painful, *31*
newborn examination, 59
scurvy, 547–9
weaning and, 72
sebaceous naevus, 506, *Plate 45*
seborrhoeic dermatitis, 35, 36
infantile, 492, *Plate 21*
seizures
following meningitis, 283
grand mal, 285, 290
masturbation mistaken for, 25
myoclonic, 287–8
neonatal, 100–2
partial (focal), 288
reflex anoxic, 289
Senning operation, 234
sentinel pile, anal fissure and, 30
septic arthritis, 480–1
versus irritable hip, 479
septicaemia
diagnosis, 351
neonatal, 96
severe combined immunodeficiency
(SCID), 440
sex-linked disorders, 131–3
sexual abuse, 345, **524–6**
genital warts and, 494
psychosexual development and, 335
recurrent UTI and, 259–60
vulvovaginitis and, 31, 525
SGA (small for gestational age), 77, **77–84**
complications of, *78*
definition, 52, 77
shellfish allergy, 506
shigellosis, 553
shingles, 358–9
shock, causes, *240*
short sightedness, 316
short stature, **386–91**
in cleido-cranial dysostosis, 484
in Down's syndrome, *119*
investigations, 387
in Turner's syndrome, 125
sick sinus syndrome, 227
sickle cell disease, *131,* **431–2,** 482, 571
failure to thrive due to, *527*
versus rheumatic fever, 570
SIDS *see* sudden infant death syndrome
Silver-Russell syndrome, 389, *391*
single gene (Mendelian) defects, 118
sinusitis, 158
sixth disease, 358
skeletal defects, in homocystinuria, 377
skeletal system, normal growth, 38
skin, structure/function, 486
skin biopsy, 487
skin cancer, 444
skin disorders, **486–509**

minor, 35–6
neurofibromatosis, *128,* **302,** *443,* 508
scleroderma, 478
Sturge-Weber syndrome, *301,* 302, 508
see also eczema; tuberous sclerosis
skin prick testing, 184
skin sepsis, in measles, 555
skinfold thickness, 39
skull fracture, 515
due to birth trauma, 112
slapped cheek syndrome, 357, *Plate 7*
sleep apnoea
due to adenoidal hypertrophy, 158
sudden infant death syndrome and, 511
sleep cycles, establishment of, 50
sleep disorders, 25–7
sleep-walking, 26
slipped femoral epiphysis, 480
small bowel atresia, 142
smallpox, 359–60
smoke inhalation, 513
smoking, 189
maternal during pregnancy, 510
smothering, in sudden infant death
syndrome, 511
Snellen's chart, 313–14
social development, 50–1
abnormal, 334–5
assessment, 44
social services, 21
social workers, 20, 21
sodium cromoglycate, in asthma
management, 185–6
sodium disorders, hypo/hypernatraemic
dehydration, 274–6
sodium valproate, as anticonvulsant, 290
soft tissue sarcomas, 446, **465–6**
solvent abuse, 349, 521
cardiorespiratory arrest due to, *240*
somatic growth, 38–9
somatic pains, 347–8
Soto's syndrome, 392
spastic diplegia, 322–3
spastic hemiplegia, 322
spastic quadriplegia, 323
scoliosis in, 483
spasticity, in cerebral palsy, 322–3
special senses, **307–18**
see also ear disorders; eye disorders
speech delay, 42, 303, 304
speech development, 44, 47, 303
Reynell Developmental Language Scale,
327
speech disorders, 302–5
speech therapy, in cerebral palsy
management, 327
spherocytosis, *128*
sphingolipidoses, 373–4
spina bifida, 144–6, 295
enuresis due to, *27*
in trisomy-18, *122*
spinal cord tethering, enuresis due to, *27*
spinal deformities, 483–4
kyphosis, 483, 550
torticollis, 483–4
see also scoliosis
spinal muscular atrophy, 300–1
respiratory failure due to, *170*
spinal tuberculosis, 563
spinal tumours, 465

spirometer, 166
splenomegaly
 assessment, 11–12
 in typhoid fever, 365
spondiloarthritis, 476
sports injuries, Osgood-Schlatter disease,
 484
squint (strabismus), **314–15**
 due to orbital tumour, 465
 in meningitis, 280
 pseudosquint, 313
 in retinoblastoma, 470
 screening for, 313
stair gates, 513, 514
stammering/stuttering, 305
Staphylococcal food poisoning, 365
Staphylococcus infections
 endocarditis, 239
 in osteomyelitis, 482
 scalded skin syndrome, 495
 in septic arthritis, 480–1
star charts
 in constipation management, 201
 in enuresis management, 27, 349
stature
 height changes at puberty, 395
 height measurement, 39, 382–5
 parental height, 387, 388, 391
 short *see* short stature
 tall child, 391–2
status epilepticus, 286
stenosis of aqueduct of Sylvius, 295
sternomastoid tumour, *111*, 112
steroid therapy
 in adrenal disorders, 415, 416–17
 in asthma management, 186
 in bronchopulmonary dysplasia
  management, 94
 failure to thrive due to, *527*
 in nephrotic syndrome, 263, 264
 osteoporosis due to, 474
 topical steroids in eczema management,
  491
 in tuberculosis, 567
Stevens-Johnson syndrome, 507
stiffness, early morning, 474–5
stillbirth, *definition*, 52
Still's disease *see* arthritis
stomatitis
 in iron-deficiency anaemia, 427
 in measles, 554
stool holding, 28, 201
strabismus *see* squint
strawberry allergy, 506
strawberry naevus, 508, *Plate 46*
strawberry tongue, 362
Streptococcus infections, 88, 95
 in developing countries, 569–71
 endocarditis, 239
 post-streptococcal nephritis, 260
 post-streptococcal osteomyelitis, 482
 post-streptococcal rheumatic fever, 476
 prevention, 570–1
 in Sydenham's chorea, 293
stridor, 159
strongyloides stercoralis, 574
Sturge-Weber syndrome, *301*, 302, 508
Stycar test, 314
subacute sclerosing encephalitis, 283–4,
 555

autism and, 345
 measles and, 357
subarachnoid haemorrhage
 neonatal, 102
 versus meningitis, 280
subdural effusion, following meningitis,
 282–3
subdural haemorrhage, 516
 following child abuse, 523
 neonatal, 101
subglottic stenosis, *88*, 160, 172
sucrose-isomaltase deficiency, 200
sudden infant death syndrome (SIDS), 15,
 510–13
 botulinum poisoning and, 365
 bronchopulmonary dysplasia and, 94
 cardiac lesions and, 226
 near-miss, 512
suffocation, sudden infant death
 syndrome and, *511*
suicide/attempted suicide, 346
sunsetting sign, *Plate 5*
'super-female' syndrome, 392
supervision order, 21
supraventricular tachycardia, 226
surfactant
 replacement therapy, 88
 role in respiratory distress syndrome,
  86, 87
 sudden infant death syndrome and, *511*
Sutton's halo naevus, 509
sweat test, in cystic fibrosis, 188
Sydenham's chorea, 293–4
syndactyly, 35
syphilis (congenital), 369
 in developing countries, 533–4, *Plate 48*
systemic lupus erythematous 262, **478**,
  Plate 12
 maternal, 227
 pleural effusion due to, *175*

tachycardia/bradycardia syndrome, 227
tachypnoea of newborn, transient, *86*, 91
taenia (tapeworm) infestations, 574
talipes (club foot), 149–50
tall child, 391–2
tantrums, 334
tapeworm, 574
Tay–Sachs disease, *131*, 373
teeth
 dental maturation, *41*, 41
 dentigenosis imperfecta, 484
 malocclusion and thumbsucking, 24
 natal, 29
teething, 29–30
 earache due to, *156*
telangiectasia, hereditary haemorrhagic,
 434
telogen effluvium, 504
temperament, differences in, 335
temperature (environmental)
 of bath, 514
 SIDS risks and, *511*
 thermoneutral environment, 85
temporal lobe epilepsy, 288–9
 treatment, *290*
tendon jerk reflexes, 6
Tensilon test, 299

tension headaches, 292
teratogenic factors, *136*
teratoma
 differential diagnosis, *450*
 sacrococcygeal, 472
 testicular, 471–2
terbutaline, in asthma management, 185
terminal illness
 analgesia, 447–8
 care during, 448
testicular feminization syndrome, 420
testis
 development, 418
 examination, 13
 maldescent, 392–4
 structure/function, 392, 418
 testicular teratoma, 471–2
 torsion of, *29*, 31, 394
 tumours, 394
tetanus
 immunization, *353*, 354–5
 neonatal in developing countries, 534
tetany
 following high phosphorus intake, 64
 in rickets, 549
tetracyclines, in acne management,
 502–3
tetralogy of Fallot *see* Fallot's tetralogy
thalassaemia, *131*, **430–1**, 571
 failure to thrive due to, *527*
 haemosiderosis in, 427, 431
theophylline, in asthma management,
 185
thermoneutral environment, 85
thermoregulation, neonatal, 84–5, 97
thiamine deficiency, in developing
 countries, 547
thoracic mass, differential diagnosis, *450*
threadworm infestation, 33, 574
 vulvovaginitis, 31
thrills, detection of, 8
throat, examination, 14
throat, disorders of, **159–62**
thrombocytopenia, 110–11
 in cancer patient, 446–7
 isoimmune, 110
 maternal idiopathic, 110
 see also disseminated intravascular
  coagulation
thrombocytopenic purpura, acute
 idiopathic, 438
thrush (candida infection), 497
 nappy rash due to, 35–6
 of throat, 161
thumbsucking, 24
thymus tumours, 189
 differential diagnosis, *450*
thyroglossal duct cysts, 164
thyroid disorders, **409–13**
 in Down's syndrome, *119*
 hyperthyroidism, **412–13**
 hypothyroidism, *107, 208*, 402, **410–13**
 short stature and, 388
thyrotoxicosis, 412–13
tibia, bowing of, 34
tic (habit spasm), 28, 293, 340, 343
tinea capitis, 495–6
tinea corporis, 496, *Plate 31*
tinea pedis (athlete's foot), 496
tobacco, abuse, 350

toddler's diarrhoea, 30, 196
Todd's paralysis, 288
toes, abnormalities of, 35
tone, assessment of, 5, 62
tonsil
    normal growth of, 38
    peritonsillar abscess, 161
    tuberculosis of, 162
tonsillectomy, 162
tonsillitis
    acute, 161
    cause of earache, *156*
    chronic, 161–2
    guttate psoriasis following, 488
TORCH infections, 97
    neonatal hepatitis syndrome due to, *208*
torsion of the testicle, *29*, 31, 394
torticollis, 483–4
total anomalous primary venous drainage, 234–5
total parenteral nutrition, in infancy, 75–6
Tourettes syndrome, 341, 343
toxic epidermal necrolysis, *versus* scalded skin syndrome, 495
toxocariasis, 573–4
    versus retinoblastoma, 470
toxoplasmosis, 366
    cerebral palsy due to, *321*
    congenital, 369
    prenatal, 77, 78, *106*
trace element requirements, of infants, 64
tracheal abnormalities, 172
    tracheo-oesophageal fistula, *86*, 139–40, 172
tracheal compression
    in leukaemia, 453
    in non-Hodgkin's lymphoma, 457, 458
tracheitis, following measles, 357
tracheomalacia, 168
    wheeze due to, *169*
transcobalamin II deficiency, 428
transient erythroblastopenia of childhood (TEC), 430
transient tachypnoea of newborn, 91
translocation, in Down's syndrome, 121
transplantation
    kidney, 266, 267–8
    liver, 212
transportation, of critically ill child, 243
transposition of great arteries, 234
transverse myelitis, 299
trauma
    birth injury, 111–12
    to bones and joints, 484
    see also accidental injury; non-accidental injury
Treacher Collins syndrome, 152
tremor, 293
triad syndrome, urinary tract abnormalities, 254
trichiniasis, 574–5
trichobezoar, 30
trichotillomania, 30, 504
trichuris trichuria, 574
tricuspid atresia, 235
tricyclic antidepressant poisoning, 519
triple vaccine, 354
    schedule, *353*
trisomy-13 (Patau's syndrome), 122–3

clinical features, *122*
    intrauterine growth retardation, 78
trisomy-18 (Edwards' syndrome), 121–2
    clinical features, *122*
    intrauterine growth retardation, 78
trisomy-21 *see* Down's syndrome
truancy, 346–7
tuberculin test *see* Heaf test; Mantoux test
tuberculosis, 181, 189–90, **555–67**
    BCG vaccination, 355–6
    BCG vaccination in developing countries, 535
    chronic septic arthritis and, 481
    diagnosis, 563–4
    failure to thrive due to, *527*
    haemoptysis due to, *167*
    malnutrition and, 545
    maternal, 537, 565
    with measles, 555
    miliary, 558, **562**
    pleural effusion due to, *175*
    prevention, 564–5
    primary infection, 558–63
    of tonsil, 162
    treatment, 565–7
    wheeze due to, *169*
tuberculous meningitis, **562**, 566, 567
tuberous sclerosis, *128*, 285, **302**
    café-au-lait patches in, 508
    de-pigmentation in, 505
    epilepsy and, 285
    tumour predisposition in, *443*
tumour lysis syndrome, 447
    in acute lymphoblastic leukaemia, 453
tumours
    adrenal gland, 417–18
    bone, 466–70
    brain, 445, 462–5
    germ cell, 471–2
    liver, 471
    lung, 189
    second, 446
    vaginal, 466
    Wilm's, 461–2
Turner's syndrome, 123–6, 390–1
    clinical features, *126*
    coarctation of aorta in, 232, 390
    delayed puberty in, 396
    horseshoe kidney in, 254
    management, 390–1
    ovarian dysgenesis in, 395
    spontaneous miscarriage and, 119
twins
    fetofetal bleeding, 105
    intrauterine growth of, 78
    premature labour, 79
    risk of SIDS in, 512
    speech delay, 303
typhoid fever, 365
tyrosinaemia, 377–8
    neonatal, *107*
    tumour predisposition in, *443*
tyrosinosis, neonatal hepatitis syndrome due to, *208*

ulcerative colitis, 203
ulcers
    Jacquet's, 492
    meatal, 31

ultrasound
    in cancer diagnosis, 450
    cardiac scans, 217–19
    in nervous system investigation, 279
    in urinary tract disorders, 248
umbilical cord, normal newborn 59
umbilical hernia, in Hurler's syndrome, 375
umbilical sepsis, 59
    in developing countries, 534
    portal hypertension due to, 212
unconjugated hyperbilirubinaemia, 106
Unna's naevus, 507
upper airway obstruction
    in leukaemia, 453
    in non-Hodgkin's lymphoma, 457, 458
urea cycle disorders, 378
ureteric duplication, 253
ureterocoele, 254
urethral syndromes, 259–60
urinalysis, 246–8, 351
urinary tract disorders, **246–72**
    see also urinary tract infection
urinary tract infection, **257–60**
    antibiotic treatment, *259*
    crying and, *29*
    enuresis and, *27*
    information leaflet on UTI prevention, *258*
    laboratory findings, *352*
    neonatal, 96
    pain on micturition and, 31
    symptoms, 246, 257
    urethral syndromes, 259–60
    vesicoureteric reflux, 259
urine
    collection techniques, 257–8
    microscopy, 246–8, 351
    pH and osmolality, 246–7
urticaria 506, *Plate 40*
    in Henoch–Schönlein purpura, 261–2
    papular, 500, *Plate 35*
    pigmentosa, 506–7, *Plate 41*
uveitis, in leptospirosis, 365

vaccination programmes, 18, **353–6**
vaginal adenocarcinoma, 444
vaginal bleeding, due to sexual abuse, 525
vaginal discharge, in neonates, 31
vaginal examination, newborn, 59
vaginal tumour, 466
varicella (chickenpox), **358–9**
    in cancer patient, 448, 454
    cerebellar ataxia and, 292
    chickenpox pneumonitis, 179
    vaccine, 356
vehicle accidents, 514, 515
ventricular spetal defect, 229–30
    in Down's syndrome, *119*
    heart sounds in, 9
    recurrence risk for siblings, *133*
    in trisomy-13, *122*
ventricular tachycardia, 227
verbal dyspraxia, 304
verrucae, 493
vertigo, 307–8
vesicoureteric junction obstruction, 252–3
vesicoureteric reflux, 257, **259**

Vincent's angina, 161
viral infections
    acute gastroenteritis due to, 552
    common cold, 32, 157
    encephalitis, 283–4
    gastroenteritis, 194
    infectious diseases, **356–62**
    meningitis, 280–1, **282–3**
    pleurisy, 174
    prenatal, 78
    of skin, 493–5
    see also pneumonia
virilizing adrenal tumours, 417
vision, anatomical pathways, 312
visual assessment, 312–14
    in newborn, 62
visual defects *see under* eye disorders
visual development, 50
vitamins
    B group deficiency, 428
    deficiency in developing countries,
        546–52
    E deficiency, 199
    hypervitaminosis D, 380
    infant requirements, 64
    K deficiency and haemorrhagic disease
        of newborn, 110–11
    supplements in liver disease, 208
    supplements to breast milk, 64
vitiligo, 505
vocal cord paralysis, 162
vomiting, 191–3
    causes of acute, *192*
    due to gastro-oesophageal reflux, 192
    due to pyloric stenosis, 192–3
    during chemotherapy, 477
    in infancy, 74
von Gierke's disease, 372
von Recklinghausen's disease, 302
von Willebrand's disease, *128*, 437–8
vulva, newborn examination, 59

vulvovaginitis, 31
    masturbation and, 25
    sexual abuse and, 31, 525
    threadworm infestation and, 33

Waardenbury's syndrome, de-
    pigmentation in, 505
walking
    delay in, 42, 325
    skills aquistion, 49
ward of Court, 21
warts, 493–4
    genital, 494
    plane, 493, *Plate 25*
    plantar, 493, *Plate 24*
warty epidermal naevus, 507, *Plate 44*
water requirements, normal 273–4
Waterhouse–Friderichsen syndrome, 366,
    416
weakness, 297–300
    causes, 297
weaning, 72–3
    in developing countries, 537
Wechsler Intelligence Scale for Children
    (WISC), 327
weed killer poisoning, 520
weight
    at birth, 52, 77
    normal weight gain, 39
    see also low birth weight; obesity
Werdnig–Hoffman disease, *93*, 300–1
West's disease, 286
wheeze, 169
    causes, *169*
whey, 64, 70
whipworm, 574
white reflex, retinopathy of prematurity
    and, 113
whooping cough *see* pertussis

Wickham's striae, 489
Wiedemann-Beckwith syndrome,
    hypoglycaemia due to, *405*
William's syndrome, 380
Wilm' tumour, **461–2**
    abdominal distension due to, *193*
    chromosome abnormalities, 443, 461
    cure rate, 450, 461–2
    treatment, 445, 450, 461–2
Wilson–Mikity syndrome, *86*, 94–5
Wilson's disease, 212, 293
    tumour predisposition in, *443*
Wiscott–Aldrich syndrome, 440
    tumour predisposition in, *443*
witch doctors, 530
Wolff–Parkinson–White syndrome, 226
Wolman's syndrome, neonatal hepatitis
    syndrome due to, *208*
Wood's light, 487
    hypopigmentation illuminated by, 505
    scalp ringworm fluorescence, 496, *Plate
    29*
word deafness/blindness, 304
World Health Organization
    ICD-9 system, 39
    immunization targets, 353

X-rays *see* radiography
xanthomata, in von Gierke's disease, 372
xeroderma pigmentosa, 444

yolk sac tumours, 472

Zellweger's syndrome, neonatal hepatitis
    syndrome due to, *208*
zinc deficiency, dermatitis due to, 492
Zoster immune globulin, 359